Although all intensive-care specialties have come to rely heavily on technology, neonatology has depended on new technology to a greater extent than most for its development and success. No neonatal patient lies in bed alone; each is constantly under surveillance for heart rate, blood pressure, or some combination of these and other variables. Fetal patients, too, are under close surveillance with ultrasound imaging and Doppler measurements of blood-flow patterns. During labor, fetal patients are often continuously monitored with electrical measurement of heart rate and beat-to-beat variability, usually in conjunction with maternal measurements of uterine contractions, amniotic pressure, and arterial pulse saturation. Clinicians can no longer live without these monitors and machines, but may need to live better with them.

This book sets out to provide perinatologists and neonatologists with an understandable explanation of the principles and applications of commonly used technologies. It aims also to stimulate a more critical review of the available biotechnology and its rational use. Each self-contained chapter is written by a physician, a bioengineer, or a physicist, and together they present a clear account of the technology underlying the principal imaging modalities, tissue oxygenation measurement, electrical monitoring, ventilators and incubators, and the measurement of blood flow and bilirubin levels. Each technical description is followed by a brief review of the practical uses of the technology and an evaluation of its risks and benefits, including cost-effectiveness.

The key to this book is simplicity and clarity of exposition, making it a readily available and comprehensive reference for clinicians regarding the major technologies that have been applied in the diagnosis of fetal and neonatal pathology and in the support of the patient. Its many diagrams and illustrations provide a strong visual emphasis that will add further to its appeal to a broad clinical readership in perinatal and neonatal medicine.

*Physiological monitoring
and instrument diagnosis in
perinatal and neonatal medicine*

Physiological monitoring and instrument diagnosis in perinatal and neonatal medicine

Edited by

Yves W. Brans, M.D.
Wayne State University School of Medicine

William W. Hay, Jr., M.D.
University of Colorado School of Medicine

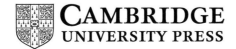

CAMBRIDGE UNIVERSITY PRESS

Published by the Press Syndicate of the University of Cambridge
The Pitt Building, Trumpington Street, Cambridge CB2 1RP
40 West 20th Street, New York, NY 10011-4211, USA
10 Stamford Road, Oakleigh, Melbourne 3166, Australia

First published 1995

Printed in the United States of America

Library of Congress Cataloging-in-Publication Data
Physiological monitoring and instrument diagnosis in perinatal and
neonatal medicine / edited by Yves W. Brans, William W. Hay, Jr.
p.   cm.
Includes index.
ISBN 0-521-41951-4 (hc)
1. Perinatology – Apparatus and instruments. 2. Neonatology –
Apparatus and instruments. 3. Fetal monitoring. 4. Neonatal
intensive care – Apparatus and instruments. I. Brans, Yves W.
II. Hay, William W.
[DNLM: 1. Monitoring, Physiologic – in infancy & childhood.
2. Monitoring, Physiologic – instrumentation. 3. Diagnostic Imaging –
in infancy & childhood. WB 142 P578 1995]
RG628.P48   1995
618.3'2075 – dc20
DNLM/DLC
for Library of Congress   94-26723

A catalog record for this book is available from the British Library.

ISBN 0-521-41951-4 hardback

This book is dedicated to the memory of the late Yves Brans:
friend,
physician,
teacher,
scientist,
scholar.
His past efforts shall be part of the future.

W.W.H.

Contents

Contributors

Bertil Axelsson, Ph.D.
Karolinska Institutet, Stockholm, Sweden

Henrietta S. Bada, M.D.
University of Tennessee Health Science Center, Memphis, TN

Yves W. Brans, M.D. (deceased)
Wayne State University Medical School, Detroit, MI

Jane E. Brazy, M.D.
University of Wisconsin, Madison, WI

Julia Brockway Curlander, M.D.
University of Colorado Health Sciences Center, Denver, CO

Robert A. Darnall, M.D.
Dartmouth Medical School, Dartmouth-Hitchcock Medical Center, Lebanon, NH

Robert A. deLemos, M.D.
University of Southern California School of Medicine, Los Angeles, CA

Michael M. Donnelly, B.E.
University of Cincinnati School of Medicine, Cincinnati, OH

Zia Q. Farooki, M.D.
Children's Hospital of Michigan, Detroit, MI

Willem P. F. Fetter, M.D., Ph.D.
Sophia Hospital, Zwolle, The Netherlands

Olof Flodmark, M.D., Ph.D.
Karolinska Institutet, Stockholm, Sweden

Linda A. Harrison, M.D.
University of Kansas Medical Center, Kansas City, KS

William W. Hay, Jr., M.D.
University of Colorado Health Sciences Center, Denver, CO

Peter Herscovitch, M.D.
National Institutes of Health, Bethesda, MD

Alan Hill, M.D., Ph.D.
British Columbia's Children's Hospital, Vancouver, British Columbia, Canada

Richard A. Humes, M.D.
Children's Hospital of Michigan, Detroit, MI

Michael F. Insana, Ph.D.
University of Kansas Medical Center, Kansas City, KS

Osman Ipsiroglu, M.D.
Kark-Franzens Universität Graz, Graz, Austria

Frans F. Jöbsis van der Vliet, Ph.D.
Duke University Medical Center, Durham, NC

Harry N. Lafeber, M.D., Ph.D.
Free University Hospital, Amsterdam, The Netherlands

Michael H. LeBlanc, M.D.
University of Mississippi School of Medicine, Jackson, MS

Karel Maršál, M.D., Ph.D.
Malmö General Hospital, Malmö, Sweden

Joseph C. McGowan, Ph.D.
University of Pennsylvania School of Medicine, Philadelphia, PA

Michael R. Neuman, Ph.D., M.D.
Metro Health Medical Center, Cleveland, OH

Rangasamy Ramanathan, M.D.
University Children's Hospital, Vienna, Austria

Elke H. Roland, M.D.
British Columbia's Children's Hospital, Vancouver, British Columbia, Canada

Rudolf Rudelstorfer, M.D.
County Hospital, Wels, Austria

George Simbruner, M.D.
Dr. von Haunersches Kinderspital, Munich, Germany

Håkan Stale, M.D., Ph.D.
University of Lund, Malmö, Sweden

K. L. Tan
National University of Singapore Hospital, Singapore

Margot J. Taylor, Ph.D.
Hospital for Sick Children, Toronto, Ontario, Canada

Elizabeth H. Thilo, M.D.
University of Colorado Health Sciences Center, Denver, CO

Michael Weindling, B.Sc., M.D.
University of Liverpool Maternity Hospital, Liverpool, UK

Akio Yamanishi
Minolta Camera Co., Ltd., Osaka, Japan

Itsuro Yamanouchi, M.D.
Okayama National Hospital, Okayama, Japan

Yoshitada Yamauchi, M.D.
Okayama National Hospital, Okayama, Japan

Preface

WILLIAM W. HAY, JR., M.D.

I remember four issues that came up during my discussion with Yves Brans when he asked me to write a chapter for a book on perinatal biomedical technology. First, Yves recognized that we were in the midst of an explosion in new instrumentation in perinatal medicine, as in nearly all fields of medicine, and a reference describing how such instruments work and should be used was not available. Second, and most practically, Yves thought that people practicing "perinatal medicine" needed a single book to which they could refer when questions about technology came up. Third, Yves believed that by understanding how an instrument works, one can better appreciate its strengths and limitations and thus put the instrument to more rational use. He believed that students and trainees and physicians and nurses all need to know how various instruments work and that this knowledge can help improve their use for appropriate diagnosis and therapy. Fourth, Yves felt optimistic, even excited, that modern technology had launched a significant leap in our capacity to care for and improve outcomes for newborn infants, particularly those born sick or preterm, and their mothers. He wanted to crystallize this optimism and excitement about this new level of medical technology and practice in this book.

It was the last point that most caught my attention. After all, I had felt the same sort of excitement as I had watched the evolution from painful and harmful arterial "sticks," through often inaccurate and cumbersome transcutaneous Po_2 sensors, to continuous, noninvasive oxygen monitoring by pulse oximetry (but hopefully not ending there). As part of this process, physicians and nurses and respiratory therapists now can better know a baby's oxygenation, more often, more accurately, and with less pain and injury. I felt that this process represented a significant and truly beneficial advance in perinatal biomedical technology. In order to deal with a clinical problem, basic physics, electronics engineering, ingenuity, and entrepreneurial venture and marketing all were combined to improve an important aspect of medical care for newborn infants. Pulse oximetry now is almost universal in neonatal intensive-care units (as well as in many other intensive-care settings in modern hospitals). Babies and the makers of the pulse oximeters have all profited.

It was the spirit of the advancement, as well as the benefit, that especially excited me. It gave me great hope for the future. It showed me that fundamental curiosity to break things apart and learn how they work could generate knowledge that would allow new things to be put together, in new ways, to improve care and outcomes for infants and their mothers. Surely this is good. And this spirit of excitement from the mixing of basic science and applied science to benefit future perinatal patients is fundamental to being a doctor, or a nurse, or any other health professional. Fiscal realities may, from time to time, impose limitations, but it is to be hoped that they will never halt the process or diminish the excitement of continuing technical advancements in biomedicine, for some of today's "high-tech" extravaganzas *will* be tomorrow's standard methods of care. Future generations of infants and their mothers will be obvious beneficiaries. But we shall all benefit from technical advancements, as much by the process as by the practical outcomes.

Acknowledgments

Dr. Richard Barling and Ms. Laura Wise at Cambridge University Press deserve credit for seeing to it that this book got finished.

Mr. Eric Deltour, nephew of Yves Brans, was most generous and helpful in making the necessary arrangements to allow Dr. Hay to step in as co-editor and complete the preparation of submitted chapters.

Ms. Judy Lee, staff assistant in Dr. Hay's office, deserves credit for carrying out so many of those chores that are necessary but often unrecognized and unappreciated parts of the editing process.

Publisher's note

This book was conceived and initiated by the late Yves W. Brans. Following his sudden death during the book's preparation, the editorial role was assumed by William W. Hay, Jr., to whom Cambridge University Press is deeply indebted for the timely completion of the text. As an Introduction, Dr. Hay has elected to adapt an article first published as the Introduction to *Clinics in Perinatology: Newer Technologies and the Neonate* (September 1991). We thank W. B. Saunders Company for permission to reprint this article.

At Dr. Hay's request, the book is dedicated to the memory of Yves W. Brans.

Editor's note

We considered it reasonable, as well as probable, that readers of this book would want each chapter to be complete, so that they could read a particular chapter to understand just that technology. Frequent references to other locations in the book, therefore, would be distracting and even confusing. For this reason, there is overlap among some details throughout the book. For example, Doppler principles and measurements of blood flow are discussed several times, as are the principles of detecting oxygen transport in blood and electrical signaling.

We also thought that the many color pictures would be worth the price; shades of gray simply do not convey the feeling of "being there," watching blood flow and metabolism actually taking place.

Introduction: Biomedical technology: to use or not to use?

YVES W. BRANS, M.D.

Technology of ever-increasing sophistication has pervaded every facet of society during the past 30 years, and there is no indication that the process will slow down in decades to come. Developments in transistors and cheap silicon microchips, coupled with the impetus given to miniaturization by the space programs, have resulted in an economic paradox. As the sophistication and power of technical devices have increased, their cost has decreased drastically during a period in which the more basic commodities have increased in price, both in terms of actual currency and corrected for the rate of general inflation. Yet, as consumer demand for relatively cheap high-tech devices has grown, so has the appetite for much more expensive technologies. Biomedical technology has more than followed this overall trend and, in so doing, actually has contributed to inflation and budgetary deficits by increasing medical costs out of proportion to most other costs incurred by today's society. In his 1989 presidential address to the Pacific Coast Obstetrical and Gynecological Society, Figge (1990) pointed out that annual expenditures for health care in the United States had risen from $12.7 billion in 1950 ($82 per capita) to $132.7 billion in 1975 ($653 per capita), $425 billion in 1985 ($1,721 per capita), and $618 billion in 1988 ($2,618 per capita). Projections indicate that expenditures will reach $1.9 trillion (some $8,000 per capita) by the end of the decade (Figures I.1 and I.2) (Sorkin, 1986). Medical technology is

Adapted by permission of W. B. Saunders Company from *Clinics in Perinatology: Newer Technologies and the Neonate* (September 1991).

said to have accounted for 15% to 25% of the increased costs of hospital care during the past 10 years, but when corrected for general inflation, the proportion is closer to 60% to 70% of the increase (Altman and Blendon, 1979; Figge, 1990). Whether the financial cost of increased (improved?) medical technology has been justified by increased benefits in both survival and quality of life is arguable. Emotionally, both the medical community and the public at large would answer the question in a resoundingly positive manner, but the question has not been appraised dispassionately. Such an appraisal is beyond the scope of this introduction. Lacking the needed data, we must confine ourselves to general remarks that perhaps will stimulate a more critical review of the available biotechnology and of its rational uses.

Although all intensive-care specialties have come to rely heavily on technology, neonatalogy has depended on new technology to a greater extent than most of its development and for its success. The invention of infant incubators marked the beginning of a new era in pediatrics (LeBlanc, 1991), but it was the simultaneous availability of mechanical ventilators and a better understanding of the respiratory pathophysiology of the premature baby that allowed a quantum leap in neonatal survival for ever-smaller babies. In the past 20 years, a host of electronic monitors have become available to provide instant information on a variety of body functions, from cardiac and respiratory rates to cerebral metabolism. Some 12 years ago, in an issue of *Clinics in Perinatology*, we compiled a relatively complete listing of all equipment available to nurseries (Brans,

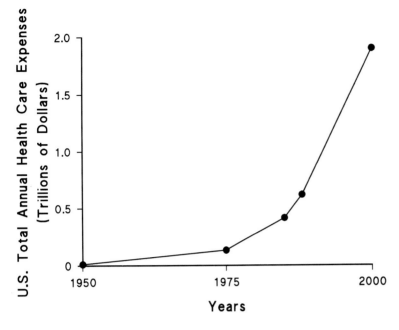

Figure I.1. Total annual expenditures (in trillions of U.S. dollars) for health care in the United States from 1950 to 1988 and estimated to the year 2000.

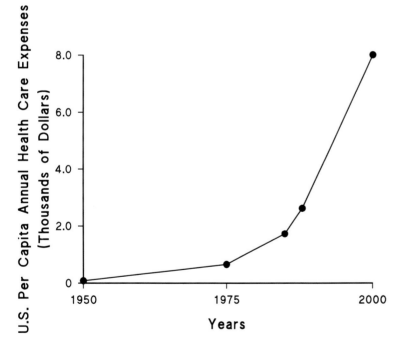

Figure I.2. Annual expenditures per capita (in thousands of U.S. dollars) for health care in the United States from 1950 to 1988 and estimated to the year 2000.

1983). It occupied 17 pages of small print. Today a similar undertaking probably would require close to an entire volume. Once upon a time, premature babies were left pretty much to their own devices to survive. So long as they breathed, attention was focused on keeping them warm and fed. A warm en-vironment was provided by a variety of more or less sophisticated boxes (aka incubators). "Monitoring" was provided by nurses who checked body tem-perature, color, heart rate, and respiration of their little charges periodically, in addition to feeding them. Today, a neonatal intensive-care bed has become a maze of electrical cords, wires, and catheters that lead to an array of instruments stacked upon one another or cluttering up the floor space around the incubator. The little patient is sometimes literally lost, in more ways than one, in the midst of all this technology. Graphs, trends, bar diagrams, and numbers are displayed on a bewildering array of dials, graph papers, screens, and liquid-crystal windows. Of course, every single one of these devices "talks" to us in a variety of beeping sounds; some are meant to be reassuring, and some shriek in a. arm to summon their human masters, and increasingly fail to elicit more than a lackadaisical response, if any. Their major contribution sometimes appears only to be to the general noise level of an environment that neonatologists generally agree should be peaceful and quiet. Who has not observed an irritable baby segregated in the corner of a neonatal unit, with overhead lights turned off and a blanket draped over the hood of the incubator to provide "quiet time," whereas a few feet away telephones ring, computers clatter, and alarm bells sound from all directions?

How and why have we reached this situation, and has it all been for the better?

WHY USE BIOMEDICAL TECHNOLOGY?

To improve care and diagnostic ability

Improvements in the care of infants and the diagnostic ability of physicians would be the universal claim and, to a large extent, an accurate one for the use of this technology. Neonates seldom suffer from disease entities, at least not in the sense that we talk about diseases in older patients. They simply have difficulties in adapting to the extrauterine environment, either because they are required to do so before they are ready or because their intrauterine environment or, more seldom, the birth process has compromised their ability to adapt. In order to assist this adaptation, or correct the problems that prevent self-adaptation, the physician must be able to determine what is going on deep inside the body. Traditional means of physical diagnosis fail in the case of a newborn. Symptoms are nonexistent because the baby is unable to communicate. Physical signs or characteristics of the neonate reduce the validity of the usual tenets of physical diagnosis – inspection, palpation, percussion, and auscultation – mostly to that of inspection, although even those findings often are too unspecific to be of much assistance. Therefore, there is an inherent need to rely on technological methods to break the communication barrier between patient and physician. To the physi-

cian used to dealing with older children and adults, measurements as mundane as the determination of blood pressure require electronic technology in order to amplify signals too weak to be detected with a stethoscope. The same applies to noninvasive measurement of intracranial pressure.

Assessment of the most basic metabolic and physiological process – oxygenation – is based on technology once removed from what matters: determination of tissue oxygenation and metabolism. The relation between what we measure (the partial pressure of oxygen in arterial blood, Pao_2) and the availability of oxygen to cells is tenuous enough. Yet attempts have been made repeatedly to substitute capillary blood sampling (Pco_2) for the more elusive arterial samples. Many years passed before neonatologists realized that static measurements of an ever-changing physiological variable had limited use. Much recent technology has been aimed at facilitating this assessment. Systems have been designed to measure Pao_2 by means of indwelling arterial electrodes that should provide continuous measurements of absolute values, as well as trends in relation to time and extraneous events. For the best part of 20 years, these systems have failed to provide sufficiently accurate results. Newer methods are promising, but they remain to be tested clinically with sufficient rigor. A great deal of effort was expended in devising methods to assess blood oxygenation without recourse to either blood sampling or indwelling, invasive cannulas. Transcutaneous determinations of the partial pressures of oxygen ($Ptco_2$) and carbon dioxide ($Ptcco_2$) resulted. Numerous $Ptco_2$ and $Ptcco_2$ monitors were commercialized and validated against the respective arterial values. Some makes and models of instruments were more successful and reliable than others, but on the whole this technology served us well for a decade. There were drawbacks, but they were rather minor, except for the babies who perhaps needed such technology most – those with chronic lung disease in whom the reliability of transcutaneous monitors became problematic. More recently, transcutaneous monitoring, at least for oxygenation, has been supplanted by pulse oximetry (Hay, Thilo, and Curlander, 1991). Although undeniably this is extremely useful to determine if a neonate's Pao_2 is sufficiently high, it fails to determine whether or not a premature infant's Pao_2 is too high, and it places the baby at increased risk for the retinopathy of prematurity. At this point, we are two steps removed from measuring tissue oxygenation. This dilemma illustrates the problem with many electronic monitors: They assess a physiologic variable, but the numbers they yield are one or more steps removed from what we really wish to monitor. This limitation is often ignored by the clinician. On the other hand, advanced biotechnology now enables us to assess cerebral oxygenation and metabolism directly with the help of nuclear magnetic-resonance spectroscopy (Hope and Moorcraft, 1991) and, probably of greater general applicability, near-infrared spectroscopy (Brazy, 1991). These methods are still experimental, but their clinical applications cannot be far in the future. Every indication so far suggests that they may be invaluable to the practitioner if used appropriately and within stated limits.

The dilemma of measurements that are several steps removed from, or tenuously related to, physiologically significant values is neither new nor specific to neonatology or electronic monitoring. Examples of similar problems abound in conventional clinical pathology. Serum concentrations of potassium often are monitored religiously, and yet clinical correlations between the extracellular concentration of a mostly intracellular ion and symptoms have repeatedly been demonstrated to be nonexistent. In newborns, this assessment is complicated by the impossibility of obtaining unhemolyzed blood samples through narrow-gauge needles or catheters, let alone from heel punctures. The same problem applies to calcium, for which we persist in determining serum concentrations of total calcium, which have no clinical correlates, rather than those of ionized calcium, which do. Yet the latter can now be measured with little more difficulty and as much accuracy as those of total calcium. Habit is ingrained deeper than common sense. A dichotomy has evolved in our clinical practice. At one end of the spectrum is the up-to-date high technology that is available and that we are so proud of; at the other end are the old, mundane, "routine" methods. Often, neither is used properly.

Diagnostic methods based on high technology can be invaluable to make noninvasive diagnoses based on "viewing" inner organs. One only needs to mention ultrasonography, computerized axial tomography, nuclear magnetic-resonance imaging, positron-emission tomography, radioactive scanning, and others. Yet each of these has specific indications, uses, and abuses that need to be learned.

To decrease the workload of caretakers

Although electronic monitors cannot replace a thinking nurse or physician, monitors do assist their work and allow them to watch more than one patient at a time. In these times, when very few intensive-care units are able to provide the 1 : 1 or 1 : 2 nurse-to-patient ratio that is required, electronic monitors play an extremely important role and may benefit both the nursing staff and the patients. They provide continuous readouts of important physiological parameters that otherwise would have to be measured periodically by the nurse, and they supposedly warn the nurse when the measured values fall outside the acceptable range, suggesting that there may be a problem with the patient. That usefulness holds only so long as the following criteria are met:

1. The monitor records a useful variable. There has been a proliferation of instruments that monitor various aspects of the functioning of mechanical ventilators. Although possibly useful for specific research applications, the clinical applicability or usefulness of these instruments is questionable.
2. The monitor records the variable accurately. This tenet is fulfilled to varying degrees by various makes and types of monitors, and the personality quirks of each instrument must be learned through experience.
3. The nurse or other caretaker is fully cognizant of the limitations of the monitor. This is often the main problem. Proper in-service training of the nursing staff about how to use a new instrument is often lacking. Frequently, this "chore" is left to the sales representative of the manufacturing company, who is either unaware of the limitations or is naturally loath to reveal them. A complicating factor is that any one intensive-care unit often uses a variety of models that are supposed to function according to the same specifications but do not. The usual rapid turnover of nursing staff only complicates matters.
4. The various alarms with which the monitor is endowed do not produce too many false alarms. Because electronic monitors are unthinking instruments, functioning according to various algorithms, unable to differentiate between really abnormal situations and artifactual conditions, they alarm frequently. Nurses and physicians have an understandably low frustration threshold for nuisance alarms and tend to shut off the alarming systems completely. In response to the manufacturers' liability consciousness and the well-meaning but bureaucratically inclined minds of the Food and Drug Administration (FDA) and the Underwriters Laboratory (UL), most alarming devices either cannot be shut off or can be shut off only for a limited period of time (30 seconds to 5 minutes), after which they reactivate.

When one considers that each baby in a 12-bed unit may be connected to a monitoring system that contains as many as 12 to 20 different alarms, the resulting mayhem is understandable. It takes a well-trained and experienced nurse to diagnose not only which baby's alarm is sounding off but also which instrument it originates from. We have suggested semiseriously that each neonatal intensive-care unit position should be equipped with a board of lights showing what instrument is alarming, and what for. Of course, each board should include an alarm in case the entire board stops functioning. The result is that the well-trained and experienced nurse also develops a remarkably selective deafness to alarms, which defeats the well-meaning minds of FDA and UL underwriters. Walking into an average intensive-care unit, one is struck by the concert of alarms acting as background music, matched only by the apparent insouciance of the nursing staff. In their defense, one must say that experienced nurses do have a sixth sense that tells them when a baby needs attention without the help of sound effects, and that will always remain the triumph of humans over machines. On the other hand, intempestive alarms may result in excessive and possibly harmful interventions on the part of less experienced caretakers (physician, nurse, or parent).

In short, electronic monitors assist the nursing staff greatly, but they are no substitute for adequate numbers of well-trained nurses.

To improve documentation

Electronic monitoring, especially trend recordings, can be invaluable to document a specific element in the condition of a patient for days on end, to indicate what goes wrong when, and sometimes to provide an explanation for an untoward event. In the early days of transcutaneous monitoring, Dr. Lucey often cited the vivid example of a small premature neonate whose $Ptco_2$ would decrease periodically without any obvious reason. Finally, thanks to the continuous recording, it was found that the $Ptco_2$ would decline each time a telephone placed near the baby's incubator rang. Aversion to a telephone's shrill ring is not necessarily a response conditioned by past experience. In fact, continuous transcutaneous Po_2 and Pco_2 tracings compose one of the considerable advantages of the technology. They provide lasting records that can be reviewed periodically. The neonatologist, on arriving in the morning, can see at a glance what happened to a baby during the night. Also, they can provide records of events during surgery, especially if carefully annotated by the staff permanently on site. Some instruments also provide a histogram that indicates during what proportion of a given period of time the baby had excessively high or low $Ptco_2$ or $Ptcco_2$ (AAP, 1985). Secondarily, these tracings may also be very helpful in documenting the use of the monitor, for billing purposes. Pulse oximeters may also be connected to strip-chart recorders, but such a recorder is not normally included with the basic instrument, whereas the vast majority of transcutaneous monitors do have a built-in recorder. Cost considerations often lead nurseries to dispense with the recorder for pulse oximetry, but in our opinion this constitutes a misguided sense of economy. Trend recorders for cardiorespiratory and blood-pressure monitors, on the other hand, are expensive and usually not worth the investment.

To protect against medical liability

In this era of high risk of professional liability, extensive monitoring, especially with devices that provide lasting documentation, and reliance on high-tech diagnostic methods have been used as means to protect oneself against the eventuality of a suit for medical liability. This constitutes monitoring or testing for the sake of the record rather than for the good of the patient. Ethically, it must be condemned as unnecessary and unjustified. Financially, it is impossible even to guess at the cost implications of such practice, but they must be considerable. Legally, although it is tempting to believe that such indiscriminate (i.e., without good presumptive reason) testing might be protective of the physician and the institution, evidence is lacking that it protects anyone. Realistically, this practice is here to stay, but it should at least be tempered with common sense. Should a computed tomography (CT) scan or more esoteric diagnostic tests be performed in any term newborn with low Apgar scores in the hope that an abnormality seen early after birth might "prove" that an insult had occurred long before birth, thereby exculpating the obstetrician being sued for a birth-related injury? The pitfalls and the shaky scientific foundation of such reasoning are obvious. Should every premature baby who experienced episodes of apnea and bradycardia or who was treated with methylxanthines while in the nursery have a sleep pneumogram before going home? Should the respiratory status of such a baby be monitored at home? Despite the overwhelming evidence that sleep pneumograms, as practiced currently, do not predict the risk of a life-threatening event or sudden infant death occurring at home (AAP, 1985; Hunt and Brouillette, 1987; Hunt, 1991) and that home monitoring has had no effect on the incidence of sudden infant death syndrome, many physicians feel obligated to use these technologies "just in case."

The same scenario applies to the increasingly uneasy relations between physicians and professional review organizations (PSROs). The troublesome fact in this case is that this pits physicians against physicians, or their appointed representatives (in the case of many PSROs). Highly qualified medical specialists see their everyday decisions questioned by other physicians, often less qualified in the specific specialty, on grounds established by some unknown bureaucrats. A common scenario reads as follows: A premature baby had a choking spell during feeding 10 days before discharge from the hospital; the physician failed to do a sleep pneumogram; therefore the PSRO will disallow reimbursement for the entire hospitalization and penalize the physician with x number of "points." The result is at best a bureaucratic hassle for the physician who has to explain his or her actions, or lack thereof – a euphemism for educating the PSRO physician. At worst, qualified physicians may be penalized for perfectly legitimate actions.

To impress other physicians, patients, and visitors

To impress others is only an extension of the preceding reason, except that the targets extend from lawyers and PSRO physicians to other physicians to whom one refers patients (a medical equivalent of "keeping up with the Joneses"), patients or their families, and visitors. In today's society, high technology has developed an aura quite independent of its usefulness or efficacy, until eventually its risks become public knowledge. Then, those who have used it are blamed for not knowing what was unknown, but what they should have known anyway (e.g., oxygen and retinopathy of prematurity in the 1950s and 1960s). The patient is perceived to have a right to state-of-the-art technology, whether he or she needs it or not.

RISKS AND PITFALLS OF BIOMEDICAL TECHNOLOGY

Although the avowed purpose of all technical advances (improvements?) is to improve delivery of care and diagnostic capabilities, there invariably are risks attendant to any new technology. First, there is a danger that technology may supersede our rational processes and the natural development of intuition that comes only from long practice of observational skills. The great physicians of the past made their mark in medicine by their powers of observation. Their diagnostic acumen was based on their ability to extract pertinent information with their eyes (inspection), fingertips (palpation and percussion), ears (auscultation), and often sense of smell. Today, the art of physical diagnosis has been all but forgotten and is barely taught in American medical schools, having been replaced by reliance on laboratory tests and ancillary examinations. Yet, appropriate teaching of biomedical technology and its uses and misuses is lagging far behind technical advances. Figge (1990) stated it best: "mastery of the technology becomes the student's preeminent aim in contrast to the traditional personalized involvement. Technology will always eventually win out over the more humanistic approach in medicine. After embracing the skills of technology, the abandonment of traditional 'hands-on' care frequently follows." In other words, we are creating a generation of technicians instead of the caring, humane physicians who are needed desperately. An even larger proportion of physicians choose to specialize in technical fields, and many of those who remain in primary-care specialties would find themselves at a distinct disadvantage in any situation in which they had to rely solely on their five senses. In intensive-care subspecialties, which should by definition encourage an understanding of physiology and medical practices based as much as possible on scientific sense, physicians have become slaves of technology. They react excessively to numbers and images, without integrating them with their intuitive and scientific understanding of the patient. If technological results do not fit in with the clinical assessment of the patient, technology is not necessarily right. Both points of view need to be reassessed before jumping to conclusions.

Second, technology can be misused, most commonly because of imperfect understanding of the indications and limitations of the methods. CT scanning should not be used in lieu of ultrasonography, nor magnetic-resonance imaging in lieu of CT scanning, unless the more complex technology is clearly expected to provide better resolution or a more accurate diagnosis. As a rule, sophisticated tests should not be performed "for the record," but should be used only if they are intended to be acted on and to change the management of the patient.

Third, as discussed earlier, biomedical technology is expensive. Its unrestricted use is unconscionable in an increasingly cost-conscious society. If we do not discipline ourselves, others will do it for us, and we will more than likely bemoan their decisions.

Fourth, however benign high technology may appear, the risk that it could prove harmful to the patient, by omission or by commission, must never be ignored. Medical history is replete with examples. *Primum non nocere* remains the order of the day, in this case translating into "do not expose patients to what they do not need."

BIOMEDICAL TECHNOLOGY AND THE FUTURE

Everything said previously needs to be said in order to avoid a natural tendency to become complacent and to take existing and future technology for granted. Yet all the negatives and potential negatives cannot outweigh the contributions that technology has made to medicine. It behooves us not to accept every new technique and every claim blindly: Technology exists, and therefore let us use it. Rather, the medical profession should be guided by three principles.

Use high technology intelligently

Instead of rushing to use whatever was suggested in the last issues of our favorite medical journals, we must think about the scientific foundations of a new technique and assess its potential, or wait for others in more than one setting (confirmatory evidence) to do so for us. It is new, but is it better than what we already use? The technology is more advanced, but does it really yield better, more useful results than older, simpler, cheaper techniques? Finally, physicians must be educated or must educate themselves to the costs of their practices, from the apparently simplest laboratory test (Why does it cost $3.00 to $6.00 for a clinical chemistry laboratory to measure a hematocrit?) to the most esoteric high-tech examination or monitoring technology. A patient should not be deprived of a test or monitoring that is needed, but it should always be remembered that someone ultimately will have to pay for it.

Use self-restraint

Acquisition of expensive technology should be a well-thought-out process. The availability of the technology in a nearby hospital should not be an incentive to acquire it in one's own institution. In fact, it might be a deterrent, or at least cause some serious thought regarding the advisability of duplicating expensive facilities. In a word, "regionalization" may be a fiscally sound approach. The track records for CT scanning, magnetic-resonance imaging, extracorporeal membrane oxygenation, and many other surgical procedures are not encouraging in this respect, but that should not prevent us from trying. In some instances, duplication cannot be helped, especially when the transfer of patients between facilities involves risks or costs of its own. The determination of cost-effectiveness can be misleading; there are too many different ways of accounting for costs, as well as determining effectiveness. The process should be subjected to the same rules of intellectual probity as any other research project.

Perform adequate research

Physicians, nurses, and hospital administrators are besieged by sales representatives who all claim that their products are better than those of their competitors, and that is fair in any commercial enterprise. What we must be careful to do is to keep our distance from the game. We have the right and the obligation to demand the data behind any claims. FDA or UL approval helps but is not sufficient in itself, as the criteria used by those organizations are not necessarily the criteria that are relevant to our specific application of the product. Requesting "loaners" for a limited time to evaluate the performance of an instrument in the setting in which it will be used is appropriate and should be encouraged. Better performance in a laboratory does not ensure greater reliability in a clinical setting. We must beware of companies that refuse to do this, companies whose only offer is to sell us an instrument with a refund guarantee; chances are they have something to hide. Above all, when evaluating an instrument, we must be sure to compare its performance to that of another instrument designed for the same purpose. Comparing apples and oranges is seldom conclusive. Finally, is it cost-effective and worth the investment?

Too many technologies introduced into neonatal intensive-care nurseries, and there to stay, have not been properly validated. Now these technologies will never be questioned, on the grounds that it would be unethical to deprive a patient of the potential benefits of this technology. The big question is where funding is to come from. This echoes the concern voiced elsewhere by LeBlanc (1991), who takes a distinctly pessimistic view. It is true that research into specific applications of biomedical technology is not held in high favor by agencies responsible for giving grants. There are, however, federal programs and private foundations that fund such projects, especially if there is a stated goal to demonstrate cost-effectiveness and a reasonable chance of drawing conclusions that can be extrapolated to the entire country. I rather tend to believe that there has been a dearth of well-designed projects submitted to the appropriate funding agencies. The medical community generally has been loath to enter into projects that do not entail high visibility and are thought to benefit industry rather than medicine or science. In my view, this is a shortsighted outlook. Symbiosis between industry and science–medicine has existed for a long time and can be highly beneficial to both.

There ought to be greater pressure put on manufacturers of high technology to support a reasonable amount of research into the performance of their instruments in the field. They stand to make a great deal of money from the sales of their instruments, and yet they are reluctant to support research, especially if it involves comparison with a competitor's model. Occasionally they may provide an instrument free of charge or at discount for testing, but they balk at paying research costs (personnel and supplies). We propose a national industrial fund contributed to by all manufacturers of biomedical equipment, but administered independently of them. This fund could then disburse money for independent field research and testing on the basis of competitive grant applications. It could thereby ensure that proper testing of instruments and performance comparisons of similar instruments would be done under conditions that would ensure credibility to the results.

CONCLUSION

The past 30 years have seen tremendous advances in biomedical technology that have dramatically changed the practice of medicine in general and of neonatology in particular. All changes have not been for the best, however. The price tag has been especially steep, but there have been adverse effects on the quality of medicine as well. The reasons we rely on high technology, with its risks and pitfalls, and our future handling of decisions regarding using or not using biotechnology, deserve careful consideration, including financial factors that physicians have traditionally been loath to address. If the medical profession is to avoid becoming enslaved to technology, our future decisions must be better informed, more rational, and based on more scientific facts than they have been in the past. Above all, physicians must avoid becoming mere technicians at the expense of the traditional humanistic approach to patient care.

REFERENCES

AAP (1985). American Academy of Pediatrics Task Force on Prolonged Infantile Apnea: Prolonged infantile apnea: 1985. *Pediatrics* 76:129–31.

Altman, S. H., and Blendon, R. (eds.). (1979). Medical technology: the culprit behind health care costs? In *Proceedings of the 1977 Sun Valley Forum on National Health*. DHEW publication no. (PHS)79-3216. Washington, DC: U.S. Government Printing Office.

Brans, Y. W. (1983). Equipment available for nurseries. *Clinics in Perinatology* 10:263–79.

Brazy, J. E. (1991). Near infrared spectroscopy. *Clinics in Perinatology* 18:519–34.

Figge, D. C. (1990). The tyranny of technology: presidential address. *American Journal of Obstetrics and Gynecology* 162:1365–9.

Hay, W. W., Jr., Thilo, E., and Curlander, J. B. (1991). Pulse oximetry in neonatal medicine. *Clinics in Perinatology* 18:441–72.

Hope, P. L., and Moorcraft, J. (1991). Magnetic resonance spectroscopy. *Clinics in Perinatology* 18:535–48.

Hunt, C. E. (1991). Cardiorespiratory monitoring. *Clinics in Perinatology* 18:473–98.

Hunt, C. E., and Brouillette, R. T. (1987). Sudden infant death syndrome: 1987 perspective. *Journal of Pediatrics* 110:669–78.

LeBlanc, M. H. (1991). Thermoregulation, incubators, radiant warmers, artificial skins and body hoods. *Clinics in Perinatology* 18:403–22.

Sorkin, A. L. (1986). *Health Care and the Changing Economic Environment* (pp. 5, 75). Lexington, MA: Heath.

PART I

Imaging

Nowhere in perinatal medicine has technology made a more prominent appearance than in the techniques of imaging; some, in fact, have called it *the* technical revolution. For the first time, live, moving fetuses with beating hearts, moving circulation, kicking and grasping extremities, and a myriad of structural malformations and deformations have been seen, for important diagnostic issues as well as the delight of parents seeing their "almost new" baby. But this revolution began with the newborn infant. Computed tomography (CT) scans defined clear pictures of normal anatomy and structural abnormalities, and ultrasound investigations of the brain revealed intracranial hemorrhage, previously known only at autopsy. And flow Doppler ultrasound (echocardiography) has virtually eliminated the need for cardiac catheterization (and even auscultation!) in newborn infants, allowing accurate and noninvasive diagnosis of cardiac and vascular anat-

omy, as well as myocardial contractility, cardiac output, and blood-flow shunts. Although the fine resolution in all of these techniques could be improved, the fuzziness of current images is just waiting for the right computer-generated subtraction–enhancement software to produce crystal-clear pictures.

What's next? If CT and/or magnetic-resonance imaging (MRI) could be combined with magnetic-resonance spectroscopy (MRS), positron-emission tomography (PET) scanning, and Doppler flow, we would have a firsthand look at metabolism taking place. Projected developments of devices that can allow real-time imaging of metabolism, oxygen consumption, blood supply, and so forth, are not just science fiction, and not even far-fetched. This book is full of technologies that not long ago were considered miraculous: "If it can be imagined, it can be done."

1

Ultrasonography

MICHAEL F. INSANA, Ph.D.
LINDA A. HARRISON, M.D.

INTRODUCTION

In attempting to maximize the benefit and minimize the risk, a physician must consider many factors when requesting a diagnostic procedure for a patient. In medical imaging, it is essential that the diagnostician understand the basic interactions between the probing radiation and the tissues of the body and the fundamental trade-offs that must be made when selecting instrumentation for a procedure, if the greatest amount of diagnostic information is to be obtained at the lowest cost and least risk to the patient. This is particularly true for ultrasonography, where the quality of the ultrasound image is as much a function of the sonographer's ability and the patient's physiology as it is a function of the instrumentation.

To use ultrasound most effectively, it is important to understand its limitations. The principal advantage of ultrasound as an imaging modality is its ability to provide information noninvasively concerning anatomy and blood flow in real time, at relatively low cost, and with little or no risk to the health of the patient and sonographer. The principal disadvantage is its limited access to many parts of the body. However, perinatal patients present unique opportunities to overcome some of the access limitations encountered in older patients. The fetal lung and neonatal brain are examples of structures that can be investigated with ultrasound, whereas such structures normally are impenetrable in older patients because of the presence of bone and air.

The purpose of this chapter is to describe the principles and applications of medical ultrasonography related to perinatal medicine. It is intended to provide the reader with a basis for deciding when ultrasound is the most appropriate tool in a given clinical situation. Particular emphasis is placed on factors that affect the many trade-offs among image quality features that are necessary to most effectively use ultrasonography.

BASIC IMAGE FORMATION

High-frequency sound waves (typically 1–10 MHz) are introduced into the body by pressing a vibrating source (transducer) onto the skin surface (Figure 1.1a). These waves interact with the tissues in which they travel, producing the scattered pressure waves that generate echo signals (Figure 1.1b). Because one transducer is used both to transmit acoustic pulses and to receive echo signals, the basic method for acquiring data is often referred to as a *pulse–echo imaging technique*.

For each position of the transducer, echo signals are detected and demodulated, and the resulting amplitudes, or A-mode signals, are stored (Figure 1.1c). The echo amplitude at a particular time t_1 depends on the properties of the tissue encompassed by the acoustic pulse at the axial position z_1. Time and distance are related by the pulse–echo equation

$$t_1 = \frac{2z_1}{c} \qquad (1.1)$$

where c is the speed of sound in the medium. Although the speed of sound varies for different tissues, imaging systems assume an average value of $1{,}540 \text{ m} \cdot \text{s}^{-1}$ throughout the body. Consequently, echoes from structures located 5 cm below the skin surface, for example, will be received 65 μs (0.000065 s) after the transmission of the pulse.

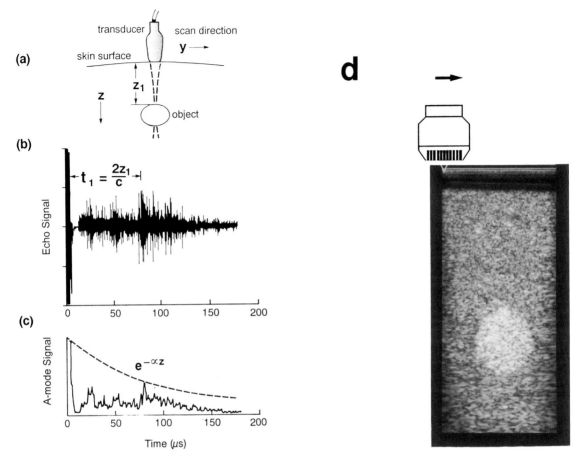

Figure 1.1. (a) Ultrasound transducer scanning a tissuelike medium. Also shown are the corresponding radiofrequency echo signal (b), A-mode signal (c), and B-mode images (d) and (e). The same phantom was scanned with a 5-MHz linear array (d) and with a 5-MHz phased array (e).

The transducer element is then moved laterally, along the y axis in Figure 1.1a, before the process is repeated and a second pulse is transmitted. For each position along y, an A-mode echo signal is recorded and converted into pixel brightness values or B-mode image signal; that is, echo amplitudes are mapped into gray-scale pixel values. B-mode signals are stored in a scan converter, which also formats the data for display on a television monitor. If A-mode signals are obtained by linearly translating transducer elements along the y axis, a rectangular image format is used, as shown in Figure 1.1d. If signals are recorded by rotating transducer elements or electronically steering the beam (as discussed later) through the sector angle φ, a sector image format results, as shown in Figure 1.1e. Selecting a transducer type automatically determines the image format.

Each complete scan resulting in an image is called a frame. Current instruments generate 10 to 60 B-mode frames per second, so that the monitor can display a continuously changing image. For this reason, ultrasound is considered to be a real-time imaging modality. The largest number of lines per frame is needed to provide the maximum information density, and the highest frame rate possible is needed to avoid distorting the appearance of fast-moving reflectors, such as heart valves. Limitations on these parameters are ultimately determined by the speed of sound in the body. We can extend the mathematical relationship between the depth in the body and the time an echo is received, equation (1.1), and compute the time necessary to generate one frame. If Z is the maximum depth of penetration and N is the number of A lines per frame, then the time needed to generate one complete frame T is

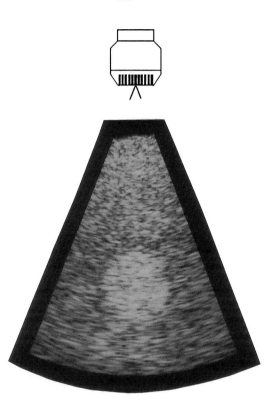

Figure 1.1 (cont.).

$$T = \frac{2ZN}{c} \qquad (1.2)$$

Recognizing that the frame rate $R = 1/T$, we can use equation (1.2) to find the following expression:

$$c = 2ZNR \qquad (1.3)$$

Equation (1.3) tells us that the product of the total path length that sound travels, $2Z$, the image line density, N, and the frame rate, R, can be no larger than the speed of sound in the body, c. So, for example, to penetrate 20 cm into the body and maintain a frame rate of 30 frames per second, the number of lines per frame is limited to 128. To increase the frame rate, therefore, requires a reduction in the field of view (FOV) and/or in lateral information density (but not lateral resolution, which is determined by the transducer-beam geometry, as discussed later). Typically, the operator chooses a FOV to include just the region of interest, and the imaging system software adjusts other parameters accordingly. Some systems, however, allow the oper-ator to vary the line density at the expense of the frame rate.

TRANSDUCERS AND IMAGE QUALITY

Often the term *ultrasound transducer* refers to the scanhead – the entire hand-held device a sonographer applies to the skin surface to produce an image. The active elements of a transducer account for only a small part of the device and are made of a piezoelectric material, usually lead zirconate titanate (PZT) or equivalent ceramic material. Piezoelectric materials convert electrical energy into mechanical vibrations, and mechanical vibrations back into electrical energy. Therefore, the same device is used both to transmit and to receive acoustic energy. To transmit acoustic pulses, a short-duration alternating-current (ac) voltage is applied to opposite surfaces of elements (Figure 1.2). The piezoelectric properties of the material cause the surfaces to vibrate in response to the applied volt-

(a)   **(b)**

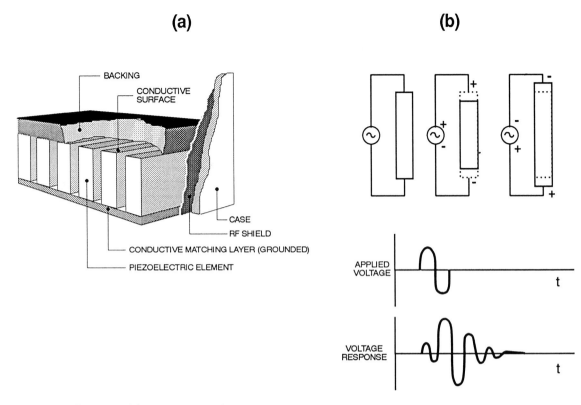

Figure 1.2. Illustration of the construction and operation of an array of piezoelectric transducer elements.

age. In effect, the active element "rings" when struck with an electrical "hammer." After transmission, the same elements are switched to the receive mode to listen for vibrations caused by echoes returning from the body. The response of the piezoelectric material to vibration is to generate a voltage that is the echo signal used to form the image. Elements are mechanically and electrically damped to shape the transmission pulse and thereby determine the *axial resolution* and *sensitivity* of the transducer. Matching layers are applied to the element surface to reduce reflections at the skin surface and enhance image sensitivity. In general, high sensitivity is possible at the expense of axial resolution.

The piezoelectric elements in a transducer are cut into particular shapes that will determine the resonant frequency and produce a beam with specified focal characteristics and beam geometry. The shape of the elements and, for arrays, the order in which signals are transmitted and received determine how the acoustic energy is distributed spatially on "transmit" and the directional sensitivity of the same elements on "receive." This information is summarized by the transducer *directivity function*.

Flexibility in forming the beam is important to real-time imaging, where it is necessary to transmit and receive signals in many directions to acquire the large number of scan lines in an image frame. Options currently used by commercial manufacturers are illustrated in Figures 1.3 and 1.4.

Before describing the different transducer types, it is important to briefly define the properties of image quality that must be considered when designing and selecting a transducer for imaging. *Image quality* can be defined in terms of the quality and uniformity of spatial resolution and gray-scale resolution. Spatial resolution refers to the ability of the system to display two closely spaced structures as discrete targets (Figure 1.5a). The main lobe of the transducer beam directivity function determines the lateral component of spatial resolution, and the pulse length (or, equivalently, system bandwidth) determines the axial component. Gray-scale resolution refers to the ability of the system to display regions of different but similar tissue types as discrete regions (Figure 1.5b), as well as to differentiate low-contrast structures in a mixed field of strong and weak reflectors (Figure 1.5c). The transducer prop-

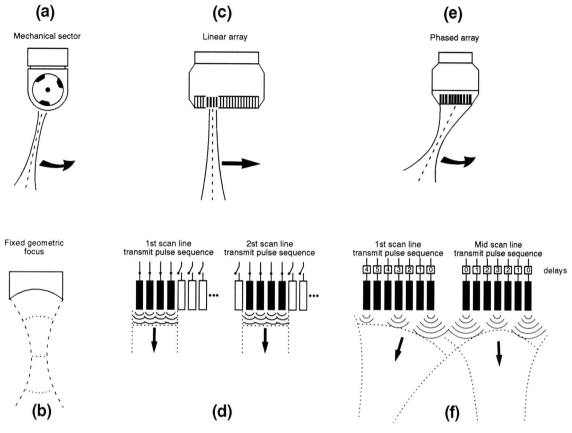

(a) Mechanical sector

(c) Linear array

(e) Phased array

(b) Fixed geometric focus

(d) 1st scan line transmit pulse sequence / 2st scan line transmit pulse sequence

(f) 1st scan line transmit pulse sequence / Mid scan line transmit pulse sequence / delays

Figure 1.3. Operations of three types of clinical transducers are diagrammed. Although an unfocused linear array is shown, current implementations are usually focused.

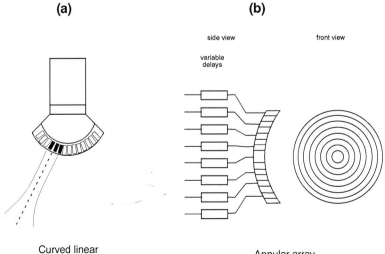

(a) Curved linear array

(b) side view / variable delays / front view / Annular array

Figure 1.4. Curved linear-array and annular-array transducers are illustrated.

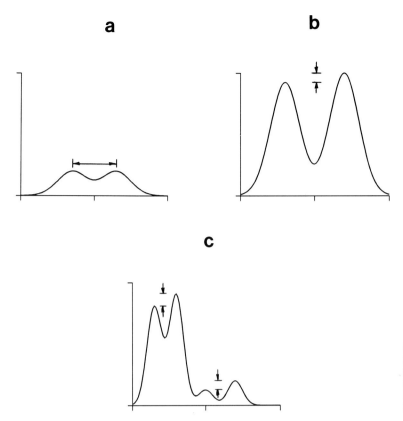

Figure 1.5. One-dimensional examples of imaging tasks that challenge specific aspects of image quality in ultrasound: (a) spatial resolution, (b) low-contrast gray-scale resolution, (c) high-contrast gray-scale resolution.

erty that dominates gray-scale resolution is the magnitude of the main lobe of the beam compared with that of the side lobes. An overall system property important for determining gray-scale resolution is the *dynamic range* – the ratio of the smallest echo amplitude that just saturates the display to the smallest echo amplitude that produces a signal on the display at the threshold of detection. The following discussion of the different transducer designs necessarily involves a discussion of the trade-offs among the features that define image quality.

In one implementation of mechanical sector transducers (Figure 1.3a), three fixed-focus circular elements are mechanically rotated to sweep out a sector field. Often three different elements are used in one scanhead to allow the operator to quickly change between resonant frequencies. High-frequency mechanical sector transducers provide higher spatial resolution than that obtained at low frequencies, but at the expense of field uniformity. Mechanical sector transducers are sensitive detectors that can achieve high spatial resolution for a fixed, limited depth of field (Figure 1.3b). To more completely control the focusing properties of transducers, array technology was developed.

The principles of *array transducers* are well known from the fields of optics, radar, and sonar (Goodman, 1968). These principles are used by manufacturers to specify array designs that can be expected to produce the highest image quality consistent with the available technology. In radiology applications, including obstetrics, many of the tasks require superior gray-scale resolution, whereas in cardiology high frame rates and high spatial resolution are emphasized. The following discussion is skewed toward radiology applications.

High spatial and gray-scale resolution is possible when the array contains a large number of piezoelectric elements, spaced one-half of the resonant wavelength ($\lambda/2$) apart, where each element has an independent channel (i.e., there is an independent pulser and receiver for each element). Large numbers of elements form the large aperture needed for superior lateral resolution. An element spacing of $\lambda/2$ minimizes the *grating lobes* inherent with arrays and therefore provides high-quality gray-scale resolution. Grating lobes are peaks in acoustic sensitivity, adjacent to the main imaging lobe of the transducer sound beam, that act to clutter the image and reduce contrast (Figure 1.6). They

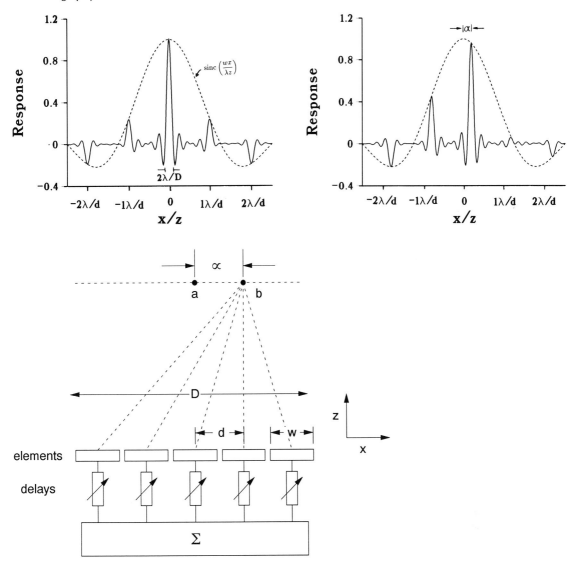

Figure 1.6. The graphs at top are the far-field beam patterns that result from steering the beam of a phased array to points a and b in the diagram at bottom. Beam pattern directivity for the array is indicated by the solid line in each graph, and the directivity for a single element is indicated by the dashed line. The width of the main lobe of the beam, $2\lambda/D$, where λ is the wavelength of sound and D is the aperture size, is a measure of the lateral resolution for the array. Grating lobes (solid line) are spaced at intervals of λ/d, where d is the spacing between elements. Properties of side lobes (dashed line) are determined by the size of the elements w, axial distance z, and the wavelength. The highest-quality beam properties are obtained when a phased array is steered straight ahead ($\alpha = 0$), because the aperture is maximum and grating lobes are minimum.

are consequences of segmenting the aperture to enable electronic focusing and steering. It should be noted that large-aperture transducers with coarsely spaced elements exhibit high spatial resolution (narrow main lobe) but often have poor gray-scale resolution because of large grating lobes. Currently, high-end imaging systems use 48, 96, or 128 channels.

Modern array transducers dynamically focus the beam by properly delaying the phase of each receive channel before summing the echo signals. It is also possible to steer and focus the transmit pulse electronically at multiple depths, but this requires that the system transmit more than one pulse per scan line. The price paid for multiple transmit foci is a loss in frame rate. These features are the beamforming function of the system (Macovski, 1979).

Some manufacturers *apodize* the array, that is,

electronically vary the sensitivity of each element, with different weighting functions on transmit and receive. If properly implemented, apodization will reduce side lobes – increasing gray-scale resolution – while increasing the width of the main lobe of the transducer beam – slightly reducing (lateral) spatial resolution. Apodization is most useful when the imaging task demands high-contrast gray-scale resolution (Figure 1.5c), because grating lobes and side lobes clutter the image, filling in cystlike structures and obscuring small variations in echo amplitudes. Another function of apodization is to maintain a constant *f* number for the transducer (often *f*/2). The *f* number is the ratio of focal length to aperture size. The full aperture is used to focus deep in the body, but to focus on superficial structures the system automatically reduces the aperture size by using fewer elements and channels. The result is an image with a more uniform image texture throughout the FOV. A significant increase in computational power made possible by advances in high-speed integrated circuits over the past 10 yr has allowed manufacturers to take full advantage of array technology and thereby dramatically improve the quality of ultrasonography (Maslak, 1985).

One-dimensional arrays. Linear-array transducers use more elements than channels to form a beam. Voltage pulses are applied to a subset of adjacent elements both to transmit pulses and to receive echo signals. Small delays in transmitting and receiving signals with each element may be used to electronically focus the beam. Element groups are activated sequentially, as shown in Figures 1.3c and 1.3d, to produce scan lines that step linearly across the image frame. This method is the electronic equivalent of moving a single-element transducer linearly across the field, as described in the previous section. Because of large apertures and minimal grating lobes, linear-array technology offers very high image quality in applications where the large transducer "footprint" does not limit access to the body (e.g., obstetrics).

Phased-array transducers use a constant number of elements and channels for each scan line to produce a sector image. Electronic delay circuits are used to both focus and steer the beam across the field, as shown in Figures 1.3e and 1.3f. A significant advantage of phased arrays over linear arrays is the smaller footprint that allows unobstructed access to many more regions in the body (e.g., the fontanelle or intercostal spaces). For this reason, phased-array technology dominates the cardiology market. The major disadvantages of phased arrays occur at large steering angles. There is a reduction in spatial reso-

lution because the smaller effective aperture at larger steering angles produces a wider main lobe. At or beyond the focal length, the size of the "speckle" spots is a general indicator of spatial resolution. Therefore, by comparing the average speckle spot size in Figure 1.1d (linear array) with that in Figure 1.1e (phased array) it is possible to observe qualitatively the differences in spatial resolution between the two transducer types. There is a reduced sensitivity for phased arrays compared with linear arrays because the directivity for the main lobe is reduced at large steering angles, and also an increase in the relative magnitude of grating lobes, as illustrated at the top of Figure 1.6.

Curved linear arrays embody an attempt to obtain the advantages of linear and phased arrays while minimizing their disadvantages. Curved linear arrays operate in a manner similar to a linear array, but the elements are arranged along an arc whose radius of curvature is designed for specific clinical applications (Figure 1.4a). Curved linear arrays have footprints smaller than those of most linear arrays, but larger than those of most phased arrays, and uniform spatial resolution similar to that of linear arrays. The curved shape of the array elements provides some passive apodization, because the outer elements of the active group pass through more attenuating lens material than the inner elements.

Two-dimensional arrays. In spite of all the signal-processing magic available to array technology, one-dimensional (1-D) arrays cannot overcome a fundamental limitation – 1-D arrays can be focused only in the two dimensions of the scan plane. In the elevation direction, perpendicular to the scan plane, the geometry of the elements provides a fixed mechanical focus and a small aperture. As a result, the thickness of the tomographic slice is large and nonuniform, and therefore the partial-volume effects that pose difficulties for x-ray computed tomographic (CT) imaging by reducing image contrast for small structures are also present in ultrasound imaging using 1-D arrays. Two-dimensional (2-D) arrays are needed to adaptively focus the beam in three dimensions. A partial solution currently available commercially is the annular-array transducer (Figure 1.4b). Similar to the mechanical sector transducer, the annular array has a circular aperture and is mechanically steered. But unlike mechanical sectors, the piezoelectric element is cut into annual rings, which makes it possible to electronically focus in three dimensions. Eight annular elements are typically used, which can result in an image quality close to that of linear 1-D arrays but inferior to that

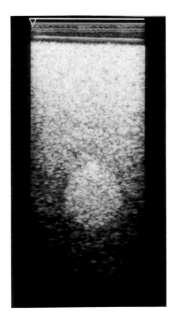 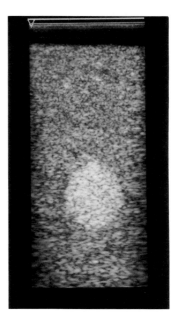

Figure 1.7. Linear-array images of a tissuelike attenuating phantom material are shown without (left) and with (right) the use of depth-gain compensation.

of a true 2-D array. Although there is a significant improvement in the out-of-plane lateral resolution, the size of the footprint and long-term durability have been problems with some annular arrays.

In summary, each type of transducer emphasizes certain features important to overall image quality. Therefore, the choice of transducer technology greatly depends on the imaging task. For obstetrical applications, where often there is free access to the tissues of interest, linear and curved linear arrays are chosen for their overall high image quality. For pediatric applications, access to the body may be more of a problem, and annular arrays are often more useful. Where access is most limited, phased arrays are the transducers of choice.

THE PHYSICS OF ACOUSTIC INTERACTIONS

When choosing an imaging modality, it is essential to know the mechanisms of interactions between the probing radiation and the tissue. The contrast in x-ray imaging is due primarily to differences in the atomic numbers and mass densities of normal and diseased tissues. Contrast in magnetic-resonance imaging reflects differences in the number density and the local chemical environment of hydrogen nuclei. Contrast in ultrasound imaging is determined by the composition and fluctuations in elastic properties of the medium, as described later. To select an imaging modality to answer a specific diagnostic question, the diagnostician must first interpret potential disease conditions in the terms previously described, that is, to understand how disease changes the physical properties of body tissues to produce the image contrast required for detection. In this section, we review the basic processes by which ultrasound interacts with tissue.

There can be no image contrast without an acoustic interaction, and all interactions attenuate (i.e., remove energy from the transmitted pulse). Therefore, it is important to understand how biological tissues attenuate sound in order to interpret the image. (Note that the ultrasound image displays reflected mechanical energy, unlike x-ray imaging, which displays transmitted electromagnetic energy.)

The most obvious effect of attenuation is the exponential reduction in signal strength with time (depth), as illustrated in the A-mode signal in Figure 1.1c and in the B-mode image in Figure 1.7. Attenuation is often characterized by the exponential parameter – the attenuation coefficient α. In imaging, the loss of signal strength usually can be recovered (if the electronic noise is small) by amplifying the echo signals from deep in the body more than those from near the skin surface. The proper use of this depth-gain compensation (DGC) feature, present on all imaging systems, is illustrated in Figure 1.7. Attenuation can also indicate diagnostically significant changes in tissues, if the interactions between ultrasound and the body are well understood.

Attenuation may be broadly divided into two processes: absorption and scattering. Absorption is the transformation of acoustic energy into heat and is the principal component of attenuation (90–95%) (Lyons and Parker, 1988). Scattering is the redirection of all or part of the acoustic energy, and it is a much smaller component of attenuation (5–10%). Through these two processes of interaction we receive information about the material composition and elastic structure of a tissue. This information may be recognized qualitatively in the B-scan image and quantitatively through signal-processing methods.

Absorption greatly depends on the composition of the tissue (e.g., fat and glycogen contents greatly affect the attenuation of liver). At one time it was thought that ultrasound absorption measurements might provide a "signature" for characterizing many different tissues. (Attenuation measurements were used to provide that information, because attenuation is dominated by absorption processes.) In vivo measurements in liver, for example, proved to be highly variable, even among normals. Therefore, quantitative estimates of attenuation/absorption were thought to have little or no diagnostic value. Recently, it has been shown that total lipid and glycogen contents are dominant factors influencing attenuation in liver (Garra et al., 1987; Tuthill, Baggs, and Parker, 1989), to the point that the time of day and diet must be taken into account to understand the apparently large variations in normal values reported in the literature. That is, normal daily fluctuations in liver contents can produce variations in attenuation on the order of those caused by disease. Once these factors are understood and properly taken into consideration, attenuation measurements could provide quantitative diagnostic information not available with imaging.

The scattering properties of tissue are determined by the macroscopic and microscopic anatomy and movement of tissues. In many situations we do not yet know which microanatomical structures interact with sound, although we do know that if an object scatters sound, its density and/or compressibility are different from those of the surrounding medium. Notable examples of macroscopic scatterers are bone and gas-filled tissues. In both cases, the density and compressibility vary from those of the surrounding soft tissues to such a large degree that the incident pulse cannot penetrate, but is mostly reflected at the boundary. Because of poor penetration, ultrasonography has been used very little in assessing the adult head, lungs, and gastrointestinal tract.

Of greater interest is the weaker scattering from the fine structure of soft tissues, the scattering that

produces the characteristic speckle patterns observed in all images. The elastic properties of collagen make it the most likely source of soft-tissue scatter, although the net water and fat contents can also be significant factors (Bamber, Hill, and King, 1981). It is important to realize that whereas the appearance of acoustic speckle depends on the tissue architecture, the speckle spots in the image (Figure 1.7) do *not* correspond one-to-one with the sources of scattering (Wagner et al., 1983). Average properties of the microscopic structure of a tissue can be estimated from the radio-frequency echo signals – the inverse-scattering problem – as many researchers are currently investigating (Greenleaf, 1986). Currently, physicians must rely on the exquisite pattern-recognition abilities of the human eye–brain system to detect the subtle changes in image texture that result from alterations in tissue architecture due to disease, although there is evidence that even trained observers have only limited ability to visually detect such changes (Wagner, Insana, and Brown, 1985). Gray-scale imaging is most sensitive for observing boundaries, such as blood vessels, heart valves, and organ surfaces, and for detecting changes in the average scattering strength (echogenicity) of large regions (e.g., determining if a mass is cystic or solid).

In summary, B-mode images describe the reflective (backscatter) properties of tissue, as determined by the spatial variation in elastic properties. The brightness of the image is reduced by absorption processes in tissues, and the positions of structures within the image vary with the speed of sound. In addition, changes in the speed of sound between two types of tissues, such as perinephric fat layers ($c = 1,450$ m·s^{-1}) and renal cortex ($c = 1,570$ m·s^{-1}), can refract or "bend" the sound beam to produce a wide range of image artifacts. Absorption and speed are determined by the type and quantity of tissue components, such as lipid and water. Accurate interpretation of ultrasound images requires an understanding of the underlying processes of sound–tissue interactions.

DOPPLER ULTRASOUND

Doppler ultrasound, based on the Doppler effect, is a noninvasive method for describing blood flow. The Doppler effect concerns the change in the frequency of echo signals caused by motion of the scatterers. For transmitted sound waves of a single frequency, the relationship between the change in frequency and the velocity of scatterers is given by the equation

$$f_D = f_r - f_i = \frac{2f_i v \cos\theta}{c} \qquad (1.4)$$

where f_D is the Doppler frequency given by the difference between the reflected (f_r) and incident (f_i) sound frequencies, c is the speed of sound in the medium, and θ is the angle between the directions of the incident sound waves and the movement of scatterers with velocity v (Figure 1.8, top; see color plates following page 121). The factor cos θ tells us that the only component of scatterer motion detected is that parallel to the incident sound beam. The component of flow perpendicular to the beam axis is not detected. The Doppler frequency f_D is positive when the flow is toward the transducer, and negative when the flow is away from the transducer. The greatest sensitivity for Doppler measurements occurs for angles between 30° and 60–70°. More shallow angles lead to low sensitivity because of refraction and critical angle artifacts, whereas steeper angles yield low sensitivity because the factor cos θ is small. Equation (1.4) also shows that the magnitude of the frequency shift is proportional to the speed of scatterer motion and the frequency of sound transmitted. To produce large values for f_D and yet obtain sufficient penetration in attenuating tissues, the frequency range for medical applications typically is 2–10 MHz.

The first Doppler units used continuous-wave (CW) Doppler methods: A sinusoidal wave (mostly one frequency) is transmitted continuously with one transducer aperture and received simultaneously with another adjacent aperture. Because f_D is typically $10^{-3} \times f_i$, the Doppler signal is in the kilohertz frequency range and is detectable as audible sound. The human ear is a sensitive spectral analyzer that can differentiate between sound waves of different frequencies sensed simultaneously. Later Doppler units have augmented the audible signal with a visual presentation of the same spectral information displayed as a time-varying trace (Figure 1.8, middle; color plate, following page 121). The horizontal axis represents time, and the vertical axis frequency. The gray-scale intensity on the trace signifies the relative contribution of each frequency at a given time. Intense high-frequency echoes appear as bright areas near the top of the vertical axis, and intense low-frequency echoes appear as bright areas near the bottom. Doppler spectra are computed from the echo signals using a signal-processing method known as the fast Fourier transform (FFT).

Doppler ultrasound is most often used to describe blood flow (Taylor and Holland, 1990). Specifically, changes in the frequency of sound scattered by red blood cells (RBCs) moving in a vessel are used to estimate their velocity. However, RBCs move at different speeds within vessels, so that a Doppler spectrum, even a CW Doppler spectrum, has many frequency components. The velocity profile is fairly uniform in normal *large* blood vessels, so that the Doppler spectrum, displayed as the width of the time trace in the example of Figure 1.8 (middle), is narrow; that is, most of the Doppler signal occurs near one frequency, because most of the RBCs have the same velocity. The Doppler spectrum is broader in normal *small* vessels, where there is greater variability in RBC speed. Spectral broadening can occur under normal and diseased conditions when there are steep velocity gradients, curvature to the vessels, and in-line turbulent flow. Doppler spectra for each vessel have characteristic patterns that are recognized by trained observers. Pathological conditions that alter blood flow may be detected as changes in these characteristic patterns. It is important to understand that blood flow and average velocity are not equivalent. It is necessary to consider the distribution of RBC velocities within the vessel to accurately relate velocity and flow using Doppler spectra.

CW Doppler techniques provide high sensitivity but no spatial resolution. Signals obtained at each instant of time using CW methods indicate motion at all depths along the beam. If, instead, we transmit broadband pulses and then electronically switch on and off ("gate") the echo signals, we can isolate a region for analysis using one pulse–echo transducer. These pulsed Doppler techniques, which trade off signal sensitivity (less energy transmitted and received) to obtain spatial resolution, are useful for combining simultaneous Doppler measurements with B-mode imaging to form a duplex Doppler system. Duplex Doppler systems make it possible to view the anatomy while precisely placing the gated region for Doppler measurements at the desired location.

There are several decisions that the sonographer must make to minimize the limitations of pulsed Doppler methods. The greatest value of f_D (the highest blood velocity) that contributes to the echo signal determines the minimum number of Doppler pulses that must be transmitted into the body per second – the pulse repetition frequency (PRF). The reason for this is as follows: All pulsed Doppler instruments currently estimate f_D by measuring the phase shift between echoes from sequential pulses. This technique is equivalent to sampling f_D at the PRF. Sampling theory shows us that the PRF must be at least twice that of the largest Doppler frequency (PRF $\geq 2f_{Dmax}$) to avoid spectral distortions known as *aliasing*. Aliasing is the phenomenon that occurs when a continuous process (e.g., blood flowing in the body) is undersampled (e.g., the PRF is too low). When aliasing occurs, the measured spectrum does not accurately represent the velocity profile within the vessel; not only is the high-frequency information lost, but also it is "folded back" onto the low frequencies, distorting the entire spectrum. Imaging systems provide the operator with the capability to adjust the PRF, image size, and other parameters necessary to avoid aliasing. The lowest PRF that avoids aliasing is known as the Nyquist frequency.

Duplex Doppler can be implemented in many different ways. The system can sweep out one B-mode image frame (128 lines) and then switch to provide as many as 128 Doppler pulses. The gaps that occur in the Doppler signal by interleaving frames must then be eliminated. Alternatively, the system can interleave lines of image data and Doppler data within a frame, which gives the impression of simultaneous acquisition but has the drawback of halving the Doppler PRF and increasing the possibility of aliasing. The method of interleaving lines can be achieved only with arrays that can be electronically steered in arbitrary directions. Mechanical sectors are limited to interleaving frames.

There are other concerns when implementing duplex Doppler. To generate B-mode images we want to use short-duration (broadband) pulses to attain high spatial resolution in the axial direction. For Doppler we want long-duration (narrowband) pulses (typically 3–15 cycles) to maximize Doppler sensitivity by transmitting as much power as possible at the frequency of interest and avoiding the frequency-dependent attenuation losses of broadband transmission. Because the same transducer is used for both tasks, the manufacturers must be able to quickly switch between broadband and narrowband electronics for each transmit and receive channel, where there are as many as 128 on current systems. Also, systems that use linear arrays often steer the Doppler pulse, as with a phased array. As described in the previous section, electronically steering the beam places grating lobes into the sensitive portion of the directivity function, which degrades Doppler resolution. Consequently, grating lobes can be a factor with linear arrays as well as phased arrays, when used for Doppler measurements.

Color-flow Doppler imaging is a multigated, pulsed Doppler method that displays velocity data in an image format on top of the B-scan image, using color (Figure 1.8, bottom) (Kisslo, Adams, and Belkin, 1988). Instead of interrogating one small gated region, as described earlier, color-flow Doppler pulses probe a large FOV with many small gates. Regions of blood flow away from and toward

Table 1.1. *Indications for obstetrical sonography in 2nd and 3rd trimesters*

Gestational dating
Inaccurate dates
Date/uterine-size discrepancy
Fetal well-being
Document life
Fetal growth–possible intrauterine growth retardation
Exclude fetal anomalies
Previous child with an anomaly
Maternal diabetes
Advanced maternal age
Increased maternal serum AFP
Amniotic fluid volume abnormality
Exposures to potential teratogens
Exclude placental abnormality
Placenta previa
Suspected uterine anomaly
Suspected pelvic mass
Guidance system for:
Diagnostic tests (e.g., amniocentesis, chorionic villous biopsy, fetal blood sampling)
Fetal therapy (e.g., fetal blood transfusion)

the transducer usually are indicated by the colors blue and red, respectively, although most systems allow the operator to choose the colors displayed. The color hue usually specifies the mean Doppler frequency or velocity, as indicated by the color bar in Figure 1.8. Other colors (e.g., green) may be used to display the width of the spectrum (velocity variance) to indicate turbulence or other disturbed flow patterns. The folding-back of high velocities onto low velocities that occurs with aliasing appears in color-flow images as islands of one color in a sea of mostly another color.

An advantage of color-flow imaging over duplex Doppler is its ability to describe the spatial distribution of blood flow over an extended two-dimensional area. Having a global description of blood flow within the spatial context of the surrounding anatomy makes it easier to guide placement of the pulsed Doppler gate and accurately obtain more detailed flow information. Hence, color-flow imaging and duplex Doppler are adjunct rather than competing procedures. A disadvantage of color-flow imaging is that less spectral information is available – only the mean and variance of the spectrum are indicated. The first two moments of the velocity distribution are usually measured using faster autocorrelation methods (Kasai et al., 1985) instead of the more computationally intensive FFT methods of duplex Doppler.

Sonographers should be aware that color-flow imaging systems filter signals to improve the appearance of the image overall, but nonetheless alter the flow information. Most systems use high-pass fil-

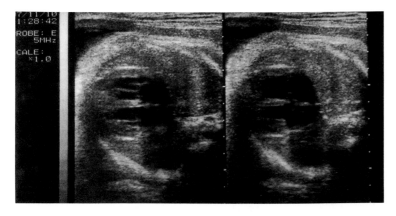

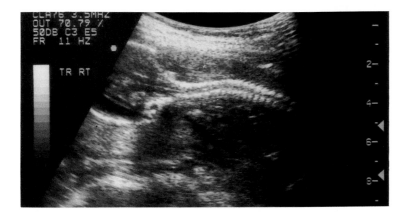

Figure 1.9. Uniform resolution throughout the field of view is demonstrated in (top) a 5-MHz linear-array side-by-side image of the fetal heart and in (bottom) a 3.5-MHz curved linear-array image of the upper spine in another fetus.

ters to suppress low-frequency signals due to unwanted body motion. Breathing and heart-wall motions produce a flash artifact that appears as a periodic flash of color over part or all of the image. Since much of this information is at frequencies below that of blood flow, low-frequency wall filters are used to reject the lowest-frequency Doppler signals. Also, the higher intensity of body-motion artifacts, as compared with that of blood flow, has been used to reject these unwanted signals. For some patients, however, flash artifacts occur within the blood-flow bandwidth and intensity, so that these artifacts cannot be completely suppressed without also distorting the velocity profile. Most systems build in some spatial filtering to blend together the Doppler gates and give the color image a smoother, more nearly continuous appearance. The image processing must be understood if one is to accurately interpret color-flow data.

CLINICAL APPLICATIONS

Ultrasound has a well-established place in perinatal medicine, providing a safe and effective means of diagnosis and guidance for interventional procedures. The following is a brief summary intended to demonstrate clinical applications in light of the foregoing discussion of image quality and acoustic interactions.

Obstetrics. There are numerous indications for obstetrical sonography in the second and third trimesters; the most common are listed in Table 1.1. Sonography serves as an effective diagnostic tool in the evaluation of the fetus, placenta, and uterus. Maternal abnormalities can also be evaluated, although the adnexal structures are more difficult to evaluate as the uterus enlarges in the second and third trimesters.

Obstetrical sonography after the first trimester is performed transabdominally using the highest-frequency transducer compatible with adequate penetration, usually 5 or 3 MHz. The enlarged uterus provides an acoustic "window" that allows the use of transducers with large footprints. Excellent low-contrast resolution with a large FOV is achieved with linear and curved linear arrays, as illustrated in Figure 1.9. Annular arrays also provide high-quality

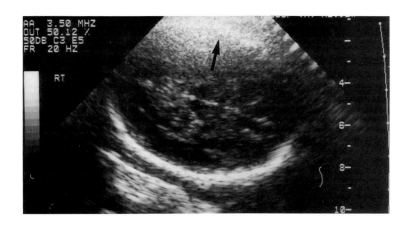

Figure 1.10. This 3.5-MHz annular-array image of a fetal head at 29 wk gestational age illustrates loss of information in the near field, with poor visualization of the calvarium closest to the transducer (arrow).

low-contrast resolution, except in the near field of the transducer beam (Figure 1.10). Transvaginal transducers, which are invaluable in the first trimester, may also be indicated later in pregnancy, particularly in the evaluation of placenta previa. Transvaginal imaging is safe and more accurate for the diagnosis of placenta previa than is transabdominal imaging (Farine et al., 1989; Leerentveld et al., 1990). The transvaginal technique places the internal cervical os closer to the transducer and improves resolution by allowing the use of high-frequency (5 or 7.5 MHz) probes.

The standards adopted by the American Institute of Ultrasound in Medicine (AIUM) (Leopold, 1986) and the American College of Obstetrics and Gynecology (ACOG, 1988) define the minimum goals of an obstetrical exam. Important components of obstetrical sonography are estimation of gestational age and assessment of fetal growth. The use of ultrasound, including Doppler, for identifying growth-retarded and small-for-gestational-age babies is an important area of research. The use of duplex Doppler and waveform analysis allows evaluation of placental resistance, which increases in a number of abnormal maternal and fetal conditions, including intrauterine growth retardation (Trudinger and Ishikawa, 1990). A reduction or, in the most severe cases, a reversal of the diastolic component of the umbilical arterial waveform can be observed as the resistance in the placenta increases. In the normal pregnancy, resistance in the fetal cerebral circulation is higher than that in the umbilical artery, manifest as a lower diastolic flow component (Figure 1.11). However, in compromised fetuses, an increase in diastolic flow may be seen in the cerebral arteries, likely reflecting a hemodynamic redistribution favoring flow to the brain when overall flow is compromised (Van Den Wijngaard et al., 1989;

Veille and Cohen, 1990). Detection of abnormal waveforms from the cerebral and umbilical arteries appears to be most important in identifying fetuses at risk for fetal distress. The Doppler parameters may indicate abnormality before other methods of fetal monitoring are able to detect fetal distress (Beattie and Dornan, 1989; Bekedam et al., 1990). As our comprehension of fetal hemodynamics in both normal and abnormal pregnancies improves, the role of obstetrical Doppler will undergo further refinement and expansion.

The guidelines of the AIUM and ACOG for obstetrical sonography were established both to ensure uniformity and to improve detection of major congenital anomalies on routine examinations performed for other indications. Identification of the fetal cerebral ventricles (Figure 1.12), cisterna magna, spine, stomach, urinary bladder, renal area, four-chamber heart, and the umbilical cord insertion site serves as an effective means of screening for major anomalies. More intensive or targeted examinations of specific organ systems may be indicated in some patients, particularly those with a history of a previous congenital anomaly or with increased maternal serum concentrations of α-fetoprotein (AFP) (Figure 1.13). In targeted exams, the sonographer's scanning technique is crucial for accurately detecting anomalies and defining their extent.

The neonate. Ultrasound is a proven diagnostic imaging modality in many neonatal applications; some of the many indications are listed in Table 1.2. The advantages of ultrasound in the newborn include its safety and ability to obtain portable studies without sedation in the neonatal intensive-care unit. The developing skeleton offers windows for ultrasound imaging not available beyond the newborn period, allowing visualization of the neonatal head, spinal

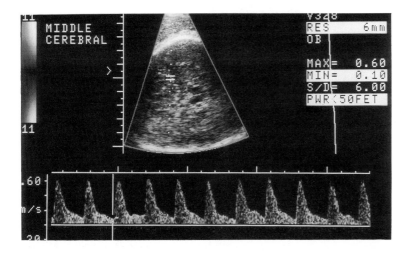

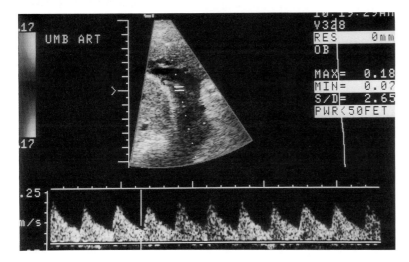

Figure 1.11. A normal spectral waveform (top) from a fetus at 33 wk gestation is obtained using duplex Doppler from the fetal middle cerebral artery. This contrasts with the normal waveform from the umbilical artery on the same fetus (bottom), which shows a significantly higher proportion of flow during diastole.

cord, and hip. In the neonate, transducers with small footprints (e.g., phased arrays and tightly curved linear arrays) are essential. The shallow depth of the structures being imaged allows the use of high-frequency transducers, which yield high-quality images.

The anterior fontanelle and, to a lesser extent, the posterior fontanelle provide windows for imaging the neonatal brain. The broadest application of this technology has been for the detection and follow-up of intracranial hemorrhage, primarily in premature infants. The vascularized region of the germinal matrix that regresses during normal gestation is the site of bleeding in premature infants. The highest incidence occurs in fetuses of less than 32 wk gestational age, with 90% of bleeds occurring in the first 5 d of life (Rumack et al., 1985). The clinical diagnosis of intracranial hemorrhage is unreliable; therefore, most experts recommend routine screening of premature infants by ultrasound (Lazzaru et al., 1980). Ultrasound readily demonstrates central intracranial hemorrhage and can be used in the initial diagnosis for grading the extent of hemorrhage (Figure 1.14) and in the follow-up of infants for sequelae of hemorrhage.

Periventricular leukomalacia (PVL), another form

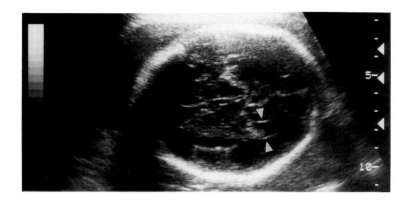

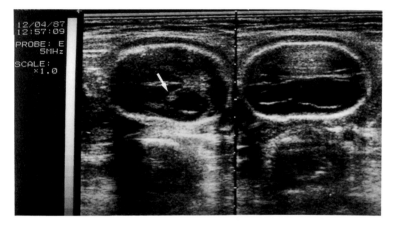

Figure 1.12. Normal cerebral ventricles (top) are seen in this fetus of 31 wk gestational age. Measurements of ventricular size should be made from the walls of the lateral ventricles (arrowheads) at the level of the atrium, with normal being less than 10 mm throughout pregnancy. An example of ventriculomegaly (bottom) in a fetus with Dandy-Walker malformation. Note the "dangling" choroid plexus (arrow), which lies dependently along the lateral wall of the ventricle. Artifacts from the calvarium obscure visualization of the cerebral hemisphere closest to the transducer.

of neuropathologic abnormality in the premature infant, can also be diagnosed by ultrasound. PVL represents necrosis of cerebral white matter in a watershed, periventricular distribution (Volpe, 1989). Initially, areas of increased echogenicity are seen adjacent to the lateral ventricles, and, with time, small cysts develop in the infarcted white matter. Other uses of intracranial ultrasound in the neonate include evaluation of congenital malformations (Figure 1.15), hydrocephalus, intracranial neoplasms, and infections.

Ultrasound is the procedure of choice for the initial imaging of the neonatal abdomen in a number of clinical situations. The gallbladder, bile ducts, liver, spleen, kidneys, and major vessels are all accessible to sonographic imaging. An important indication

for abdominal ultrasound is a palpable mass. Sonography allows identification of the anatomic location of the mass and determination of whether the mass is solid or cystic, and often it can provide a specific diagnosis (Figure 1.16).

Duplex and color-flow Doppler expand the diagnostic capabilities of ultrasound. They provide valuable information regarding vessel patency and the vascularity of masses, which is helpful in the evaluation of hepatic masses in the neonate. They also facilitate the distinction between a cystic mass and a dilated vessel, such as a vein-of-Galen aneurysm. Doppler ultrasound simplifies evaluation for aortoiliac or inferior vena caval thrombosis, which can complicate the use of umbilical vascular catheters. It is also helpful in the neonate with acute renal fail-

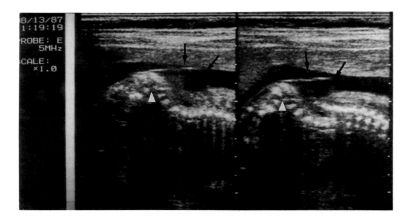

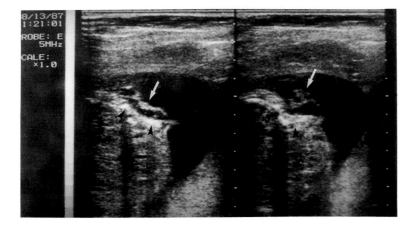

Figure 1.13. Evaluation of the spine of a fetus of 26 wk gestational age, in a patient with elevated maternal serum AFP, revealed a large myelomeningocele beginning at the thoracolumbar junction. A longitudinal parasagittal image (top) shows the myelomeningocele as a cystic mass posterior to the spine (arrows). Also note the abnormal kyphosis of the lower lumbar spine (arrowhead). Splaying of the posterior ossification centers (arrowheads) is seen at the level of the myelomeningocele (arrow) on transverse view (bottom).

Table 1.2. *Indications for neonatal ultrasound*

Head ultrasound[a]	Skin anomalies overlying sacrum	Hematuria
Prematurity	Chest ultrasound[a]	Pyuria
Abnormal facies	Suspected cardiac or great-vessel	Palpable mass
Cephalocele/meningocele	anomalies	Neonatal jaundice
Increasing head circumference	Suspected diaphragmatic hernia	Suspected umbilical artery/venous catheter thrombosis
Birth trauma	Suspected bronchopulmonary	
Unexplained cardiac failure	foregut malformation	Extremity ultrasound
Spine ultrasound[a]	Suspected diaphragmatic paralysis	Birth trauma
Spina bifida	Abdominal ultrasound[a]	Hip click
Segmentation fusion anomalies	Neonatal ascites	Limp/cold extremity
of the bony spine	Oliguria/annuria	Focal soft-tissue swelling

[a]May also be performed to evaluate suspected abnormal fetal findings in prenatal scans.

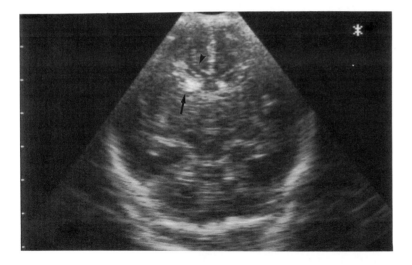

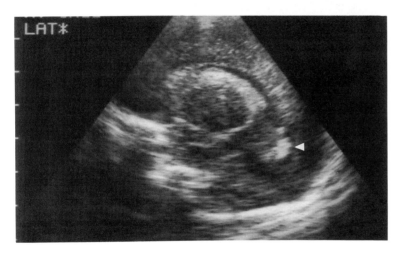

Figure 1.14. An example of a grade II hemorrhage in a neonate born at 26 wk gestational age is shown in a coronal image through the anterior fontanelle (top). An area of echogenic hemorrhage (arrow) is seen inferior to the right lateral venticle (arrowhead). A right parasagittal image (bottom) shows echogenic intraventricular hemorrhage layering in the dependent occipital horn (arrowhead).

ure to exclude renal venous or the rarer renal arterial thrombosis.

In summary, ultrasonography is invaluable in the fetus as a safe means of documenting fetal life and health, diagnosing fetal structural abnormalities, and guiding invasive techniques. In the neonate, ultrasound is the initial procedure of choice in a variety of clinical situations, allowing accurate evaluation of the neonatal head, abdomen, and musculoskeletal system.

SAFETY CONSIDERATIONS

In earlier sections we discussed the importance of spatial and gray-scale resolution to image quality. In each case, the highest image quality – and presumably the greatest patient benefit – is achieved by concentrating large amounts of acoustic energy into small volumes of tissue. This is precisely the situation where we expect the greatest possibility of undesirable *bioeffects* from ultrasound exposure. Therefore, the wisest use of ultrasound involves a

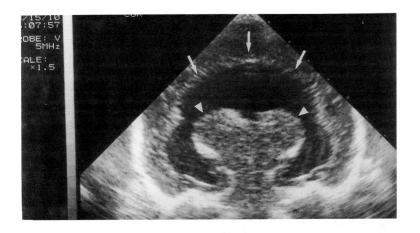

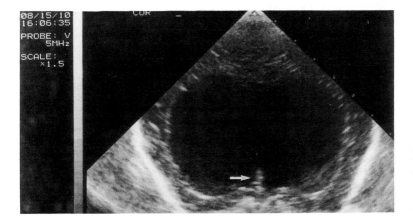

Figure 1.15. A neonate with holoprosencephaly shows (top) partially fused thalami (arrowheads) surrounded by a dilated monoventricle (arrows) and (bottom) partial formation of a falx (arrow) on coronal images obtained through the anterior fontanelle.

consideration of ultrasound exposure to maximize the benefit-to-risk ratio. The concept of the maximum benefit-to-risk ratio has been described by the National Council on Radiation Protection and Measurement (NCRP, 1983), with the recommendation that "users should strive to obtain the most medically significant information possible while producing the least ultrasonic exposure to the patient." Although we do not yet have enough information to compute this ratio, the emphasis has been shifting away from minimizing exposure and toward maximizing diagnostic information. Kremkau (1989b) has raised some interesting questions regarding the benefit of higher exposures. Using simplified calculations, he has shown that only small (~5%) improvements in imaging properties (e.g., depth of penetration, dynamic range, sensitivity, and spatial resolution) can be expected for a 100% increase in exposure, raising the question whether or not the increased risk of bioeffects and distortions due to nonlinear propagation outweigh the benefits.

It is well known that exposure to ultrasound of very high intensities is capable of damaging tissues. For example, the mechanical effects of cavitation are the basis for shock-wave lithotripsy therapy, and the thermal effects of ultrasonic hyperthermia are useful for treating some tumors. Mechanical and thermal mechanisms are the predominant bioeffects. Laboratory studies, however, offer no independently confirmed evidence to suggest that low-intensity diagnostic exposures are hazardous through these or any other mechanisms. In addition, decades of widespread clinical exposures have not revealed any adverse bioeffects. What keeps the ultrasound community continuously searching for bioeffects is the possibility of subtle genetic damage.

Risk assessment is currently based on ultrasonic exposure measurements, more specifically intensity measurements. The most appropriate intensity

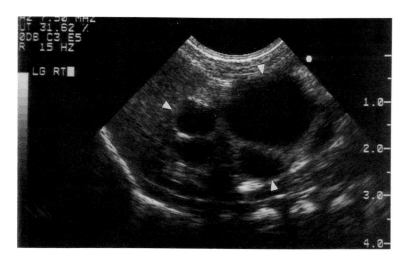

Figure 1.16. A multicystic dysplastic kidney was diagnosed with ultrasound in this neonate with a palpable abdominal mass. This longitudinal image of the right upper abdomen shows a right renal fossa mass with multiple, noncommunicating cysts (arrowheads) of varying sizes.

Table 1.3. *FDA list of highest known acoustic-output values for "preenactment" ultrasound devices used for fetal, neonatal cephalic, and pediatric imaging (focused transducers only)*[a]

I_{SPTA}	I_{SPPA}	I_{SPTP}
0.046 W·cm^{-2}	65 W·cm^{-2}	460 W·cm^{-2}

[a]In situ intensities are listed, meaning that free-field intensities (measured in water) have been adjusted to account for attenuation of the intervening tissues, as described in appendix D of CDRH/FDA (1985). The equation used is $I = I_w \exp(-0.23\alpha f z)$, where I is the in situ intensity, I_w is the intensity measured in water, α is the slope of the attenuation coefficient versus frequency (0.3 dB · cm^{-1} · MHz^{-1} was used), f is the center frequency of the transducer in megahertz, and z is the depth of focus in centimeters.
Source: Data from CDRH/FDA (1985).

measure depends on many factors (AIUM/NEMA, 1981; CDRH/FDA, 1985), including beam shape, focusing, pulse duration, and PRF. Three intensity measures commonly used are the spatial peak–temporal average intensity I_{SPTA}, the spatial peak–pulse average intensity I_{SPPA}, and the spatial peak–temporal peak intensity I_{SPTP}. These quantities have been discussed in detail elsewhere (AIUM/NEMA, 1981; CDRH/FDA, 1985; Kremkau, 1989a). Table 1.3 lists acoustic output values for diagnostic imaging devices used for perinatal applications, as summarized by the FDA (CDRH/FDA, 1985).

There is a move under way to replace the current instrumentation output limitations with a display of the information necessary for the sonographer to make an informed decision as to the proper levels necessary for each exam. The premise is that the minimum output necessary to obtain the required diagnostic information should always be used. In essence, responsibility is being shifted away from regulatory agencies and toward practitioners. At least two display parameters have been proposed to reflect the potential for bioeffects (AIUM/NEMA, 1991): A mechanical index is designed to be an indicator of mechanical effects such as cavitation, and thermal indices for soft tissue and bone are designed to be indicators of thermal mechanisms. The mechanical index is defined as the peak, in situ, rarefaction pressure at each point along the beam, divided by the square root of the center frequency. The thermal index is the ratio of the total in situ acoustic power to that required to raise the tissue temperature by 1°C. Since the temperature increases for bone and soft tissue are different, a separate thermal index could be reported for each.

CONCLUSIONS

Ultrasonography is a very flexible and diverse imaging modality. Operators are required to make many informed decisions to achieve maximum diagnostic information. When ultrasound is indicated, the operator should interpret clinical findings in terms of acoustics–tissue interactions and select the appropriate transducer–signal-processing combination for the task at hand. The industry trend is for manufacturers to provide sonographers with an increasing number of options for approaching a clinical exam. While increasing the sonographer's responsibility, the added flexibility will increase the opportunities for this already important imaging modality.

REFERENCES

ACOG (1988). Technical bulletin 116. American College of Obstetrics and Gynecology.

AIUM/NEMA (1981). *Safety standard for diagnostic ultrasound equipment.* NEMA, 2101 L Street, N.W., Washington, DC 20037.

(1991). *Standard for realtime display of thermal and mechanical indices of diagnostic ultrasound equipment.* American Institute of Ultrasound in Medicine, 11200 Rockville Pike, Suite 205, Rockville, MD 20852-3139.

Bamber, J. C., Hill, C. R. & King, J. A. (1981). Acoustic properties of normal and cancerous human liver. II. Dependence on tissue structure. *Ultrasound in Medicine and Biology* 7:135–44.

Beattie, R. B., & Dornan, J. C. (1989). Antenatal screening for intrauterine growth retardation with umbilical artery Doppler ultrasonography. *British Medical Journal* 298:631–5.

Bekedam, D. J., Visser, G. H. A., Van Der Zee, A. G. J., Snijders, R. J. M., & Poelmann-Weesjes, G. (1990). Abnormal velocity waveforms of the umbilical artery in growth retarded fetuses: relationship to antepartum late heart rate decelerations and outcome. *Early Human Development* 24:79–89.

CDRH/FDA (1985). *510(k) guide for measuring and reporting acoustic output of diagnostic ultrasound medical devices.* CDRH, HFZ-132, Rockville, MD 20857.

Farine, D., Fox, H. E., Jakobson, S., & Timor-Tritsch, I. E. (1989). Is it really a placenta previa? *European Journal of Obstetrics & Gynecology and Reproductive Biology* 31:103–8.

Garra, B. S., Insana, M. F., Shawker, T. H., & Russell, M. A. (1987). Quantitative estimation of liver attenuation and echogenicity: normal state versus diffuse liver disease. *Radiology* 162:61–7.

Goodman, J. W. (1968). *Introduction to Fourier Optics.* New York: McGraw-Hill.

Greenleaf, J. F. (ed.). (1986). *Tissue Characterization with Ultrasound,* 2 vols. Boca Raton, FL: CRC Press.

Kasai, C., Namekawa, K., Koyano, A., & Omoto, R. (1985). Real-time two-dimensional blood flow imaging using an autocorrelation technique. *IEEE Transactions on Sonics and Ultrasonics* SU-32:458–64.

Kisslo, J., Adams, D. B., & Belkin, R. N. (1988). *Doppler Color Flow Imaging.* New York: Churchill Livingstone.

Kremkau, F. W. (1989a). *Diagnostic Ultrasound: Principles, Instruments, and Exercises,* 3rd ed. Philadelphia: W. B. Saunders.

(1989b). Clinical benefit of higher acoustic output levels. *Ultrasound in Medicine and Biology* 15:69–70.

Lazzaru, A., Ahmann, P., Dykes, F., Brann, A. W., Jr., & Schwartz, J. (1980). Clinical predictability of intraventricular hemorrhage in preterm infants. *Pediatrics* 65:30–4.

Leerentveld, R. A., Gilberts, E. C. A. M., Arnold, M. J. C. W. J., & Wladimiroff, J. W. (1990). Accuracy and safety of transvaginal sonographic placental localization. *Obstetrics and Gynecology* 76:759–62.

Leopold, G. R. (1986). Antepartum obstetrical ultrasound examination guidelines. *Journal of Ultrasound in Medicine* 5:241–2.

Lyons, M. E., & Parker, K. J. (1988). Absorption and attenuation in soft tissues. II. Experimental results. *IEEE Transactions on Ultrasonics, Ferroelectric, and Frequency Control,* UFFC-35:511–21.

Macovski, A. (1979). Ultrasonic imaging using arrays. *Proceedings of the IEEE* 67:484–95.

Maslak, S. H. (1985). Computed sonography. In *Ultrasound Annual,* ed. R. C. Sanders & M. C. Hill (pp. 1–16). New York: Raven Press.

NCRP (1983). *Biological Effects of Ultrasound,* National Council on Radiation Protection and Measurement report no. 74. Bethesda: NCRP Publications.

Rumack, C. M., Manco-Johnson, M. L., Manco-Johnson, M. J., Koops, B. L., Hathaway, W. E., & Appareti, K. (1985). Timing and course of neonatal intracranial hemorrhage using real-time ultrasound. *Radiology* 154:101–5.

Taylor, K. J. W., & Holland, S. (1990). Doppler US: Part I. Basic principles, instrumentation, and pitfalls. *Radiology* 174:297–307.

Trudinger, B. J., & Ishikawa, K. (1990). Use of Doppler ultrasound in the high-risk pregnancy. In *Duplex Doppler Ultrasound,* ed. K. J. W. Taylor & D. E. Strandness, Jr. (pp. 124–8). New York: Churchill Livingstone.

Tuthill, T. A., Baggs, R. B., & Parker, K. L. (1989). Liver glycogen and water storage: effect on ultrasonic attenuation. *Ultrasound in Medicine and Biology* 15:621–7.

Van Den Wijngaard, J. A. G. W., Groenenberg, I. A. L., Wladimiroff, J. W., & Hop, W. C. J. (1989). Cerebral Doppler ultrasound of the human fetus. *British Journal of Obstetrics and Gynecology* 96:845–9.

Veille, J.-C., & Cohen, I. (1990). Middle cerebral artery blood flow in normal and growth-retarded fetuses. *American Journal of Obstetrics and Gynecology* 162:391–6.

Volpe, J. J. (1989). Current concepts of brain injury in the premature infant. *American Journal of Roentgenology* 153:243–51.

Wagner, R. F., Insana, M. F., & Brown, D. G. (1985). Progress in signal and texture discrimination in medical imaging. *Proceedings of the SPIE: Application of Optical Instrumentation in Medicine XIII* 535:57–64.

Wagner, R. F., Smith, S. W., Sandrik, J. M., & Lopez, H. (1983). Statistics of speckle in ultrasound B-scans. *IEEE Transactions on Sonics and Ultrasonics* SU-30:156–63.

2

Echocardiography

RICHARD A. HUMES, M.D.
ZIA Q. FAROOKI, M.D.

INTRODUCTION

Diagnostic ultrasound has become the most important clinical tool for evaluation of fetal and newborn hearts. Echocardiography (ultrasound of the heart) has evolved tremendously since its inception in the early 1960s. Whereas most new technologies in pediatric cardiology tend to be modified or borrowed from those developed for adult cardiology, echocardiography is, in many ways, ideally suited for the pediatric heart (Sanders, 1990; Snider and Serwer, 1990). M-mode echocardiography, with its unidimensional view of the heart, was replaced in the mid-1970s by two-dimensional imaging of cardiac structures. Improvements in image processing have greatly enhanced the imaging of intracardiac structure and anatomy. The concomitant development of Doppler echocardiographic techniques and color-flow imaging has added the dimension of blood-flow measurement to the echocardiographic examinations of the 1980s and 1990s (Hatle and Angelsen, 1985). Cardiac catheterization has been largely replaced by echocardiography as the primary diagnostic test for evaluation of infants with congenital heart disease (Huhta et al., 1987). The addition of computer-enhanced imaging, as well as digital signal processing, has improved the resolution of the image enough that diagnostic studies in the fetus can be routinely performed with high quality by 18 wk of gestation. In the latter part of the 1980s and early 1990s, newer transducers that can be placed nearer the infant heart (as in transesophageal exams) and nearer the fetal heart (as in transvaginal exams) have further increased the diagnostic ability of this test. The future of echocardiography appears to be that of a rapidly advancing technology. The continuing development of modalities such as three-dimensional reconstruction and measurement of volumetric flow, as well as other technologies yet to be developed, will ensure that ultrasound as a diagnostic tool will continue to play a major role in our understanding of cardiac anatomy and function.

PHYSICAL PRINCIPLES OF ULTRASOUND

The term *ultrasound* refers to sound waves above the audible range, typically frequencies greater than 20,000 cycles per second (cps) (1 cps = 1 hertz = 1 Hz). The frequencies used in medical diagnostic ultrasound are generally 2–10 megahertz (1 MHz = 1,000,000 Hz). The advantages of this high-frequency ultrasound are that (1) it can be directed and focused as a beam of many ultrasound waves, (2) it obeys laws of reflection and refraction and, (3) it will be reflected by objects of relatively small size (Feigenbaum, 1986). Ultrasound will propagate extremely well through fluid media such as the heart and blood vessels. It will not pass well from fluid to gaseous media. The heart can be imaged only from locations on the chest and abdomen where the transducer is reasonably close to the chest wall and the sound waves are free from interference by overlying ribs or lung tissue. Therefore, the results of ultrasound examination will be poor over areas of the chest with underlying lung or when the lung is hyperexpanded, such as is seen in the premature, ventilated infant.

Ultrasound is transmitted in longitudinal waves consisting of regions of rarefaction and compression that can be described by the formula $v = f \times w$, where v is the velocity of sound through the medium, f is frequency, and w is the wavelength of the sound. From a practical standpoint, two points must be separated by more than one wavelength to be resolved on the image. Because wavelength and frequency are inversely related, the higher the frequency of ultrasound used for diagnostic purposes (and conversely the shorter the wavelength), the greater will be the resolution of small structures (Feigenbaum, 1986).

Sound will travel faster through a more dense medium, such as a solid. The velocity of sound in soft tissue is relatively constant at $1{,}540$ m $\cdot$ s^{-1}. However, sound will not pass unimpeded through every tissue. The amplitude and intensity of a sound are decreased as it passes through any medium. This reduction is referred to as *attenuation* and is expressed in the following equation: attenuation (in decibels, dB) = attenuation coefficient (dB $\cdot$ cm^{-1}) $\times$ path length (cm) (Kremkau, 1989). The attenuation coefficient is a property of the medium or tissue through which the sound is passing and is affected by absorption (conversion of acoustic energy into heat), reflection, and scatter. The attenuation coefficient is also related to the frequency of the sound, such that higher frequencies are attenuated more rapidly than lower frequencies (just as the low bass notes of the orchestra will be more easily heard in the back of the auditorium than the high notes of the flute).

Herein lies a fundamental conflict in the physics of diagnostic ultrasound. The use of a higher frequency of sound (and lower wavelength) will allow greater resolution and finer detail of imaging. However, higher-frequency ultrasound will be attenuated more rapidly and will not penetrate as deep into tissues. The practical solution to this conflict is the development of multiple transducers of different frequencies that can be alternated, depending on the depth and size of the area of interest. High-frequency transducers using sound in the range of 7–10 MHz can be used for imaging structures near the skin, such as vascular structures or the neonatal heart. Medium- to low-frequency transducers (5–2.5 MHz) must be used in older patients or for deeper penetration. More recent attempts at electronically altering the transmitted frequency of a given transducer have shown some improvement in the versatility of some devices, but have not changed the basic physical conflict (Kremkau, 1989; Snider and Serwer, 1990).

Another important physical property of a medium is its acoustic impedance. Impedance is deter-

mined by the density and stiffness of a medium and is defined as the product of the density (in kilograms per cubic meter) and the propagation speed of sound (in meters per second) (Kremkau, 1989). Sound traveling through a uniform homogeneous medium will be attenuated with distance, but will not be reflected. When a sound wave encounters a difference in acoustic impedance, some sound waves will pass through the boundary area (refracted wave), and some will be reflected backward (reflected wave). Diagnostic ultrasound depends on these characteristics of sound and tissue, because biological tissues are heterogeneous and therefore contain many interfaces, with different acoustic impedances, between the different tissue layers. The reflection of the sound wave can be detected as it returns to the source, and it will ultimately produce the ultrasound output signal. The degree of reflection versus refraction of the ultrasound will be determined by the relative mismatch of acoustic impedances at the boundary area, as well as by the incident angle between the ultrasound wave and the boundary. Cardiac structures are ideally suited to ultrasound imaging because of natural differences between the impedance values of cardiac muscle and valves and the value for the blood within the chambers. These differences allow excellent imaging of cardiac structures, because the density of the soft tissue of the heart is significantly different from that of blood, allowing good edge definition of epicardial and endocardial surfaces, but not so dense that it reflects all ultrasound and does not allow imaging of underlying cardiac and thoracic structures. The angle of incidence of the ultrasound beam will affect the image, such that objects that present an impedance boundary more nearly perpendicular to the ultrasound source will reflect more sound directly back toward the source. This will increase the strength of the returned signal from objects that are oriented more nearly perpendicular to the ultrasound beam, and relatively less signal from objects oriented parallel to the beam. Because the heart can be imaged only from certain areas free of underlying rib and lung, the angle of incidence to the ultrasound beam often is not ideal to produce good images of all cardiac surfaces. The complete ultrasound examination utilizes multiple views from multiple locations to develop the best composite pictures of the heart.

Imaging modalities

The basic elements necessary to produce an ultrasound image include a transmitter (a device that can

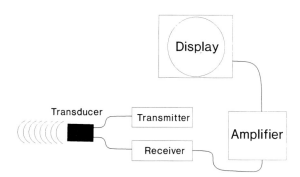

Figure 2.1. Schematic representation of the components necessary for diagnostic ultrasound: a transducer (from which the ultrasound signal is both sent and received), a transmitter capable of modifying the outgoing signal, and a receiver that can translate the incoming signal. This electronic signal then passes through an amplifier to a display device, which is a form of cathode-ray tube such as a television monitor.

regulate the ultrasound signal), a receiver to recognize the returning reflected signal, an amplifier, and a display device (Figure 2.1). The transducer is used to both send and receive the ultrasound signal. Features of transducer design will be discussed in a later section. As stated previously, the characteristics of the transmitted ultrasound signal will greatly affect the quality and quantity of the returned echo signal. Once the echo signal is received, different types of signal processing may be employed to produce the clinically useful forms of ultrasound images that make up the echocardiogram, that is, M-mode images, two-dimensional images, and Doppler images.

M-mode imaging

A stationary beam of ultrasound directed at a target will produce reflections from that target of varying intensities, depending on the acoustic impedance, the depth of the target, and the wavelength of the ultrasound. In order to receive and interpret those signals, the beam of ultrasound is turned off intermittently so that the transducer can function as a receiver. On a standard oscilloscope, the intensity of the reflection will be displayed as the height or amplitude of the signal. Because the reflected signals from various depths take finite but variable times to return to the transducer, the complete signal from a complex object will be displayed as a series of "spikes" of varying amplitude and spacing on the screen. This type of signal was the first type of ultrasound signal, and it was designated the A mode (Figure 2.2). This signal can be modified elec-

tronically to convert the spike into a dot on the screen, with the intensity of the dot proportional to the amplitude of the spike. This second-generation modification of the ultrasound signal was called the B mode (for brightness mode). The oscilloscope or cathode-ray tube can then be modified to "sweep" its information across the screen, which introduces an element of time. With standard M-mode (or motion-mode) echocardiography, the depth information is displayed along the vertical y axis, and the time or sweep is displayed along the horizontal x axis, usually sweeping from left to right across the screen. When the heart is the target, the effect of this is to produce a tracing of the motion of the epicardial and endocardial surfaces of the heart over time. A standard electrocardiogram signal is often displayed simultaneously to allow for timing of the cardiac events of contraction and relaxation (Feigenbaum, 1986). To produce this type of ultrasound signal, the transmitted ultrasound is sent in intermittent pulses and turned off between pulses to allow for reception of the echo signal. Standard M-mode signals repeat the pulses 1,000 to 2,000 times per second (the "pulse repetition frequency"). The pulses last 1.5–2 μs, which results in the transducer being in the receiving mode more than 98% of the time. This allows extremely sensitive reception of the reflected signals. In the standard M-mode tracing, the depth of origin of the reflected signal is calibrated automatically because the speed of sound in the tissue is known. Therefore, the resulting tracing will accurately display changes in dimensions, such as the internal left ventricular dimension, over time. Measurements can then be made to estimate the size and function of intracardiac chambers, which will be discussed later.

Two-dimensional imaging

The M-mode image represents a one-dimensional (depth) or ice-pick view of the heart, using a single narrow pulse of ultrasound. This allows excellent axial (along a line) resolution of structures, but no lateral resolution of adjacent structures. If the M-mode transducer is moved laterally, or if multiple M-mode transducers are placed side by side, and the sweep of the oscilloscope is eliminated, then a second dimension (the lateral dimension) can be introduced into the image. Two types of transducers have been developed to produce such two-dimensional images: (1) mechanical, in which a single crystal or series of crystals is oscillated or swept through an arc to produce the image; (2) electronic, in which multiple crystals in a bank are fired se-

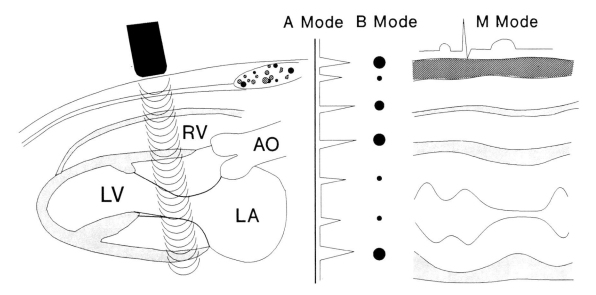

Figure 2.2. An ultrasound beam is passed through the heart from a left parasternal transducer location. In the A mode this produces a series of spikes on the oscilloscope at various levels as the ultrasound beam is reflected back from the surfaces of the heart. The B mode is produced by electronically converting the amplitude of the A-mode spike into varying levels of brightness, thereby producing a series of dots on the screen that will move and change as the heart beats. "Sweeping" the signal across the screen produces a one-dimensional view of the cardiac structures as they move. This motion mode or M mode can be timed (by using the sweep speed of the oscilloscope) and is clinically useful for timing and measuring cardiac structures.

quentially to produce an electronic sweep through the image (Snider and Serwer, 1990). Two-dimensional imaging has revolutionized the diagnostic capabilities of ultrasound in much the same way that computed tomography (CT) has affected radiology. The two-dimensional echocardiogram produces a planar view of the beating heart instantaneously, in "real time." The early two-dimensional scanning has been improved with up-to-date electronic processing to provide extremely sensitive resolution of small structures. Currently, lateral resolution is possible for differences of less than 1 mm.

Doppler echocardiography

The Doppler effect, first described by Christian Johann Doppler in 1842, is a change in the frequency of a wave as a result of motion of either the receiver or the source of the wave. Doppler, an astronomer, was describing the spectral shift of light from stars as they moved toward or away from the earth. His principles have been put to many practical uses. The Doppler principle applied to sound waves states that sound moving away from the listener (or receiver) will have a decreasing frequency (and longer wavelength), whereas sound moving toward the listener will have an increasing frequency (and shorter wavelength). The best-known example of this is the change in the sound of a train whistle as the train approaches a trackside observer, passes, and then moves away (Figure 2.3). There is no moving source of sound within the human body, so the technique as applied in clinical ultrasound is similar to that of the policeman at a speed trap to catch motorists with his radar gun. In that case, radio waves of a given frequency are "bounced" off moving cars. The change in frequency between the signal sent and the returning signal is termed the "Doppler shift," and from that the speed of the car can be calculated. In clinical application, the moving targets for the Doppler ultrasound are the blood cells within the heart and blood vessels (Figure 2.4). The Doppler shift can be expressed by the following equation: $f_D = f_r - f_t$. That is, the Doppler frequency (or shift) f_D is the difference between the received (f_r) and transmitted (f_t) frequencies. Another way of expressing this is

$$f_D = 2f_t \frac{v \cos \theta}{c}$$

where v is the velocity of the moving target (blood), c is the speed of sound in the medium, and θ is the angle between the beam of ultrasound and the direction of motion of the target. Therefore, the velocity of the target can be expressed as

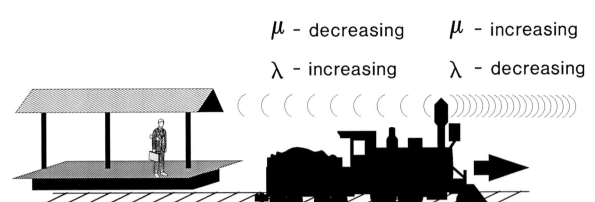

μ - decreasing μ - increasing

λ - increasing λ - decreasing

Figure 2.3. The whistle sound from a moving train illustrates the Doppler effect. The sound from the train as it moves away from the listener will exhibit a lower frequency (or pitch) μ and a longer wavelength λ. Conversely, the sound of the approaching train whistle will have an increased frequency and shorter wavelength.

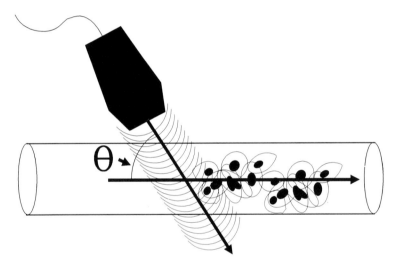

Figure 2.4. Doppler ultrasound uses moving blood cells as "targets" and analyzes the Doppler shift of the returning (reflected) signal to calculate the speed of the cells. This calculation is affected by the angle of incidence θ between the Doppler beam and the path of the blood cells.

$$V = \frac{f_D \cdot c}{2f_t \cos \theta}$$

The transmitted or carrier frequency f_t is a known constant, and the Doppler shift f_D can be measured with good accuracy. This equation demonstrates two important features of Doppler evaluation of blood flow: (1) velocity varies with the cosine of the angle between the Doppler signal and the target path, and (2) the transmitted frequency and velocity have an inverse relationship. Higher velocities are easier to resolve when using a *lower* transmitted frequency. This is important from a practical stand-point, because we have already noted that better resolution of the two-dimensional image is achieved with *higher* transmitted frequencies. The magnitude of the Doppler shift is on the order of a few kilohertz, which places this signal in the audible range. The signal usually is evaluated both as an audible sound and by means of a visual display. To produce the visual display, the shifted frequencies are subjected to a fast Fourier transform (FFT) and are converted on the screen as calibrated velocities of blood flow. The angle of incidence θ is assumed to be zero (and thus $\cos \theta = 1$), unless a correction factor is supplied manually into the echo computer. Blood

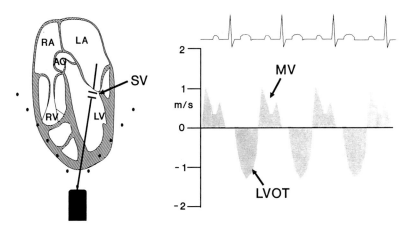

Figure 2.5. The pulsed Doppler sample volume is placed just distal to the mitral valve orifice. The characteristic Doppler tracing produces a signal above the zero line (toward the transducer) from the mitral valve in diastole and a systolic velocity away from the transducer resulting from flow out of the left ventricle toward the aortic valve.

flow should therefore be measured along a line that parallels the direction of blood movement. This is done from a practical standpoint by using multiple transducer positions on the patient's chest. In practice, angles of incidence to blood flow that are less than 20° do not change the cosine function significantly. However, flow that is at an angle of more than 20° from the Doppler beam can introduce significant error. Also important to note is that flow that is directly perpendicular to the Doppler signal will not be detected (cos 90° = 0). The standard visual display of the Doppler signal indicates velocity (in meters or centimeters per second) as well as direction relative to the source of sound. A baseline or line of zero Doppler shift is designated, and all velocities appearing above the line represent flow *toward* the transducer, whereas velocities displayed below the line represent flow away from the transducer (Figure 2.5) (Nishimura et al., 1985).

Doppler modalities

Continuous-wave Doppler. The Doppler modalities that are used in clinical ultrasound can be divided into two types: continuous-wave and pulsed-wave Doppler. The continuous-wave Doppler transducer employs two crystals, one for transmitting and one for receiving. Therefore, a constant beam of Doppler ultrasound is sent along a line, and all returning signals are continuously recorded. The advantage of this continuous sampling is that continuous-wave Doppler can detect virtually any velocity because of its infinite sampling rate. The disadvantage of continuous-wave Doppler is that it is range-insensitive (Reeder et al., 1986).

Thus, continuous-wave Doppler is an excellent modality for high-velocity jets of blood, such as those in stenotic valves or small ventricular septal defects. The continuous-wave signal is a composite signal of all velocities along the path of the beam. Care must be taken in the alignment of the Doppler beam to ensure that only the area of interest lies in the path of the beam. The normal velocity of blood across valves has little clinical importance; in clinical cardiology, it is the pressures and flows inside heart chambers that are commonly used to describe the severity of different lesions. Obstruction to flow, such as in aortic valve stenosis, will result in increased left ventricular systolic pressure, while aortic pressure remains normal. The result is a gradient, or pressure drop, across the stenotic aortic valve during systole. The greater the gradient (assuming normal left ventricular function), the more severe the stenosis (Nishimura et al., 1985; Reeder et al., 1986).

The human body will automatically regulate the heart to maintain normal blood pressure and cardiac output. This means that the amount of blood moving across a normal aortic valve during systole is the same amount that moves across the stenotic valve. Because the area of the stenotic valve is less than that of the normal valve, the blood must move faster across the stenotic valve to maintain a normal car-

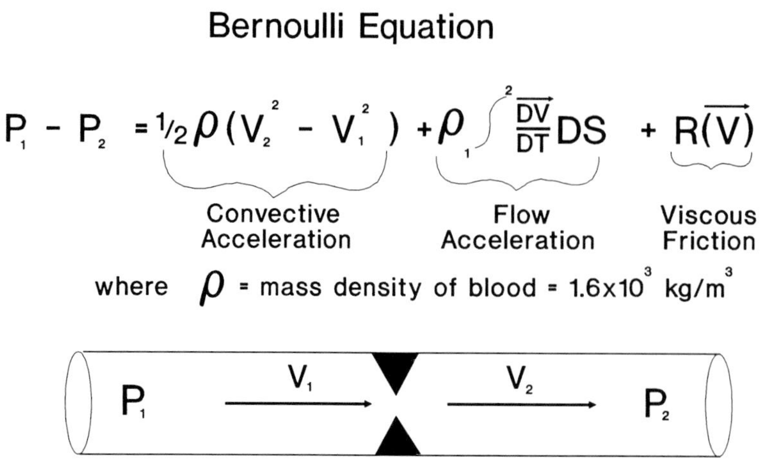

Bernoulli Equation

$$P_1 - P_2 = \tfrac{1}{2}\rho(V_2^2 - V_1^2) + \rho\int_1^2 \overrightarrow{\frac{DV}{DT}} DS + R(\overrightarrow{V})$$

| Convective Acceleration | Flow Acceleration | Viscous Friction |

where ρ = mass density of blood = 1.6×10^3 kg/m^3

Figure 2.6. The Bernoulli equation describes the relationship between changes in pressure and velocity of a fluid as it moves through a narrowed area: P_1, pressure proximal to narrowing; P_2, pressure distal to narrowing; V_1, velocity of fluid proximal to narrowing; V_2, velocity of blood distal to narrowing.

diac output. It is this concept that brings together the ideas of Doppler velocity and changes in pressure or flow.

The Bernoulli equation is a complex fluid-dynamics principle that relates flow and pressure (Figure 2.6). The final modified Bernoulli equation $\Delta P = 4V^2$ is simple to apply to most velocities and gives an accurate measure of the pressure drop across an orifice. To get to this simplified modification of the formula, one must assume that the elements of flow acceleration and viscous friction are negligible. This holds true for most clinical circumstances. The next assumption is that $V_1 \ll V_2$. This is true with moderate to severe stenosis, but becomes less so as milder stenosis (and hence lower velocities or V_2) is encountered.

Pulsed Doppler. The course of blood flow through the chambers of the heart is a series of twisting turns through chambers and valves of varying caliber. To accurately identify the blood velocity at any one point within the heart requires separation of discrete signals from within the chambers. The design, and hence the advantage, of pulsed Doppler incorporates the concept of range-gating into the Doppler signal: A pulse of Doppler ultrasound is sent out, and the receiver is turned on only at a specific time to receive reflected signals from a certain distance away (assuming a constant speed). This "opening of the gate," to let only certain signals in, is termed *range-gating*. This process is repeated multiple times in "pulses" at a rate called the pulse repetition frequency (PRF). Each pulse must be sent and

received before the next one can be sent, to obtain an unambiguous signal from the target area of interest. Pulsed Doppler is therefore affected by depth, because the greater the depth, the longer it will take for the signal to return. Specifically, the maximum detectable frequency shift is equal to one-half the sampling rate or PRF. This is called the Nyquist limit. The carrier frequency (transducer frequency) also affects this, as noted earlier. Lower-frequency transducers can detect higher velocities at a given depth. Pulsed-wave Doppler is less useful for higher-velocity flow. If the Nyquist limit is exceeded by a given signal, the velocity cannot be displayed in an unambiguous fashion. These higher peak velocities are received and displayed ambiguously in the opposite direction. This phenomenon is called aliasing. Aliasing can be reduced by shifting the baseline of the receiver and emphasizing only returning signals from one direction. This baseline shift effectively eliminates some aliasing and can double the effective PRF. Another technique is simply to increase the PRF directly. This is called high-PRF Doppler. To do this, some signals are sent before all of the returning signals are back. This reduces the aliasing but introduces some potential errors, as Doppler shift may be detected from more than just the area of interest, because the gate must be left open more of the time to accept the greater number of returning signals.

Color-flow Doppler. The development of fast, compact microprocessors has led to an extension of the pulsed-wave Doppler technique called color-flow

Doppler or color-flow imaging (Miyatake et al., 1984). The modality has evolved from pulsed Doppler much as two-dimensional imaging evolved from M-mode tracings. Rather than examining a single point of interest, the Doppler beam is swept rapidly and repeatedly through an area. Flow is then displayed directly over the two-dimensional imaging, and color encoding is used in the display. Just as with other forms of Doppler, velocity and directional information is displayed. Although any color may be used, a standard convention has been employed by most manufacturers that displays flow away from the transducer in shades of blue and flow toward the transducer in shades of red or orange (this can be remembered by use of the mnemonic BART, *blue away, red toward*).

This color Doppler display follows the same basic principles as pulsed Doppler. That is, if the Nyquist limit is exceeded, color aliasing will occur. In this case, aliasing produces color ambiguity, where blue becomes red, or vice versa. With very high velocities, the procedure often will produce a multicolored or mosaic pattern of colors that is distinctive and easy to see.

Color Doppler is somewhat different from other pulsed Doppler because of the great amount of information that must be processed to display the flow in real time. The velocity information is not subjected to FFT, because that would be too slow to produce an image. Rather, a process known as autocorrelation is used, where estimates of mean velocity along each sample line are obtained using a minimum number of samples. Increasing the size or depth of the sample will require more time for the internal computer processing the information to produce a visual display. This degrades the image by slowing the frame rate of sampling. Clearly, significant compromises in the quantitative nature of color Doppler must be made in order to produce an image that simulates the flow of blood through the heart. This results in information that is, at best, semiquantitative under current constraints. Nevertheless, the advent of color Doppler has proved extremely useful in the assessment of normal and abnormal hearts by virtue of producing a visual display of blood flow. This has been invaluable for the detection of flow in small shunt lesions, such as patent ductus arteriosus and ventricular septal defect, as well as for detecting and measuring the abnormal flow produced by valvular stenosis and regurgitations.

INSTRUMENTATION

The ultrasound signal is produced by passing an electrical signal through a piezoelectric crystal, causing it to vibrate at a higher rate and produce the ultrasound wave. The crystal element can be used as both a transmitter and receiver of the ultrasound signal. The elements that produce the ultrasound are placed together in a hand-held device that can be placed on the patient's chest, called a transducer. Transducer design is a critical factor in the production of quality ultrasound images. A design for a *pediatric* transducer probe additionally requires sensitivity to the size of the patient.

Ultrasound produced by a single small element will propagate outward in a series of waves in a circular fashion (Figure 2.7). If multiple small elements are placed side by side, the multiple circular wavelets from all the transducers will combine to produce a linear waveform directed away from the transducer. In fact, this type of transducer is in clinical use and is called a linear-array transducer. The advantage of multiple small elements in linear array is that they produce fine image resolution, because each of the crystals can be used to send and receive along a given line of reference. This transducer is often used in abdominal and obstetrical imaging. Unfortunately, imaging of the heart requires multiple planar views *between the ribs*. A large linear transducer would encounter signal artifacts from the underlying ribs and would be impractical for small neonates.

The first attempt to provide a smaller transducer for neonates led to a variety of mechanical scanning probes. In such designs, a small single crystal or two or three crystals could be rotated or oscillated through an arc, producing a sector of interest (hence the early name for two-dimensional echocardiography: sector scan). A sufficiently rapidly moving crystal can produce an excellent image, displayed on the screen as a wedge of 80° to 90°. The advantages of this type of transducer are that it is relatively inexpensive and can be made as a small probe, with a relatively small "footprint" on the patient's chest. The disadvantages of mechanical scanning included initial difficulties with incorporating Doppler modalities such as color-flow and continuous-wave Doppler into the probe capability, as well as failure of the moving parts. Many of those disadvantages have been eliminated by improved technology, and many mechanical transducers are now able to perform all parts of the echo exam.

Most of the ultrasound scanners in use today are electronically controlled phased-array transducers. In this design, multiple crystals are arrayed in a small bank. Instead of firing all the crystals simultaneously, as in a linear array, the elements are activated sequentially. This allows the ultrasound beam to be steered in a certain direction and shaped and

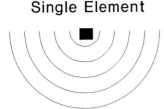

Single Element

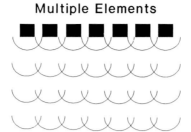

Multiple Elements

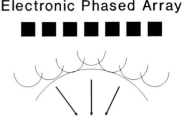

Electronic Phased Array

Figure 2.7. *Left:* A single ultrasound crystal will send out a series of circular waves like a stone thrown into a pool of water. *Middle:* Multiple crystal elements placed side by side firing simultaneously will produce a wavefront that will move out from the transducer in a linear fashion.

Right: In electronically steered phased-array transducers, the timing of the firing of the crystals allows shaping and steering of the ultrasound wavefront, to allow the ultrasound beam to be directed.

focused to certain depths. The advantage of this arrangement is the high fidelity of the images that multiple crystals allow, without the need for a large bank of crystals and a large-size footprint. Thus, a transducer can be made to fit reasonably between the ribs. Because of the multiple crystals, simultaneous imaging and Doppler are possible. The absence of moving parts results in a reliable transducer with a low failure rate. The major disadvantage of phased-array systems is their high cost.

Transducer size plays a significant role in the quality of the ultrasound signal. As the ultrasound beam travels outward from the transducer, the beam remains essentially parallel for a given distance and then begins to diverge. The point of divergence marks the boundary between the near field and far field. For practical purposes, the ultrasound signal is best when one images within the near field. The length of the near field (and hence the optimum depth of imaging) varies with the square of the radius of the Doppler beam and inversely with the wavelength. Thus, the optimal transducer to have the largest near field would be a high-frequency (lower-wavelength) transducer with a larger aperture or footprint. But, of course, we have already mentioned that a large transducer has problems imaging between ribs. The engineering of transducers, particularly those suited for neonatal use, requires decisions involving a series of trade-offs.

The "ideal" pediatric echocardiogram machine

The wide range of disease entities seen in neonatal and pediatric cardiology requires a full-feature machine capable of performing M-mode, two-dimensional, and Doppler studies, including color-flow imaging. The importance of color-flow imaging and the precision that it adds to the neonatal exam cannot be overemphasized. A range of transducers of different frequencies (7, 5, 3 MHz) is necessary because of the variety of patient sizes one encounters in pediatrics. The field of digital image processing and storage is an advancing technology that improves the fidelity of the recording. Internal storage and playback features that can acquire a "loop" of cardiac cycles are useful to allow the examiner to slow down the image (particularly with rapid neonatal heart rates) for detailed examination.

The most important feature of the pediatric machine is not a high-technology hardware item: Without a skilled operator, the best machine will yield no answers. The extreme variety of heart problems seen in the field of congenital heart disease set this role distinctly apart from its counterpart in the adult world. The pediatric sonographer must be more than just a skilled technician. Sonographers who receive no feedback from physicians regarding outcomes and diagnoses will never be able to acquire high-quality studies of complex hearts. The pediatric cardiologist must be more than just a "reader" of ultrasound pictures. He or she must also have good technical skills in obtaining the ultrasound images. Physicians must find time for a team approach at the bedside. The overall skill of this team must be a blend of applied knowledge of congenital heart disease and excellent technical skill in image acquisition.

NORMAL ECHOCARDIOGRAPHIC EXAMINATION

The complete echocardiographic examination involves the use of all of the ultrasound modalities: M-mode and two-dimensional imaging, Doppler examination, and color-flow imaging. Each of these modalities plays a distinct role in the diagnostic and functional assessment of the heart. The approach to the patient must be systematic and rigorous, to avoid missing important defects. Excellent and comprehensive reviews of the techniques of pediatric and fetal echocardiographic examination are available (Solinger, Elbl, and Minhas, 1974; Tajik et al., 1978). We shall briefly describe the chronology of the technique used in our laboratory: The patient must be comfortable, quiet, and cooperative. This may require the use of innovative toys, milk or glucose-water feedings, or sedation. The entire examination can be performed with the baby in the lap of the mother. The operator should ensure clean hands and clean equipment. In patients with open wounds or fresh incisions, a sterile gel medium should be used to make airless contact. In cases of premature or sick neonates, it is important to maintain thermal regulation. Excessive pressure in the subcostal region of the premature infant can result in marked bradycardia. The operator should be comfortably positioned before starting the examination. A transducer with highest frequency should be used initially (5–7 MHz). It is our policy to perform a two-dimensional (2-D) directed M-mode examination first, to be followed by complete 2-D study and finally the Doppler examination. This method ensures a complete, very methodical approach to the study.

M-mode examination

The two-dimensionally directed M-mode examination is carried out by first examining the left ventricle. In our laboratory we begin by imaging the heart in a parasternal short-axis plane (as discussed later) at the level of the midventricle. The M-mode cursor is placed between the papillary muscles just below the level of the mitral valve, and an M-mode recording is obtained. A recording of the aortic-valve M-mode is then obtained by tilting the transducer cephalad toward the aortic valve. Additional M-mode recordings of the mitral, tricuspid, and pulmonary valves may also be obtained. However, these latter techniques are somewhat antiquated and unnecessary with the advent of Doppler. In our laboratory, these are omitted.

Two-dimensional examination

Ultrasound examination of the heart is performed by obtaining a series of planar sections of the moving cardiac structures. This examination is in contra-

distinction to other planar imaging modalities, such as CT scanning or magnetic-resonance imaging (MRI), which use external reference points to orient the imaging. Very few truly sagittal, coronal, or transverse images of the heart have traditionally been displayed. Rather, the heart and great vessels provide their own axis along which the images are obtained – thus the terms *long axis*, referring to an imaging plane oriented through the major dimension of the heart, and *short axis*, which images the minor dimension (often the cross-sectional plane) of the heart. Additionally, many newer, oblique planes of imaging are now in standard use. The advantage of choosing this technique for imaging is that the cardiac structures can be better seen in their relationships to important surrounding or nearby structures (e.g., the aortic valve with the mitral valve). The major disadvantage is that standard reference positions, such as right, left, caudad, and cephalad, may not be truly applicable to many images.

The complete 2-D examination is accomplished by imaging the heart from four areas or "windows": (1) left parasternal area, (2) apical area, (3) subxiphoid (subcostal) area, and (4) suprasternal area. A detailed description of the techniques and anatomic features of all echocardiographic imaging planes is beyond the scope of this chapter. Rather, we present a systematic methodology for obtaining a complete study. The approach that we use in our laboratory is outlined in Table 2.1. Imaging of the heart, particularly in the presence of complex congenital heart disease, can produce many very interesting pictures. It is easy for even the experienced examiner to become interested in an anomalous area of the heart and forget to obtain other, standard views.

The method that we use has four steps, which should be followed in order to avoid omission of some of the exam:

1. Perform M-mode exam from parasternal area.
2. Perform complete 2-D study in sequence: parasternal → apical → subcostal → suprasternal.
3. Perform color-flow and pulsed Doppler exam in sequence: suprasternal → subcostal → apical → parasternal.

Perform continuous-wave (CW) exam on all areas of color or pulsed Doppler signal aliasing.

4. Stand back and answer the following questions:
   (a) Have I identified all of the normal cardiac structures and great vessels?
   (b) Have I identified/measured all areas of shunt?

Table 2.1. *Systemic approach to echocar-diographic examination*

I. Perform different echo modalities separately
   A. M mode (5% of exam)
   B. Two-dimensional imaging (75% of exam)
   C. Doppler/color-flow imaging (20% of exam)
II. Obtain standard two-dimensional view from each location
   A. Left parasternal area
      1. Long axis
         a. LV long axis
         b. RV inflow
         c. RV outflow
      2. Short axis
         a. Base
         b. Midventricle
         c. Apex
   B. Apical area
      1. Four-chamber
      2. Five-chamber
   C. Subxiphoid area (subcostal)
      1. Four-chamber
      2. RV inflow/outflow
      3. Caval view
   D. Suprasternal area
      1. Long axis: aorta
      2. Short axis: aorta, pulmonary veins
III. Obtain Doppler/color-flow examination from each location
   A. Suprasternal area
      1. Ascending aorta
      2. Descending aorta
      3. Superior or inferior vena cava
      4. Pulmonary arteries
      5. Pulmonary veins
   B. Subxiphoid area
      1. Atrial septum
      2. Right ventricular outflow tract
      3. Ventricular septum
      4. Caval connections
   C. Apical area
      1. Atrioventricular valves
      2. Aortic valve (five-chamber)
      3. Atrial septum
      4. Ventricular septum
   D. Parasternal area
      1. Ventricular septum
      2. Pulmonary valve, branch arteries, ductus arteriosus
      3. Aortic valve
      4. Mitral valve
      5. Atrial septum

(c) Have I identified/measured all areas of valvular stenosis/insufficiency?

(d) Have I identified how the blood enters and leaves the heart?

The relative emphasis on each part of the exam should be heavily weighted toward the 2-D exam, roughly 75% of the recorded study, with the Dop-pler exam about 20%, and the M-mode exam 5%. It is a common mistake for many technician/sonographers (physicians too!) to record far more Doppler images than are needed. The most important part of the examination for congenital heart disease is the 2-D image. The use of this segmental approach to thinking, in combination with a methodical detailed approach to the performance of the study, will produce consistently accurate diagnoses of both simple and complex heart defects.

Figures 2.8–2.14 (2.13 and 2.14 are color plates, following page 121) demonstrate schematically the images that should be obtained from a systematic approach to the 2-D echocardiographic examination.

Doppler examination

The normal Doppler examination is an interrogation of all heart valves, septa, and great vessels, looking for hemodynamic abnormalities, shunts, or narrowing (Sahn, 1989; Silverman and Schmidt, 1989). This employs a combination of color-flow imaging, to visually scan for abnormalities, and conventional pulsed and CW Doppler, to examine the hemodynamic effects quantitatively. The Doppler exam begins at the end of the 2-D exam and proceeds in the reverse of the previous order, using the same echocardiographic windows. Color-flow imaging permits visualization of flow, identification of laminar versus turbulent flow, and sizing of the orifice through which the disturbance is flowing. The color-flow Doppler examination helps to identify areas of shunt and disturbed flow. It can also be used to better define flow through areas that are poorly seen on the 2-D image. Once these areas are identified, pulsed-wave Doppler and/or CW Doppler are used to obtain the recordings for spectral analysis. All areas of color-flow or pulsed-wave aliasing should be examined with CW Doppler, and peak velocities should be recorded. After completing the examination in the suprasternal and high parasternal areas, we move on to the left parasternal, apical, and subcostal regions and perform the Doppler examination in the views mentioned for 2-D examination.

Contrast echocardiography

Rapid injection of glucose-water, saline, the patient's own blood, or indocyanine dye into the vascular system (especially when agitated before injection) will result in creation of microcavitations that can be easily recorded by the 2-D ultrasound beam

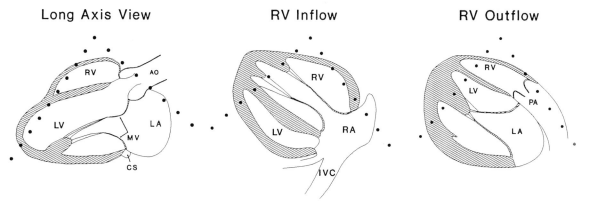

Figure 2.8. Parasternal long-axis views. The transducer is placed in the left parasternal position at the third or fourth intercostal space, with the plane of section oriented along a plane connecting the right shoulder and left hip. This produces the long-axis view (left) of the left ventricle (LV) and demonstrates all left-side heart structures (LA, left atrium; MV, mitral valve; CS, coronary sinus; AO, aorta; RV, right ventricle). Slight angulation of the transducer toward the left hip will produce the RV inflow view (middle), identifying the tricuspid valve and RV. Tilting the transducer back through the long-axis view and continuing to tilt toward the left shoulder will produce the RV outflow view (right), demonstrating the pulmonary valve and main pulmonary artery (PA).

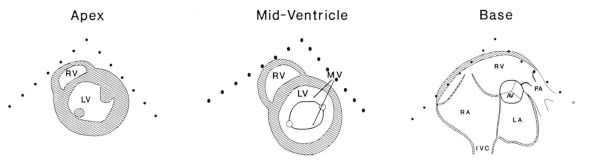

Figure 2.9. Parasternal short-axis views. With the transducer in the same position on the chest as in Figure 2.8, the transducer is rotated 90° clockwise to produce a cross-sectional or short-axis view of the heart. This plane can be moved caudally to the apex or cranially to the base of the heart. A cross section toward the apex of the LV reveals the LV cavity, papillary muscles, mitral chordae, muscular ventricular system, and part of the right ventricle (left). A similar section at the mid-LV cavity region shows the mitral valve leaflets, right ventricular inflow region, mid–muscular ventricular system, and part of the right ventricular outflow region (middle). A cross-sectional view at the level of the aortic root shows the aortic leaflets (AV), left atrium, atrial septum, tricuspid valve, membranous ventricular septum, right ventricular inflow and outflow regions, and the origin of the coronary arteries (right). Slight anterior and leftward tilt will reveal the pulmonary valve and main pulmonary artery. A short-axis cross section obtained from under the left clavicle will reveal the bifurcation of the pulmonary arteries.

as a dense cloud of echoes (Bommer et al., 1984). Although this technique has been partly replaced by color-flow Doppler, it continues to be useful in many patients in whom there is difficulty with echo windows or imaging.

QUANTITATIVE ECHOCARDIOGRAPHY

Echocardiography permits quantitative evaluation of the structure and function of the cardiovascular system.

Evaluation of structures

Two-dimensional imaging, complemented by M-mode recordings of the cardiac chambers, valves, and great vessels, allows precise measurements of these structures. The rates of growth of cardiac structures have been related to somatic growth, body surface area, age, and body weight in many excellent studies (Epstein et al., 1975; Henry et al., 1978; Roge et al., 1978; Gutgesell and Rembold, 1990). The degree of hypoplasia or dilation can

Four-Chamber

Five-Chamber

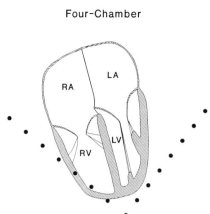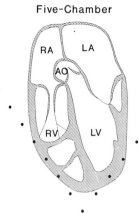

Figure 2.10. Apical views. Placement of the transducer at the area of the apical impulse produces a four-chamber view of the heart (left). In this position, one visualizes the posterior or inlet ventricular septum separating the tricuspid and mitral valves. The septal leaflet of the mitral valve inserts more cephalad onto the septum than the corresponding tricuspid valve leaflet. This identifies the morphologic left ventricle, which also has less muscular trabeculation than the right ventricle. The morphologic right ventricle contains a thick muscle bundle near its apex, the moderator band. The ventricular septum displayed in this plane consists of the inlet portion superiorly and the trabecular septum inferiorly. The atrial septum is very thin and parallel to the ultrasound beam in this plane and may show false dropout in the area of the fossa ovalis. The left atrium with its appendage, the left lower pulmonary vein, and the right upper pulmonary vein are frequently imaged. The right atrium is also well seen in this plane. Slight anterior angulation of the transducer will reveal the membranous ventricular septum, aortic valve, ascending aorta, and left ventricular outflow region in what has been called a "five-chamber" view (right).

Four-Chamber   RV Inflow/Outflow   Caval View

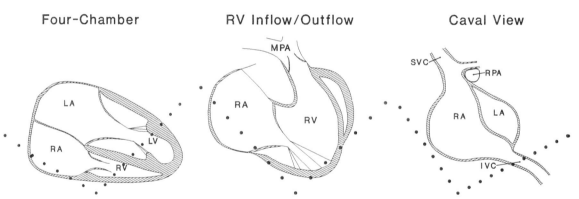

Figure 2.11. Subcostal views. The subcostal examination is begun with a transverse, cross-sectional view of the abdomen in the subxiphoid area (not shown). This view reveals the vertebral column, inferior vena cava (IVC), abdominal aorta, liver, and stomach, and will help determine the abdominal visceral situs. The spleen frequently can be imaged. The transducer is then rotated 90° to obtain the long axis of the IVC and the abdominal aorta. The pulsatility of the abdominal aorta should be noted to aid in ruling out significant coarctation of the aorta. The transducer is then rotated 90° clockwise and tilted superiorly to produce a four-chamber view of the heart (left). The atrial septum can be imaged well from this view, and the flap of the foramen ovale should be identified. The left atrium, right superior pulmonary vein, and left pulmonary veins are frequently visualized in this plane. The right ventricular cavity may appear foreshortened in the subcostal four-chamber view. Varying degrees of counterclockwise rotation will provide a view of the right ventricle inflow, right ventricular cavity, outflow tract, pulmonary valve, and main pulmonary artery and its branches (middle). A view of both cavae can be obtained by directing the sector along the long axis of the IVC and then tilting the sector toward the right (right). The subcostal examination is an extremely useful part of the echocardiographic examination of the newborn. In adult patients, because of problems with distance from the heart, such images often are poor in quality. For this reason, many technicians trained primarily in adult cardiology neglect this important set of views. In the sick neonate, ventilatory support will hyperexpand the lungs and impair visualization of the heart from standard chest views. Hyperventilation and air trapping will also push the heart caudally, which will make the subcostal views that much better.

Long Axis

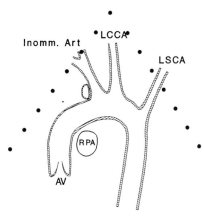

Short Axis

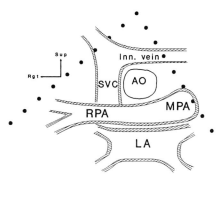

Figure 2.12. Suprasternal views. The arch is better imaged in the neonate because often a large thymus is present that can provide a better ultrasound medium than the air-filled lung. High left and right parasternal (or infraclavicular) views are also technically easier in younger patients. This discussion includes the views obtained from the suprasternal notch and highest right and left parasternal regions. The transducer is placed in the suprasternal notch, with the neck slightly hyperextended, with the plane of section between the right medial clavicular head and the left scapula. A long-axis view of the aorta and its branches is obtained (left). Left parasternal views may be superior for visualizing the descending aorta, whereas right parasternal views may be better for seeing the ascending aorta. Each brachiocephalic vessel should then be identified (Innom. Art, innominate artery; LCCA, left common carotid artery; LSCA, left subclavian artery). Clockwise rotation of approximately 45% and slight anteroposterior tilting of the transducer from this position produces the short-axis view of the aorta and a crab-type view of the left atrium, with all pulmonary veins (right). A long-axis view of the right pulmonary artery, left innominate vein, and superior vena cava is also seen. Abnormal courses of the pulmonary veins usually are well demonstrated in this plane. The suprasternal views probably are the most clinically crucial views to obtain in the sick neonate. Congenital problems of the aortic arch and great vessels often involve ductal-dependent lesions, which can produce significant and serious problems in the neonatal period. Once again, these images often are technically poor in adults, and adult-trained sonographers often are not used to obtaining all the views necessary for accurate diagnosis of arch abnormalities.

therefore be easily assessed. Multiple formulas have been used in attempts to calculate the volumes of the atria and the ventricles (Silvermen et al., 1980a; ASE, 1989). The myocardial thickness, mass, and distribution of hypertrophy can also be reliably evaluated.

Evaluation of ventricular function

The most commonly used and easily obtained criterion (Gutgesell et al., 1977) for assessment of systolic left ventricular function (LVF) is the shortening fraction (SF):

$$SF = \frac{LVEDD - LVESD}{LVEDD}$$

where LVEDD is left ventricular end-diastolic dimension, and LVESD is left ventricular end-systolic dimension. SF is load-dependent but is independent of age, sex, and heart rate. The normal mean value is 0.36, with a range of 0.28–0.44. It reflects the extent of shortening in the minor axis of the left ventricular cavity during systole.

Another parameter, the mean velocity of circumferential fiber shortening (V_{cf}), can be obtained as follows:

$$V_{cf} = \frac{SF}{ET}$$

where ET is ejection time. Normal values for V_{cf} are 1.5 ± 0.04 circumferences per second for neonates and infants, and 1.3 ± 0.03 for children ages 2–10 yr. Because ET is highly rate-dependent, it can be corrected for heart rate: $ET_c = ET \div \sqrt{RR}$ (RR = RR interval in seconds). Therefore,

$$\text{mean } V_{cf_c} = \frac{SF}{ET_c}$$

(c = corrected). The normal value is 0.98 ± 0.07 circumferences per second.

The ventricular *ejection fraction* (EF) is a measure of function that originated in the catheterization laboratory. This can be derived from the shortening fraction or from tracings of 2-D volumes. The former method usually employs a squared or cubed formula that is not easily reproducible. The latter method, though more accurate, is time-consuming and depends on good endocardial edge definition in certain views. EF can be derived from the following formula:

$$EF = \left[\frac{(LVEDD)^2 - (LVESD)^2}{(LVEDD)^2}\right] \times 100$$

The normal range is 55–80%.

The distance between the most anterior portion of the anterior mitral leaflet (E point) and the ventricular septum has been called the E point–septal separation (EPSS) and appears to reflect left ventricular dysfunction (Massie et al., 1977). EPSS can be normalized to chamber size by dividing by end-diastolic dimension (EDD), and in normal children it is 0.8 ± 0.06.

Measurement of the left ventricular mass can also have a role in determining the prognoses of courses for some disease states. This methodology has been described, but is beyond the scope of this chapter (Collins, Kronenberg, and Byrd, 1989).

The ventricular wall stress correlates with the ventricular afterload and can be calculated (Douglas et al., 1987) as

$$\text{wall stress } (g \cdot cm^{-2})$$
$$= \frac{\text{ventricular pressure} \times \text{dimension}}{\text{wall thickness}}$$

Specifically, meridional wall stress is derived by the following formula:

$$\text{wall stress } (g \cdot cm^{-2})$$
$$= \frac{0.334P \times LVEDD}{LVPW(1 + LVPW/LVEDD)}$$

where P is left ventricular systolic pressure (mm Hg), and LVPW is left ventricular posterior wall thickness (cm).

Cardiac output can be calculated by a combined 2-D and Doppler study that allows estimation of flow across any orifice. For example,

$$\text{cardiac output} = \text{stroke volume (SV)}$$
$$\times \text{heart rate (HR)}$$

where SV = 2-D cross-sectional area (2-D CSA) × mean velocity (Doppler).

In practical terms, the cardiac output can be obtained by Doppler interrogation of the left ventricular outflow tract (LVOT) combined with an accurate measurement of the diameter of the LVOT during systole (Sahn, 1985a).

Methods for measuring ventricular diastolic function have also been developed during the past 5 yr

(Snider et al., 1985; Spirito et al., 1986; Appleton, Hatle, and Popp, 1988; Feigenbaum, 1989; Riggs et al., 1989). The relaxation characteristics of the ventricles can be evaluated by M-mode or Doppler echocardiography. Studies of isovolumic relaxation and the rapid-filling phase and atrial-contraction phase of diastole have contributed greatly to our understanding of ventricular function. However, clinical application of many of these semiquantitative measures is still under investigation.

Evaluation of stenotic areas

Application of a modified Bernoulli equation to stenotic jets provides an accurate description of the pressure gradient across a stenotic orifice. Most clinical experience with a pressure gradient or pressure drop has come from data obtained during catheterization. Doppler gradients and catheterization gradients are not always identical. Doppler velocimetry provides a measure of instantaneous velocity over time. The highest or peak velocity represents the peak instantaneous velocity across the orifice. If the Bernoulli equation is applied to this number, one obtains the peak instantaneous pressure gradient. Catheterization measurements of this gradient generally reveal the difference between two peak pressures, but the peaks may not (and in some cases rarely do) occur at the same time. Measurement of the area under the Doppler velocity curve divided by the ejection time provides the *mean* Doppler velocity. This correlates well with the catheter-obtained peak aortic valve pressure gradient. The Doppler-derived peak instantaneous gradients across the pulmonary valve and subaortic regions correlate better with the catheter-derived peak systolic gradients. Pressure gradients are dependent on the size of the orifice and the amount of flow through the orifice. In the presence of a significant restriction, one depends on normal ventricular function to force blood through the narrow orifice. Therefore, the area of flow (valve area) may be a better indicator of the severity of obstruction, as it is a physical parameter that is independent of these variables. This can be derived from the continuity equation, which states that the volume of blood moving across a stenotic valve is equal to the amount of blood just proximal to the valve. In Doppler terms, flow is estimated as velocity times the area of the tube or orifice. Thus, $A_1V_1 = A_2V_2$, where A_1 is the area proximal to the valve, V_1 is the mean velocity proximal to the valve, A_2 is the valve area, and V_2 is the velocity across the valve. Because V_1 and V_2 are easily measured by Doppler, and A_1

can be measured by 2-D examination, A_2 can be calculated:

$$A_2 = A_1 \frac{\times V_1}{V_2}$$

The mitral valve area (MVA) can be calculated from an even simpler equation:

$$\text{MVA (cm}_2) = \frac{220}{\text{PHT}}$$

where PHT (the pressure half-time) is the time between the initial peak velocity and the peak velocity divided by 1.4. PHT is less than 60 ms in normal patients (Gonzales, Child, and Krivokapich, 1987; Wranne, Ask, and Lloyd, 1990). A simplified modification of this formula is as follows:

$$\text{MVA (cm}^2) = 750 \div \text{AT}$$

where AT (acceleration time) is the time between the peak E velocity (the E-wave is the first portion of the biphasic mitral inflow signal recorded by Doppler) and the point of intersection of the line drawn along the downslope of the E velocity and the baseline.

Quantification of valvular regurgitation

Quantification of valvular regurgitation by color-flow imaging has been extensively evaluated (Cooper et al., 1989; Yoshida et al., 1990). Measurements of the length and width, as well as the area under the jet, provide an estimate of the severity of regurgitation. The usual picture of regurgitation jets provided by color-flow imaging can be dependent on many factors, including gain, depth, and image quality. One must understand that color-flow imaging can, at best, provide only a semiquantitative measure of regurgitation and that these technical pitfalls may limit its accuracy. The size of the jet at its origin also correlates with the severity of regurgitation. An estimation of the degree of valvular regurgitation is best expressed simply in terms such as mild, moderate, or severe. There is no existing "gold standard" to which the findings from ultrasound techniques can be reliably compared. As with many other qualitative measures, a number of clinical factors must all be evaluated to develop the best noninvasive *estimate* of valvular regurgitation.

Evaluation of pulmonary artery pressure

Semiquantitative measures

Assessment of pulmonary artery pressure is an important step in evaluating newborns, who may have varying degrees of pulmonary disease. A rising pulmonary artery (PA) pressure will change the normal configuration of the Doppler spectral recordings of PA antegrade flow (dome-shaped) to a spike-and-dome-shaped flow pattern (Silverman, Snider, and Rudolph, 1980b). Notching of the decelerating limb of the PA systolic flow tracing is predictive of PA hypertension in 50% of cases, but can also be seen in idiopathic dilation of the pulmonary artery with normal pressure (Hatle, Angelsen, and Tromsdal, 1981).

The PA systolic time intervals recorded by M-mode or Doppler methods have been used to estimate the PA pressure (Hirschfeld et al., 1975). The ratio of the PA preejection period (PEP) to the ejection time (ET) does not consistently correlate with PA pressure.

The right ventricular isovolumic contraction time obtained by M-mode or Doppler methods can be used to predict mean PA pressure with the use of established tables (Burstin, 1967). The acceleration time (AT), in the form AT/ET and PEP/AT, has also been used in adults, but data in children are limited.

The curvature of the ventricular septum at end-systole, as seen on 2-D short-axis view, provides an estimate of the right ventricular (RV) pressure (King et al., 1983). If the circular contour of the left ventricle (LV) is preserved, the RV pressure is predicted to be less than 50% of the LV pressure. Increasing RV hypertension (RV pressure between 50% and 100% of LV pressure) results in flattening of the ventricular septum at end-systole. Suprasystemic RV pressure results in reversal of the septal curvature, with convexity toward the LV.

Quantitative measures

The Doppler examination may yield the most accurate noninvasive measure of pulmonary pressures. Application of Bernoulli equation

$$\text{gradient} = 4 \times (\text{peak velocity}^2)$$

to the measurable jets of tricuspid regurgitation, pulmonary regurgitation, ventricular septal defect (VSD), or ductus arteriosus (if present) allows an accurate calculation of gradients across their orifices. If the blood pressure (BP) or right atrial (RA) pressure is known, RV or PA pressure can be calculated by this simple, reliable, reproducible method. For example:

Cuff BP = 100/60 mm Hg
Peak jet velocity through VSD = 4 m · 5^{-1}
Peak gradient between LV and RV = $4 \times 4^2 = 64$ mm Hg

LV systolic pressure $=$ 100 mm Hg
RV systolic pressure $=$ 100 $-$ 64 mm Hg
PA systolic pressure $=$ 36 mm Hg

Another example is as follows:

Cuff BP $=$ 100/60 mm Hg
Peak tricuspid regurgitation jet velocity $=$ 4 m $\cdot$ 5^{-1}
Peak gradient between RV and RA $=$ 4 $\times$ 4^2 $=$
64 mm Hg
Estimated or measured RA pressure $=$ 5–10 mm
Hg
PA systolic pressure $=$ 64 $+$ (5–10) $=$ 69–74 mm
Hg

FETAL ECHOCARDIOGRAPHY

Fetal echocardiography offers exciting new applications for all of the previously described techniques of echocardiography (Allan et al., 1980, 1981, 1984a; Kleinman and Donnerstein, 1985; Kleinman, Huhta, and Silverman, 1988; Reed, 1989; Huhta, Helton, and Wood, 1989; Wheller, Reiss, and Allen, 1990). The development of higher-quality scanners with fine resolution allows the sonographer to see most of the cardiac structures with great precision at early gestational ages. Congenital cardiac defects have an incidence of 0.8% among all live births, and 2.7% among stillbirths, making this an important source of perinatal morbidity and mortality. Ultrasound examination of all fetuses is close to becoming a routine test in obstetrical practice. Specific examination for cardiac disease should combine two elements: (1) identification of the fetus at greater risk for congenital heart disease and (2) performance of the test by a professional with experience in imaging congenital cardiac malformations.

The risk factors for congenital heart disease can be subdivided into maternal and fetal. Maternal risk factors include a family history of congenital or inheritable heart disease, diabetes mellitus, or certain other maternal diseases such as systemic lupus erythematosus or phenylketonuria, as well as exposure to potentially teratogenic agents such as birth-control pills, lithium, anticonvulsants, or amphetamines. Risk factors specific to the fetus usually involve a detected abnormality, such as a known chromosomal abnormality or a detected cardiac abnormality or rhythm disorder (Nyberg and Emerson, 1990).

The fetal echocardiogram can involve a lengthy procedure lasting up to an hour. All of the previously described echo modalities may be used, including color-flow imaging, pulsed-wave and CW Doppler, and M-mode imaging, with no known del-

eterious side effects to the fetus (Sahn, 1985b). A complete evaluation of the fetal heart can best be performed between 18 and 20 wk of gestation. At that stage of cardiac development, the fetal heart is quite small and may be located far away from the abdominal wall. However, it is surrounded by airless lung tissue and amniotic fluid, so that excellent images frequently are obtained. A 5-MHz transducer usually is adequate and is preferable to get the most detailed pictures of the heart. The higher-frequency transvaginal probes currently being used may allow accurate identification of cardiac structures as early as 14 wk of gestation. The fetus may be quite mobile, and great patience may be required to complete an adequate examination. During the last few weeks of gestation, the amount of amniotic fluid will be less, and the ribs will have calcified, so that the examination may become more difficult. The fetus may move under the transducer unexpectedly and produce a spectrum of unorthodox images that may be difficult to recognize. The most useful initial step is to obtain an overall cranial–caudal view of the fetus so that the head, spine, and abdomen can be located. A cross-sectional view of the fetal trunk then provides a point from which cranial-to-caudal sweeps can be obtained.

Four-chamber view. The four-chamber view has been described as the most important overall scanning view, for many reasons: The ventricles can be identified by the insertions of the atrioventricular (AV) valves and the position of the atrial septum (Figure 2.15). Many significant cardiac defects will produce discrepancies in the sizes of the cardiac chambers that can be seen in this view. Absence or hypoplasia of either AV valve is often part of a serious cardiac disorder that can be easily detected from this view. This view does not provide good visualization of the great arteries and semilunar valves and should not be the only view obtained. The four-chamber view permits visualization of right and left atria and ventricles, atrial septum, inlet ventricular septum, and pulmonary veins. A Doppler evaluation from this view helps assess stenosis or regurgitation of AV valves. The hepatic veins and inferior vena cava can be visualized with slight caudal angulation. Anterior angulation will produce a "five-chamber" view, bringing the aortic valve into view in continuity with the mitral valve.

Abdominal short-axis view. This view helps localize the side of the inferior vena cava (IVC), abdominal aorta (AO), liver, and stomach. If the IVC and AO are located on the same side of the spine, asplenia

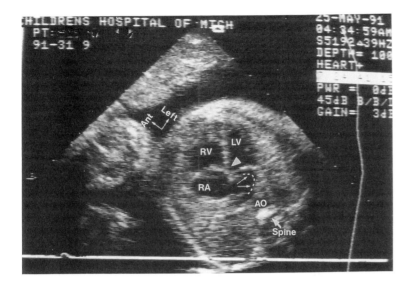

Figure 2.15. In this four-chamber view of the fetal heart, two-equal size atria and ventricles can be seen. The right ventricle (RV) is distinguished from the left ventricle (LV) by the more apical displacement of the tricuspid valve (arrowhead) and the bowing of the fossa ovalis into the left atrium (arrows and dotted line) caused by the fetal right-to-left shunt at this level. The aorta (AO) and spine are also demonstrated, and the heart can be seen to be in the left chest; RA, right atrium.

(bilateral right-sidedness) should be suspected. Absence of a suprahepatic portion of the IVC is suggestive of polysplenia (bilateral left-sidedness). Abnormal positions of abdominal organs frequently are associated with complex heart defects.

Aortic short-axis view. A cephalad angulation with leftward tilt will produce a short-axis view of the aortic root along with a long-axis view of the pulmonary artery. The right ventricular inflow and outflow tracts can be well seen, and slight angulation of the transducer may bring into view the right pulmonary artery and the ductal continuation of the main pulmonary artery into the descending aorta.

Caval axis view. The long axis of the superior and inferior venae cavae can be imaged along the right side of the spine. Slight tilt of the transducer to the opposite side of the spine will display the thoracic aorta, which can be traced cephalad to the aortic arch or the ductus arteriosus.

Long and short axes of the left ventricle. With the sector oriented along an axis between the right shoulder and left hip, the classic long axis of the left ventricle can be recorded (Figure 2.16). A 90° rotation of the transducer along this axis will produce a short-axis view of the left ventricle. The ventricular dimen-

sions, myocardial thickness and function, inferior vena cava, aortic valve, and ventricular septum can be interrogated in these planes.

Aortic arch and ductal view. Minimal rotation and cephalad angulation from the left ventricular long-axis view may display the aortic arch to varying degrees (Figure 2.17). The origin of brachiocephalic vessels identifies the aorta. Slight tilting from this plane will also display the ductal continuation into the descending aorta. This has been referred to as the "ductal arch" which originates more anteriorly in the chest and has a more acute curve (hockey stick) than the aortic arch (candy cane).

EVALUATION OF FETAL HEART RHYTHM

An abnormal fetal heart rhythm can be easily detected and evaluated using ultrasound modalities (Kleinman et al., 1983; Allan et al., 1984b; Chan et al., 1990). Rhythm abnormalities may be classified as tachycardia (>200 bpm), bradycardia (<100 bpm), or irregular. Accurate determination of the rate alone often will provide the diagnosis, because the possibilities are limited. Of potentially greater importance is an evaluation of heart structure and function in the setting of fetal dysrhythmia. Sustained fetal tachycardia or bradycardia may lead to

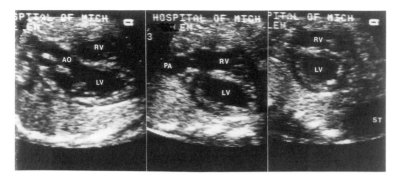

Figure 2.16. *Left:* The long axis of the left ventricle (LV) is shown, with the aorta (AO) and mitral and aortic valves. *Center:* Slight rotation of the transducer will produce a right ventricular (RV) outflow view and identify the main pulmonary artery (PA). *Right:* Continued rotation of the transducer, 90° from the long-axis view, will produce a short-axis (cross-sectional) view of the heart at the midventricle level.

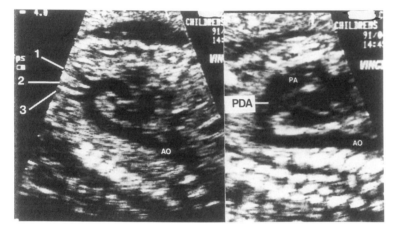

Figure 2.17. *Left:* Often the entire fetal aortic arch can be well seen, and the three bracheocephalic vessels identified (1, innominate artery; 2, left common carotid artery; 3, left subclavian artery; AO, descending aorta). *Right:* A very slight angulation from the arch view will demonstrate the course of the ductus arteriosus (PDA) from the main pulmonary artery (PA) into the descending aorta. Care must be taken not to confuse this "ductal arch" with the real aortic arch. Identification of bracheocephalic vessels is useful in making this distinction.

heart failure and fetal hydrops. The presence of significant structural heart disease with dysrhythmia, particularly bradycardia, carries a dire prognosis.

Very fast (>250–300 bpm) fetal tachycardia is virtually always supraventricular in origin. Very slow bradycardia (<80 bpm) commonly indicates complete heart block. Complete heart block should be suspected in cases of maternal lupus or congenital heart defects, such as an atrioventricular canal or corrected transposition. In either case, the echocardiogram can be used to investigate the relation between atrial and ventricular activities. An irregular heart rate is most commonly due to premature atrial

contractions. This rhythm usually is benign, even in the presence of structural heart disease. However, a potential exists for the development of supraventricular tachycardia, with frequent premature atrial beats. Atrial activity should be identified first. An M-mode recording of the right or left atrial contraction (wall motion) can be used to identify the atrial rate (Figure 2.18, color plate, following page 121). The atrial contraction can also be seen on the M-mode recording of the tricuspid and mitral valves. Pulsed Doppler recording of the right-to-left shunt across the foramen ovale has also been used as a marker for atrial contractions. The antegrade

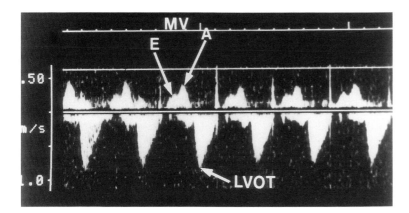

Figure 2.19. Pulsed-wave Doppler sample volume near the mitral valve, with recording of mitral valve inflow (above the centerline) and left ventricular outflow tract (LVOT) flow. The E wave of the mitral signal reflects early diastolic filling, and the A wave occurs with atrial contraction. Ventricular contraction is indicated by the LVOT signal. A normal 1 : 1 rhythm relationship is clearly demonstrated by Doppler techniques in this fetus.

flow across the tricuspid and mitral valves recorded by pulsed or continuous-wave Doppler will also be reflective of atrial contractions (Figure 2.19). Left ventricular wall motion and the opening of an aortic valve recorded on the M-mode echo can be used as indicators of ventricular contraction. Flow in the left ventricular outflow tract, ascending aorta, or pulmonary artery recorded by Doppler can also be used as an indicator of ventricular contraction. Once the atrial and ventricular activities are delineated, their interrelationship should be deduced. The simplest method of establishing atrioventricular synchrony is to place the Doppler in the area of the left ventricular outflow tract, with a large sampling gate, in such a way that mitral inflow and left ventricular outflow tract velocities are simultaneously recorded. Both M-mode and Doppler techniques can be used to deduce fetal rhythm abnormalities. M-mode is superior to Doppler for detecting mechanical events as wall contraction. Because flow does not always follow a mechanical event (such as a blocked premature beat), Doppler derivation of the rhythm may be limited in these instances.

CONCLUSIONS

Echocardiographic techniques can provide a thorough and often complete assessment of cardiac structure and function in the fetus, neonate, and infant. This noninvasive test can be performed at the bedside, with no risk to even the critically ill infant. The complexity of the images, the spectrum of disease, and the rapidly changing technology demand a skilled examiner at the bedside. Echocardiographic examinations in the newborn nursery are used to evaluate patients for the possibility of congenital heart disease, as well as to evaluate the consequences of prematurity and other diseases unique to the newborn infant. The expanding field of fetal echocardiography requires a close relationship among the pediatric cardiologist, perinatologist, obstetrician, and neonatologist to provide a new vista on care for the fetus and mother.

REFERENCES

Allan, L. D., Crawford, D. C., Anderson, R. H., and Tynan, M. J. (1984a). Echocardiographic and anatomical correlations in fetal congenital heart disease. *British Heart Journal* 52:542–8.

(1984b). Evaluation and treatment of fetal arrhythmias. *Clinical Cardiology* 7:767–73.

Allan, L. D., Tynan, M., Campbell, S., and Anderson, R. H. (1981). Identification of congenital cardiac malformations by echocardiography in midtrimester fetus. *British Heart Journal* 46:358–62.

Allan, L. D., Tynan, M. J., Campbell, S., Wilkinson, J. L., and Anderson, R. H. (1980). Echocardiographic and anatomical correlates in the fetus. *British Heart Journal* 44:444–51.

Appleton, C. P., Hatle, L. K., and Popp, R. L. (1988). Relation of transmitral flow velocity patterns to left ventricular diastolic function: new insights from a combined hemodynamic and Doppler echocardiographic study. *Journal of the American College of Cardiology* 12:426–40.

ASE (1989). American Society of Echocardiography, Committee on Standards, Sub-committee on Quantitation of Two-dimensional Echocardiograms: Recommendations for quantitation of the left ventricle by two-dimensional echocardiography. *Journal of the American Society of Echocardiography* 2:358–67.

Bommer, W. J., Shah, P. M., Allen, H., et al. (1984). The safety of contrast echocardiography: report of the committee on contrast echocardiography for the American Society of Echocardiography. *Journal of the American College of Cardiology* 3:6–13.

Burstin, L. (1967). Determination of pressure in the pulmonary artery by external graphic recordings. *British Heart Journal* 29:396–404.

Chan, F. Y., Woo, S. K., Ghosh, A., Tang, M., and Lam, C. (1990). Prenatal diagnosis of congenital fetal arrhythmias by simultaneous pulsed Doppler velocimetry of the fetal abdominal aorta and inferior vena cava. *Obstetrics and Gynecology* 76:200–4.

Collins, H. W., Kronenberg, M. W., and Byrd, B. F. (1989). Reproducibility of left ventricular mass measurements by two-dimensional and M-mode echocardiography. *Journal of the American College of Cardiology* 14:672–6.

Cooper, J., Nanda, N., Philpot, E., and Fan, P. (1989). Evaluation of valvular regurgitation by color Doppler. *Journal of the American Society of Echocardiography* 2:56–67.

Douglas, P. S., Reichek, N., Plappert, T., Muhammed, A., and Sutton, M. G. (1987). Comparison of echocardiographic methods for assessment of left ventricular shortening and wall stress. *Journal of the American College of Cardiology* 9:945–51.

Epstein, M. L., Goldberg, S. U., Allen, H. D., et al. (1975). Great vessel, cardiac chamber, and wall growth patterns in normal children. *Circulation* 51:1124–9.

Feigenbaum, H. (1986). *Echocardiography*, 4th ed. Philadelphia: Lea & Febiger.
    (1989). Echocardiographic evaluation of left ventricular diastolic function. *Journal of the American College of Cardiology* 13:1027–8.

Gonzales, M. A., Child, J. S., and Krivokapich, J. (1987). Comparison of two-dimensional and Doppler echocardiography and intracardiac hemodynamics for qualification of mitral valve stenosis. *American Journal of Cardiology* 60:327–32.

Gutgesell, H. P., Paquet, M., Dugg, D. F., et al. (1977). Evaluation of left ventricular size and function by echocardiography. Results in normal children. *Circulation* 56:457–62.

Gutgesell, H. P., and Rembold, C. M. (1990). Growth of the human heart relative to body surface area. *American Journal of Cardiology* 65:662–8.

Hatle, L., and Angelsen, B. (1985). *Doppler Ultrasound in Cardiology: Physical Principles and Clinical Applications*, 2nd ed. Philadelphia: Lea & Febiger.

Hatle, L., Angelsen, B. A. J., and Tromsdal, A. (1981). Noninvasive estimation of pulmonary artery systolic pressure with Doppler ultrasound. *British Heart Journal* 45:157–65.

Henry, W. L., Ware, J., Gardin, J. M., et al. (1978). Echocardiographic measurements in normal subjects. Growth-related changes that occur between infancy and early childhood. *Circulation* 57:278–85.

Hirschfeld, S., Meyer, R., Schwartz, D. C., Korfhagen, J., and Kaplan, S. (1975). The echocardiographic assessment of pulmonary artery pressure and pulmonary vascular resistance. *Circulation* 52:642–50.

Huhta, J. C., Glasow, P., Murphy, D. J., Gutgesell, H. P., Ott, D. A., McNamara, D. G., and Smith, E. O. (1987). Surgery without catheterization for congenital heart defects: management of 100 patients. *Journal of the American College of Cardiology* 9:823–9.

Huhta, J., Helton, G., and Wood, D. C. (1989). Color Doppler in the fetal examination. *Echocardiography*.

King, M. E., Braun, H., Goldblatt, A., Liberthson, R., and Weyman, A. E. (1983). Interventricular septal configuration as a predictor of right ventricular systolic hypertension in children: a cross-sectional echocardiographic study. *Circulation* 68:68–75.

Kleinman, C. S., and Donnerstein, R. L. (1985). Ultrasonic assessment of cardiac function in the intact human fetus. *Journal of the American College of Cardiology* 5:845–945.

Kleinman, C. S., Donnerstein, R. L., Jaffe, C. C., DeVore, G. R., Weinstein, E. M., Lynch, D. C., Talner, N. S., Berkowitz, R. L., and Hobbins, J. C. (1983). Fetal echocardiography. *American Journal of Cardiology* 51:237–43.

Kleinman, C. S., Huhta, J. C., and Silverman, N. H. (1988). Doppler echocardiography in the human fetus. *Journal of the American Society of Echocardiography* 1:287–90.

Kremkau, F. W., (1989). *Diagnostic Ultrasound: Principles, Instruments, and Exercises*, 3rd ed. Philadelphia: W. B. Saunders.

Massie, B. M., Schiller, N. B., Ratshin, R. A., and Parmley, W. W. (1977). Mitral-septal separation: new echocardiographic index of left ventricular function. *American Journal of Cardiology* 39:1008–11.

Miyatake, K., Okamato, M., Kinoshita, N., Izumi, S., Owa, M., Takao, S., Sakakibara, H., and Nimura, Y. (1984). Clinical applications of a new type of realtime two-dimensional Doppler flow imaging system. *American Journal of Cardiology* 54:857–68.

Nishimura, R. A., Miller, F. A., Callahan, M. J., Berassi, R. C., Seward, J. B., and Tajik, A. J. (1985). Doppler echocardiography: theory, instrumentation, technique, and application. *Mayo Clinic Proceedings* 60:321–43.

Nyberg, D. A., and Emerson, D. S. (1990). Cardiac malformations. In *Diagnostic Ultrasound of Fetal Anomalies*, ed. D. A. Nyberg, B. S. Mahony, and D. H. Pretorius (pp. 300–41). Chicago: Year Book.

Reed, K. L. (1989). Doppler ultrasound studies of human fetal blood flow. *Circulation* 80:1914–17.

Reeder, G. S., Currie, P. J., Hagler, D. J., Tajik, A. J., and Seward, J. B. (1986). Use of Doppler techniques (continuous-wave, pulsed-wave, and color flow imaging) in the non-invasive hemodynamic assessment of congenital heart disease. *Mayo Clinic Proceedings* 61:725–44.

Riggs, T. W., Rodriguez, R., Snider, R., Batton, D., Pollock, J., and Sharp, E. (1989). Doppler echocardiographic evaluation of right and left ventricular diastolic function in normal neonates. *Journal of the American College of Cardiology* 5:700–5.

Roge, C. L., Silverman, N. H., Hart, P. A., et al. (1978). Cardiac structure growth pattern determined by echocardiography. *Circulation* 57:285–90.

Sahn, D. J. (1985a). Determination of cardiac output by echocardiographic Doppler methods: relative accuracy of various sites of measurement. *Journal of the American College of Cardiology* 9:663–4.

(1985b). Resolution and display requirements for ultrasound Doppler/evaluation of the heart in children, infants and the unborn human fetus. *Journal of the American College of Cardiology* 5:125–95.

(1989). Applications of color flow mapping in pediatric cardiology. *Cardiology Clinics* 7:255–64.

Sanders, S. P., (1990). Echocardiography. In *Fetal and Neonatal Cardiology*, ed. W. A. Long (pp. 301–29). Philadelphia: W. B. Saunders.

Silverman, N. H., Ports, T. A., Snider, A. R., et al. (1980a). Determination of left ventricular volume in children: echocardiographic and angiographic comparisons. *Circulation* 62:548–57.

Silverman, N. H., and Schmidt, K. G. (1989). The current role of Doppler echocardiography in the diagnosis of heart disease in children. *Cardiology Clinics* 7:265–97.

Silverman, N. H., Snider, A. R., and Rudolph, A. M. (1980b). Evaluation of pulmonary hypertension by M-mode echocardiography in children with ventricular septal defect. *Circulation* 61:1125–32.

Snider, A. R., Gidding, S. S., Rocchini, A. P., Rosenthal, A., Dick, M., Crowley, D. C., and Peters, J. (1985). Doppler evaluation of left ventricular diastolic filling in children with systemic hypertension. *American Journal of Cardiology* 56:921–6.

Snider, A. R., and Serwer, G. A. (1990). *Echocardiography in Pediatric Heart Disease*. Chicago: Year Book.

Solinger, R., Elbl, F., and Minhas, K. (1974). Deductive echocardiographic analysis in infants with congenital heart disease. *Circulation* 50:1072–96.

Spirito, P., Maron, B. J., Bellotti, P., et al. (1986). Noninvasive assessment of left ventricular diastolic function: comparative analysis of pulsed Doppler ultrasound and digitized M-mode echocardiography. *American Journal of Cardiology* 58:837–43.

Tajik, A. J., Seward, J. B., Hagler, D. J., Mair, D. D., and Lie, J. T. (1978). Two-dimensional real-time ultrasonic imaging of the heart and great vessels: technique, image orientation, structure identification, and validation. *Mayo Clinic Proceedings* 53:271–303.

Wheller, J. J., Reiss, R., and Allen, H. D. (1990). Clinical experience with fetal echocardiography. *American Journal of Diseases of Children* 144:49–53.

Wranne, B., Ask, P., and Lloyd, D. (1990). Analysis of different methods of assessing the stenotic mitral valve area with emphasis on the pressure gradient half-time concept. *American Journal of Cardiology* 66:614–20.

Yoshida, K., Yoshikawa, J., Yamaura, Y., Hozumi, T., Akasaka, T., and Fukaya, T. (1990). Assessment of mitral regurgitation by biplane transesophageal color Doppler flow mapping. *Circulation* 82:1121–6.

Computed tomography

BERTIL AXELSSON, Ph.D.
OLOF FLODMARK, M.D., Ph.D.

INTRODUCTION

Clinical evaluation of the neonatal central nervous system is difficult. It is particularly difficult to make reliable predictions about neurological outcome in a severely ill newborn with the potential for serious disease or damage to several different organ systems. Neuroradiological investigation of the distressed newborn has emerged as a very important adjunct to clinical evaluation of the neonate. Routine imaging has developed in two main directions: computed tomography (CT) and, later, ultrasonography. Ultrasonography has many advantages, as the equipment is portable, inexpensive, and usually more readily available. The examination can be performed at bedside, in the incubator, but is limited to the first few months of life, and some parts of the brain are poorly visualized. Ultrasonography is very operator-dependent, and the quality of the study is intimately related to the skill and experience of the sonologist, as well as his or her knowledge of the anatomy and abnormalities of the neonatal brain. Ultrasonography is the imaging method of choice for the immature neonate, despite its shortcomings. Although cranial CT scanning may provide additional information in the premature neonate, it is rarely done in routine practice. The situation is quite different in assessing the mature neonate suspected of having suffered hypoxic/ischemic damage to the brain. Although ultrasonography may be quite useful, CT should remain the primary mode of imaging in the term neonate.

CT is not suited to investigate the unborn fetus, as it is necessary to properly position and immobilize the patient to be able to obtain a useful study.

This is, of course, impossible with the patient in utero. Other imaging methods, particularly ultrasonography, but also magnetic resonance imaging, are far better in this situation. Although recent developments toward faster CT scanners have allowed other parts of the neonate to be investigated successfully, CT currently is used almost exclusively to investigate the neonatal central nervous system.

CT has been in clinical use since the mid-1970s and is now a well-established, routine radiological procedure. Initially the procedure was termed computerized axial tomography (CAT). However, modern equipment allows scanning in planes other than the axial plane, and the word "axial" has been dropped from the name. The name commonly accepted and used today is simply "computed tomography." There are some basic differences between conventional radiographic images presented on film and CT images. The conventional film can be regarded as a presentation of the findings from measurements of the transmission of roentgen rays through the object being investigated. This results in a mapping of the three-dimensional distribution of attenuation properties on a two-dimensional film. The attenuation properties of a substance depend on its atomic composition, its density, and the energy of the roentgen rays.

The findings from transmission measurements performed in several directions are used to calculate a CT image describing the attenuation properties in a transverse section through the object. The CT image thus is dependent not only on the investigated object and the measurement procedure but also on how the calculations are performed. CT offers several advantages over conventional radiography,

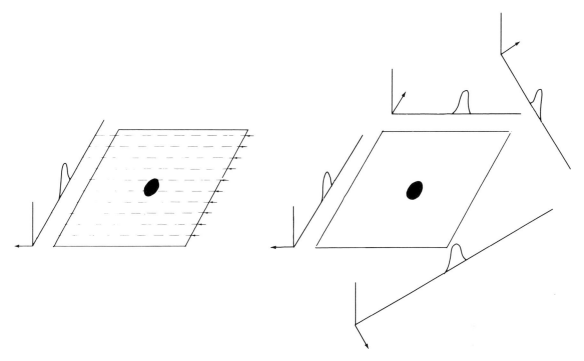

Figure 3.1. *Left:* Illustration of the measurement technique using a simplified model with a high-attenuation substance at the center of the investigated object. Attenuation measurements are performed along several lines to form the projection data for this direction. *Right:* Similar measurements are performed in several directions through at least 180°. Some examples of the measured profile data are given.

such as improved contrast resolution and elimination of disturbing interferences from regions other than those being studied. However, the technique also has some limitations. The advantages and limitations of CT will be discussed later, but to understand the method it is necessary to have a basic understanding of the algorithm used to calculate the image. Therefore, a short description of this algorithm will follow.

FILTERED BACK-PROJECTION

The data used to calculate the transverse-section image are obtained from measurements of the transmission of roentgen rays along several lines in one direction, as shown in Figure 3.1 (left). The measured value associated with a certain line in one projection thus indicates the total attenuation of roentgen rays in all substances along that line through the object. The figure illustrates a simplified situation, with a highly attenuating substance in the center and nonattenuating surroundings. To obtain enough data for an accurate calculation of a transverse-section image, measurements have to be per-

formed in several directions through at least 180°. Some examples of measurement profiles obtained in different directions are seen in Figure 3.1 (right).

In the calculation of the image, measurement data in the profile are back-projected onto the matrix that is used to map the attenuation properties within the section being investigated. The measurement data associated with a certain line in one profile are back-projected to all matrix elements (pixels) along that line in the image matrix (Figure 3.2, left). The back-projection procedure is repeated using profile data for all the directions in which measurements were performed (Figure 3.2, right). In the example used here, all lines with high attenuation values are back-projected through the pixels in the center of the image. This results in a higher value in these pixels than in the surrounding pixels, and thus an image roughly describing the actual attenuation properties described in Figure 3.1 (left) is obtained. However, as can be seen from Figure 3.2 (right), the highly attenuating central part appears blurred as compared with the actual situation, and also pixels that represent zero attenuation contain nonzero values. These problems can be counteracted by a mathe-

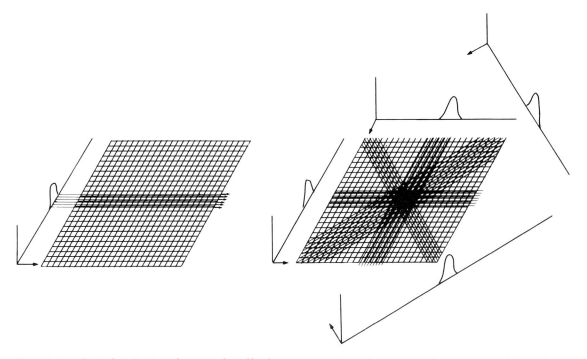

Figure 3.2. *Left:* Back-projection of measured profile data from one direction onto the image matrix. *Right:* Back-pro- jection of data from several directions gives a blurred image of the investigated object.

matical filtration of the measured profile data before back-projection. The result of such a filtration in the example used here is illustrated for one profile in Figure 3.3 (left). In the filtered profile, the high attenuation values in the center are surrounded by negative values on both sides. Both positive and negative values are back-projected as described earlier. The negative "tails" serve to reduce the blurring of the central high-attenuation part and to restore pixels representing nonattenuating substances to zero values. The final result after back-projection of filtered profiles from several directions is illustrated in Figure 3.3 (right).

The method described here, filtered back-projection, is the method used in almost all CT equipment. These mathematical methods have been known for a long time (Radon, 1917), but their implementation in a radiological technique depended on the availability of fast computers capable of handling the large number of calculations involved. More detailed descriptions of the technique have been presented (Brooks and Di Chiro, 1975, 1976; Edholm, 1975; Gordon, Herman, and Johnson, 1975).

When the calculated image is presented, the value associated with each pixel does not represent the attenuation coefficient. Instead, the attenuation coefficient is transformed to a CT number or Hounsfield unit (HU) using the following formula. The CT number thus represents the attenuation coefficient (μ) relative to the attenuation coefficient of water (μ_w):

$$\text{CT number} = \frac{\mu - \mu_w}{\mu_w} \times 1{,}000$$

EQUIPMENT

To allow calculation of high-quality images, large numbers of measurements have to be performed with great accuracy and in a reasonably short time. A model of the measurement system used in most modern CT scanners is shown in Figure 3.4. The radiation emitted from the x-ray tube is shaped into a thin slice (fan beam) by lead diaphragms. Slice widths typically can be chosen between 1 and 10 mm. The amount of radiation that is transmitted through the object is measured by the detector. To allow measurements along several lines, as discussed earlier in connection with back-projection, the detector is separated into a large number of measurement channels. Separate measurements are performed for each channel. The x-ray tube and de-

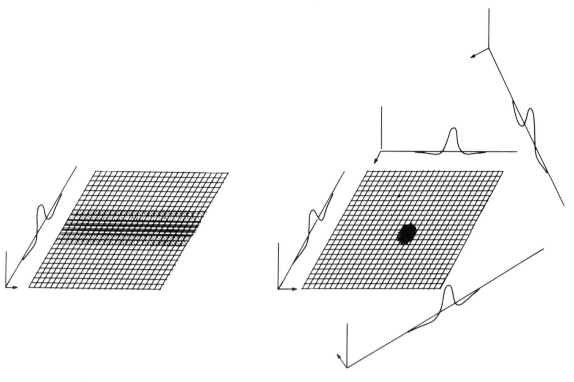

Figure 3.3. *Left:* Filtered projection data for one direction are back-projected onto the image matrix. *Right:* After back-projection of filtered projection data from several directions, the blur is reduced, and pixels representing zero attenuation are restored to zero values.

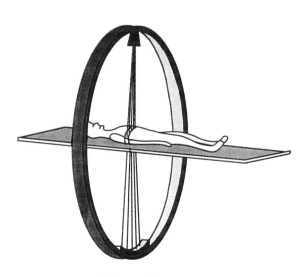

Figure 3.4. Simplified model of the measurement system. The x-ray tube and detector array are rotated around the patient during measurement.

tector are mechanically aligned and rotate simultaneously around the object during acquisition of data to allow measurements in different directions.

The shortest scan time, for a single scan, is limited mainly by the time it takes to rotate the x-ray tube–detector package around the object, but also to some degree by the need to make accurate measurements in each direction used. The shortest scan times usually are around 1–2 s with 270° rotation. The longest scan time, 6–8 s, can be used for more accurate measurements. When several consecutive scans are performed, other problem arise because of the huge amount of data that must be handled, the accumulation of heat in the x-ray tube, and the time needed to accurately reposition the patient table. The scan cycle time for consecutive slices typically is 15–20 s for the first 20–30 scans. A longer pause between scans is needed for the purpose of cooling the tube when larger numbers of consecutive scans are being obtained.

The scan cycle time can be shortened if, as in some types of equipment, the x-ray tube–detector package is continually rotated in the same direction, rather than changing the direction of rotation between each scan. However, this presents other problems related to the transmission of power and data. Scanning of a volume with a craniocaudal dimension of up to 15 cm can be accomplished in 15 s with simultaneous continuous rotation and continuous movement of the patient table (spiral CT).

The type of detector most often used is an ion chamber filled with xenon gas under high pressure. The ion chamber is divided into 400–800 detector elements. In other types of equipment an array of crystal detectors is used instead of the ion chamber. This increases the detection efficiency but sometimes creates problems due to instability. It is, in all equipment, essential that the actual detection efficiency of each detector element be known, so that the transmission measurements can be corrected accordingly. This is accomplished by daily control measurements (calibration).

Ultrafast CT scanners have recently become available. The detector package (or both the radiation source and the detector package) is stationary in these constructions. Thus, one must use a large number of detector elements, so that a full circle, or at least the major part of a circle, around the patient will be covered. In the fastest equipment, the x-ray tube is replaced by an electron accelerator and an anode ring in a semicircle around the patient. The electron beam is electronically directed to move the focus, where the roentgen rays are produced, from one side of the ring to the other, allowing measurements in different directions. The scan time using this type of equipment can be less than 0.1 s.

The positioning of the patient, using the computer-controlled patient table, can be performed with an accuracy of about 0.5 mm. The positioning for the scans is usually chosen from a planar, digital image obtained by moving the patient table, during exposure, through the gantry while the x-ray tube and detector are held stationary. To adjust the scan plane correctly, the gantry can also be tilted $\pm 20°$.

The calculated digital images from the CT scanner are displayed for evaluation on a video screen. The presented image is produced by translation of the CT number of each pixel into gray-scale levels. The translation is controlled by adjustment of the image "window." The window level is used to determine which CT number is to correspond to the center of the gray scale, and manipulation of the window width is used to determine the range of CT numbers. Pixels with CT numbers outside the window will be either black or white.

Digital data from the CT examination can be stored in digital form on a magnetic tape or an optic laser disc. Both the acquisition data and the pixel values from the reconstructed image can be stored. However, reconstruction of an image using a different algorithm or different matrix is possible only if complete acquisition data are stored. Because that would occupy a large space on the storage medium, usually only the reconstructed images are stored.

Documentation of the study for clinical use is usually done by creating a hard copy of the image as it appears on the video screen. This is accomplished either by exposure of a video monitor image on a film or by using the information from the video image to modulate a laser beam sweeping across the film.

IMAGE QUALITY

Image quality is not a well-defined concept, and several parameters are used to describe its different aspects. The most useful parameters are spatial resolution and contrast resolution. The following discussion will concern mainly these two parameters.

It is essential to make measurements with high spatial resolution, to enable calculation of images that can depict very small details. Thus, there should be a small distance between each measurement line in a projection, and measurements should be performed in a large number of projections. The distance between the measurement lines is, in most types of equipment, defined by the number of detector channels and the maximum field of view and thus is not variable. Typical line spacing for modern equipment is about 0.6 mm at the center of the image field. High-spatial-resolution measurements can be accomplished in equipment with fewer detector channels by moving the x-ray tube closer to the patient and the detector array away from the patient (i.e., a magnification technique). This technique reduces the field of view and is associated with a higher radiation dose.

In most types of equipment the number of measurement projections is the same for all scan times, except during the shortest scanning time. Scans of 1 or 2 s are usually performed with less than 360° rotation and thus with fewer projections. Conversely, an increased number of projections obtained during a longer scan time can enable more accurate measurements.

Spatial resolution is also greatly affected by how the reconstruction of the image is performed. High spatial resolution is achieved by using "sharp" filters in the filtration of the measured projection data. Sharp filters result in sharp delineation of high-con-

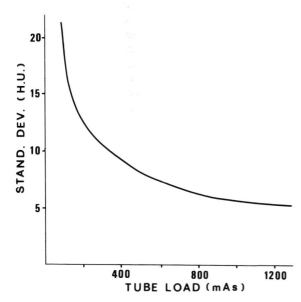

Figure 3.5. Noise in the image (presented as the standard deviation for a small area) as a function of the tube load. Increasing the tube load above about 600 mA will result in only a minor reduction of the noise for this equipment.

crease the accuracy of the transmission measurement. Thus the total accuracy is affected mainly by the tube load (milliampere-seconds) in turn determined by the exposure per projection and the number of projections. An increased acceleration potential (kilovolts) will also increase the output and at the same time increase the transmission of radiation through the object. However, the differences in the attenuation properties between, for instance, muscle and fat will decrease with an increase in kilovolts (acceleration potential), and that will cause less contrast in the measured projection data. Furthermore, an increase in the amount of radiation will also result in a higher absorbed dose to the patient, while the noise level will be only slightly decreased, as compared with a more moderate exposure (Figure 3.5). The noise level is also affected by the filtration of the projection data. A "soft" filter decreases the small statistical variations in the measurement data and thus also the noise in the reconstructed image. However, sharp edges between, for instance, bone and soft tissue will be softened. The best large-area low-contrast resolution that can be obtained with modern equipment is about 0.3% contrast. In comparison, the contrast resolution for a conventional film/screen system is about 2%.

Spatial resolution and contrast resolution are also greatly affected by the width of the transverse section (slice thickness). Most of the radiation emitted from the x-ray focus is blocked by the lead diaphragm defining the slice width of a thin slice (1–2 mm). In a thicker slice (8–10 mm), a larger amount of radiation is allowed to pass the lead diaphragms, and therefore a larger amount of radiation is reaching the detector elements, resulting in a decrease in the noise level. Thus, thick slices allow better contrast resolution. However, smaller details are more difficult to visualize in thick slices, because of volume averaging. Volume averaging occurs when a blurred image is seen of a sharp edge, as a sharp edge is likely to pass through several adjacent pixels of the typical dimension $(1 \times 1 \times 10 \text{ mm}^3)$ in a thick slice.

In summary, an image with the highest possible spatial resolution is obtained when the acquisition is performed with a large number of projections, a small distance between measurement lines, and a thin slice. The filtered back-projection should be performed with a sharp filter and small picture elements. Conversely, an image with the best possible contrast resolution is obtained using acquisition with a high tube load (milliampere-seconds) and a

trast edges in the image. The "noise" level in the image will then increase, as the noise represents small focal variations in measured data. The accuracy in the back-projection calculations is higher for small objects than for large objects, because the image is divided into smaller pixels. Thus, the spatial resolution for a large object can be increased by reconstructing a selected part of the object (zoom reconstruction). The best high-contrast spatial resolution that can be obtained using modern equipment is about 0.5 mm with zoom reconstruction, whereas the spatial resolution in an image of a large object is about 1 mm without zoom. The spatial resolution in conventional radiography using a standard film/screen combination is about 0.1 mm.

Contrast resolution is affected mainly by the noise level in the image, which in turn is partly dependent on the noise level in the measured projection data. Noise in the projection data is due to statistical variations in the signals from the detector elements. These variations are reduced if the amount of radiation reaching the detectors is increased. For a certain thickness of the object, the amount of radiation is affected by the output from the x-ray tube and by the slice thickness. The output is usually increased by increasing the x-ray tube current (milliamperes), and an increased number of projections also will in-thick slice, and the reconstruction should be performed using a soft filter and slightly larger pixels. Thus, it is virtually impossible to get an image that simultaneously shows both very high spatial resolution and very good contrast resolution.

ARTIFACTS

Artifacts are disturbances in the image caused by deficiencies in the measurement procedure or the image calculations. It is important to understand the origin and appearance of such artifacts to avoid misinterpretation of the images. Malfunction of the detector system usually results in streaks or rings in the image. With the reconstruction procedure in mind, it is obvious that a "bad" measurement from one detector channel in one projection will result in a sharp line across the image. If one detector channel gives bad results in all projections, that will result in a ring in the calculated image due to overlap of the "bad" line from all projections. The magnitude of the ring artifact will be larger if the bad line is close to the center of rotation. Sometimes detector problems can be eliminated by a renewed calibration of the detector channels. Ring artifacts are more commonly seen when scanning small objects, such as the neonatal skull. A "center artifact" is a specific type of ring artifact (Figure 3.6). The center artifact is usually easy to recognize as a small area with, most commonly, low attenuation. However, in some cases the center artifact may mimic an anatomic abnormality, particularly for the untrained interpreter. This artifact is found in a location of the image corresponding to the center of the gantry. With proper positioning of the head in the gantry, the artifact will be found at or near the center of the image. Although ring artifacts usually can be eliminated by carrying out frequent calibrations of the detectors, the center artifact may be inherent to the equipment and impossible to eliminate completely.

As described earlier, the detectors in the CT scanner record and measure the radiation transmitted through the object in the gantry. The amount of radiation must be adjusted to the proper range of measurements to assure proper function of the detectors. A small object, such as an infant's skull, will absorb and scatter less radiation than an adult head. Thus, the output of the x-ray tube must be reduced to avoid overload of the detectors. Some CT scanner systems will indicate to the operator that "over-ranges" have occurred. However, overload of the detectors may be seen only as artifacts in the image. An overload of the detectors will create an error in calculation of the image, and areas in the image will be assigned lower CT values than the "true" attenuation. This artifact will influence the entire image, but will be more obvious in some parts of the image if the object is placed asymmetrically in the gantry. The combination of excessive radiation and an asymmetric position of the head in the gantry will have the most serious effects on image quality. The resulting artifact is known as "shading" and is seen as a gradient over the entire image (Flodmark, 1987). This artifact can be very difficult to detect and frequently is misinterpreted as representing an abnormality, even by trained neuroradiologists lacking specific experience with scanning of the neonatal head (Figure 3.6). Thus, it is of utmost importance that the head be placed centrally in the gantry. This is true for all CT scanners, even those with software specifically designed to move the image on the screen to offset asymmetric location of the object in the gantry.

The use of an x-ray tube as the radiation source causes some problems, because the emitted roentgen spectrum contains radiation of various energies, ranging from an energy corresponding to the acceleration potential to an energy approximately one-third of that. For a thin object, both the low- and high-energy parts of the beam will influence the transmission measurement. However, a thick or highly attenuating object will completely or almost completely absorb or block the radiation of low energy, and the transmission measurement will be more influenced by the high-energy part of the beam. This "beam hardening" will cause falsely high results in the transmission measurements. Without correction for beam hardening, a cupping effect will be seen, with, for instance, artificially high CT values close to the skull (Di Chiro et al., 1978). Beam hardening also causes broad streaks between areas of highly attenuating matter, such as cortical bone. These artifacts can interact with similar artifacts that are due to incomplete correction for the distribution of scattered radiation. It is generally not possible to remove these artifacts from the reconstructed image, although various methods to reduce them have been discussed (Nielsen, 1984).

Dental fillings or other artificial matter that causes extremely high attenuation will cause artifacts in the image, because virtually no radiation will be transmitted. This artifact is star-shaped, with its center at the object.

Because the reconstructed image is obtained using measurement values from all projections, movement of the patient during acquisition usually will render the image useless. Short scan times, or reconstruction using data from only 180° rotation,

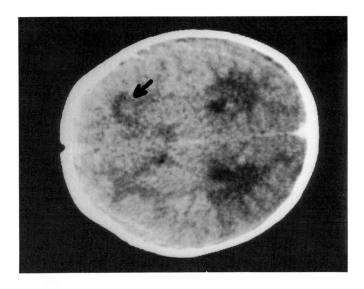

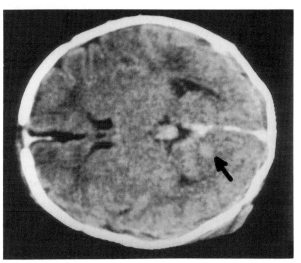

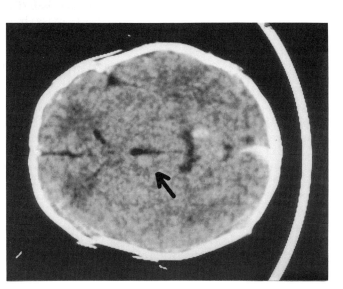

Figure 3.6. Shading artifact. Three images obtained using the same equipment on the same day, but of three different asphyxiated neonates without any pathological findings in the CT scans. Note the center artifact (arrow) seen in all three images. *Left:* The center artifact is located close to the center of the image, indicating correct placement of the neonate's head in the center of the gantry. *Middle:* The center artifact is located in the right posterior aspect of the image (arrow). Note the apparent decreased attenuation, "shading" in the anterior left aspect of the image. *Right:* The center artifact is located in the left anterior aspect of the image (arrow), and the corresponding shading artifact is found in the right posterior part of the image. These artifacts, found in two of the neonates, we initially assumed to represent abnormalities.

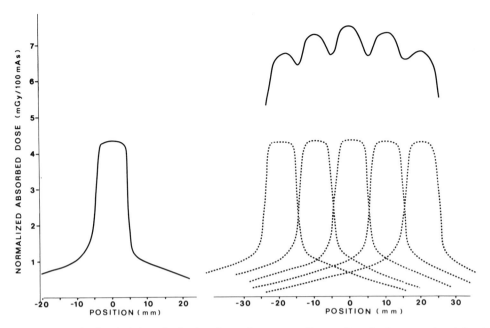

Figure 3.7. *Left:* Absorbed-dose distribution along a line perpendicular to the scan plane. Measurement at the center of a 10-mm slice. *Right:* Absorbed-dose distribution for several adjacent slices (broken curves) and the absorbed-dose distribution for the total examination (solid curve).

may be used if it is difficult to immobilize the patient.

ABSORBED DOSE

The success of the examination is dependent not only on the quality of the images produced but also on the radiation-dose burden necessary to obtain those images. The absorbed dose in an organ is the amount of energy absorbed from the radiation per unit mass of tissue. The measurement unit for the absorbed dose is the gray (Gy), where 1 Gy = 1 J · kg^{-1} (1 cGy = 1 rad).

Figure 3.7 (left) illustrates an example of the distribution of absorbed dose along a line perpendicular to the scan plane. The shape of the "tails" on both sides of the investigated slice will depend on the effectiveness of the collimation of the radiation beam and on the scattered radiation. Several adjacent slices are obtained in most clinical situations. Therefore the absorbed dose will be higher than is indicated in Figure 3.7 (left), because of the overlap of the tails from adjacent slices (Figure 3.7, right). There is greater overlap because of the smaller distance between slices, and thus a greater increase in absorbed dose, when thin slices are used, as compared with thicker slices (Moström and Ytterbergh, 1987). This is in addition to the already relatively high absorbed dose because of the increased output needed to get acceptable noise levels when thin slices are used.

The distribution of the absorbed dose in the investigated volume is quite different from that in conventional radiography, because of the rotation of the x-ray tube around the object during exposure. This results in a circular symmetric distribution, with the highest absorbed dose in the periphery and slightly lower doses in the center. The absorbed dose to a patient depends on the exposure parameters used and on the number and width of the slices. An increase in the tube load with 50% will cause an increase of the absorbed dose with about 50%. However, as shown in Figure 3.5, the gain in image quality, mainly contrast resolution, that can be achieved by an increase in tube load is limited if the tube load is already relatively high. A standard examination of the head might give a skin dose of 40–60 mGy, with the absorbed dose in the center being 30–50 mGy. By way of comparison, the skin dose for a single anteroposterior standard film is about 2 mGy. An examination with several adjacent thin slices might give a skin dose of 70–80 mGy in the investigated area. For pediatric patients, the exposure parameters used in examination of the abdomen are similar to those used for the head.

Two types of risk must be considered with respect to radiation exposure. For deterministic effects, such as formation of cataract in the lens of the eye, there is a threshold with regard to absorbed dose below which the risk is considered to be zero. For radiation doses well above the threshold, the risk is 1, and thus such a dose is certain to cause the effect. The lowest radiation dose that has been reported to cause a cataract is about 2 Gy (Merriam, Szechter, and Focht, 1972; Otake and Schull, 1990). For protracted irradiation, the threshold is considerably higher (10–15 Gy).

For stochastic effects, such as induction of cancer and induction of hereditary defects, it is considered that there is no threshold and that the risk is linearly related to the dose. Usually, the main focus of attention is the carcinogenic risk. The risk of inducing fatal cancer is considered to be about 0.005% per mGy (ICRP 60, 1991).

These risk estimates are based on a uniform whole-body irradiation and the average age distribution of the population. For routine x-ray examinations, where only a part of the body is irradiated, a risk estimate must be based on the absorbed dose to the radiosensitive organs involved and on the age distribution of the patients. The risk factor for small children is considered to be a few times higher than for the average population. Risk estimates obtained from such calculations show very large uncertainties and should be used with great care. However, even a very rough calculation will show that the radiation-dose burden from CT examinations in general is not small compared with those for most conventional x-ray examinations.

It should be noted that the distribution of the absorbed dose and the associated estimation of the risks strongly depend on the examination procedure and the equipment used (Nishizawa et al., 1991). Therefore, risk estimates used in discussions about justification or optimization of certain examinations should be based on "local" data. It should further be noted that the radiation-associated risk usually is quite small and therefore should not inhibit the use of such examinations, provided they are properly indicated.

Sometimes, particularly when studying pediatric patients under sedation, it might be suitable that a person (professional or relative) remain in the examination room during the procedure. The absorbed dose to that person, properly shielded using a lead-rubber apron and standing about 2 m away from the gantry, usually would be below 0.05 mGy, less than the absorbed dose from environmental sources over a period of a week.

SPECIAL APPLICATIONS

Acquisition and reconstruction of several adjacent slices essentially will give the attenuation data for the three-dimensional volume being examined in the form of CT numbers for small volume elements. Because all data are available, images representing the attenuation data in any plane can be formed. It is also possible to form images of curved slices, as, for instance, to reproduce a panoramic view of the jaw. The spatial resolution in the craniocaudal direction is, however, dependent on the slice width. To get good, detailed resolution, thin slices are needed. However, if a rather large distance is covered with thin slices, this will result in a higher radiation-dose burden, as discussed earlier.

With the standard technique, the CT numbers are dependent both on the atomic composition and on the density of the tissue. If two acquisitions with different acceleration potentials (kilovolts) are performed, the measurement results can be combined to enable calculation of CT numbers dependent only on atomic composition. This can be used to estimate the mineralization of the skeleton.

The geometric accuracy of the presented images is very high. This is an inherent property of the reconstruction technique. Accurate measurements of distances, areas, and volumes are thus possible, provided digital data are used for these measurements. However, that is not necessarily the case if the same measurements are made on hard copies of the reconstructed images, as such images may have been distorted in the copying unit used to produce them.

CLINICAL TECHNIQUE AND APPLICATIONS

The distressed newborn, particularly if born prematurely, is in a very fragile physiological state. Handling of the neonate should be kept to a minimum. Whenever possible, imaging should be done at cribside using real-time ultrasonography. However, when the ultrasound findings are inadequate, it becomes necessary to transport the neonate to the radiology department for a CT scan or magnetic-resonance imaging. Transportation must be performed in such a way that ongoing therapy and body temperature can be maintained. Thus, transportation of a distressed neonate should be done using a fully equipped transport incubator. The room temperature in the CT room should be between 24°C and 26°C. The neonate's body temperature can be maintained during the procedure, which takes between 10 and 20 min, depending on equipment, by using a heating lamp or by wrapping the neonate in a rubber blanket with circulating warm water. A physician or nurse with knowledge of neonatal resuscitation, wearing suitable protection, must be present in the gantry room at all times.

Interpretation of CT images of the neonatal brain is difficult. Thus, every precaution must be taken to avoid improper technique that might cause artifacts in the images. The neonate's head must be placed centrally in the gantry. This is extremely important, in order to avoid the shading artifact (Figure 3.6). Moving an off-center image on the screen, as is possible with most modern CT scanners, will not prevent the artifact, but will make its detection even more difficult. A proper headrest should be used, as the tabletop usually will give edge artifacts when a very small object, such as an infant's head, is imaged lying directly on the table. Similar artifacts can be caused by intravenous lines passing through the gantry, by a scalp needle, or by the loose ends of sticky tape or velcro bands used to immobilize the head. Optimal spatial and contrast resolutions in scanning the neonatal brain are achieved by using thin slices (4–5 mm) and a soft reconstruction filter. A zoom reconstruction should be used, and the image reconstructed to the full matrix. Electronic magnification should be avoided, as this procedure will increase pixel size and reduce the apparent spatial resolution.

As detailed earlier, the radiation dose will increase as thinner slices are used. If this is a concern, it is possible to reduce radiation by not obtaining contiguous slices, but using a double table move after each slice. If subsequently deemed necessary, the interjacent images can then be obtained at the end of the procedure. However, the entire brain should be examined, particularly the posterior fossa. It is not acceptable to omit scanning of significant parts of the brain in order to reduce radiation exposure to the neonate, provided the study is properly indicated. Direct exposure of the lens of the eye can be avoided by using a scanner plane about 20° above the canthomeatal line.

Intravenously administered contrast material is rarely indicated in the neonate, as contrast is not indicated in studying the asphyxiated neonate, the most common reason for a neonatal CT scan. Only rare cases of congenital tumors may warrant contrast injection. If used, less toxic, nonionic contrast medium should be used, at a dose of 900 mg VI per kilogram body weight. Sedation is rarely necessary in order to obtain a good study without motion artifacts in a neonate. Feeding prior to the study is sufficient in most cases, though ongoing seizures may

require additional medication in order to obtain a diagnostic study.

Careful assessment of brain-tissue attenuation is the foundation of neuroradiological diagnosis of hypoxic/ischemic brain damage in neonates. Hence, it is of utmost importance that the CT equipment provide reliable information about attenuation values in the images. Regularly performed calibrations, at least daily, can assure correct digital information. However, interpretation of images is, in clinical practice, most often done from hard copies, without the benefit of digital information. It is therefore important to ensure correct adjustment of the camera used to produce these images. Furthermore, the images must be photographed using standard settings for window width and level, selected specifically for neonatal imaging. The water content in the neonatal brain is normally high, resulting in lower tissue attenuation, and the difference in attenuation between white and gray matter is normally less obvious than in the adult brain. It is therefore important always to interpret images obtained at a reduced window width of 60–80 HU and a window level of 25–30 HU. These values correspond to the attenuation normally found in the neonatal brain.

Hypoxic/ischemic damage to the neonatal brain will cause cerebral edema, with increased water content in brain tissue and hence a further decreased brain-tissue attenuation. These changes, if the damage is extensive, will be quite widespread and will involve most parts of the supratentorial brain. The most common pitfall in performing and interpreting neonatal brain CT scans is the error of adjusting the viewing parameters (window width and level) in such a way that most of the brain will appear to have a "normal" appearance, so that the image will "please the eye." Areas of normal brain tissue will then appear abnormally dense and may mimic fresh hemorrhage or calcifications. Such errors can lead to serious misinterpretation of the imaging data and are best avoided by directly measuring brain-tissue attenuation in the image on the video display. This is of particular importance if the findings are to be used for scientific publication. Failure to do so will prevent the results from being used by other scientists and will raise the possibility of erroneous conclusions being drawn and published (Shewmon et al., 1981; Aicardi & Goutieres, 1984). When digital data are unavailable, the radiologist must first establish that the hard-copy images were obtained using the correct window width and level before radiological interpretation is done. Variations in film contrast due to instability of the video/laser camera or of the film-processing unit may, for similar reasons, make comparison between studies performed on different occasions difficult.

REFERENCES

Aicardi, J., and Goutieres, F. (1984). A progressive familial encephalopathy in infancy with calcifications of the basal ganglia and chronic cerebrospinal fluid lymphocytosis. *Annals of Neurology* 15:49–54.

Brooks, R. A., and Di Chiro, G. (1975). Theory of image reconstruction in computed tomography. *Radiology* 117:561–72.

(1976). Principles of computer assisted tomography (CAT) in radiographic and radioisotopic imaging. *Physics in Medicine and Biology* 5:689–732.

Di Chiro, G., Brooks, R. A., Dubal, L., and Chew, E. (1978). The apical artifact: elevated attenuation values toward the apex of the skull. *Journal of Computer Assisted Tomography* 2:65–70.

Edholm, P. (1975). Image construction in transversal computer tomography. *Acta Radiologica* [suppl.] 346:21–38.

Flodmark, O. (1987). The neonatal brain. In *Syllabus: A Categorical Course in Diagnostic Radiology – Neuroradiology* (pp. 43–54). Oak Brook, IL: Radiological Society of North America.

Gordon, R., Herman, G. T., and Johnson, S. A. (1975). Image reconstruction from projections. *Scientific American* 233:56–68.

ICRP 60 (1991). *1990 Recommendations of the International Commission on Radiological Protection.* Oxford: Pergamon Press.

Merriam, G. R., Szechter, A., and Focht, E. F. (1972). The effects of ionizing radiation on the eye. *Frontiers of Radiation Therapy and Oncology* 6:346–85.

Moström, U., and Ytterbergh, C. (1987). Spatial distribution of dose in computed tomography with special reference to thin-slice techniques. *Acta Radiologica* 28:771–7.

Nielsen, B. (1984). Measurement of background signals due to scattered and off-focal radiation on CT-scanners. *Acta Radiologica* 25:73–9.

Nishizawa, K., Maruyama, T., Takayam, M., Ukada, M., Hachiya, J.-I., and Furuya, Y. (1991). Determinations of organ doses and effective dose equivalents from computed tomographic examination. *British Journal of Radiology* 64:20–8.

Otake, M., and Schull, W. J. (1990). Radiation-related posterior lenticular opacities in Hiroshima and Nagasaki atomic bomb survivors based on the DS 86 dosimetry system. *Radiation Research* 121:3–13.

Radon, J. (1917). Ueber die Bestimmung von Functionen durch ihre Intergralwärte längs Gewisser Männigfaltigkeiten. *Berichte über die Verhandlungen der königlich sächsischen Gesellschaft der Wissenschaften zu Leipzig. Matematisch-Physische Klasse* 69:262–77.

Shewmon, D. A., Fine, M., Masdeu, J. C., and Palacios, E. (1981). Postischemic hypervascularity of infancy: a stage in the evolution of ischemic brain damage with characteristic CT scan. *Annals of Neurology* 9:358–65.

4

Magnetic resonance

JOSEPH C. McGOWAN, Ph.D.

INTRODUCTION

In the 20 yr since the suggestion by Lauterbur (1973) that magnetic resonance might be used to create images of anatomic structures in humans, development of the technology has proceeded at a phenomenal rate. Today, magnetic resonance imaging is the method of choice for a wide variety of diagnostic applications, and the use of magnetic resonance spectroscopy for in vivo study is commonplace. These techniques can be completely noninvasive and are apparently risk-free. The usefulness of the magnetic resonance (MR) study reflects its inherent flexibility, which has been demonstrated in the imaging of dynamic processes, in biochemical analysis, and in applications covering all parts of the body. MR techniques offer many current and potential advantages over competing modalities in the practice of neonatal and perinatal medicine.

FUNDAMENTAL PRINCIPLES

Nuclear magnetic resonance (NMR) refers to the enhanced absorption of energy that occurs when certain nuclei are exposed to radio-frequency energy at a particular frequency. The effect was first described and observed in particle beams by Rabi, Millman, and Kusch (1937). Bloch and Purcell independently elucidated the principles of NMR in 1946 (Bloch, 1946; Bloembergen, Purcell, and Pound, 1948), for which they shared a Nobel prize in 1952.

All NMR techniques exploit a quantum-mechani-

John S. Leigh, Ph.D., and Jane McGowan, M.D., reviewed numerous versions of the manuscript for this chapter and provided many valuable suggestions. Their contributions are very much appreciated.

cal property of some nuclei called "spin." The spin quantum represents an inherent angular momentum, and there is a particular, quantized energy associated with each spin state. Because each nucleus is a charged particle with angular momentum, a magnetic moment μ also exists. In the simplest case relevant to MR, there are precisely two spin states, which can be referred to as $\pm$ ½ or simply as "up" and "down." In the presence of an external magnetic field, these spin states will exhibit a difference in energy level, which scales linearly with the magnitude of the magnetic field. An individual nucleus can experience a transition between spin states by emitting or absorbing energy, but these transitions occur only when the amount of energy involved is exactly the correct amount, given by Planck's law:

$$\Delta E = h\nu \qquad (4.1)$$

where ΔE is the energy of transition, ν is frequency, and h is Planck's constant. The energy is in the form of a time-varying electromagnetic (EM) field. Equation (4.1) indicates that in order to cause a spin-state transition to a higher energy level, the EM field must be applied at the correct frequency. Conversely, energy emitted due to a transition to a lower energy state will be characterized by the same *resonance frequency*. The resonance frequency ν can be found with the use of the Larmor equation:

$$\nu = \gamma B_0 \qquad (4.2)$$

where B_0 is the strength of the magnetic field, and γ is the gyromagnetic ratio, a fundamental property of each nucleus. For example, the gyromagnetic ratio for a single proton (the nucleus of the hydrogen atom) is approximately 4,258 hertz (Hz) per gauss (G). Assuming a magnetic-field strength of 1.5 tesla (T) (i.e., 15,000 G), equation (4.2) gives a value of

63.87 MHz for the resonance frequency, corresponding to channel 3 in the television range of radio-frequency (rf) emissions.

The mechanism of MR can be summarized with a thought experiment in which a sample containing a population of identical nuclei is placed in a magnetic field. We assume that the nuclear spins are characterized by the lower-energy "spin-down" condition. In the first part of the experiment we apply rf energy at the proper frequency, as predicted by equation (4.2), causing the nuclei to absorb energy and undergo a transition to the spin-up state. We then turn off the rf energy. Subsequently, we observe that the nuclei emit rf energy at precisely the resonance frequency as they undergo a transition back to the lower-energy spin-down state. This simple description, based in quantum mechanics, underlies all of magnetic-resonance spectroscopy (MRS) and magnetic-resonance imaging (MRI). However, the quantum-mechanical descriptions of most important MR phenomena are quite complex and beyond the scope of this book. For additional information, the reader should consult any of several comprehensive texts and review articles on these subjects (Abragam, 1961; Moore, 1984; Koutcher and Burt, 1984; Ernst, Bodenhausen, and Wokann, 1987).

Precession and relaxation

In classical physics, there is no precise analogy to nuclear spin. However, the time-dependent behavior of ensembles of nuclear spins is accurately represented by theories of classical mechanics. We shall make use of these ideas to provide a description of nuclear precession and relaxation.

As mentioned earlier, each nucleus that possesses spin has associated with it a magnetic moment. By summing the magnetic moments associated with many nuclei that make up a sample, we arrive at the net magnetic moment, or magnetization, **M**. This vector quantity can be treated as a classical physics parameter (Koutcher and Burt, 1984; Ernst et al., 1987). That is, it can assume a continuum of magnitudes and can point in any direction. The remainder of this chapter will rely primarily on classical arguments, which are sufficient to account for most of the observed phenomena.

Some important behaviors of the net magnetization of a sample in a magnetic field are illustrated by a gyroscope in a gravitational field. Referring to Figure 4.1 (top), if the gyroscope is set spinning and then suspended in alignment with the gravitational field, no motion, save the intrinsic rotation about the gyroscope's axis, will occur. If, however, the gy-

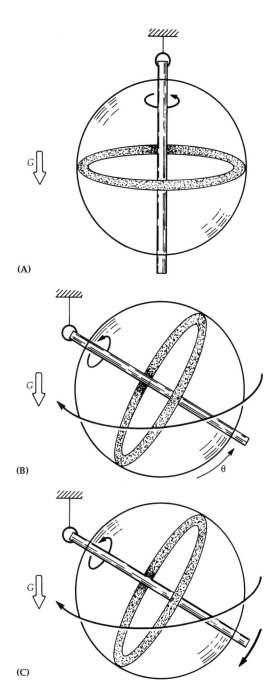

(A)

(B)

(C)

Figure 4.1. A spinning gyroscope is suspended in alignment with the gravitational field (top). If the gyroscope is displaced by the application of a force, it will continue to rotate about its physical axis but will also precess about the direction of gravity (middle). If the intrinsic rotation of the gyroscope were to remain constant, the angle θ between gravity and the axis of the gyroscope would not change. In a real gyroscope, the rotational velocity decreases, and θ approaches zero (bottom).

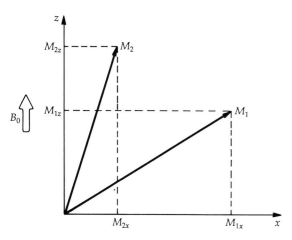

Figure 4.2. A relaxing magnetization vector (**M**) is viewed in a rotating reference frame that removes its rotational component. Two time points (M_1 and M_2) are shown. T_1 relaxation corresponds to the increase of the longitudinal (z) component of magnetization over time (M_{1z} to M_{2z}), and T_2 relaxation corresponds to the decrease in transverse (x) magnetization (M_{1x} to M_{2x}).

roscope is displaced so that its axis of rotation is no longer aligned with the gravitational field, the gyroscope will *precess* (rotate about an axis) with respect to the direction of the gravitational field (Figure 4.1, middle). If the intrinsic rotation (energy state) of the gyroscope were to remain constant, this precession would continue until an additional force was applied. However, a real gyroscope loses energy as it spins down, so that the angle between the axis of rotation of the gyroscope and the direction of gravity continuously decreases toward zero (Figure 4.1, bottom). In a similar manner, the magnetization vector **M** is preferentially aligned with the direction of the external magnetic field. If displaced from that alignment because of the absorption of energy, it will precess at a frequency equal to the Larmor frequency, given by equation (4.2). In fact, the hydrogen nuclei in our bodies spend most of their time precessing innocuously (at a rate of approximately 2 kHz) about the direction of the earth's magnetic field (5×10^{-5} T).

Consider spin magnetization that has been displaced from its equilibrium state because of absorption of energy. When the rf field is no longer applied, the magnetization will begin to approach the lower-energy (equilibrium) orientation by emitting energy. This process, exponential in nature, is termed *relaxation* and is characterized by two relaxation times, T_1 and T_2. Figure 4.2 illustrates these two characteristic times with the use of a rotating reference frame, allowing the magnetization vector

to be viewed without its rotational component. The longitudinal relaxation time (T_1) describes the loss of energy from the sample to the environment and is also referred to as the spin-lattice relaxation time, whereas the transverse relaxation time (T_2) describes the exchange of energy between spins. The T_2 relaxation process is seen as a result of small variations in the precession velocity of spins, causing the spins to get out of phase with one another or to lose phase *coherence*. It is apparent that T_1 must always be as long as or longer than T_2, because the longitudinal magnetization cannot be fully restored until all of the transverse magnetization has disappeared. Thus, T_1 can be considered an upper limit for T_2, a limit that is approached in some aqueous solutions. In biological tissue, however, T_2 is observed to be shorter than T_1 by an order of magnitude.

The T_1 and T_2 relaxation times appear in the *Bloch equations*, a set of three differential equations that describe the time-dependent behavior of the magnetization (Bloch, 1946). Although Bloch's use of these relaxation terms was entirely empirical, they have been spectacularly successful in describing observed MR phenomena (Moore, 1984).

Acquisition of an MR signal

We have seen that in order to perform an MR experiment we require a sample residing in a magnetic field, a means of applying energy to the sample, and a means of detecting energy that is emitted from the sample. The application and detection of energy are accomplished by tuned rf coils, a single one of which can serve both purposes, as is often the case in practice. Figure 4.3 shows a diagram of how this might be accomplished in a horizontal-bore MR instrument. The sample is depicted after it has been placed within the magnetic field, and its magnetization **M** is aligned with B_0 in the z direction. The rf coil is placed adjacent to the sample, with the axis of the coil at right angles to the orientation of the B_0 field. If a sinusoidal current (with frequency equal to the resonance frequency) is applied to the coil, a second magnetic field (B_1) is established that exerts a torque on a magnetization vector, causing it to precess about the *effective magnetic field* that exists as the combination of B_0 and B_1. Under that condition, the angle of the precession relative to the B_0 direction increases linearly with time. Let us assume that we apply rf power for the exact time required for **M** to rotate 90°, and then we turn the power off. The magnetization **M** is said to have been flipped into the x–y plane, where it immediately begins to precess. In a manner analogous to

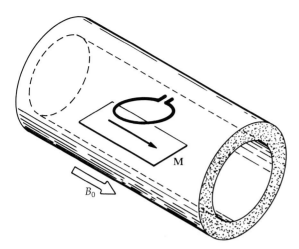

Figure 4.3. A horizontal-bore MR instrument. The sample is placed at the center of the magnetic field, adjacent to the rf coil. Under the influence of the B_0 field, the sample magnetization (**M**) will align with the axis of the magnet.

a simple electric generator, this magnetic dipole turning within a conducting loop induces a voltage in the coil, which is measured as the MR signal. At the same time, the value of **M** approaches its equilibrium state of alignment with B_0 through relaxation. Note that, as shown in Figure 4.4, only the x–y component of **M** induces a voltage in the coil. Therefore, an MR signal is present only when **M** is not aligned with B_0. The plot of the signal intensity over time is known as the *free-induction decay* (FID) and is given by the following equation:

$$M_{xy} = M_0 e^{-t/T_2} (\cos 2\pi \, \nu t + \phi) \qquad (4.3)$$

where M_0 is the equilibrium value of **M**, M_{xy} is the transverse component of **M**, with magnitude proportional to the number of spins in the sample, ϕ is the phase angle, and t is time.

MAGNETIC RESONANCE SPECTROSCOPY

The term *magnetic resonance spectroscopy* (MRS) refers to the use of MR techniques to elucidate the properties of a sample that can be assumed to be spatially homogeneous. In order to obtain an MR spectrum, a FID is collected as described in the previous section, which can be plotted as shown in Figure 4.5 (top). These data represent the decaying magnetization in the time domain. Computer application of the Fourier transform to the FID results in a frequency-domain representation of the same data (Figure 4.5, bottom). The form of this line, the Fourier transform of a decaying exponential, is Lorentzian. The Lorentzian line is characterized by three

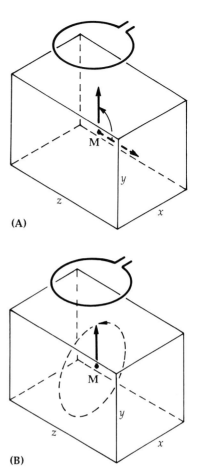

(A)

(B)

Figure 4.4. The sample in Figure 4.3 is shown inside the stationary magnet (not pictured). When a sinusoidal current is applied to the rf coil, a B_1 field is established that changes the direction of the effective magnetic field experienced by **M**. The magnetization is allowed to precess about the new effective field until it is aligned with the y axis (top), whereupon the rf energy is turned off. The magnetization will then precess about B_0, and the transverse (x–y) component of the magnetization will induce a voltage in the coil.

parameters: center frequency, height, and width at half-height (line width). The center frequency is the Larmor frequency, and the area under the curve, which can be obtained from the height and line width, corresponds to the number of nuclear spins that contribute to it. The transverse relaxation time can be obtained from the line width as follows:

$$T_2 = \frac{1}{\pi \Delta \nu_{1/2}} \qquad (4.4)$$

where $\Delta \nu_{1/2}$ is the width at half-height, in hertz, and T_2 is given in seconds. Recall that T_2 relaxation represents a loss of coherence, or dephasing of spins. This results from small variations in the effective

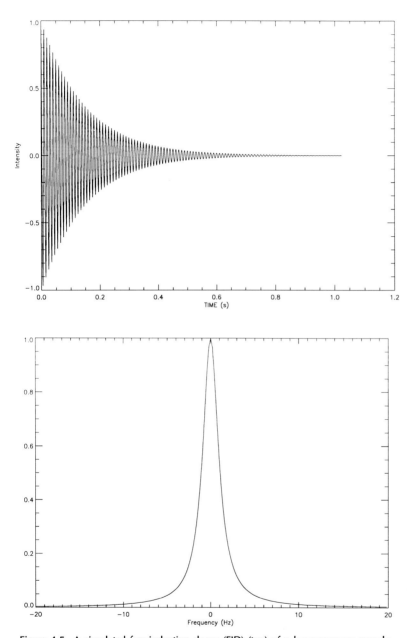

Figure 4.5. A simulated free-induction decay (FID) (top) of a homogeneous sample following a 90° pulse. T_2 is simulated as 150 ms. The Fourier transform of the FID yields a frequency-domain representation (bottom) consisting of a single Lorentzian line.

static field that occur because of the molecular environment. Dephasing of spins with respect to spins in different parts of the sample will also result from inhomogeneity of the static field due to local differences in magnetic susceptibility, as well as imperfect magnet construction. The T_2 given by equation (4.4) is the expected value using a completely homogeneous magnet, so that there is no contribution to T_2 relaxation from static B_0 inhomogeneities. The presence of inhomogeneity results in additional loss of coherence of the nuclear spins and observed shortening of T_2. Therefore, an additional parameter T_2^* is defined as the observed value of T_2, which includes effects of a spatially variant static field.

The analysis given thus far would predict that all MR spectra should resemble Figure 4.5 (bottom); that is, they should consist of only one spectral line. That is not the case, in part because of the existence of the phenomenon known as the "chemical shift."

Chemical shift and Fourier transform MR

Equation (4.2) predicts that all nuclei of a given nuclide will resonate at the same frequency when under the influence of a given B_0 field. In fact, the resonance frequency is affected very slightly by the nature of its chemical environment, as was first observed by Proctor and Yu in 1950. This occurs because the magnitude of the magnetic field experienced by individual nuclei differs from the magnitude of the external B_0 field. The deviation is due to small perturbations resulting from the presence of electrons, other nuclei, and other molecules. We have observed that random variations of this type lead to T_2 relaxation through loss of coherence. In contrast, systematic variations in the chemical environment lead to the appearance of multiple spectral lines. Thus, variations in the effective B_0 field give rise to differences in resonance frequencies that are observed to exist between identical nuclei residing in different chemical environments, and these are called "chemical shifts." The magnitude of the chemical shift is expressed in terms of a reference frequency as a dimensionless, field-independent parameter δ, given by

$$\delta = \frac{\nu_x - \nu_{ref}}{\nu_{ref}} \cdot 10^6 \qquad (4.5)$$

where ν_x is the measured resonance frequency of the sample, and ν_{ref} is the reference frequency. The units of δ are parts per million (ppm). An example of the presence of chemical shifts is found in MRI of the human body, where the majority of MR-visible spins arise from the protons of either tissue water or lipids. The lipid proton spins are characterized by a resonance frequency that, at 1.5 T, is 220 Hz removed from the water proton resonance. This difference corresponds to a chemical shift of 3.5 ppm. Discriminating between the two proton resonances can be important in diagnostic imaging, and MR techniques of "fat suppression," which take advantage of the chemical shift to allow selective attenuation of the lipid signal (Dixon, 1984), are continually being refined.

It is the existence of chemical shifts that makes MR such a valuable tool for chemical and biochemical analysis, and the Fourier transform makes acquisition of the chemical-shift information feasible. One can imagine the possibility of conducting many experiments on the same sample using different frequencies of excitation in order to obtain spectral information for all possible resonances. The need for such tedious methods is obviated by Fourier transform MR, in which a sample is excited with a range of frequencies, causing the different components of the sample to respond in accordance with their specific magnetic environments. The FID collected in this manner is a complex sinusoid representing the sum of many different sinusoids, and effectively containing the information from a continuum of experiments over the frequency range of excitation. The transform of this FID yields the individual frequency components, corresponding to spectral lines for each spectrally distinct component of the sample.

An example of the information that can be obtained using MRS is given in Figure 4.6. This spectrum results from excitation of the phosphorus nuclide in normal neonatal piglet brain. Seven individual resonances make up the spectrum, including phosphocreatine (PCr), inorganic phosphates (P_i), phosphomonoesters (PME), phosphodiesters (PDE), and the α, β, and γ phosphorus atoms of adenosine triphosphate (ATP). A more detailed discussion of the phosphorus spectrum will be provided later.

Spectral complexities

We have thus far restricted our discussion to isolated nuclei with only two possible energy states, that is, to nuclei with spin $\frac{1}{2}$. A few more complex situations are clinically relevant. These include coupled spins, spins undergoing chemical exchange, and values of spin angular momentum greater than $\frac{1}{2}$.

Spin-spin coupling, or J coupling, is an important parameter arising from interactions of nuclei with bonding electrons. Recall that a resonance peak or line in an MR spectrum corresponds to a particular resonance frequency as well as to an energy of transition. In the relatively simple case of two coupled nuclear spins, the effect of J coupling is to split the single resonance peak of each of the nuclei into two peaks equally displaced from the center frequency of the nucleus. This occurs because of the two possible transition energy values for each nucleus that accompany the presence of bonding electrons in two orientations. Additional possible transitions resulting from more complex coupling may result in the splitting of peaks into triplets, quartets, or higher multiplets. The observed splitting can be useful in the identification of specific peaks, such as that of lactate, but also may tend to complicate spectral analysis by making individual resonances more difficult to detect and resolve.

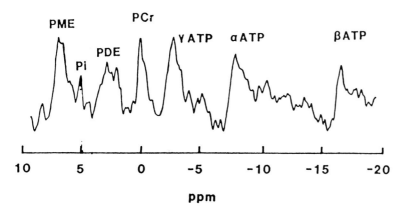

Figure 4.6. A phosphorus (^{31}P) spectrum from the brain of a newborn piglet in vivo. Labeled peaks correspond to phosphomonoesters (PME), inorganic phosphates (P$_i$), phosphodiesters (PDE), phosphocreatine (PCr), and the γ, α, and β phosphorus nuclei of adenosine triphosphate (ATP). This spectrum was obtained at 2.7 T in a horizontal-bore superconducting magnet (60 acquisitions, TR = 4.0 s).

MRS is useful for study of the dynamics of molecules, such as those that are involved in chemical exchange systems. The most ubiquitous application of MR to an exchange process has exploited the relationship between the frequency separation of the ^{31}P resonances of PCr and P$_i$. The PCr resonance, which has been shown to be unaffected by pH (Moon and Richards, 1973), is often used as a reference for phosphorus spectroscopy. The P$_i$ resonance is a population average of primarily two species, H$_2$PO$_4{}^-$ and HPO$_4{}^{2-}$, whose relative proportions depend on pH. These species undergo exchange of phosphorus atoms that is so rapid that the single resonance line observed for P$_i$ is actually an average of the two resonances, which are displaced from one another by chemical shift. Therefore, the observed chemical shift of the P$_i$ resonance reflects the relative concentrations of those species, and consequently the intracellular pH.

We have seen that a resonance peak in an MR spectrum represents the energy level of a transition between two spin states and that for the simplest nuclei that exhibit the MR phenomenon, only two states exist in the system. Examples of such nuclei are the hydrogen nucleus (proton) and the ^{31}P nucleus, which are, to date, the most important from the standpoint of biomedical MRS. As discussed earlier, J coupling represents the addition of energy states to the system, which results in the splitting of spectral lines. Another example of a situation where a single nuclide will be represented by multiple spectral lines is the case of nuclei with spin greater than $\frac{1}{2}$, examples of which are included in Table 4.1.

These nuclides have multiple energy levels that lead to signals that are somewhat more complex.

Spatial localization

Table 4.1 lists the MR properties of various nuclei of biomedical interest. Using these numbers, one can compare studies of different nuclei and estimate the volume of tissue required to provide a reasonable signal-to-noise ratio with scan times appropriate for human or animal study. Taking as a reference the volume from which an individual signal is obtained (voxel) for a high-quality MRI study, where the signal arises from protons associated with water molecules, the voxel size for a phosphorus MRS study with the same magnetic-field strength and acquisition time must be five orders of magnitude larger to achieve equivalent sensitivity (Lenkinski and Schnall, 1991). Similarly, it can be shown that detection of proton-containing metabolites such as N-acetyle aspartate (NAA) requires a sample volume approximately four orders of magnitude larger than the water proton volume. Consider that a high-resolution MR image can be acquired using voxels measuring 8/256 × 8/256 × 0.3 cm^3, or 3 × 10^{-4} cm^3, with 7 min of imaging time. An approximately equivalent signal-to-noise ratio would be achieved in the same time with the use of 30-cm^3 voxels for phosphorus, and 2-cm^3 voxels for NAA.

There are two principal means by which an MRS examination can be localized to a volume of interest. The first is through the use of *surface coils*, the geometric design of which determines the dimensions

Table 4.1.

Nuclide	Spin	Frequency (at 1.5 T, in MHz)	Physiological concentration	Sensitivity relative to ^{1}H in water
^{1}H	½	63.89	$110 \, mol \cdot l^{-1}$	1.00
^{1}H	Metabolites[a]	63.89	$1-12 \, mmol \cdot l^{-1}$	2.4×10^{-6}
^{23}Na	3/2	16.89	$80 \, mmol \cdot l^{-1}$	0.13
^{31}P	½	25.85	$10-50 \, mmol \cdot l^{-1}$	8.3×10^{-2}
^{13}C	½	16.06	$10 \, mmol \cdot l^{-1}$	2.5×10^{-4}

[a]Proton-containing metabolites such as those detected with water-suppressed proton MRS.

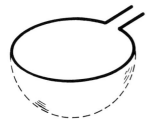

Figure 4.7. A surface coil consisting of a circular current loop will establish a B_1 field that diminishes with distance. The B_1 profile in an adjacent sample is approximately hemispherical, with depth of penetration equal to the radius of the coil.

of the excited region. For example, a surface coil consisting of a circular current loop excites a hemispherical region, with the depth of penetration approximately equal to the radius of the coil (Figure 4.7). Surface coils do not provide uniform excitation of the sample volume, as the rf field (B_1) is attenuated by distance, as illustrated in Figure 4.8, a MR image acquired with a surface coil.

Alternative means of spatial localization for a spectroscopic examination make use of B_0 field *gradients*, such as those used for MRI. These techniques can be employed with surface coils, as discussed earlier, or with *volume coils*, which excite a cylindrical region in which the sample is placed. Gradients are discussed in more detail in the MRI section of this chapter. In brief, the use of field gradients in conjunction with sequences of rf pulses allows the excitation of selected lines, planes, or volumes. Many techniques exist for spatially localized spectroscopic examinations, including the stimulated echo-acquisition mode (STEAM) (Frahm et al., 1989), point-resolved spectroscopy (PRESS) (Bottomley, 1984), image-selected in vivo spectroscopy (ISIS) (Ordridge, Connelly, and Lohman, 1986), and Hadamard spectroscopic imaging (Bolinger and Leigh, 1988). These techniques, which represent

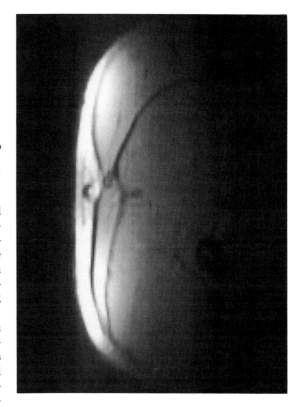

Figure 4.8. A cross-sectional MR image of a human leg at midcalf level, demonstrating the B_1 profile of a surface coil with circular current loop. (Image courtesy of Glenn Walter.)

only a sample of methods in current use, differ in terms of complexity, the maximum amount of signal available, and the exclusivity of excitation of the volume of interest. There is no single optimal method, and selection of the appropriate means for spatial localization is highly dependent on sample geometry, time available for study, hardware limitations, and other factors.

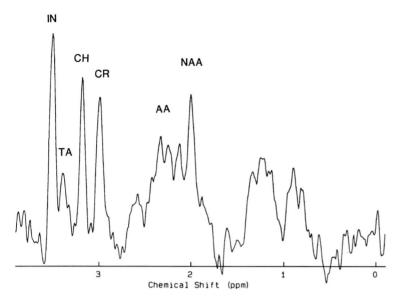

Figure 4.9. A proton (^{1}P) spectrum from the brain of a normal preterm newborn. Labeled peaks correspond to *myo*-inositol (IN), taurine (TA), choline (CH), total creatine (CR), glutamate, glutamine, and GABA (amino acids, AA), and *N*-acetyl aspartate (NAA). The spectrum was obtained using the STEAM localization technique, with chemical-shift selective water suppression in a 1.5-T clinical MR scanner. Acquisition parameters included TR = 2.0 s, TE = 19 ms, and 128 acquisitions.

Proton MRS and solvent suppression

A subfield of MRS that offers the potential for examination of a great many biochemical metabolites is proton spectroscopy. Unlike conventional MRI, which relies on the water proton for its signal, proton MRS incorporates solvent-suppression techniques that are designed to allow the observation of protons that are not associated with water. These proton-containing metabolites include NAA, PCr, lactate, *myo*-inositol, taurine, choline, and others (Michaelis et al., 1991). The resonance lines associated with these metabolites are chemically shifted away from the water resonance, but the natural abundance of water protons, at approximately 100 mol · l^{-1}, compared with millimolar concentrations of metabolites, makes simultaneous detection of both a challenging dynamic-range problem. Solvent-suppression techniques, designed to address this problem, destroy the coherence of the water proton spins through the use of selective rf pulses and field gradients or, alternatively, excite only the protons that are being sampled (Haase and Frahm, 1985). Solvent suppression relies on accurate adjustment of the static field (shimming) to minimize inhomogeneity over the region of interest. This can be simplified and accelerated with the use of auto-

mated shimming techniques (Schneider and Glover, 1991).

Figure 4.9 shows a proton spectrum from a normal preterm infant at 33 wk of postconceptional age (PCA), who was born at 26 wk PCA. This spectrum was acquired using the STEAM technique for spatial localization within a volume coil, combined with chemical-shift selective pulses for solvent suppression. It was acquired in 4 min as the average of 128 acquisitions using a cubic voxel 1.5 cm on a side. The prominent lines in this spectrum include NAA, total creatine (sum of creatine and phosphocreatine), choline, *myo*-inositol, and a peak corresponding to glutamate, glutamine, and GABA (amino acids). Taurine is also seen as a relatively small peak.

Quantitation in MRS

The results of spectroscopic studies are often reported in terms of the change in one peak area relative to another, or as a change in peak-area ratios (Bruhn et al., 1992a). Increasingly, however, absolute quantitation of metabolite concentrations is attempted. Absolute quantitation is useful in order to eliminate site dependence, to allow comparison of MRS results with those from other modalities, and to increase the sensitivity of the examination to the situation in which two concentrations might change simultaneously. Unfortunately, there are many factors that can affect the peak area independently of concentration, including relaxation effects, J coupling, accurate selection of the volume of interest, and the presence of signal originating from outside of the voxel. These potential sources of error must be addressed for accurate quantitation. Several techniques have been proposed for determination of metabolite concentrations, including the extraction of reference tissue samples and the use of external or internal (exogenous or endogenous) markers (Wray and Tofts, 1986; Tofts and Wray, 1988). Some of these methods have been applied in vivo in a small number of studies, but the most appropriate method for any individual application remains a matter of controversy.

MAGNETIC-RESONANCE IMAGING

An MR image could be abstractly envisioned as the result of acquisition of FIDs for each volume in a thin slab that is to be studied. Application of the Fourier transform to each FID would yield a single Lorentzian line (assuming that the water proton is the nuclide of interest) whose area would correspond to the density of water protons in that location. The image could be formed by constructing a two-dimensional map of the slab such that the gray-scale value assigned to each point on the map would correspond to the peak area for its spatial equivalent volume in the slab. Fortunately, the use of field gradients and multidimensional Fourier transform techniques makes the actual acquisition of an MR image much simpler than the procedure as outlined here, although this description serves to reinforce the fact that the identical physical principles are exploited in MRS and MRI.

Field gradients and slice selection

It can be seen from equation (4.2) that resonance frequency varies directly with B_0 field strength. Thus it is possible to encode spatial information in the frequency detected in the MR experiment through the use of equipment designed to vary the static magnetic-field strength along a particular axis. Consider an MR scanner with static B_0 field oriented in the z direction, as shown in Figure 4.10. A linear field gradient is established by positioning two current loops along the axis of B_0, with the center of the magnet midway between the coils. When current is passed through the loops in appropriate directions, two addi-

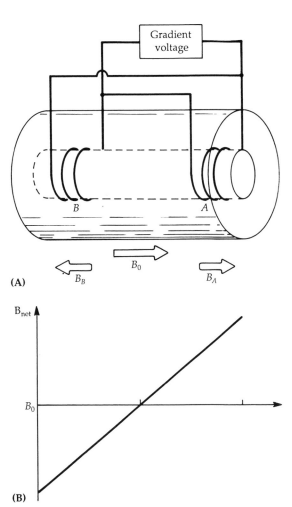

Figure 4.10. An MR scanner with static field B_0 and field gradient coils A and B. Application of gradient voltage produces gradient magnetic fields B_A and B_B. The effective magnetic field (B_{net}) is obtained by adding, at each location along the z axis, the contribution from all three fields. As shown in the graph (bottom), B_{net} increases with increasing z and is equal to B_0 at the magnet center, where B_A cancels B_B.

tional magnetic fields are generated along the B_0 axis, equal in magnitude but opposite in orientation. The net B_0 at any point along the axis is the sum of both of these fields and the static field, establishing a gradient of resonance frequency in the z direction. In practice, gradient coils are installed in the three orthogonal directions x, y, and z, allowing manipulation of resonance frequencies in three dimensions.

A gradient can be used for slice selection, a process by which only spins that occupy specified positions along the gradient axis are excited. This is ac-

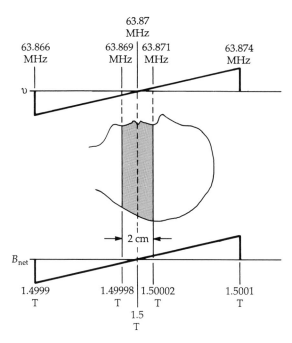

Figure 4.11. Application of rf excitation with a range of frequencies in conjunction with a field gradient is used for slice selection. The example depicts a 2-kHz-wide excitation bandwidth, applied with a gradient that changes the B_{net} field by $0.2 \; G \cdot cm^{-1}$. The rf excitation corresponds to the resonance frequencies of protons experiencing fields of 1.49998–1.50002 T, a range of 0.4 G. This results in excitation of a slice 2-cm thick that is centered on the magnet center.

complished by applying rf excitation with a specified frequency range while the gradient is turned on. As diagrammed in Figure 4.11, the range of excitation frequencies corresponds to a range of spatial positions that make up the selected slice. Subsequent repetition of this procedure with the y (or x) gradient will allow selection of the intersection of two slices. A final excitation with the remaining gradient will select a volume corresponding to the intersection of three slices. In this manner, one can obtain an image of a region of interest by simply repeating the three excitations for each point in the region. This technique, known as the sensitive-point method, is the basis for all spatial-localization schemes (Hinshaw, 1974, 1976; Ernst et al., 1987).

Another consideration regarding field gradients that is of interest to the physician prescribing an MR examination is that they are the sources of the audible noise that accompanies the operation of the scanner. Specifically, the sound, described as "tapping" or "banging," results from the rapid energization and deenergization of the gradient coils.

Imaging with a spin-echo technique

Combinations of rf pulses and the application of gradients are known as pulse sequences, and many simple and complex variations exist. There is an important class of these techniques that take advantage of the fact that the observed decay of signal during acquisition may be primarily due to spatial inhomogeneities, that is, T_2^* effects, as opposed to intrinsic T_2 decay. The T_2^* effects differ from the pure T_2 relaxation effects in that they are reversible. Recall that the exponential decay of transverse magnetization does not represent a loss of energy from the spin system, but rather a loss of coherence between the oscillations of individual spins due to small variations (static or dynamic) in the effective static magnetic field. This is also referred to as dephasing of spins. As first observed by Hahn (1950), and subsequently refined by Carr and Purcell (1954), it is possible to reverse the static dephasing process by application of a second rf pulse following the initial excitation pulse, creating what is known as a *spin echo*. The spin echo appears in time as two FIDs placed back-to-back, building to a maximum intensity and then decaying with characteristic time T_2^*. This procedure is illustrated in Figure 4.12, which also serves to describe two experimental parameters that determine the nature of the contrast in MR images derived with spin echoes: echo time (TE) and repetition time (TR). The echo time is the measure of time between excitation and acquisition, which is equal to twice the time between the excitation and inversion pulses. The repetition time is measured between successive excitation pulses. An important feature of the spin-echo experiment is that it separates the time point of maximum signal from the original acquisition, allowing time for other pulse-sequence events to occur between excitation and acquisition. Referring to Figure 4.12, the spin-echo experiment is begun with the application of an rf pulse that rotates the spin magnetization 90° into the x–y plane. At this point, T_1 and T_2 relaxation processes commence, with the T_2 relaxation being described by the loss of signal due to the dephasing of individual spins. As diagrammed in the figure, this dephasing results from the small differences in static field experienced by the spins, making the individual spin vectors appear to rotate at different speeds. After a time TE/2, a second rf pulse is applied that is twice the strength of the first, resulting in an inversion (or 180° rotation) of the spin magnetization. The effect of the 180° pulse on the spin vectors is to reverse the dephasing process, so that the spins re-

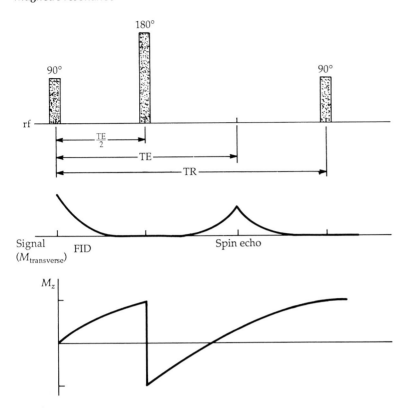

Figure 4.12. A spin-echo pulse sequence consisting of an excitation pulse (90°) and an inversion pulse (180°). The echo time (TE) is defined as twice the time between the excitation and inversion pulses, and the repetition time (TR) is defined between subsequent excitations (top). The signal strength decays due to T_2^* effects (dephasing), which are reversed by the inversion pulse, leading to a relative maximum of signal strength known as the spin echo (middle). The longitudinal magnetization (M_z) is zero following the 90° pulse and then increases exponentially toward its equilibrium value (normalized to 1.0) with time constant T_1 until it is inverted by the 180° pulse, after which it again undergoes T_1 relaxation.

gain their original phase at time TE. As the spins rephase, the signal strength builds to a maximum value that is the spin echo, and then the spins once again dephase. This sequence of pulse, invert, and detect (acquire) the echo can be played out along with the application of gradients and other rf pulses. The remainder of the TR time allows for partial restoration of equilibrium magnetization in preparation for the next excitation.

Many variations of this technique exist, and it can be shown that it is not necessary that the excitation be achieved with a 90° pulse. In fact, any two pulses in succession will produce a spin echo, a fact that must be taken into consideration when any pulse sequence with multiple rf excitations is employed (Frahm et al., 1989).

In order to obtain an MR image using spin ech-oes, the two-dimensional Fourier transform method is most commonly employed (Edelstein et al., 1980). The spin-echo imaging sequence consists of a series of spin-echo experiments, accompanied by the use of gradients in all three directions for slice selection, frequency encoding, and phase encoding. The slice-selection gradient is turned on during the initial rf excitation pulse, as described earlier. The phase-encoding gradient is applied during the TE time period (when the rf is off) and establishes a phase differential between spins along the axis of that gradient. In successive excitations, the duration of the phase-encoding gradient is kept constant while its amplitude is varied. The frequency-encoding gradient is applied on an axis perpendicular to the phase-encoding axis during the acquisition of the signal, establishing a specific resonance frequency for each point along its axis. The sequence is repeated with different amplitudes of the phase-encoding gradient, and the number of such acquisitions determines the spatial resolution of the image in the phase-encoding direction. In the frequency-encoding direction, the limiting spatial resolution is determined by characteristics of the rf receiver. The frequency encoding and phase encoding imparted to the signal are decoded using a two-dimensional Fourier transform, which is a straightforward digital signal-processing technique.

Contrast in the MR image

Unlike conventional x-ray imaging, where the contrast is essentially derived from differences in the attenuation of radiation, MRI offers the ability to manipulate the contrast mechanism and therefore the appearance of the image. This is, of course, a two-edged sword, for although an important advantage of MRI over x-ray is its ability to demonstrate contrast between adjoining soft tissues, it is possible to make diverse tissues appear isointense on an MR image by manipulation of the experimental parameters. Thus it is essential that the imaging parameters of TE and TR be known and understood when interpreting an MR image. For example, consider an image obtained by performing multiple acquisitions (each with different phase encoding) using a value of TR that is long compared with T_1, and a value of TE that is short compared with T_2. The objective of this timing is to ensure that essentially complete restoration of equilibrium magnetization is established before the next pulse is applied. An image acquired in this way is said to be proton-density-weighted, as the contrast will result primarily from differences in the numbers of proton spins contributing to the signal reflected in each pixel intensity. Relaxation effects have little influence on such an image, as the short TE minimizes T_2 effects, while the long TR minimizes T_1 effects.

Another alternative is to set TR to be shorter than T_1, while maintaining TE short. The resultant contrast still will have little to do with T_2, but differences in T_1 will have a pronounced effect on the signal strength reflected in the pixel intensities. The reason for this is that tissue regions with long T_1 values will not fully recover to the equilibrium magnetization state before the excitation pulse for the subsequent acquisition is given. Because the maximum transverse magnetization (i.e., the maximum MR signal) immediately following the pulse is equal to the longitudinal magnetization immediately preceding the pulse, a smaller signal will be detected in

regions of longer T_1. Thus the contrast in the short-TR, short-TE image will primarily result from differences in T_1, such that regions of relatively long T_1 will be hypointense, whereas regions of relatively short T_1 will be hyperintense. This type of image is referred to as T_1-weighted.

It is straightforward to extend these ideas to obtain an image with T_2 weighting. To do so requires a TE on the order of T_2 or longer than T_2, allowing significant T_2 relaxation to occur before acquisition of the signal. The effects of T_1 are minimized as in the proton-density image by using a long TR. In this case, hypointense areas on the image indicate short T_2 values, whereas regions of long T_2 will experience less loss of signal during the TE period and consequently will be hyperintense.

The three types of images that have been described are obtained in many clinical MRI examinations. Images with T_1 weighting are most useful for determining anatomic structure, providing excellent delineation of fat, fluids, soft-tissue structures, and bone. Images with T_2 weighting have been found to be useful for diagnosis of many disorders affecting soft tissue. For example, malignant tumors often are bright on T_2-weighted images, as compared with surrounding normal tissue. The proton-density-weighted image may provide minimal additional information, but usually is obtained concurrently with the T_2-weighted image and requires no additional expenditure of imaging time.

Gradient echoes and rapid imaging techniques

The image quality available with MRI represents a compromise between acquisition time and spatial resolution. Because of inherent limitations imposed by the sensitivity of the experiment, often it is possible to improve quality by repeating acquisitions and averaging the results. Of course, some examinations are limited by patient motion, either voluntary or involuntary, that may tend to reduce the time available for examination and/or the TR for scans that make up the examination. Rapid imaging techniques offer methods to decrease the time required to perform an MR examination, sometimes at the expense of signal strength.

In the preceding sections, the spin-echo technique was discussed as a means to refocus the individual spin magnetizations in order to counteract the effects of small field inhomogeneities, as well as a method to maximize signal strength while allowing time within the pulse sequence for spatial encoding and slice selection. Modern superconducting magnets can achieve field homogeneity to such an extent that it may not be necessary to employ a spin-echo technique to accomplish the former objective. However, it may still be necessary to use an echo-type technique in order to manipulate the spin magnetizations to encode specific information. This can be accomplished with gradient echoes, which are achieved through the use of dephasing and rephasing gradients in a manner somewhat analogous to the spin-echo technique (Frahm, Haase, and Matthaei, 1986; Haase, Frahm, and Matthaei, 1986). The gradient-echo technique offers the opportunity to exchange signal strength for speed, resulting in several advantages when the strength of the available signal is not limiting. First, the second rf pulse is eliminated, negating any effects of inaccuracies in the inversion pulse. Second, the excitation pulse need not be a 90° pulse, and in practice often is on the order of 10–15°. The advantage here is the rapid recovery of magnetization prior to the subsequent excitation, as well as the reduced excitation pulse width. The following equation can be used to predict the effect of reduced flip angles on the steady-state magnetization:

$$M_{xy} = M_0 \frac{1 - E_1}{1 - E_1 \cos \beta} \sin \beta \quad (\text{with } E_1 = e^{-TR/T_1})$$

$$(4.6)$$

where M_{xy} is the steady-state maximum value of transverse magnetization, M_0 is the equilibrium longitudinal magnetization and is proportional to proton density, and β is the flip angle (Ernst et al., 1987).

Through the use of equation (4.6), one can predict the optimal flip angle that will maximize signal strength for given values of TR and T_1. This is called the Ernst angle and is equal to arccos (E_1) (Ernst et al., 1987). For example, an imaging experiment with TR = 3 s and a sample characterized by $T_1 = 1.5$ s would produce maximum signal if the flip angle used were 82°, whereas a sequence with TR = 0.5 s would correspond to an optimal flip angle of 44°.

Other methods exist to reduce the imaging time while still obtaining contrast reflective of differences in relaxation times, some of which can be applied to spin- and gradient-echo techniques. Examples include methods that collect fewer data than the standard examination, such as the use of a smaller number of phase-encoding steps with the same field of view, resulting in coarser spatial resolution in the phase-encoding direction. A related method uses the same spatial resolution in the phase-encoding direction, but a smaller field of view. Alternatively,

the number of equivalent acquisitions for averaging purposes can be reduced at the expense of image quality, and the inherent redundancy of the information content of the two halves of the echo can be eliminated to achieve a half-Fourier image. Finally, hybrid applications of the spin-echo techniques employ one acquisition with a succession of spin echoes and individual phase encoding for each echo (Hennig, Nauerth, and Freidburg, 1986).

The fastest methods for MRI are those that acquire all of the necessary data using only one excitation. So-called echo-planar imaging (EPI) and other single-shot techniques accomplish this objective through the use of rapidly varying gradients that create a series of (gradient) echoes, each with slightly different phase encoding. All of the spatial information is obtained before the T_2^* decay makes the signal indistinguishable from the noise, and data for an entire image can be acquired in less than 50 ms.

Other contrast mechanisms

The vast majority of clinical MRI studies are designed to develop contrast based on differences in relaxation times. However, other applications of MRI have been developed and continue to be developed, including magnetic-resonance angiography (MRA), magnetization-transfer imaging (MTI), and imaging based on perfusion. Contrast can also be provided or enhanced through administration of exogenous agents, which are used routinely in some adult and pediatric MR studies.

MRA involves the use of MR techniques to visualize blood flow and, indirectly, blood-vessel integrity or stenosis. Flowing blood can be visualized with MR by several methods, including time-of-flight and phase-contrast techniques (Dumoulin and Hart, 1986; Wehrli et al., 1986; Dumoulin et al., 1988, 1989; Keller, Drayer, and Fram, 1989). These methods establish contrast between flowing and nonflowing spins through an encoding of flow with magnetic "tagging," so that flowing spins have the highest signal strength, or by subtraction of images with and without flow encoding. Although MRA is finding increasing use in adult radiology as an alternative to conventional invasive angiography, reported applications of MRA in newborns (Lewin et al., 1989; Connelly et al., 1993) have been sparse to date.

MTI expands the measured parameters in an MR study beyond proton density, T_1, and T_2 by exploiting the interaction in biological tissues between endogenous macromolecular components and components in the aqueous phase. The exchange of protons between water and macromolecules provides an additional relaxation mechanism, leading to characterization of the sample in terms of exchange constants and intrinsic relaxation times of the observed water protons as well as protons bound to macromolecules. The magnetization-transfer (MT) effect is induced by applying rf irradiation such that protons bound to macromolecules will preferentially experience saturation; that is, their magnetization will be held at or near zero magnitude (Wolff and Balaban, 1989). The exchange of these spins into the water proton pool will decrease the measured magnetization of water protons, leading to a lower signal intensity and, consequently, hypointensity on an MR image when compared with the intensity on a control image acquired without the MT pulses. Contrast in MTI is difficult to interpret, in that it may represent differences in exchange rates as well as relaxation times and proton densities. However, tissue is generally hypointense on MTI when compared with body fluids, and diverse tissues often can be differentiated (McGowan, Schnall, and Leigh, 1994). Applications of MTI include studies of cartilage (Morris and Freemont, 1992), hepatic tumors (Outwater et al., 1992), and demyelinating disease (Dousset et al., 1992). MT methods have also found application as a novel method for MRA (Pike et al., 1992).

MR techniques can also be used to provide images of tissue perfusion, particularly in brain (Belliveau et al., 1990, 1991; Rosen et al., 1990; Detre et al., 1992; Williams et al., 1992; Zhang et al., 1992). This has led to the establishment of a new field of MR study known as functional imaging (Belliveau et al., 1991). Using ultrarapid scanning methods, including echo-planar imaging (discussed earlier), images can now be produced that will demonstrate regional brain activity during specific behaviors (Belliveau et al., 1991). These techniques have yet to be applied in neonates, but the potential for a completely noninvasive functional neurological examination will certainly be of interest to practitioners of neonatal/perinatal medicine.

The final contrast mechanism to be discussed is administration of exogenous materials, analogous to various tracers and dyes used in conventional x-ray studies. These materials provide contrast in a way fundamentally different from that of other radiographic contrast media, acting indirectly by altering the relaxation properties of the nuclei under observation. That is, the agents themselves are not detected, but their effects are observed. Contrast agents appropriate for MR use contain paramag-

netic ions that produce a shortening of observed T_1 in water protons (Koutcher et al., 1984). The most common of these is gadolinium, a rare-earth element containing seven unpaired electrons. In the presence of paramagnetic ions, T_1 relaxation is enhanced and dominated by interactions between the nuclei and the unpaired electrons, allowing the paramagnetic ions to function as a sink for magnetization (Dwek, 1973). The effect of this modulation in observed relaxation times is to make regions that are affected by the contrast agents hyperintense on short-TR, short-TE scans. T_2 can also be shortened by the presence of microscopic magnetic dipoles that create inhomogeneities into the static field, leading to dephasing of spins. MR contrast agents are used for screening and characterization of cerebral lesions, in a manner analogous to the use of iodinated contrast agents in computed tomography (CT) scans. They are also increasingly used in the body (e.g., for detection of liver metastases).

SAFETY

Safety considerations in the MR examination can be divided into three broad categories: static magnetic-field effects, time-varying gradient fields, and rf energy deposition. Additional safety considerations accompany the use of exogenous contrast agents.

No harmful bioeffects of static fields up to 2 T have been reported in humans (Schaefer, 1988). However, the presence of a strong magnetic field is of concern because of the great attractive force of the magnet for ferromagnetic objects. The hazards posed by the static field thus fall into the categories of displacing or applying force to metal objects within the body, such as pacemakers, and attraction of potential missiles from outside of the magnet toward the magnet center. Internal objects are seldom of concern with neonatal patients, but extreme care must be taken to avoid the introduction of ferromagnetic items into the MR scanner area, in order to prevent serious injury to a patient in the scanner. These include pieces of monitoring equipment, such as temperature probes, as well as supporting equipment, such as needles, hemostats, and the poles used to hold containers of intravenous fluids. The danger is compounded by the invisibility of the magnetic field and by the fact that the force applied to an object in the field increases dramatically as the distance between the object and the magnet decreases.

Rapidly changing magnetic fields due to the use of field gradients are of potential concern because of the voltages that they induce in conducting media.

For example, visualization of magnetophosphenes (flashes of light seen by people exposed to rapidly varying magnetic fields) demonstrates that nerve and/or retinal cells can be directly excited by these field variations. However, currents and current densities resulting from induced voltages in MR equipment as currently used are small compared with the values necessary to cause this effect (Lovsund et al., 1980), and therefore they are not presently considered of significance (Schaefer, 1988).

Heating of tissue due to the application of rf energy is described in terms of the specific absorption rate (SAR) and is controlled in modern MR equipment through hardware and software constraints. The guidelines of the United States Food and Drug Administration (FDA) call for justification whenever rf electromagnetic fields result in SARs that exceed $0.4 \text{ W} \cdot \text{kg}^{-1}$ averaged over the whole body or 2 $\text{W} \cdot \text{kg}^{-1}$ averaged over 1 g of tissue (FDA, 1982). Justification can be established by ensuring that a rise in core temperature will not exceed 1°C and that temperatures will not exceed 38°C in the head, 39°C in the trunk, and 40°C in the extremities. Although the effects of excessive heating are potentially serious (Wyndham et al., 1965), power deposition in the MR examination has not reached levels of concern in imaging experiments to date. Excess heat is dissipated by humans through respiration, as well as, in older children and adults, perspiration, tending to reduce or eliminate the observable effects. Furthermore, localized heating within the body can be mitigated by normal blood flow, which tends to diffuse heat rapidly. The findings from human studies of temperature rises in MR scanning led investigators to conclude that no thermally induced ill effects resulted following a 20-min scan at 4 $\text{W} \cdot \text{kg}^{-1}$ (10 times the FDA guideline) in normal adult volunteers (Schaefer, 1988).

A safety issue that has yet to be fully addressed by MR researchers is whether or not MR is contraindicated in pregnant women. At present it is uncommon for such studies of mother or fetus to be performed, although no untoward effects are anticipated, nor have any been reported from MRI exposure to the fetus when studies have been performed (Dinh, Wright, and Hanigan, 1990). A criterion that has been used for application of MR in pregnant patients is a medical need for an imaging study where alternate imaging modalities would involve exposure to ionizing radiation (Kanal, Shellock, and Talagala, 1990). Based on the widespread use of MR in humans and experimental animals, as well as the documented exposure of health-care workers to MR scanners with no reported ill effects, it seems unlikely that any danger to mother or fetus will be presented by MR studies. The potential for increased diagnostic information regarding mother and fetus through MR examination may be exploited in the future.

The effects of exogenous contrast agents have been examined in both adult and pediatric populations, and these agents have been found to demonstrate a high safety margin when compared with iodinated contrast media. Their use is not recommended in pregnant women, however, as one agent (gadopentetate dimeglumine, Gd-DTPA) has been shown to cross the placenta and appear within the fetal bladder during MR imaging (Kanal et al., 1990).

Potential health effects must continue to be evaluated as new MR techniques evolve. For example, it is becoming more common in research practice to scan human subjects at fields of 4 T. The limits on SAR are approached by some applications of MTI, and new gradient designs are in development for rapid imaging techniques. Some of these applications will involve operation under conditions that have not been analyzed to date, and it is expected that further research into safety issues will be driven by the perceived clinical need for advancements in the technology.

SPECIAL CONSIDERATIONS IN MR EXAMINATION OF HIGH-RISK NEONATES

Examination of a high-risk neonate in the MR scanner poses a number of challenges, among them adequate support and monitoring to ensure the well-being of the baby. In addition, proper positioning and preparation of the infant are essential to the outcome of the study.

Candidates for MR study include patients in neonatal intensive-care units who may require ventilatory support, supplemental oxygen, feeding, and intravenous fluids. Mechanical ventilation with many commercial ventilators is complicated because of their inclusion of ferromagnetic components. Operation of this equipment may be affected by the magnetic field, and the ventilator itself is a potential missile hazard unless properly secured. It may be feasible to provide tubing and valving so that the ventilator can be located a suitable distance from the magnet. Alternatively, manual ventilation can be provided. Supplemental oxygen is often available in the MR scan room. Intravenous fluids and continuous feeding can be provided by pumps located outside of the scan room, with the use of sufficient tubing. Proper operation of the pump when it is within the influence of the magnetic field (even outside of the scan room) should always be verified. It is also important, particularly in very small babies, to provide a source of heating in order to maintain temperature stability. Unfortunately, most commercial heating equipment for infants is unsuitable for use in the magnet. Items that have been found to be useful in this regard are polymer heating pads that undergo a phase transition at body temperature, providing an isothermal environment for several hours when the baby is properly swaddled and insulated. It is also possible to use warm-water recirculating units and bottles. Self-contained isolettes that are designed to be compatible with MR equipment have been constructed and may become commercially available because of increased interest in MR studies of neonates.

Monitoring equipment compatible with MR scanners is available and can provide pulse oximetry, blood pressure, and electrocardiogram data while scanning is in progress. End-tidal CO_2 detectors are available that can be configured to detect apnea. Sound monitoring may also be provided through microphones in the scan room and in the bore of the magnet. In addition, a physician may remain in the scan room during scanning if it is necessary to continuously observe the patient. Although visualization inside the bore of a long magnet may be difficult, some rf coil designs incorporate windows and see-through plastic construction to enhance observation. Thus, adequate support and monitoring systems are available to ensure the safety and well-being of most infants who are stable enough for transport to the scanner.

It may not be necessary to sedate very young infants for MR study, although sedation is indicated for some older children and is standard practice for neonatal MR imaging at some institutions. Alternatively, infants can be fed shortly before the scan, transported to the scanner, and then swaddled tightly and insulated well to keep them warm. If they are properly prepared and made comfortable, they usually will sleep through the study, in spite of the noise from the gradient switching. We have used this method at the University of Pennsylvania in term and preterm newborns, and only rarely has patient motion led to failure to obtain an adequate study.

CLINICAL APPLICATION OF MAGNETIC-RESONANCE SPECTROSCOPY

This section will be confined primarily to ^{31}P and ^{1}H spectroscopy, which together account for the vast majority of MRS studies in adults as well as in neonates. Studies have also been performed using the ^{23}Na (Berendson and Edzes, 1973), ^{13}C (Lauterbur, 1970; Shulman, 1987), and ^{19}F (Joseph et al., 1985) nuclei, and they may lead to perinatal research or clinical applications in the future.

^{31}P spectroscopy

The ^{31}P spectrum (Figure 4.6) contains peaks representing key components of cellular energy metabolism and has been used to study cellular energetics in skeletal muscle (Radda, Bore, and Rajagopalan, 1983) and brain. This technology was first applied to the study of newborn infants in 1983 (Cady et al., 1983; Younkin et al., 1984). A prominent peak in the spectrum is due to PCr, a high-energy phosphorus compound that acts as a buffer to changes in adenosine triphosphate (ATP) through the creatine kinase equilibrium (Meyer, Sweeney, and Kushmerick, 1984). The PCr/P_i ratio provides an estimate of metabolic reserve, when corrected for pH, as calculated from the spectral separation of the P_i and PCr peaks (Chance et al., 1985, 1986). It has been suggested that as PCr/P_i falls below unity, the system is approaching its limit for the synthesis of ATP. With persistence of this condition, recovery is increasingly less likely, leading to metabolic collapse (Chance, Smith, and Nioka, 1987). The ^{31}P spectrum also contains three peaks corresponding to ATP that remain relatively constant under all but the most severe metabolic challenges, reflecting the inherent regulation of the concentration of this substance. The peak assigned to phosphodiesters (PDEs) is primarily made up of phosphatidylcholine and phosphatidylethanolamine resonances, which are thought to reflect turnover of the cell membrane. This peak has been suggested to be a marker of brain catabolic activity (Younkin et al., 1988). The phosphomonoester (PME) peak, composed of phosphorylethanolamine and sugar phosphates (Gyulai, Bolinger, and Leigh, 1984), is significantly more prominent in the neonatal brain spectrum, as compared with the adult, and has been shown to fall with maturation in rats (Tofts and Wray, 1985). Because it is also elevated in rapidly growing neoplasms (Marris et al., 1985), it has been suggested that the compounds contributing to this resonance reflect rapid membrane synthesis (Marris et al., 1985; Hubesch et al., 1990).

Boesch et al. (1989) reported that the phosphorus spectrum varies with brain development in neonates and infants. In their study of 40 neonates, infants, and children up to 6 yr of age, the ratio of

PME to PDE decreased during development, while the ratio of PCr to β-ATP increased. The observed changes in the PME/PDE ratio were found to reflect lipid metabolism and were suggested as a potential maturation index. Additionally, a difference was observed between the areas of the α- and β-ATP peaks that was correlated with age and the PCR/β-ATP ratio.

The effects of cerebral hypoxia on the appearance of the ^{31}P spectrum have been extensively studied in animal models, and to a lesser degree in human infants. These effects result from a decrease in the maximal rate of ATP synthesis, causing the metabolic reserve of the tissue to be reduced. Thus, there is a decrease in the spectral PCr/P$_i$ ratio. If hypoxia is profound, there is an accumulation of lactate that decreases the intracellular pH, changing the chemical shift of the P$_i$ resonance. Metabolic collapse and cell death are indicated by the disappearance of the PCr peak and finally the ATP peak. Serial MRS data following episodes of severe asphyxia demonstrated that some infants who initially had normal MR spectra subsequently developed severe cerebral atrophy, suggesting that brain injury evolves over time (Hope et al., 1984). Azzopardi, Wyatt, and Cady (1989) demonstrated in a study of infants of gestational ages from 27 to 42 wk who had experienced cerebral hypoxia-ischemia that observation of PCr/P$_i$ below normal (1.18 ± 0.17 in their study) was highly suggestive of a poor prognosis, with a positive predictive value of 96% for death or major impairment. Hamilton et al. (1986) concluded that MRS was helpful to assess the extent of suspected brain injury in neonates; their study included term and preterm infants with cerebral ultrasound echodensities.

During seizures, the maximal rate of ATP synthesis is not altered, but the increased electrical activity is associated with an increase in ATP consumption. As a result, the PCr/P$_i$ ratio decreases to maintain the steady-state ATP concentration (Petroff et al., 1985; Schnall, Yoshizaki, and Leigh, 1988), but lactate production does not increase, so there is no accompanying change in intracellular pH.

Cerebral infarction can be demonstrated by values of intracellular pH (Levine et al., 1989) that are higher than normal, but no significant change in metabolite ratios has been reported. This may be due to the rapid utilization of the phosphate pool in association with cerebral ischemia, resulting in the affected area being devoid of phosphate. A quantitative study of mature cerebral infarcts in adults indicated that whereas the relative concentrations of phosphorus metabolites remained the same, their

absolute concentrations were decreased (Levine et al., 1989).

^{1}H spectroscopy

Proton spectroscopy allows the observation of some metabolites reflected in the phosphorus spectrum, as well as non-phosphorus-containing metabolites. It also offers a significant advantage over phosphorus spectroscopy in the area of spatial localization. To illustrate, localized phosphorus spectroscopy with current technology may be limited to regions encompassing an entire hemisphere of a neonatal brain, whereas with proton spectroscopy it is feasible to obtain data (using similar rf coil, magnet, and time expenditure) from volumes smaller than 1 cm^3. This allows proton spectroscopy to sample specific functional brain regions and makes possible chemical-shift imaging, a hybrid technique where many spectra are gathered simultaneously and used to construct images reflecting peak areas, that is, relative concentrations, of the constituents of the proton spectrum (Brown, Kincaid, and Ugarbil, 1982; Haselgrove et al., 1983).

One of the most prominent peaks in the solvent-suppressed ^{1}H brain spectrum (Figure 4.9) has been assigned to NAA (Michaelis et al., 1991). The function of NAA has not been clearly elucidated, but its presence at high levels is associated primarily with neuronal tissue (Nadler and Cooper, 1983). Another strong resonance is associated with the $-CH_3$ group common to creatine and PCr, that is, the total creatine pool. This peak has been found to remain stable under pathological conditions and may serve as a useful reference for changes in other peaks. In close proximity to the Cr-PCr peak is the resonance assigned to choline, a compound important to cell membrane synthesis and often found to be elevated in malignant tumors. These peaks are characterized by relatively long values of T_2, and usually are the only peaks observed with spectroscopic studies that require TE values of 100 ms or longer. Lactate, if present in sufficient concentration, will be observed as a doublet due to J coupling, but is not typically observed in the normal brain spectrum. Performance of an examination with shorter echo time (e.g., 20 ms), though increasing the demands on machine performance, will result in greater signal strength and allow the observation of metabolites with shorter T_2 values, which include *myo*-inositol and taurine, and smaller peaks from glutamine, glutamate, and GABA (Michaelis et al., 1991).

Although proton spectroscopy has only recently been applied in pediatric studies, initial results indicate that ratios of peak areas of proton-containing metabolites may vary with age and abnormalities. Published results provide normative data for spectroscopy with both long (Peden et al., 1990; van der Knapp et al., 1990) and short echo times (Ross, Kreis, and Ernst, 1992). In addition, Peden et al. (1990) have reported that the NAA/creatine and NAA/choline ratios correlate with clinical outcome in infants with hypoxic-ischemic encephalopathy. In the neonate, absolute quantitation of proton-containing metabolites through the use of tissue extracts has been investigated by Hüppi et al. (1991), who used representative autopsy data to calibrate peak amplitudes. The use of the water protons as an internal reference was applied by Kreis, Ernst, and Ross (1993), who reported the age dependence of metabolite concentrations, as well as T_1 and T_2 relaxation. Specifically, they found that concentrations of *myo*-inositol and choline decreased with age, whereas NAA and creatine/PCr increased, although on different time scales.

Proton MRS has been applied to the study of metabolic disorders, including the cerebrohepatorenal syndromes of Zellweger, pseudo-Zellweger, and neonatal adrenoleukodystrophy. These are autosomal recessive disorders characterized by lack of peroxisomes or loss of peroxisomal function. Spectroscopic study of patients with these disorders revealed decreased levels of NAA, as evidenced by decreased ratios of NAA/creatine and NAA/choline and elevated cerebral glutamine (Bruhn et al., 1992b). Increased cerebral glutamine was also reported by Connelly et al. (1993) in ornithine carbamoyltransferase deficiency, where sufficient glutamine was present to allow observation in a long-TE study. Patients with chronic hepatic encephalopathy were studied by Kreis et al. (1992), who reported reductions in choline and *myo*-inositol levels coupled with elevated brain glutamine concentrations in this population.

Proton MRS may be of value in assessing damage due to infarcts. For example, in a study of adult stroke victims, the NAA resonance was found to be decreased, and lactate was visible in the spectrum (Bruhn et al., 1989).

CLINICAL APPLICATION OF MRI

It is well known that MRI is an exquisitely sensitive technique for delineation of morphology, most often through the use of T_1-weighted imaging. For example, in brain images obtained with T_1 weighting, cerebrospinal fluid (CSF), with its long T_1, is typically the darkest component, providing precise an-

atomic orientation. Imaging with T_1 weighting is also useful for delineation of fat, visualization of paramagnetic contrast agents, and detection of subacute hematoma and fluids with a high protein content. In neonatal brain tissue, gray matter and white matter are distinguished through differences in T_1 relaxation times, as well as proton density, with the gray matter appearing hyperintense in comparison with white matter. As the brain develops, water content lessens, reducing relaxation times, and myelination proceeds in white matter, with the result that gray–white contrast is reduced and finally reverses to demonstrate the characteristic adult brain appearance, with gray matter hyperintense to white matter. Figure 4.13 shows examples of T_1-weighted sagittal images of normal term and preterm infant brains.

T_2-weighted imaging exhibits high sensitivity to many pathological processes, including edema, infarction, demyelination, infection, neoplasm, and most fluid collections (Heard, Wolpert, and Runge, 1992). In areas exhibiting these conditions, the T_2 relaxation time is increased, possibly because of the addition of more mobile protons, leading to a hyperintense appearance on T_2-weighted imaging. The long T_2 value of CSF also makes it appear hyperintense to brain tissue. Gray–white-matter contrast is the opposite of that seen in T_1-weighted imaging, with gray matter hypointense to white. Again, in adults, the opposite contrast pattern is observed on T_2-weighted imaging owing to myelination and proton density changes. One notes that gray–white contrast is, in general, reversed between infants and adults, and between T_1-weighted and T_2-weighted scans. These instances underscore the necessity for understanding the method of acquisition when interpreting an MR image.

When planning an MRI study for an infant, it is desirable to increase TR and TE over the values appropriate for adult studies in order to account for the greater water content of the infant brain, with attendant longer relaxation times. Examples of T_2-weighted axial images of brain in term and preterm newborns are shown in Figure 4.14, and some of the specific pathological features most often encountered in neonatology are summarized next.

MRI of congenital malformations of the central nervous system (CNS)

MRI has become recognized as the diagnostic modality of choice for evaluation of a wide range of congenital anomalies (Lee, 1989), including anatomic deformities, infarction, and defects of myeli-

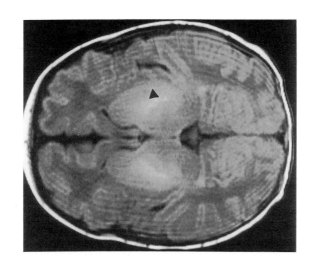

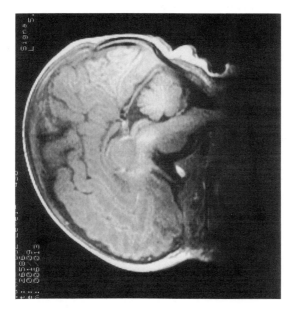

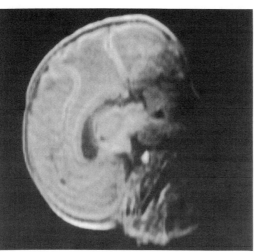

Figure 4.13. MR images of normal preterm (PCA = 30 wk) (left) and term (middle, right) infants with T_1 weighting. These images demonstrate the progress of gyration and sulcation, as well as the pattern of gray-matter–white-matter contrast. Unmyelinated white matter is hypointense to gray matter on these images, the reverse of the normal adult pattern. CSF is most hypointense in the image, and myelinated white matter is seen in the region of the internal capsule on the axial image (right, arrow). Acquisition parameters included TR = 500 ms, TE = 20 ms, and slice thickness 5.0 mm.

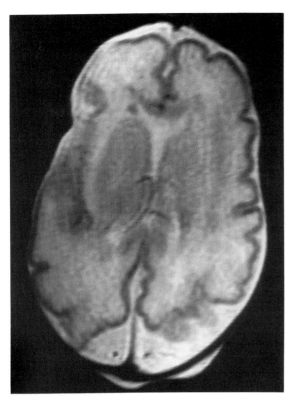

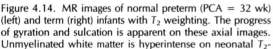

Figure 4.14. MR images of normal preterm (PCA = 32 wk) (left) and term (right) infants with T_2 weighting. The progress of gyration and sulcation is apparent on these axial images. Unmyelinated white matter is hyperintense on neonatal T_2- weighted images, with gray matter less intense and myelinated white matter still less intense, as is demonstrated on the term-infant image (right). Acquisition parameters included TR = 3.0 s, TE = 120 ms, and slice thickness 5.0 mm.

nation. For example, agenesis of the corpus callosum is better demonstrated with MRI than with CT (Han et al., 1985). MRI clearly demonstrates the associated findings of separation of the lateral ventricles, upward extension of the third ventricle, and absence of the septum pellucidum (Cohen, 1986).

Disorders of dorsal induction or neurulation such as Arnold-Chiari malformation (Longridge and Mallinson, 1985; Spinos et al., 1985), anencephaly, lipomeningocele (Han et al., 1983; Modic et al., 1983), and meningomyelocele are well visualized with MRI. The observed contrast between gray and white matter is useful in diagnosis of migrational disorders such as agyria, pachygyria, polymicrogyria, schizencephaly, and gray-matter heterotopia (Heard et al., 1992).

Gray–white-matter contrast can be used to assess the progress of myelination, which normally occurs during the time period from birth to about 2 yr of age. Over this time period, the gray–white-matter contrast observed in the neonate disappears, and then reverses, as a result of myelination, as well as changes in brain water content that influence relaxation times. T_1 changes precede those in T_2 (Fagan and Byrd, 1990; Heard et al, 1992). The normal regional progress of myelination, visualized with MRI as increased hyperintensity of white matter on T_1- weighted scans and increased hypointensity on T_2- weighted scans, proceeds from central to peripheral, from inferior to superior, and from posterior to anterior (Barkovich et al., 1988; Hayakawa et al., 1991; Konishi et al., 1991).

MRI has also been found valuable in detecting abnormalities of the pituitary stalk and pituitary gland in cases of growth-hormone deficiency (Carlier et al., 1991; Maghnie et al., 1991; Argyropoulou et al., 1992; Ochi et al., 1992) and in diagnosis of optic-nerve hypoplasia (Brodsky and Glasier, 1993).

MRI of hypoxic-ischemic CNS injury

Cerebral hemorrhage, whether intraventricular (IVH) or periventricular (PVH), is a common sequela of prematurity that typically is diagnosed by cerebral ultrasound. However, additional information can be gained with the use of MRI, including the precise extent of bleeding, as well as differentiation among acute, subacute, and chronic hemorrhages (Gomori and Grossman, 1988). Secondary hydrocephalus can be accurately seen, and communicating and noncommunicating hydrocephalus distinguished, and porencephalic cysts can be detected at the site of resolving intraparenchymal hematoma. Subdural hematoma and subarachnoid hemorrhage are also easily visualized with MRI, as is atrophy resulting from cerebral infarction (Smith and Bauman, 1991).

Another application of MRI is found in periventricular leukomalacia (PVL). This disorder is seen as focal areas of increased T_1 and T_2 relaxation times that are adjacent to the ventricles. Late sequelae of PVL, including focal or diffuse white-matter atrophy and abnormal or delayed myelination, are clearly defined by MRI (Ichord, 1992; Skranes et al., 1992). MRI has also been used to detect some prenatal brain disorders that otherwise would be unsuspected and undiagnosed in infants at risk for PVL (Dubowitz, Bydder, and Mushin, 1985; Van der Bor et al., 1990; Ichord, 1992).

MRI has been used to assess patterns of structural damage following severe perinatal asphyxia (Barkovich and Truwit, 1990; Barkovich, 1992; Truwit et al., 1992), and to demonstrate lesions that were not detected by CT (Pasternak, Predey, and Mikhael, 1991). In another study, age-dependent injury patterns were found, suggesting that MRI-observable changes due to profound hypoxic-ischemic encephalopathy vary with the age of the patient at the time of the injury (Steinlin et al., 1991).

MRI of the body

The majority of reported applications of MRI in neonatology have been in the brain, in part because of the high level of interest in neurodevelopment, but also because of the additional difficulties presented by imaging other areas of the body. First among the challenges to imaging in the body is motion, including some or all of respiratory, cardiac, blood-flow, and voluntary movements. Motion can properly be considered a fourth parameter measured or imaged by MRI that is exploited in some applications, such as MRA, but generally must be avoided or corrected for. Other complications include the presence of paramagnetic ions (such as in liver) that reduce relaxation times via the same mechanism as exogenous contrast agents. However, abnormalities of the cardiovascular and musculoskeletal systems, as well as of many other organ systems, have been investigated (Davids, Wenger, and Mubarak, 1993). For these purposes, techniques developed for adults generally are applicable, perhaps with minor modifications in experimental settings. These techniques can also be applied to image the fetus in utero (Dinh et al., 1990). Other applications in the CNS include diagnosis of the spinal injuries that occasionally occur in the perinatal period (Rossitch and Oakes, 1992). Additional information regarding specific adult MRI procedures with potential applicability to perinatology can be found in any comprehensive summary of MRI applications (Edelman and Hesselink, 1990; Heard et al., 1992).

EQUIPMENT

The acquisition of MR signals requires a magnet to produce a static magnetic field, an rf coil to transmit excitation pulses, the same or a separate rf coil to receive the MR signal, and one or more computers and associated electronic equipment. For an imaging experiment, as well as for some types of spatial localization in spectroscopy, field gradients are also required. Advantages of particular electronic configurations, gradient coils, and computer architectures will not be discussed, but can be easily found in the technical literature (Stetter, 1992).

Most magnets appropriate for clinical use are horizontal-bore superconducting systems of 1.5 T and greater field strengths, although less expensive units with field strengths as low as 0.15 T are also available. Bore sizes vary from 18 cm or less to 125 cm, with field strengths up to 4 T (Vine, 1990). An approximately linear increase in signal-to-noise ratio can be gained in some applications with the use of higher static fields (Koutcher and Burt, 1984), which has led to current human studies being conducted at 4 T.

With a given MR system, proper construction/selection of rf coils will have a profound influence on the quality of the study, particularly in the case of neonates, who by virtue of their small size may fall outside of the design criteria for standard rf coils. As a general rule, the maximum signal available from a properly designed coil will be obtained when its sensitive volume is equal to the volume of interest in the patient. For a given coil, a signal-to-noise ratio (SNR) advantage of $\sqrt{2}$ will also result from a quadrature design, as opposed to a linear design (Hoult, Chen, and Sank, 1984). Thus, the use of, for example, a General Electric extremity coil (GE Medical Systems, Milwaukee, WI) for neonatal head imaging will provide an increase in the SNR because of its small size compared with the adult quadrature head coil. For small infants, this improvement will outweigh the decrease in SNR that results from the linear construction of the extremity coil. Of course, care must be taken to use rf coils only for purposes that have been taken into consideration in their design and testing. Other considerations in coil selection include the choice of surface and volume coils, with surface coils offering advantages in sensitivity and ease of spatial localization, but requiring corrections for inhomogeneity. Volume-coil designs are inherently more homogeneous and may be desirable for imaging experiments. Both surface and volume coils can also be configured to provide multinuclear capabilities, such as to combine proton imaging with localized phosphorus spectroscopy (Isaac et al., 1990). The additional complexity of these designs makes construction and tuning of these coils more difficult, but their use makes possible direct comparison of imaging and spectroscopic information and minimizes patient repositioning during study.

Conclusions

MR techniques are increasingly important to the practice of neonatal-perinatal medicine, and the potential is great for the further expansion of applications. Most MR examinations of babies are currently performed using equipment designed for adults, sometimes resulting in less than optimal image quality. Therefore, it is not unreasonable to expect that, as demand increases, equipment that is more appropriate for neonatal application will become available. The areas of ultrafast imaging and functional brain mapping hold particular promise for application in babies, and increased understanding of safety considerations may permit a wider application of MR study of the fetus in utero. MR spectroscopy has the potential to provide metabolic information that is precisely correlated with anatomic structure, allowing an enhanced understanding of pathophysiology, such as disease processes leading to cerebral dysfunction. An increased understanding of the basic principles of MR by practitioners of perinatal medicine will facilitate the most effective use of this technology.

REFERENCES

Abragam, A. (1961). *Principles of Nuclear Magnetism.* Oxford: Clarendon Press.
Argyropoulou, M., Perignon, F., Brauner, R., and Brunelle, F. (1992). Magnetic resonance imaging in the diagnosis of growth hormone deficiency. *Journal of Pediatrics* 120:886–91.

Azzopardi, D., Wyatt, J. S., and Cady, E. B. (1989). Prognosis of newborn infants with hypoxic-ischemic brain injury assessed by phosphorus magnetic resonance spectroscopy. *Pediatric Research* 25:445.
Barkovich, A. J. (1992). MR and CT evaluation of profound neonatal and infantile asphyxia. *American Journal of Neuroradiology* 13:959–72.
Barkovich, A. J., Kjos, B. O., Jackson, D. E., and Norman, D. (1988). Normal maturation of the neonatal and infant brain: MR imaging at 1.5 T. *Radiology* 166:173–80.
Barkovich, A. J., and Truwit, C. L. (1990). Brain damage from perinatal asphyxia: correlation of MR findings with gestational age. *American Journal of Neuroradiology* 11:1087–96.
Belliveau, J. W., Kennedy, D. N., McKinstry, R. C., Buchbinder, B. R., Weisskoff, R. M., Cohen, M. S., Vevea, J. M., Brady, T. J., and Rosen, B. R. (1991). Functional mapping of the human visual cortex by magnetic resonance imaging. *Science* 254:716–18.
Belliveau, J. W., Rosen, B. R., Kantor, H. L., Rzedzian, R. R., Kennedy, D. N., McKinstry, R. C., Vevea, J. M., Cohen, M. S., Pykett, I. L., and Brady, T. J. (1990). Functional cerebral imaging by susceptibility-contrast NMR. *Magnetic Resonance in Medicine* 14:538–46.
Berendson, H. J. C., and Edzes, H. T. (1973). The observation and general interpretation of sodium magnetic resonance in biological material. *Annals of the New York Academy of Sciences* 204:459–80.
Bloch, F. (1946). Nuclear induction. *Physics Reviews* 70:460–74.
Bloembergen, N., Purcell, E. M., and Pound, R. V. (1948). Relaxation effects in nuclear magnetic resonance absorption. *Physics Reviews* 73:679–718.
Boesch, C., Gruetter, R., Martin, E., Duc, G., and Wuthrich, K. (1989). Variations in the in vivo P-31 MR spectra of the developing human brain during postnatal life. *Radiology* 172:197–9.
Bolinger, L., and Leigh, J. S. (1988). Hadamard spectroscopic imaging (HSI) for multivolume localization. *Journal of Magnetic Resonance* 80:162–7.
Bottomley, P. A. (1984). Selective volume method for performing localized NMR spectroscopy. U.S. Patent 4,480,228.
Brodsky, M. C., and Glasier, C. M. (1993). Optic nerve hypoplasia. Clinical significance of associated central nervous system abnormalities on magnetic resonance imaging. *Archives of Ophthalmology* 11:66–74.
Brown, T. R., Kincaid, B. M., and Ugarbil, K. (1982). NMR chemical shift imaging in three dimensions. *Proceedings of the National Academy of Sciences USA* 79:3523–6.
Bruhn, H., Frahm, J., Gyngell, M. L., Merboldt, K. D., Hänicke, W., and Sauter, R. (1989). Cerebral metabolism in man after acute stroke: new observations using localized proton NMR spectroscopy. *Magnetic Resonance in Medicine* 9:126–31.
Bruhn, H., Frahm, J., Merboldt, K. D., Hänicke, W., Hanefeld, F., Christen, H. J., Kruse, B., and Bauer, H. J. (1992a). Multiple sclerosis in children: cerebral metabolic alterations monitored by localized proton magnetic resonance spectroscopy in vivo. *Annals of Neurology* 32:140–50.
Bruhn, H., Kruse, B., Korenke, G. C., Hanefeld, F., Hänicke, W., Merboldt, K. D., and Frahm, J. (1992b).

Proton NMR spectroscopy of cerebral metabolic alterations in infantile peroxisomal disorders. *Journal of Computer Assisted Tomography* 16:335–44.

Cady, E. B., Costello, A. M. de L., Dawson, M. J., Delpy, D. T., Hope, P. L., Reynolds, E. O. R., Tofts, P. S., and Wilkie, D. R. (1983). Non-invasive investigation of cerebral metabolism in newborn infants by phosphorous nuclear magnetic resonance spectroscopy. *Lancet* 1:1059–62.

Carlier, R., Monnet, O., Idir, A. B., Halimi, P., Simon, P., Bouchard, P., Schaison, G., and Doyon, D. (1991). Anterior and posterior hypopituitarism with pituitary stalk abnormalities. *Journal of Neuroradiology* 18:49–60.

Carr, H. Y., and Purcell, E. M. (1954). Effects of diffusion on free precession on nuclear magnetic resonance experiments. *Physics Reviews* 94:630.

Chance, B., Leigh, J. S., Clark, B. J., Maris, J., Kent, J., Nioka, S., and Smith, D. (1985). Control of oxidative metabolism and oxygen delivery in human skeletal muscle: a steady state analysis of the work/energy cost transfer function. *Proceedings of the National Academy of Sciences USA* 82:8384.

Chance, B., Leigh, J. S., Kent, J., et al. (1986). Multiple controls of oxidative metabolism in living tissues as studied by phosphorous magnetic resonance. *Proceedings of the National Academy of Sciences USA* 83:9458.

Chance, B., Smith, D., and Nioka, S. (1987). Nature of ischemic injury. In Cerra F., Shoemaker WC. *Critical Care: State of the Art,* ed. F. Cerra and W. C. Shoemaker (p. 1–11). Fullerton, CA: Society of Critical Care Medicine.

Cohen, M. D. (1986). *Pediatric Magnetic Resonance Imaging.* Philadelphia: W. B. Saunders.

Connelly, A., Cross, J. H., Gadian, D. G., Hunter, J. V., Kirkham, F. J., and Leonard, J. V. (1993). Magnetic resonance spectroscopy shows increased brain glutamine in ornithine carbamoyl. transferase deficiency. *Pediatric Research* 33:77–81.

Davids, J. R., Wenger, D. R., and Mubarak, S. J. (1993). Congenital muscular torticollis: sequela of intrauterine or perinatal compartment syndrome. *Journal of Pediatric Orthopedics* 13:141–7.

Detre, J. A., Leigh, J. S., Williams, D. S., and Koretsky, A. P. (1992). Perfusion imaging. *Magnetic Resonance in Medicine* 23:37–45.

Dinh, D. H., Wright, R. M., and Hanigan, W. D. (1990). The use of magnetic resonance imaging for the diagnosis of fetal intracranial anomalies. *Child's Nervous System* 6:212–15.

Dixon, T. (1984). Simple proton spectroscopic imaging. *Radiology* 153:189–94.

Dousset, V., Grossman, R. I., Ramer, K., Schnall, M. D., Young, L. H., Gonzalez-Scarano, F., Lavi, E., and Cohen, J. A. (1992). Experimental allergic encephalomyelitis and multiple sclerosis: lesion characterization with magnetization transfer imaging. *Radiology* 182:483–91.

Dubowitz, L. M., Bydder, G. M., and Mushin, J. (1985). Developmental sequence of periventricular leukomalacia: correlation of ultrasound, clinical and NMR functions. *Archives of Disease in Childhood* 60:349–55.

Dumoulin, C. L., and Hart, H. R. (1986). MR angiography. *Radiology* 161:717–20.

Dumoulin, C. L., Souza, S. P., Walker, M. F., and Wagle, W. (1989). Three dimensional phase contrast angiography. *Magnetic Resonance in Medicine* 9:139–49.

Dumoulin, C. L., Souza, S. P., Walker, M. F., and Yoshitome, E. (1988). Time resolved MR angiography. *Magnetic Resonance in Medicine* 6:275–86.

Dwek, R. A. (1973). *Nuclear Magnetic Resonance in Biochemistry: Applications to Enzyme Systems.* Oxford: Clarendon Press.

Edelman, R. R., and Hesselink, J. R. (eds.) (1990). *Clinical Magnetic Resonance Imaging.* Philadelphia: W. B. Saunders.

Edelstein, W. A., Hutchison, J. M., Johnson, G., and Redpath, T. (1980). Spin-warp imaging and applications to human whole-body imaging. *Physics in Medicine and Biology* 25:751–6.

Ernst, R. R., Bodenhausen, G., and Wokann, A. (1987). *Principles of Nuclear Magnetic Resonance in One and Two Dimensions.* Oxford: Clarendon Press.

Fagan, S. J., and Byrd, S. E. (1990). Normal anatomy and development of the brain. In *Magnetic Resonance Imaging of Children,* ed. M. D. Cohen and M. K. Edwards. Philadelphia: B. C. Decker.

FDA (1982). Bureau of Radiologic Health, United States Food and Drug Administration guidelines for evaluating electromagnetic exposure for trials of clinical NMR systems. *Federal Register* 47.

Frahm, J., Bruhn, H., Gyngell, M. L., Merboldt, K. D., Hänicke, W., and Sauter, R. (1989). Localized high resolution proton NMR spectroscopy using stimulated echoes: initial applications to human brain in vivo. *Magnetic Resonance in Medicine* 9:79–93.

Frahm, J., Haase, A., and Matthaei, D. (1986). Rapid NMR imaging of dynamic processes using the FLASH technique. *Magnetic Resonance in Medicine* 3:321–7.

Gomori, J. M., and Grossman, R. I. (1988). Mechanisms responsible for the MR appearance and evolution of intracranial hemorrhage. *Radiographics* 8:427–40.

Gyulai, L., Bolinger, L., and Leigh, J. S. (1984). Phosphoethanolamine – the major constituent of the phosphomonoester peak observed by ^{31}P NMR in the developing dog brain. *Federation of European Biochemical Societies Letters* 178:137.

Haase, A., and Frahm, J. (1985). Multiple chemical-shift-selective NMR imaging using stimulated echoes. *Journal of Magnetic Resonance* 64:94–102.

Haase, A., Frahm, J., and Matthaei, D. (1986). Rapid NMR imaging using low flip angle pulses. *Journal of Magnetic Resonance* 67:258–66.

Hahn, E. L. (1950). Spin echoes. *Physics Reviews* 80:580–94.

Hamilton, P. A., Hope, P. L., Cady, E. B., et al. (1986). Impared energy metabolism in brains of newborn infants with increased cerebral echodensities. *Lancet* 1:1242.

Han, J. S., Benson, J. E., Kaufman, B., Rekate, H. L., Alfidi, R. J., Huss, R. G., Sacco, D., Yoon, Y. S., and Morrison, S. C. (1985). MR imaging of pediatric cerebral abnormalities. *Journal of Computer Assisted Tomography* 9:103–14.

Han, J. S., Kaufman, B., El Yousef, S. J., Benson, J. E., Bonstelle, C. T., Alfidi, R. J., Hagga, J. R., Yeung, H., and Huss, R. G. (1983). NMR imaging of the spine. *American Journal of Radiology* 141:1137–45.

Haselgrove, J. C., Subramanian, V. H., Leigh, J. S., Gyulai, L., and Chance, B. (1983). In vivo one-dimensional imaging of phosphorous metabolites by phosphorus-31 nuclear magnetic resonance. *Science* 22:1170–3.

Hayakawa, K., Konishi, Y., Kuriyama, M., Konishi, K., and Matsuda, T. (1991). Normal brain maturation in MRI. *European Journal of Radiology* 12:208–15.

Heard, G. G., Wolpert, S. M., and Runge, V. M. (1992). Congenital malformations of the brain. *Magnetic Resonance Imaging Clinical Principles*, ed. V. M. Runge (pp. 125–49). Philadelphia: Lippincott.

Hennig, J., Nauerth, A., and Freidburg, H. (1986). RARE imaging: a fast imaging method for clinical MR. *Magnetic Resonance in Medicine* 3:823–33.

Hinshaw, W. S. (1974). Spin mapping: the application of moving gradients to NMR. *Physics Letters* 48:87–8.

(1976). *Journal of Applied Physics* 47:3709.

Hope, P. L., Costello, A. M. de L., Cady, E. B., Delpy, D. T., Tofts, P. S., Chu, A., Hamilton, P. A., Reynolds, E. O. R., and Wilkie, D. R. (1984). Cerebral energy metabolism studied with phosphorus NMR spectroscopy in normal and birth-asphyxiated infants. *Lancet* 2:366–70.

Hoult, D. I., Chen, C. N., and Sank, V. J. (1984). Quadrature detection in the laboratory frame. *Magnetic Resonance in Medicine* 1:339.

Hubesch, B., Sappey-Mariner, D., Roth, K., Meyerhoff, D. J., Matson, G. B., and Weiner, M. W. (1990). P-31 spectroscopy on normal brain and brain tumors. *Radiology* 174:401–9.

Hüppi, P. S., Posse, S., Lazeyras, F., Burri, R., Bossi, E., and Herschkowitz, N. (1991). Magnetic resonance in preterm and term newborns: ^{1}H-spectroscopy in developing human brain. *Pediatric Research* 30:574–8.

Ichord, R. N. (1992). Advances in neonatal neurology. *Pediatric Annals* 21:339–45.

Isaac, G., Schnall, M. D., Lenkinski, R. E., and Vogele, K. (1990). A design for a double-tuned birdcage coil for use in an integrated MRI/MRS examination. *Journal of Magnetic Resonance* 89:41–50.

Joseph, P. M., Fishman, J. E., Mukherji, B., et al. (1985). In-vivo F-19 NMR imaging of the cardio-vascular system. *Journal of Computer Assisted Tomography* 9:1012–19.

Kanal, E., Shellock, F., and Talagala, L. (1990). Safety considerations in MR imaging. *Radiology* 176:593–606.

Keller, P. J., Drayer, B. P., and Fram, E. K. (1989). MR angiography with two dimensional acquisition and three dimensional display. *Radiology* 173:527–32.

Konishi, Y., Kuriyama, M., Hayakawa, K., Konishi, K., Yasujima, M., Fujii, Y., Sudo, M., and Ishii, Y. (1991). Magnetic resonance imaging in preterm infants. *Pediatric Neurology* 7:191–5.

Koutcher, J. A., and Burt, C. T. (1984). Principles of nuclear magnetic resonance. *Journal of Nuclear Medicine* 25:101–11.

Koutcher, J. A., Burt, C. T., Lauffer, R. B., and Brady, T. J. (1984). Contrast agents and spectroscopic probes in NMR. *Journal of Nuclear Medicine* 25:506–13.

Kreis, R., Ernst, T., and Ross, B. D. (1993). Development of the human brain: in vivo quantification of metabolite and water content with proton magnetic resonance spectroscopy. *Magnetic Resonance in Medicine* 30:424–37.

Kreis, R., Ross, B. D., Farrow, N. A, and Ackerman, Z. (1992). Metabolic disorders of the brain in chronic hepatic encephalopathy detected with H-1 MR spectroscopy. *Radiology* 182:19–27.

Lauterbur, P. C. (1970). ^{13}C nuclear magnetic resonance spectra of proteins. *Applied Spectroscopy* 24:450–2.

(1973). Image formation by induced local interactions: examples employing nuclear magnetic resonance. *Nature* 242:190.

Lee, B. C. (1989). Congenital and perinatal lesions. *Topics in Magnetic Resonance Imaging* 2:1–16.

Lenkinski, R. E., and Schnall, M. D. (1991). MR spectroscopy and the biochemical basis of neurological disease. In *Magnetic Resonance Imaging of the Brain and Spine*, ed. S. W. Atlas (pp. 1099–121). New York: Raven Press.

(1993). Magnetic resonance spectroscopy. In *imaging of Bone Tumors*, ed. M. E. Kricun (pp. 447–73). Philadelphia: W. B. Saunders.

Levine, S., Welch, K., Gdowski, J., et al. (1989). The relationship of brain pH to energy metabolism and clinical outcome in acute human cerebral ischemia. *Journal of Cerebral Blood Flow and Metabolism [Suppl. 1]* 9:357.

Lewin, J. S., Masaryk, T. J., Modic, M. T., Ross, J. S., Stork, E. K., and Wiznitzer, M. (1989). Extracorporeal membrane oxygenation in infants: angiographic and parenchymal evaluation of the brain with MR imaging. *Radiology* 173:361–5.

Longridge, N. S., and Mallinson, A. I. (1985). Arnold-Chiari malformation and the otolaryngologist: Place of magnetic resonance imaging and electronystagmography. *Laryngoscope* 95:335–9.

Lovsund, P., Nilsson, S. E. G., Reuter, T., et al. (1980). Magneto-phosphenes: a quantitative analysis of thresholds. *Medical and Biological Engineering and Computing* 18:326.

McGowan, J. C., Schnall, M. D., and Leigh, J. S. (1994). Magnetization transfer imaging with pulsed off-resonance saturation: contrast variation with saturation duty cycle. *Journal of Magnetic Resonance Imaging* 4:79–82.

Maghnie, M., Larizza, D., Triulzi, F., Sampaolo, P., Scotti, G., and Severi, R. (1991). Hypopituitarism and stalk agenesis: a congenital syndrome worsened by breech delivery? *Hormone Research* 35:104–8.

Marris, J. M., Evans, J. E., McLauglin, A. C., D'Angio, G. J., Bolinger, L., Manes, H., and Chance, B. (1985). ^{31}P nuclear magnetic resonance spectroscopic investigation of human neuroblastoma in situ. *New England Journal of Medicine* 312:1500.

Meyer, R. A., Sweeney, A. H., and Kushmerick, M. J. (1984). A simple analysis of the "phosphocreatine shuttle." *American Journal of Physiology* 246:365.

Michaelis, T., Merboldt, K. D., Hänicke, W., Gyngell, M. L., Bruhn, H., and Frahm, J. (1991). On the identification of cerebral metabolites in localized ^{1}H NMR spectra of human brain in vivo. *NMR in Biomedicine* 4:90–8.

Modic, M. T., Weinstein, M. A., Pavlicek, W., Starnes, D. L., Duchesneau, P. M., Boumphrey, F., and Hardy, R. J., Jr. (1983). Nuclear magnetic resonance imaging of the spine. *Radiology* 148:757–62.

Moon, R. B., and Richards, J. H. (1973). Determination of intracellular pH by ^{31}P magnetic resonance. *Journal of Biological Chemistry* 248:7226.

Moore, W. S. (1984). Basic physics and relaxation mechanisms. *British Medical Bulletin* 40:120–4.

Morris, G. A., and Freemont, A. J. (1992). Direct observation of the magnetization exchange dynamics responsible for magnetization transfer contrast in human cartilage in vivo. *Magnetic Resonance in Medicine* 28: 97–104.

Nadler, J. V., and Cooper, J. R. (1972). *N*-acetyl-*L*-aspartic acid content of human neural tumors and bovine peripheral nervous tissues. *Journal of Neurochemistry* 19:313–19.

Ochi, M., Morikawa, M., Yoshimoto, M., Kinoshita, E., and Hayshi, K. (1992). Growth retardation due to idiopathic growth hormone deficiencies: MR findings in 34 patients. *Pediatric Radiology* 22:477–80.

Ordridge, R. J., Connelly, A., and Lohman, J. A. B. (1986). Image-selected in vivo spectroscopy (ISIS): a new technique for spatially selective NMR spectroscopy. *Journal of Magnetic Resonance* 66:283.

Outwater, E., Schnall, M. D., Braitman, L. E., Dinsmore, B. J., and Kressel, H. Y. (1992). Magnetization transfer of hepatic lesions: evaluation of a novel contrast technique in the abdomen. *Radiology* 182:535–40.

Pasternak, J. F., Predey, T. A., and Mikhael, M. A. (1991). Neonatal asphyxia: vulnerability of basal ganglia, thalamus, and brainstem. *Pediatric Neurology* 7:147–9.

Peden, C. J., Cowan, F. M., Bryant, D. J., Sargetoni, J., Cox, I. J., Menon, D. K., Gadian, D. G., Bell, J. D., and Dubowitz, L. M. (1990). Proton MR spectroscopy of the brain in infants. *Journal of Computer Assisted Tomography* 14:886–94.

Petroff, O. A. C., Pritchard, J. W., Behar, K. L., et al. (1985). In-vivo phosphorus nuclear magnetic resonance spectroscopy in status epilepticus. *Annals of Neurology* 16:169–77.

Pike, G. B., Hu, B. S., Glover, G. H., and Enzmann, D. R. (1992). Magnetization transfer time-of-flight magnetic resonance angiography. *Magnetic Resonance in Medicine* 25:372–9.

Proctor, W. G., and Yu, F. C. (1950). The dependence of nuclear magnetic resonance frequency upon chemical compound. *Physiological Reviews* 70:717.

Rabi, I. I., Millman, S., and Kusch, P. (1937). Space quantization in a gyrating magnetic field. *Physiological Reviews* 51:652–5.

Radda, G. K., Bore, P. J., and Rajagopalan, B. (1983). Clinical aspects of ^{31}P NMR spectroscopy. *British Medical Bulletin* 40:155–9.

Rosen, B. R., Belliveau, J. W., Vevea, J. M., and Brady, T. J. (1990). Perfusion imaging with NMR contrast agents. *Magnetic Resonance in Medicine* 14:249–265.

Ross, B. D., Kreis, R., and Ernst, T. (1992). Clinical tools for the 90's: magnetic resonance spectroscopy and metabolite imaging. *European Journal of Radiology* 14:128.

Rossitch, W., and Oakes, W. J. (1992). Perinatal spinal cord injury: clinical, radiographic and pathologic features. *Pediatric Neurosurgery* 18:149–52.

Schaefer, D. J. (1988). Safety aspects of magnetic resonance imaging. In *Biomedical Magnetic Resonance Imaging*, ed. F. W. Wehrli, D. Shaw, and J. B. Kneeland (pp. 553–78). New York: VCH.

Schnall, M. D., Yoshizaki, K., and Leigh, J. S. (1988). Triple nuclear NMR studies of cat brain metabolism during seizure. *Magnetic Resonance in Medicine* 6:15–23.

Schneider, E., and Glover, G. (1991). Rapid in vivo proton shimming. *Magnetic Resonance in Medicine* 18:335–347.

Shulman, R. G. (1987). Contributions of ^{13}C and ^{1}H NMR to physiological control. *Annals of the New York Academy of Sciences* 508:10–14.

Skranes, J. S., Nilsen, G., Smevik, O., Vik, T., Rinck, P., and Brubakk, A. M. (1992). Cerebral magnetic resonance imaging of very low birth weight infants at one year of corrected age. *Pediatric Radiology* 22:406–9.

Smith, C. D., and Bauman, R. J. (1991). Clinical features and magnetic resonance imaging in congenital and childhood stroke. *Journal of Child Neurology* 6:263–272.

Spinos, E., Laster, D. W., Moody, D. M., Ball, M., Witcofski, R. L., and Kelly, D. L. (1985). MR evaluation of Chiari I malformations at .15 T. *American Journal of Roentgenology* 144:1143–8.

Steinlin, M. Dirr, R., Martin, E., Boesch, C., Largo, R. H., Fanconi, S., and Boltshauser, E. (1991). MRI following severe perinatal asphyxia: preliminary experience. *Pediatric Neurology* 7:164–70.

Stetter, E. (1992). Instrumentation. In *Clinical Magnetic Resonance Imaging*, ed. R. R. Edelman and J. R. Hesselink (pp. 355–76). Philadelphia: W. B. Saunders.

Tofts, P. S., and Wray, S. (1985). Changes in brain phosphorous metabolites during the postnatal development of the rat. *Journal of Physiology* 359:417–29.

(1988). A critical assessment of methods of measuring metabolite concentrations by NMR spectroscopy. *Nuclear Magnetic Resonance in Biomedicine* 1:1–10.

Truwit, C. L., Barkovich, A. J., Koch, T. K., and Ferriero, D. M. (1992). Cerebral palsy: MR findings in 40 patients. *American Journal of Neuroradiology* 13:79–83.

Van de Bor, M., Guit, G. S. L., Schrender, A. M., et al. (1990). Does very preterm birth impair myelination of the central nervous system? *Neuropediatrics* 21:37–9.

van der Knapp, M. S., van der Grond, J., van Rijen, P. C., Faber, J. A. J., Valk, J., and Willemse, K. (1990). Age-dependent changes in localized proton and phosphorus MR spectroscopy of the brain. *Radiology* 176:509–15.

Vine, W. (1990). Clinical diagnosis by nuclear magnetic resonance spectroscopy. *Archives of Pathology and Laboratory Medicine* 114:453–62.

Wehrli, F. W., Macfall, J. R., Shutts, D., Breger, R., and Herfkens, R. J. (1984). Mechanisms of contrast in NMR imaging. *Journal of Computer Assisted Tomography* 8:369.

Wehrli, F. W., Shimakawa, A., Gullberg, G. T., and Macfall, J. R. (1986). Time-of-flight MR flow imaging: selective saturation recovery with gradient refocusing. *Radiology* 160:781–5.

Williams, D. S., Detre, J. A., Leigh, J. S., and Koretsky, A. P. (1992). Magnetic resonance imaging of perfusion using spin inversion of arterial water. *Proceedings of the National Academy of Sciences USA* 89:212–16.

Wolff, S. D., and Balaban, K. S. (1989). Magnetization transfer contrast and tissue water proton relaxation in vivo. *Magnetic Resonance Medicine* 10:135–44.

Wray, S., and Tofts, P. S. (1986). Direct in vivo measurement of absolute metabolite concentrations using ^{31}P nuclear magnetic resonance spectroscopy. *Biochimica et Biophysica Acta* 886:399–405.

Wyndham, C. H., Strydom, N. B., Morrison, J. F., et al. (1965). Criteria for physiological limits for work in heat. *Journal of Applied Physiology* 20:37–45.

Younkin, D. P., Delivoria-Papadopoulos, M., Leonard, J. C., Subramanian, V. H., Eleff, S., Leigh, J. S., and Chance, B. (1984). Unique aspects of human newborn cerebral metabolism evaluated with phosphorus nuclear magnetic resonance spectroscopy. *Annals of Neurology* 16:581–6.

Younkin, D. P., Medoff-Cooper, B., Guillet, R., Sinwell, T., Chance, B., and Delivoria-Papadopoulos, M. (1988). In-vivo 31-P measurement of chronic changes in cerebral metabolites following neonatal intraventricular hemorrhage. *Pediatrics* 82:331–6.

Zhang, W., Williams, D. S., Detre, J. A., and Koretsky, A. P. (1992). Measurement of brain perfusion by volume-localized NMR spectroscopy using inversion of arterial water spins: accounting for transit time and cross relaxation. *Magnetic Resonance in Medicine* 25:362–371.

5

Positron-emission tomography in the newborn

PETER HERSCOVITCH, M.D.

INTRODUCTION

Positron-emission tomography (PET) is a nuclear-medicine technique for performing regional physiological measurements in vivo. The PET scanner provides tomographic images of the distribution of positron-emitting radioactive tracers by means of radiation detectors arrayed around the body. From these images, measurements of functions such as blood flow and glucose metabolism can be obtained. Conceptually, there are three components involved in PET: (1) tracer compounds of physiological interest that are labeled with positron-emitting radionuclides, (2) a PET scanner to obtain images of the concentration of positron-emitting radioactivity in the body, and (3) a mathematical model that describes the in vivo behavior of the specific radiotracer used, so that the physiological process under study can be quantitated from the tomographic measurements of regional radioactivity.

A brief review of the earlier methods used to measure brain blood flow and metabolism will demonstrate the advantages of PET. Kety and Schmidt, in the 1940s, developed the nitrous oxide method to measure cerebral blood flow (CBF) (Kety and Schmidt, 1948). Whole-brain blood flow was calculated from arterial and cerebral venous concentrations of nitrous oxide measured during inhalation of the gas. Determination of brain arterial–venous differences for glucose and oxygen permitted measurement of cerebral metabolism as well. Because that technique provided only global measurements, however, methods were subsequently developed to measure regional CBF. Those methods used exter-

nal radiation detectors to measure the clearance, from different brain regions, of freely diffusible radioactive gases, such as xenon 133, that were administered either by injection into the internal carotid artery or by inhalation (Obrist et al., 1967; Lassen and Ingvar, 1972). Subsequently, external-probe techniques using intracarotid injection of positron-emitting radiotracers were devised to measure not only CBF but also local cerebral blood volume and metabolism (Welch et al., 1975).

Those techniques, however, had several drawbacks. The variety of measurements possible was restricted to determinations of cerebral hemodynamics and metabolism. Only global measurements of metabolism could be obtained unless invasive intracarotid injections were used. Methods to obtain regional CBF measurements with external detectors had several limitations. Such detectors record radioactivity from a variable volume of brain tissue beneath the probe, and their field of view and sensitivity vary with depth. Measurements from heterogeneous tissue elements are superimposed, and the presence of underperfused tissue in the field of view may not be detected. Also, such techniques are restricted to cortical tissue; deeper structures, such as basal ganglia, cannot be studied.

Those limitations provided the impetus for PET. The first tomographs for quantitative PET imaging were developed in the mid-1970s (Phelps et al., 1975b; Ter-Pogossian et al., 1975). Subsequently, the design of tomographs has become more sophisticated, with greatly improved spatial resolution and sensitivity. Radiotracer techniques have been developed to study regional CBF, regional cerebral

93

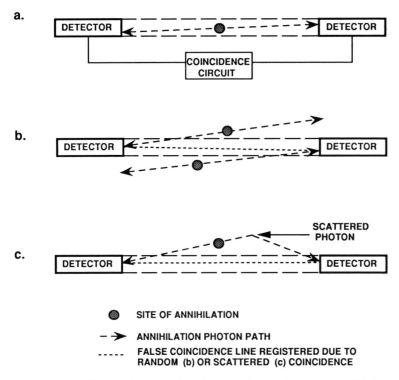

Figure 5.1. (a) The two photons resulting from a positron emission and annihilation are detected by two radiation detectors that are connected by an electronic coincidence circuit. A decay event is recorded as a coincidence line between the detectors only when both photons are detected almost simultaneously. This coincidence requirement localizes the site of the annihilation to the volume of space between the detectors. (b) A random coincidence is registered if two photons from two different positron annihilations are sensed by a detector pair within the coincidence resolving time. (c) A scattered coincidence occurs when an annihilation photon traveling in tissue is deflected, so that its direction changes. This results in incorrect positioning of the coincidence line.

blood volume, the metabolism of glucose, oxygen, and protein, the permeability of the blood–brain barrier, neuroreceptors and transmitters, tissue pH, and tissue concentrations of radiolabeled drugs. These methods have been widely applied to study both normal brain and neuropsychiatric disease (Jamieson and Greenberg, 1989; Grafton and Mazziotta, 1992). In addition, PET has been used in other organ systems, including heart and lung, and in oncology (Council on Scientific Affairs, 1988c; Shuster, 1989; Bergmann, 1991; Strauss and Conti, 1991). The use of PET in the perinatal period is less well developed, primarily because of the additional technical difficulties. Relatively few studies have been reported, but they have yielded new insights into the pathophysiology of neonatal illness and have demonstrated that PET can be used productively in this age group.

This chapter will review the basic principles of PET. Radiotracer techniques that have been used in neonates to measure regional CBF and metabolism will be described. Aspects of the methodology of special relevance to neonatal studies will be indicated. Then the literature on clinical research with PET in the neonate will be reviewed.

PET INSTRUMENTATION

Formation of the PET image

Certain radioactive atoms decay by the emission of a positron from the atomic nucleus. A positron has the same mass as an electron, but a positive charge. After its emission, the positron travels a variable distance in tissue, up to a few millimeters, losing kinetic energy. When almost at rest, it interacts with

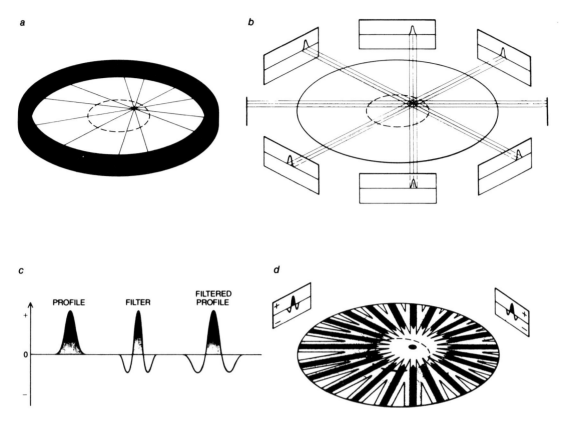

Figure 5.2. The steps in PET reconstruction are depicted in these diagrams, which illustrate the imaging of a small region of uniform radioactivity in a single tomographic plane. (a) Multiple coincidence lines are recorded by opposing detector pairs in the ring. Each line results from a positron emission and annihilation, so that the number of coincidence lines recorded by any detector pair is proportional to the amount of radioactivity between them. (b) After the "scan," the coincidence lines are sorted into parallel groups representing the profile or projection of the radioactivity distribution viewed from a different angle. These projections are then combined using the same mathematical technique as in x-ray CT (Brooks and Di Chiro, 1976) to obtain the PET image. (c) Each projection is mathematically processed by means of a special function called the filter function. (d) The modified projections are then combined by "back-projection" to reconstruct an image of the radioactivity distribution. Note that there are several other steps in reconstruction, such as corrections for attenuation, deadtime, and random and scattered coincidence counts, as described in the text. (From Ter-Pogossian et al., 1980. Copyright © October 1980 by *Scientific American*, Inc. All rights reserved. Courtesy of Dr. M. M. Ter-Pogossian and by permission of *Scientific American*.)

an electron, resulting in the "annihilation" of both particles. Their combined mass is converted into two high-energy, 511-keV photons that travel in opposite directions from the annihilation site at the speed of light. Detection of these photon pairs is used to measure both the location and amount of radioactivity. The two annihilation photons can be detected by two opposing radiation detectors connected by an electronic coincidence circuit (Figure 5.1a). This circuit records a decay event when both detectors sense the almost simultaneous arrival of the two photons. A very short time window for photon arrival, typically 5–20 ns, called the coincidence resolving time, is allowed for registration of a coincidence event. The site of the decay event is therefore localized to the volume of space between the two detectors.

In practice, several rings, with many radiation detectors per ring, are used, with opposing detector pairs in each ring connected by coincidence circuits. With each decay event, the two resulting annihilation photons are detected as a coincidence line. A computer records the coincidence events from each ring and then reconstructs a cross-sectional or tomographic image of the underlying distribution of radioactivity (Figure 5.2). The intensity of each point or pixel in the image is proportional to the concentration of radioactivity at the corresponding position in the body. To calibrate the scanner to obtain *absolute* radioactivity measurements, a con-

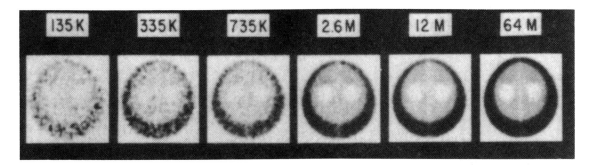

Figure 5.3. Effect on image noise of increasing the number of counts. The images are PET scans of a cylindrical phantom with chambers that have relative radiotracer concentrations of 3 in the outer rim, 1 in the large inner portion, and 0 in the two small regions. Image noise, apparent as graininess, de-creases with increasing counts (toward the right). (From Phelps et al., 1979. Courtesy of Dr. M. E. Phelps, and by permission of the Institute of Electrical and Electronics Engineers, © 1979 IEEE.)

tainer holding a uniform solution of radioactivity is imaged. The radioactivity concentration of the solution is then measured with a calibrated well counter, and the scanner calibration factor is calculated to convert PET image counts to units of radioactivity concentration (e.g., microcuries per cubic centimeter).

The reconstruction process requires a correction for the absorption or attenuation of some annihilation photons due to their interaction with tissue, which decreases the number of coincidence events detected. The amount of attenuation can be estimated using an assumed value for the attenuating properties of tissue between each detector pair. Actual measurement of attenuation is more accurate, however (Frackowiak et al., 1980). Prior to the emission scan, a separate transmission scan is performed with a source of positron-emitting radioactivity between the subject's head and the detector rings. A similar measurement is also made with nothing in the field of view of the scanner. The ratio of the two measurements gives the amount of photon attenuation between each detector pair and is used in the image-reconstruction process to correct for attenuation. This can mean a correction by as much as a factor of 5 to 6 in the center of the adult head. Because of the smaller head size and immature skull, the required correction is less in neonates, but it is still substantial.

Performance characteristics of PET scanners

Many factors in the PET imaging process have major impacts on image quality and our ability to quantitate radioactivity accurately, including image "noise," count-rate performance, random and scat-

tered counts, and spatial resolution. The PET image has inherent statistical noise because of the random nature of radioactive decay. The disintegration rate of a radioactive sample undergoes moment-to-moment variations. The resulting uncertainty in measuring the amount of radioactivity decreases as the number of counts recorded increases. Similarly, the statistical reliability of a PET measurement depends on the number of counts. The situation is more complex, however, because the value of radioactivity in any small brain region is obtained from an image reconstructed from multiple views or projections of the radioactivity distribution throughout the entire brain slice. Thus, the noise in any individual brain region is affected by noise in other brain regions and tends to be greater (Budinger et al., 1978). Excessive noise gives the PET image a "salt-and-pepper" appearance (Figure 5.3) and decreases our ability to quantitate radioactivity accurately.

Noise depends on the number of counts collected, which in turn depends on scanner sensitivity, the duration of the scan, and the concentration of radioactivity in the field of view. Scanner sensitivity is determined by its design features, such as the nature and arrangement of the radiation detectors. Although increasing the scan duration will increase counts, frequently this is not possible, either because of the short half-life* of the radiotracer or because it would not be compatible with the tracer-kinetic mathematical model that is used. Administering more radioactivity will increase counts, but this approach is limited by radiation safety considerations and also by the inability of tomographs

---

* The half-life of a radioactive nuclide is the time required for the radioactivity to decay to one-half its original value.

to operate accurately at high count rates. This count-rate limitation results from deadtime losses and from random coincidence counts, which will increase image noise. "Deadtime loss" refers to the decreasing ability to register counts as the count rate increases, because of the time required to handle each count, primarily in the electronic circuitry. Although a correction factor for deadtime count loss can be determined (Daube-Witherspoon and Carson, 1991), this correction may break down beyond a certain count rate. Also, it does not compensate for the loss in statistical accuracy that occurs because fewer counts were actually collected.

Random coincidences also limit count-rate performance. These occur when two photons from two *different* positron annihilations are sensed by a detector pair within the coincidence resolving time (Figure 5.1b), so that a false or random coincidence count is collected. The fraction of total coincidences recorded that are randoms increases linearly with radioactivity. Random coincidences add noisy background to the image. Although corrections can be made that will subtract an estimate of the false counts, the contribution to the image noise persists (Hoffman et al., 1981). Thus, for any given tomograph, the amount of radioactivity administered must be carefully selected to balance the competing effects of improved counting statistics with the "diminishing returns" due to deadtime and random coincidences. It should be noted that count-rate limitations are of less concern in neonatal PET studies than in adult studies, because the total amount of radioactivity in the scanner field of view is substantially less. This is because of the smaller brain size and because physiological parameters such as blood flow and metabolism tend to be low in ill neonates, which results in less radiotracer being taken up by brain tissue.

Another source of image noise is scatter, which occurs when an annihilation photon traveling in tissue is deflected by an electron, so that its direction changes. This results in incorrect positioning of the coincidence line (Figure 5.1c). Not only is information lost from affected coincidence lines, but also a noisy background is added to the image. This leads to an overestimation of radioactivity, especially in areas containing relatively less radioactivity. It is necessary to correct for scatter, because it can contribute up to 25% of the counts in an image. The methods that have been developed to correct for scatter vary in their complexity and effectiveness (Bergstrom et al., 1983; Hoffman and Phelps, 1986).

The concept of spatial resolution is critical to understanding quantitative PET imaging. One inter-

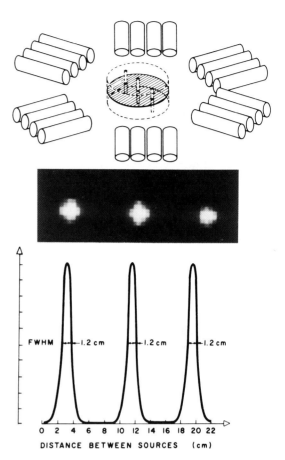

Figure 5.4. How the resolution of a PET scanner is defined and measured. Thin line sources of positron-emitting radioactivity perpendicular to the image plane are scanned (top). Because of resolution limitations, the radioactivity in each source appears blurred or spread over a larger area (middle). Scanner resolution is defined by the amount of spreading that occurs. A plot of the image intensity (bottom) shows that this spreading approximates a bell-shaped or Gaussian curve, called the line-spread function. The width of the line-spread function at one-half of its maximum amplitude (termed the full width at half maximum, FWHM) is the measure of resolution. Here the resolution is 1.2 cm. (From Ter-Pogossian et al., 1975. Courtesy of Dr. M. M. Ter-Pogossian and by permission of the Radiological Society of North America.)

pretation of "resolution" is that it is the minimum distance by which two points of radioactivity must be separated to be perceived independently in the reconstructed image. Operationally, scanner resolution is measured by imaging a thin "line source" of positron-emitting radioactivity (Figure 5.4). Spatial resolution depends on how accurately the location of a positron-emitting nucleus can be determined. The physics of positron annihilation and the detector design will both limit resolution. The annihila-

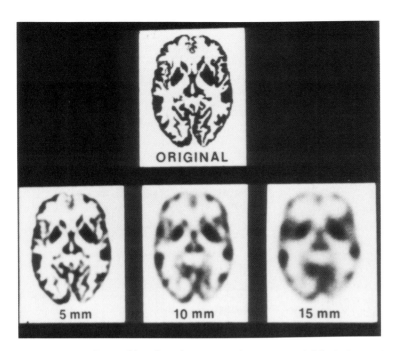

Figure 5.5. Simulation of the effect of scanner resolution on an adult brain image. At the top is an original brain image. Subsequent images simulate the effect of scanning this image with tomographs of varying resolution, from 5 to 15 mm FWHM. (From Mazziotta et al. 1981. Courtesy of Dr. J. C. Mazziotta and by permission of Raven Press.)

tion photons are produced only after the positron has traveled up to several millimeters from the nucleus. The average range the positron will travel will vary with the specific radionuclide (e.g., 1.1 mm for ^{11}C, 2.5 mm for ^{15}O) (Phelps et al., 1975a). This limits the accuracy with which one can locate the radioactive nucleus. A second factor limiting resolution is the noncolinearity of the annihilation photons. Because positrons may have residual kinetic energy at the time of annihilation, the angle between the two photons can deviate slightly from 180°. This results in a slight misplacement of the coincidence line. These combined effects can result in a resolution loss of about 1–3 mm (Phelps and Hoffman, 1976). Detector design also limits scanner resolution. The size and shape of the radiation detectors determine how accurately the position of each coincidence line is recorded, with smaller detectors providing better resolution. The resolution of commercially available, multiring scanners is 4–5 mm in the image plane (DeGrado et al., 1994; Wienhard et al., 1994), although a single-ring device with 2.6-mm resolution has been constructed (Derenzo et al., 1988).

Limited resolution will result in blurring of the PET image (Figure 5.5). More important, though, is the effect on radioactivity quantitation (Hoffman, Huang, and Phelps, 1979; Mazziotta et al., 1981). The radioactivity in a brain region will appear blurred or spread out over a larger area. Thus, in the reconstructed image, a brain region of interest will reflect only a portion of the radioactivity that was in the corresponding brain structure; in addition, some of the surrounding radioactivity will be spread into the region. As a result of this effect, termed "partial-volume averaging," a regional measurement will contain contributions both from the structure of interest and from surrounding structures. High radioactivity levels surrounded by lower values will be underestimated, and low radioactivity surrounded by high activity will be overestimated. These errors will be less when the size of the structure of interest is large with respect to scanner resolution. In a circular structure with a diameter twice the resolution and with a uniform radioactivity concentration, the radioactivity will be accurately represented in the center. However, statistical considerations limit our ability to obtain a measurement from such a small region. In general, then, it is not possible to measure pure gray-matter radioactivity, especially in cortical regions. In addition, partial-volume averaging with cerebrospinal fluid in sulci or ventricles can lead to underestimation of tissue blood flow and metabolism, especially if there is cerebral atrophy (Herscovitch et al., 1986; Videen et al., 1988). In addition to in-plane resolution, axial resolution also affects quantitation (Kessler, Ellis, and Eden, 1984). Axial resolution, measured perpendicular to the tomographic plane, can be thought of as the effective thickness of a slice. It is determined by the axial thickness of the detectors. Current tomographs have axial and transverse resolutions that are approximately equivalent (DeGrado et al., 1994; Wienhard et al., 1994).

Design of PET systems

A PET system consists of many components. There are several rings of radiation detectors mounted in a gantry. A detector typically consists of a small scintillation crystal that gives off light when energy from an annihilation photon is deposited in it. The detector is coupled to a photomultiplier tube that converts the light pulse to an electrical signal that is fed into the coincidence circuitry. Current commercially available scanners (DeGrado et al., 1994; Wienhard et al., 1994) have from 18 to 24 rings, each containing up to several hundred detectors. A tomographic slice is provided by each ring. In addition, "cross-slices" are derived from coincidences between detectors in adjacent rings. These planes are halfway between the detector rings. Therefore, 47 contiguous tomographic slices can be obtained simultaneously by a 24-ring system. Many gantries can be tilted to obtain slices in desired anatomic planes, such as parallel to the canthomeatal line. The subject rests on a special couch fitted with a head holder to restrain head movement during the scanning procedure. For neonatal studies, a specially designed support resting on the PET couch and head holder can be used. A dedicated computer is used to control the scanning process, collect the coincidence count information, and reconstruct and display the images.

The design of PET systems involves several interacting factors (Brooks et al., 1981; Hoffman and Phelps, 1986; Muehllehner and Karp, 1986; Council on Scientific Affairs, 1988b). These include the size, shape, and composition of the detector crystals, the arrangement of the crystals and photomultiplier tubes in the gantry, the design of the coincidence circuitry, and the methods for image reconstruction

and for the various corrections required. All these features affect our ability to obtain accurate measurements of regional radioactivity. Formal procedures have been devised to test scanner performance characteristics (Karp et al., 1991). These are performed when a scanner is accepted from the manufacturer, to ensure that it meets specifications, and they must be repeated at regular intervals to verify that it continues to operate within these specifications.

Scanner design is still evolving, and new developments may have an impact on neonatal studies. Scanners have been designed specifically for imaging the brain or heart in laboratory animals, such as dogs and monkeys (Cutler et al., 1992). These scanners have fewer rings, of smaller diameter, and can have higher sensitivity and resolution than standard tomographs at a lower cost. They should also be suitable for studies of the smaller brain of the neonate. A new approach to image formation is true three-dimensional volume imaging (Townsend et al., 1991). Changes in tomograph design permit coincidence counts to be collected by opposing detectors that do not have to be in the same ring or adjacent rings. Many more coincidence lines can be collected, and scanner sensitivity can be increased substantially. This improves image quality or, alternatively, permits less radioactivity to be administered while maintaining image counts. The image-reconstruction process is more complicated, however.

RADIOTRACERS FOR PET

The second requirement for PET is a radiotracer of physiological interest labeled with a positron-emitting radionuclide. A radiotracer can be a naturally occurring compound in which one of the atoms is replaced with its radioactive counterpart (an isotope), or it can be a labeled analogue that has behavior similar to the natural substance. Alternatively, it can be a synthetic substance, such as a radiolabeled drug, that interacts with a specific biological system. A key requirement is that in the amounts used, the tracer must not affect the physiological process being studied. The positron-emitting radionuclides most commonly used to synthesize PET radiotracers are ^{15}O, ^{13}N, ^{11}C, and ^{18}F. Their half-lives and examples of specific applications are listed in Table 5.1. The chemical natures of ^{15}O, ^{13}N, and ^{11}C are identical with those of their nonradioactive counterparts, which are basic constituents of living matter, as well as of most drugs. Thus, each can be incorporated into radiotracers with the same in vivo behavior as

Table 5.1. *Positron-emitting nuclides and representative radiotracers*

Radionuclide[a]	Half-life (min)	Radiotracer	Application
Oxygen-15 (^{15}O)	2.05	$C^{15}O$	Cerebral blood volume
		$^{15}O_2$	Cerebral oxygen metabolism
		$H_2^{15}O$	Cerebral blood flow
		$C^{15}O_2$	Cerebral blood flow
		^{15}O-butanol	Cerebral blood flow
Nitrogen-13 (^{13}N)	10.0	^{13}N-BCNU	Tissue and tumor drug levels
		^{13}N-amino acids	Amino acid transport
Carbon-11 (^{11}C)	20.4	^{11}CO	Cerebral blood volume
		^{11}C-butanol	Cerebral blood flow
		$^{11}CO_2$	Tissue pH
		^{11}C-deoxyglucose	Cerebral glucose metabolism
		^{11}C-3-O-methylglucose	Glucose transport
		^{11}C-N-methylspiperone	Dopamine receptor ligand
		^{11}C-raclopride	Dopamine receptor ligand
		^{11}C-nomifensine	Presynaptic dopamine uptake sites
		^{11}C-carfentanil	Opiate receptor ligand
		^{11}C-flumazenil	Central benzodiazepine receptor ligand
		^{11}C-α-methyltryptophan	Brain serotonin synthesis rate
		^{11}C-deprenyl	Monoamine oxidase distribution
		^{11}C-cocaine	Cocaine binding sites
Fluorine-18 (^{18}F)	110	^{18}F-fluorodeoxyglucose	Cerebral glucose metabolism
		^{18}F-fluorotyrosine	Protein synthesis
		^{18}F-fluoromethane	Cerebral blood flow
		^{18}F-spiperone	Dopamine receptor ligand
		^{18}F-halperidol	Dopamine receptor ligand, drug distribution
		^{18}F-GBR	Presynaptic dopamine reuptake site ligand
		^{18}F-fluorodopa	Presynaptic dopaminergic function
		^{18}F-cyclofoxy	Opiate receptor ligand
		^{18}F-fluoroestradiol	Estrogen receptor ligand
		^{18}F-setoperone	Serotonin S2 receptor ligand

[a]The standard abbreviation for the radionuclide listed is shown in parentheses.

the corresponding nonradioactive compound. ^{18}F is used to substitute for hydrogen or hydroxyl groups to synthesize analogues with characteristics similar to those of the unsubstituted compound. In addition, certain drugs contain fluorine, so that ^{18}F-labeled forms can be synthesized. These radionuclides have short physical half-lives (e.g., 2 min for ^{15}O, 110 min for ^{18}F). Thus, relatively large amounts of radioactivity can be administered to obtain images of good statistical quality, but because of rapid decay, the absorbed radiation levels are acceptable. Also, the short half-lives, especially ^{15}O, permit repeat studies in a given subject in one experimental session, because of rapid decay after each administration.

The synthesis of PET radiotracers is particularly demanding. Because of the short half-lives, on-site preparation of the radionuclides is required, by means of a cyclotron (Figure 5.6), and rapid techniques must be devised for radiochemical synthesis and purification. These must yield radiotracers that are nontoxic, sterile, and apyrogenic. The product

must be not only chemically pure but also radiochemically pure; most or all of the positron-emitting radioactivity in the product should be attached to the desired compound. A critical issue is specific activity, the amount of radioactivity per unit mass of compound. For syntheses with ^{15}O, ^{11}C, and ^{13}N, it is not possible to remove all traces of the ubiquitous stable elements from the environment. Therefore, during radiotracer synthesis, some of the compound is also produced in its nonradioactive form, lowering specific activity. This is less of a problem with ^{18}F, so that it is easier to produce higher-specific-activity compounds. Radiotracers must have specific activity sufficiently high that the amount administered will result in levels of tissue radioactivity sufficient to be measured with PET without causing physiological effects. The specific activity required depends on the potential for the compound to produce such effects. It is not critical for ^{15}O-water, but is important for ^{15}O- or ^{11}C-labeled carbon monoxide used to measure blood volume, and also for ligands that bind to neuroreceptors.

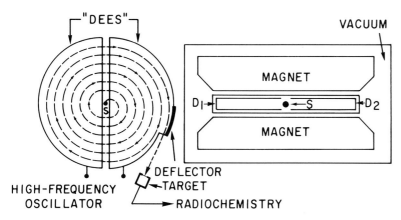

Figure 5.6. Simplified schematic diagram of a cyclotron, top (left) and side (right) views. The ion source (S) provides the particles that are accelerated. A high-frequency oscillator supplies voltage across the two "dees" that accelerate the ions in a vacuum. The deflector allows the extraction of the beam of high-energy particles. These interact in the target with stable atoms to produce positron-emitting nuclides. For example, ^{11}C is formed when nitrogen is bombarded with protons. The radionuclides that are produced are then incorporated into radiotracers for PET. (From Sorenson and Phelps, 1987. Reproduced courtesy of Dr. M. E. Phelps and by permission of W. B. Saunders Company.)

Several factors must be considered in the selection and development of new PET radiotracers (Dannals, Ravert, and Wilson, 1990; Barrio, 1991; Kilbourn, 1991). In addition to the issues noted earlier, the tracer must have the appropriate in vivo properties to permit the desired PET measurement to be made. One must consider its ability to cross the blood–brain barrier, the formation and behavior of any radioactive metabolites in blood and tissue, the ability to develop a mathematical model to describe the behavior of the tracer, and, for neuroreceptor ligands, the binding characteristics. Extensive preclinical studies often are performed. These may use tracers more easily labeled with long-lived nuclides, such as ^{3}H and ^{14}C, tissue sampling or autoradiography in animal models, and PET studies in animals. In spite of the difficulties involved, positron-emitting radiopharmaceuticals of a wide variety have been synthesized (Council on Scientific Affairs, 1988a; Kilbourn, 1990; Fowler and Wolf, 1991). To date limited numbers of these have been used in neonates: ^{18}F-fluorodeoxyglucose (FDG), and ^{15}O-labeled water, carbon monoxide, and oxygen.

GENERAL PRINCIPLES OF TRACER MODELING

A critical step in PET is the use of a mathematical model that describes the in vivo behavior of the radiotracer, that is, the relationship, over time, between the amount of tracer presented to a brain region in its arterial input and the amount of tracer in the region. With a model, one can calculate the value of the biological variable of interest, such as CBF, from measurements of radiotracer concentrations in brain and blood. The use of models allows PET to be a quantitative physiological technique, rather than only an imaging method.

Compartmental mathematical models are used in PET. These models assume that there are entities called compartments in which the tracer concentration is uniform at any instant in time and that have uniform physiological properties with respect to the tracer. The compartments can be physical spaces, such as the extravascular space, or biochemical entities, such as specific neuroreceptor binding sites. The number and nature of the compartments in a model are based on a priori knowledge of the system under study. Rate constants describe the movements of tracer between compartments. The amount of tracer that leaves a compartment is proportional to the amount that is in the compartment; the rate constant is the constant of proportionality. Usually there is more than one compartment in a model, with separate rate constants for the movements of tracer in both directions between communicating compartments. Such a model is described by one or more differential equations. These contain measurable terms, such as local brain and arterial blood radiotracer concentrations over time, and unknowns, such as rate constants or the size of a compartment, that are of physiological interest.

Several factors must be considered in developing a model. These include the transport of tracer across the blood–brain barrier, the behavior of the tracer and any of its labeled metabolites in brain, the amount of tracer in the vascular space of the brain, rather than in tissue, the presence of any labeled metabolites in blood, and the potential for alterations in radiotracer behavior if there is a local pathological process. It must be emphasized that with PET, one measures the total amount of radioactivity in a brain region. The measurement does not distinguish among the various compartments in which the tracer may be resident (e.g., intravascular versus extravascular, receptor-bound versus free in tissue), nor between the tracer and any of its radioactive metabolites. These distinctions must be made in the model. One must also take into account the physical decay of radiotracer that occurs during the study. The number of unknown variables in the model cannot be so large that it is impossible to solve the model accurately from the measured data. In some cases, there is a single unknown, and its calculation is straightforward. Often there are many unknowns, and parameter estimation techniques are used to determine their values (Carson, 1986). Simplifying assumptions may be required to limit the number of compartments and thus the number of unknown variables. The accuracy with which physiological variables can be estimated also depends on the statistical accuracy of the PET image, that is, the number of counts, as discussed earlier.

Two important components in the development of a model are error analysis and model validation. Error analysis consists in using mathematical simulations to determine the sensitivity of the model to potential sources of error. These include the effects of deviations from the model assumptions, such as the uniformity of a compartment, the effect of a local abnormality that may invalidate certain assumptions, and the effects of inaccuracies in the measurement of tissue and blood radioactivity. Several approaches can be used to validate a model. A preliminary step is to examine how well the model fits the experimental data. That is, when unknown parameters are estimated and then inserted into the model, do they predict the observed tissue radioactivity measurements? Specific experiments can also be performed. With indirect validation, the experimental environment is manipulated, and one determines whether or not the measured parameters vary as expected. For example, one can study the ability of a CBF measurement technique to follow changes in flow produced by varying arterial P_{CO_2}. Direct validation experiments consist in comparing

the measured parameter to the same physiological variable determined in an accepted but usually more invasive fashion. For example, one can compare measurements of blood flow with PET and measurements made in the same animals with radiolabeled microspheres and tissue sampling. In many cases, however, such a "gold-standard" reference technique may not exist.

Specific radiotracer methods that have been used in neonates will be discussed later. More extensive treatments of tracer-kinetics modeling can be found elsewhere (Shipley and Clark, 1972; Lassen and Perl, 1979; Sorenson and Phelps, 1987; Baron et al., 1989; Gjedde and Wong, 1990; Lammertsma and Mazoyer, 1990).

RADIOTRACER TECHNIQUES

Cerebral blood volume

To measure regional cerebral blood volume (rCBV), carbon monoxide labeled with either ^{11}C (Grubb et al., 1978) or ^{15}O (Martin, Powers, and Raichle, 1987) is administered in trace amounts by inhalation. It binds avidly to hemoglobin in red blood cells and is confined to the intravascular space. The local radioactivity in brain is directly proportional to the local red-cell content. Therefore, rCBV can be calculated from the ratio between the radioactivity concentration in brain and that in peripheral blood. Because of the behavior of blood in the brain microvasculature, however, the concentration of red cells in blood (i.e., the hematocrit) is less in brain than in peripheral large vessels. To correct for this difference, the parameter R (the ratio of cerebral hematocrit to peripheral hematocrit) is incorporated into the calculation. After a 2-min period to allow labeled carboxyhemoglobin to equilibrate throughout the blood pool (Martin et al., 1987), scan data are collected over several minutes. The rCBV, in units of milliliters per 100 g, is calculated from the tissue radiotracer concentration C_t (counts per second per gram) and the average blood radiotracer concentration C_b (counts per second per milliliter), obtained from blood samples during the scan, as follows:*

---

* Note that PET radioactivity measurements are made per cubic centimeter of tissue, but physiological measurements usually are quoted per 100 g of tissue. Therefore, it is necessary to divide tissue radioactivity measurements by the density of brain, 1.05 g · cm^{-3}. For simplicity, neither this operation nor the multiplication by 100 to convert to units of 100 g of tissue will be shown explicitly. In addition, appropriate corrections must be made for the physical decay of blood and tissue radioactivity that occurs during a PET scan (Videen et al., 1987).

$$\text{rCBV} = \frac{C_t}{C_b R} \tag{5.1}$$

A value of 0.85 has been used for R, based on an average of values obtained in both animal and human studies (Phelps et al., 1979a). Determinations of cerebral hematocrit from tomographic measurements of plasma and red-cell volumes indicate, however, that the routine use of this value may be incorrect (Lammertsma et al., 1984; Sakai et al., 1985). Although the same tracer model applied to both $C^{15}O$ and ^{11}CO, the use of ^{15}O has practical advantages. First, the shorter half-life of ^{15}O (2 min versus 20 min for ^{11}C) results in more rapid decay of the radioactive background, so that other PET determinations can be made with little delay. Second, the use of ^{15}O results in lower radiation exposure (Kearfott, 1982). Finally, the rCBV determination is often made in conjunction with measurements of CBF and oxygen metabolism that require ^{15}O-labeled tracers. Using ^{15}O for the rCBV measurement avoids having to change the cyclotron targetry. A representative image of rCBV is shown in Figure 5.7 (top left) (color plate, following page 121).

The measurement of rCBV is of interest in cerebrovascular disease in adults because it reflects vasodilation of the cerebral vasculature in response to decreased perfusion pressure, as may occur with a narrowed internal carotid artery (Powers, 1991). In addition, rCBV data may be required as part of other PET methods to correct for radiotracer located in the intravascular space of the brain, so as to determine the amount of radiotracer that actually enters tissue. This is the case in the measurement of the regional cerebral metabolic rate for oxygen (rCMRO$_2$) with ^{15}O-labeled oxygen. The rCBV method has been applied for this purpose in neonates (Altman et al., 1989), with $C^{15}O$ in air being administered by hand ventilation through an endotracheal tube.

Cerebral blood flow

Kety tissue autoradiographic method

Methods for measuring rCBF with PET are based on a one-compartment model developed by Kety to measure rCBF in laboratory animals (Kety, 1951, 1960; Landau et al., 1955; Sakurada et al., 1978). The model describes inert tracers that can diffuse freely between blood and tissue. The technique involves infusing a radioactive tracer over a brief time period T (e.g., 1 min); the animal is then killed. Frequent, timed arterial blood samples are obtained during the infusion, and regional tissue radioactivity at the end of the infusion is measured by quantitative tissue autoradiography. The rate of change of tracer concentration in any tissue region during the infusion is equal to the rate at which the tracer is transported to tissue in the arterial circulation, minus the rate at which it is washed out from tissue into its venous drainage. This concept is expressed mathematically as

$$\frac{dC_t}{dt} = fC_a - fC_v \tag{5.2}$$

where f is the tissue blood flow (milliliters per 100 g per minute), C_t the tissue radiotracer concentration (counts per second per gram), and C_a and C_v are the tracer concentrations (counts per second per milliliter) in the arterial input and venous drainage. Because it is not possible to measure C_v regionally, Kety introduced a substitution for C_v in terms of C_t and λ, the brain–blood partition coefficient for the tracer, defined as the ratio between the tissue and blood radiotracer concentrations when they are in equilibrium (i.e., $\lambda = C_t/C_v$). Its value can be determined from independent experiments based on this definition or can be calculated as the ratio of the solubilities of the tracer in brain and blood (Kety, 1951; Herscovitch and Raichle, 1985b). When there is no limitation to diffusion of the tracer across the blood–brain barrier, venous radiotracer will be in equilibrium with radiotracer in tissue, so that C_v in equation (5.2) can be replaced by C_t/λ:

$$\frac{dC_t}{dt} = f(C_a - C_t/\lambda) \tag{5.3}$$

This can be integrated and rearranged to give

$$C_t(T) = f \int_0^T C_a(t) \exp[-f/\lambda(T - t)] \, dt \tag{5.4}$$

Equation (5.4) indicates that at time T following the onset of tracer administration, the local brain radiotracer concentration $C_t(T)$ depends on the flow f, the arterial time–activity curve $C_a(t)$, and the partition coefficient. This equation is solved numerically for flow, using measured values for $C_t(T)$ and $C_a(t)$.

Equations (5.3) and (5.4) provide the basis for methods to measure rCBF with PET. The most commonly employed PET tracer for measuring rCBF is ^{15}O-labeled water ($H_2^{15}O$). It is easily synthesized in large quantities (Welch and Kilbourn, 1985). Because of the short half-life of ^{15}O (2 min), relatively large amounts of radioactivity can be used to obtain satisfactory PET images quickly, with an acceptable radiation exposure to the subject. Rapid radioactive decay permits other PET measurements to be performed with little delay. A value for λ can be calculated from the ratio of the water contents of brain and blood (Herscovitch and Raichle, 1985b). Because the water content of brain in neonates is greater than in adults, λ is greater: 1.10 ml · g^{-1}, compared with 0.91 ml · g^{-1}. The appropriate value should be used in rCBF calculations in neonates (Volpe et al., 1985).

Steady-state rCBF method

This was the earliest widely used method for measuring rCBF with PET (Jones, Chesler, and Ter-Pogossian, 1976; Subramanyam et al., 1978; Frackowiak et al., 1980). rCBF is measured while the subject inhales trace amounts of C^{15}O$_2$, which is delivered continuously in air at a constant rate. The catalytic action of carbonic anhydrase in red blood cells in the pulmonary vasculature results in rapid transfer of the ^{15}O label to water. Therefore, H$_2$^{15}O is constantly generated in the lungs and circulates throughout the body. After approximately 10 min, a steady state is reached in which the radioactivity delivered to a brain region in its arterial input equals that leaving the region by radioactive decay and by washout into the venous circulation. The distribution of radioactivity in the brain remains constant, and because the rate of change of regional radioactivity is zero, equation (5.3) can be reformulated as

$$\frac{dC_t}{dt} = f(C_a - C_t/\lambda) - \alpha C_t = 0 \qquad (5.5)$$

where α is the decay constant of ^{15}O (ln 2/half-life of ^{15}O), and the term αC_t is the loss of tracer due to decay. Solving for flow gives

$$f = \frac{\alpha}{C_a/C_t - 1/\lambda} \qquad (5.6)$$

C_a, the arterial radiotracer concentration, is determined by sampling arterial blood, and C_t, the tissue radiotracer concentration, is measured with PET. This method is particularly suited to tomographs that operate accurately only at low count rates, because the rate of radiotracer delivery can be adjusted to suit the count-rate capability. It was especially convenient for use with the early, single-ring tomographs, because multiple tomographic slices could be obtained by repositioning the patient during continued tracer inhalation. Validation studies in experimental animals showed that measured rCBF changed appropriately in response to variations in arterial Pco$_2$ (Rhodes et al., 1981) and that it

was similar to the rCBF measured with a reference microsphere technique (Steinling et al., 1985).

The advantages and limitations of the steady-state method have been extensively analyzed (Lammertsma et al., 1981, 1982; Jones, Greenberg, and Reivich, 1982; Herscovitch and Raichle, 1983; Meyer and Yamamoto, 1984). Most of the limitations arise because there is a nonlinear relationship between rCBF and tissue radiotracer concentration. At higher flow rates, a large change in rCBF will produce a relatively smaller change in brain ^{15}O concentration. Thus, errors in measuring tissue radioactivity will produce proportionately larger errors in flow measurement. Calculated flow values are also sensitive to errors in the measurement of C_a and to any difference between the value of λ used in equation (5.6) and its true value, which may vary in pathological conditions because of changes in brain water content. Because of these limitations, as well as the cumbersome inhalation method of tracer administration, and because of the development of multislice, high-count-rate scanners, the steady-state rCBF method has been largely supplanted by other methods, described later, that use bolus intravenous injection of H$_2$^{15}O.

PET/autoradiographic method

An alternative approach to measuring rCBF with H$_2$^{15}O is the adaptation to PET of Kety's tissue autoradiographic method, as embodied in equation (5.4). The method cannot be used directly in this form because scanners cannot measure the instantaneous brain radiotracer concentration $C_t(T)$. A scan must be performed over many seconds, summing enough counts to obtain a satisfactory PET image. Therefore, equation (5.4) was modified (Herscovitch, Markham, and Raichle, 1983) by an integration of the instantaneous count rate, $C_t(T)$, over the scan time, T_1 to T_2, to correspond to the summing process of tomographic data collection:

$$C = \int_{T_1}^{T_2} C_t(T)\, dT = f \int_{T_1}^{T_2} \int_0^T C_a(t) \exp[-f/\lambda(T - t)]\, dt\, dT \qquad (5.7)$$

C is the local number of counts per gram of tissue recorded by the tomograph during the scan. H$_2$^{15}O is administered by bolus intravenous injection, and a 40-s scan is obtained following arrival of radiotracer in the head (Raichle et al., 1983). Blood is sampled every 4–5 s via an arterial catheter to determine $C_a(t)$. In neonates, H$_2$^{15}O at 0.7 mCi · kg^{-1} in 0.5 ml of saline is injected intravenously, and 0.1–

0.2-ml blood samples are drawn from radial, tibial, or umbilical arterial catheters previously placed for intensive-care purposes (Altman et al., 1988). Equation (5.7) is solved numerically for flow on a pixel-by-pixel basis to convert the PET image of tissue counts to a quantitative CBF image (Figure 5.7, top right). rCBF measurements obtained with this technique have been validated in the baboon by comparison to flow measured in the same animals by intracarotid injection of radiotracer and external residue detection (Raichle et al., 1983).

The relationship between tissue counts and rCBF for the PET-autoradiographic approach is almost linear. This has several advantages (Herscovitch et al., 1983). Errors in measurement of tissue radioactivity result in approximately equivalent errors in rCBF; there is no amplification of error at high flows. Because the PET image of tissue counts closely reflects relative flow differences in different brain regions, useful information about rCBF can be obtained without blood sampling. This approach has been used in neonatal PET studies (Volpe et al., 1983, 1985; Perlman and Altman, 1992). Also, inaccuracy in the value of λ results in minimal error. A relative disadvantage is the need for frequent, accurately timed blood samples. The peripheral arterial time–activity curve is assumed to be equal to the arterial input to the brain. If this is not true, inaccuracy will occur in the calculation of rCBF. In fact, the bolus of radioactivity typically arrives at the arterial sampling site several seconds later than in brain, and there is also dispersion or smearing of the arterial curve as the tracer bolus traverses the arterial system (Iida et al., 1986). Methods have been developed to correct for these effects (Raichle et al., 1983; Iida et al., 1988; Meyer, 1989). To simplify blood sampling, automated blood-counting systems have been designed that continuously draw arterial blood through tubing past a radiation detector (Hutchins, Hichwa, and Koeppe, 1986; Nelson et al., 1990). Because they withdraw relatively large amounts of blood, however, they have not been used in neonates.

Other methods to measure rCBF

Other approaches have been described to measure rCBF, although they have been applied less frequently in clinical research, and not in neonatal studies. These methods are also derived from the Kety model and use $H_2^{15}O$ or other diffusible-flow tracers. One method involves collecting several sequential, brief images after bolus intravenous administration of tracer (Koeppe, Holden, and Ip, 1985). Parameter-estimation techniques are used to estimate both rCBF and λ from the scan data and measurements of arterial radioactivity. Another approach involves using scan data collected after $H_2^{15}O$ injection in two different forms (Huang et al., 1983; Alpert et al., 1984; Carson, Huang, and Green, 1986; Yokoi et al., 1991). The terms in equation (5.3) or (5.4) are multiplied by two time-dependent weighting functions. The resultant two equations are then solved for rCBF and λ. The weighting functions can be selected to minimize the effect of statistical noise in the PET images on the flow calculation. These methods have been less well studied than the methods described earlier and have not been validated experimentally. They do offer potential advantages, including the ability to estimate both rCBF and λ for $H_2^{15}O$, and less sensitivity to dispersion and time shifts in the arterial blood curve.

Flow tracers for PET

All these rCBF methods assume that the radiotracer is freely diffusible across the blood–brain barrier, so that the amount of tracer entering a tissue will depend only on delivery to the region, that is, the local flow. However, $H_2^{15}O$ does not exhibit this ideal behavior. At higher flow rates, there is a progressive decline in the extraction of $H_2^{15}O$ from blood by the brain (Eichling et al., 1974). This results in less tracer entering tissue than would be predicted and leads to an underestimation of rCBF, especially at higher flow values (Raichle et al., 1983). There are other tracers that do not have a diffusion limitation, such as butanol. In comparison with ^{11}C-butanol, $H_2^{15}O$ was found to underestimate rCBF by approximately 15% (Herscovitch et al., 1987). Although ^{11}C-butanol does provide more accurate rCBF estimates, its longer half-life and more complex synthesis make it a less convenient tracer. Recently, ^{15}O-labeled butanol has been developed as a flow tracer; this has the advantages of a short half-life and no diffusion limitation (Berridge, Cassidy, and Terris, 1990; Berridge et al., 1991). It should be noted, however, that the diffusion limitation of $H_2^{15}O$ is not a significant problem in neonates, because in most patients studied, rCBF has been relatively low. Therefore, there is little, if any, underestimation of flow (Altman et al., 1988).

Cerebral oxygen metabolism

Background

rCMRO$_2$ is measured using inhalation of ^{15}O-labeled oxygen ([15]O$_2$). One method, developed in conjunction with the steady-state rCBF technique, uses continuous inhalation of $^{15}O_2$ (Subramanyam et al., 1978; Frackowiak et al., 1980). Another uses a brief inhalation of $^{15}O_2$ and is a companion to the PET/autoradiographic rCBF method (Mintun et al., 1984). The principles underlying these methods are similar. Only a fraction of the oxygen delivered to the brain is extracted and metabolized, approximately 0.40 in normal adult brain. Both methods measure this fraction, termed the oxygen extraction fraction (OEF). There are essentially no stores of oxygen in the brain, and all extracted oxygen is metabolized. Therefore, rCMRO$_2$ can be determined from the product of OEF and the rate of oxygen delivery to the brain, which equals rCBF multiplied by arterial oxygen content. The tracer models describe the fate of the ^{15}O label following $^{15}O_2$ inhalation. The extracted $^{15}O_2$ is converted to ^{15}O-labeled water of metabolism, which is then washed out of the brain. Labeled water of metabolism, produced by the rest of the body and by the brain, recirculates to the brain and diffuses into and out of brain tissue. A large component of the measured radioactivity consists of intravascular $^{15}O_2$ that is not extracted. It is necessary to account for this component, so that it will not be attributed to radioactivity in tissue; that would lead to an overestimation of rOEF. Determination of this intravascular component requires an independent measurement of rCBV using $C^{15}O$. In fact, both the steady-state and brief-inhalation methods require three separate scans to measure rOEF and rCMRO$_2$: an rCBF scan, an rCBV scan, and a scan obtained with $^{15}O_2$. In addition, arterial blood samples are required to measure the components of radioactivity in blood: $^{15}O_2$ bound to hemoglobin and ^{15}O of the water of metabolism in plasma and red cells.

Steady-state method

Scanning is performed during continuous inhalation of $^{15}O_2$ in air delivered through a face mask. rCBF is measured with continuous inhalation of $C^{15}O_2$, and rCBV with $C^{15}O$. rOEF is computed from data obtained during these three scans and from measurements of blood radioactivity (Subramanyam et al., 1978; Frackowiak et al., 1980; Lammertsma and Jones, 1983; Lammertsma et al., 1983). The method has the same practical features as the $C^{15}O_2$ flow technique, being particularly suited to earlier tomographs that required low count rates or that had few slices. Validation studies in which rOEF was directly determined from the cerebral arterial–venous oxygen difference in baboons demon-

strated a 13% overestimation of rOEF, most likely because there was no correction for intravascular tracer in those experiments (Baron et al., 1981). Indirect validation experiments showed that with increasing arterial Pco$_2$, rCBF increased and rOEF decreased, while rCMRO$_2$ remained constant, as would be expected (Rhodes et al., 1981). Deviation from the steady-state requirement of constant arterial radiotracer concentration, caused by fluctuations in either cyclotron delivery of ^{15}O gases or the subject's respiratory pattern, results in inaccuracies in both rCBF and rCMRO$_2$ values with the steady-state method. These can be decreased by using multiple arterial samples or by modifying the tracer model (Senda et al., 1988). Several error analyses of the method have been reported (Lammertsma et al., 1981, 1982; Correia et al., 1985; Herscovitch and Raichle, 1985a).

Brief-inhalation method

Mintun and colleagues described a method for measuring rOEF and rCMRO$_2$ with a brief inhalation of $^{15}O_2$ in air (Mintun et al., 1984; Herscovitch, Mintun, and Raichle, 1985; Videen et al., 1987). The method also involves measurement of rCBF with intravenous H$_2$$^{15}O$ and the PET/autoradiographic approach and measurement of rCBV with inhaled $C^{15}O$. A 40-s emission scan is obtained following brief inhalation of $^{15}O_2$, and frequent arterial blood samples are collected for measurements of blood radioactivity. Representative images are shown in Figure 5.7 (bottom). As with the PET/autoradiographic technique for measuring rCBF, this method requires a tomograph capable of operating at high count rates. Simulation studies demonstrated that measurement errors in rCBV or rCBF cause approximately equivalent percentage errors in rOEF and rCMRO$_2$ determinations at high or normal levels of rCMRO$_2$, although errors are larger at low metabolic rates. The method was validated in baboons by comparing rOEF measured with PET to OEF measured by intracarotid injection of $^{15}O_2$ (Mintun et al., 1984). In those experiments, rOEF was varied over a wide range by changing arterial Pco$_2$, but rCMRO$_2$ varied little. Additional validation experiments showed that the brief-inhalation method can also be used under conditions of reduced rCMRO$_2$ (Altman, Lich, and Powers, 1991). This is of particular relevance to neonatal PET studies, in which reduced rCMRO$_2$ has been observed (Altman et al., 1989).

Both the steady-state and brief-inhalation methods for rCMRO$_2$ measurement require data from three separate scans obtained over 30–60 min. One must assume that during this time, rCBF, rCBV, and rCMRO$_2$ remain constant. In addition, the subject's head must remain in the same position, so that proper registration of the three images will be maintained. A few millimeters of head movement can result in errors in calculated rCMRO$_2$ (Correia et al., 1985). To overcome these difficulties, methods have been sought to estimate rCMRO$_2$ from a single scan obtained after ^{15}O$_2$ administration (Meyer et al., 1987; Ohta et al., 1992). These give estimates of rCMRO$_2$ from data collected over 1–3 min that are similar to those obtained with the three-scan, brief-inhalation method. This approach, if appropriately validated, could facilitate rCMRO$_2$ measurement in the neonate.

Cerebral glucose metabolism

Deoxyglucose method

The most widely used PET technique, the measurement of regional cerebral glucose metabolism (rCMRGlu) with ^{18}F-deoxyglucose (FDG), is based on the deoxyglucose (DG) method to measure rCMRGlu in laboratory animals (Sokoloff et al., 1977; Sokoloff, 1985). Sokoloff's technique uses 2-deoxy-D-[^{14}C]glucose as the metabolic tracer, and tissue autoradiography to determine local brain radioactivity. DG is an analogue of glucose that is transported bidirectionally across the blood–brain barrier by the same transport system as glucose. In tissue, DG is phosphorylated, as is glucose, by hexokinase to form ^{14}C-deoxyglucose-6-phosphate (DG-6-P). Because of its anomalous structure, however, DG-6-P cannot be metabolized further. Also, there is little dephosphorylation of DG-6-P back to DG because of the low activity of glucose-6-phosphatase in brain. As a result of this "metabolic trapping," there is negligible loss of DG-6-P. This facilitates the calculation of rCMRGlu from measurements of local tissue radioactivity. Sokoloff developed a three-compartment model consisting of DG in plasma in brain capillaries, free DG in tissue, and DG-6-P in tissue (Figure 5.8, top). Three rate constants describe the movement of tracer between compartments. An operational equation was derived to calculate rCMRGlu (Figure 5.8, bottom). It contains terms readily measured in laboratory animals: the tissue radiotracer concentration at a single time point, the arterial plasma concentration of DG measured over time, and the plasma glucose concentration. The equation also contains the three rate constants and an additional factor, the lumped constant

(LC), all of which must be specified. The LC corrects for the fact that DG, rather than glucose, is used as the tracer. It accounts for the differences between glucose and DG in transport across the blood–brain barrier and in phosphorylation.

Neither the rate constants nor the LC can be routinely determined in each experimental animal or condition. It was found possible, however, to use standard values for these terms in the operational equation. Calculation of the rate constants requires multiple measurements of tissue radioactivity in animals killed at different times after DG administration. Their values, determined in a separate group of animals, were found to be uniform in gray and white matter. Thus, mean gray- and white-matter values are used. The rate constants, however, can vary in different experimental conditions. A strategy was developed to minimize the error associated with using standard values. The terms in the operational equation containing rate constants approach zero with increasing time. Therefore, a 45-min delay between DG injection and animal death was chosen to minimize this error. A longer period was avoided in order to reduce loss of DG-6-P from tissue due to the small amount of glucose-6-phosphatase activity in brain and because of difficulty in maintaining a physiological steady state. The measurement of the LC in animals on a regional basis would be very difficult. Theoretical arguments demonstrated, however, that the LC should be constant and uniform throughout brain under normal physiological conditions. Therefore, a method was developed to measure the LC of whole brain from the ratio between the brain arterial–venous extraction fraction of DG and that of glucose. The whole-brain LC value, which is species-dependent, is used in the operational equation to calculate rCMRGlu.

The PET FDG technique

The DG method was subsequently adapted for PET (Phelps et al., 1979b; Reivich et al., 1979; Huang et al., 1980). DG was labeled with ^{18}F (110 min half-life) to produce FDG. In the brain, FDG is phosphorylated to FDG-6-P, which is metabolically trapped in the tissue. In order to obtain PET images from the entire brain with the early, single-slice tomographs, it was necessary to scan well beyond the 45-min interval used in experimental animals, and dephosphorylation of FDG-6-P, although small, became more important. To account for this, a fourth rate constant was added to the model. The four rate constants were calculated in a group of normal subjects from serial PET images obtained after FDG adminis-

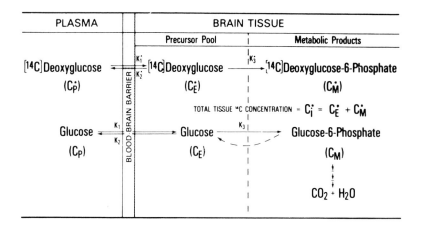

Operational Equation of the Deoxyglucose Method

$$\text{rCMRGlu} = \frac{C_p}{LC} \cdot \frac{C(T) \; - \; k_1^* \exp[-(k_2^* + k_3^*)T] \int_0^T C_p^*(t) \exp[(k_2^* + k_3^*)t] \; dt}{\int_0^T C_p^*(t) \; dt \; - \; \exp[-(k_2^* + k_3^*)T] \int_0^T C_p^*(t) \exp[(k_2^* + k_3^*)t] \; dt}$$

$$= \frac{\text{Plasma glucose}}{\text{Lumped constant}} \cdot \frac{\text{Tissue radioactivity at time } T \; - \; \text{Free DG in tissue at time } T}{\text{Total amount of FDG entering tissue}}$$

Figure 5.8. *Top:* Diagrammatic representation of Sokoloff's three-compartment model used to measure rCMRGlu with DG. The compartments consist of DG in the plasma in brain capillaries, DG in brain tissue, and DG-6-P in tissue. Three rate constants describe the movement of tracer between compartments, two (k_1^*, k_2^*) for the bidirectional transport of DG across the blood–brain barrier between plasma and tissue, and one for the phosphorylation of DG to DG-6-P (k_3^*). The lower portion of the figure shows the metabolic fate of glucose, and the upper portion that of DG. In the adaptation of this model to PET, ^{18}F-labeled DG is used, and a fourth rate constant, k_4^*, is added to account for dephosphorylation of DG-6-P back to DG. (From Sokoloff et al., 1977. Courtesy of Dr. L. Sokoloff and by permission of Raven Press.)
Bottom: Operational equation for the deoxyglucose (DG) method of Sokoloff used to measure rCMRGlu. The equation expressed in words aids in understanding the model. $C(T)$ is

the tissue radioactivity concentration measured at time T at the end of the experiment, typically 45 min after DG administration. The concentration of free DG in tissue at time T is calculated from the plasma concentration of DG over time [$C_p^*(t)$] and the rate constants. The difference between these two terms in the numerator equals the local concentration of DG-6-P that has been formed. The denominator represents the amount of DG delivered to tissue. Therefore, the ratio on the right-hand side of the equation represents the fractional rate of phosphorylation of DG. Multiplying this by the plasma glucose concentration (C_p) would give the rate of glucose phosphorylation if DG and glucose had the same behavior. Because that is not the case, the lumped constant (LC) must be included to account for the difference. In the adaptation of this model to PET using FDG, a fourth rate constant (k_4^*) is included to account for dephosphorylation of DG-6-P, and the operational equation is more complex.

tration. Average gray- and white-matter values were computed for use in the operational equation. Originally, a value for the LC was selected so that the average whole-brain CMRGlu measured with FDG would equal that determined by earlier investigators with the more invasive Kety-Schmidt technique (Phelps et al., 1979b). The LC was subse-

quently measured in humans from determinations of steady-state arterial and internal-jugular-vein concentrations of FDG and glucose (Reivich et al., 1985). To implement the FDG method, PET images are obtained starting about 45 min after intravenous injection of 5–10 mCi of tracer. Blood samples are collected to measure the concentrations of glucose and FDG in plasma as a function of time. Either peripheral arterial blood is sampled or venous sampling is performed from a hand heated to 44°C to "arterialize" venous blood (Phelps et al., 1979b). Scan duration typically is 5–10 min. Even with current multislice tomographs, the subject is often repositioned in the axial direction by a fraction of the slice thickness (e.g., one-half) to further increase axial sampling. The operational equation, with standard values for the four rate constants and LC, is used to generate images of rCMRGlu from the image of tissue counts and the blood measurements.

Application of the DG technique in pathological conditions

The accuracy of using standard values for the rate constants and LC, especially in pathological conditions, has been the subject of considerable discussion (Cunningham and Cremer, 1985; Ingvar and Siesjö, 1985; Baron et al., 1989). The originators of the method noted that these parameters may change in abnormal conditions (Sokoloff et al., 1977; Sokoloff, 1985) and that use of incorrect parameter values results in inaccurate calculation of rCMRGlu. There has been much further work that has yielded a better understanding of the method. As noted earlier, the mathematical form of the operational equation lessens the impact of errors in the rate constants. In pathological conditions such as ischemia (Wienhard et al., 1985; Hawkins, Phelps, and Huang, 1986; Nakai et al., 1987) or tumor (Graham et al., 1989), however, the use of standard rate constants can result in substantial error. Several investigators have suggested alternative formulations of the operational equation to decrease its sensitivity to the rate constants. They have also refined the methods used to calculate rate constants from sequential tomographic images, especially in pathological conditions (Brooks, 1982; Hutchins et al., 1984; Wienhard et al., 1985; Lammertsma et al., 1987). Experiments in both animals and humans have demonstrated that the LC also changes in pathological states. In acute cerebral ischemia and in postischemic tissue in the cat, the LC increased by a factor of more than 1.5 (Nakai et al., 1987; Greenberg et al., 1992). In the presence of recent cerebral infarction in human brain, it is increased 3–6-fold (Gjedde et al., 1985). In other conditions in which the tissue demand for glucose exceeds the supply, such as hypoglycemia (Suda et al., 1990) and seizure (Ingvar and Siesjö, 1985), the LC is increased, and in hyperglycemia it is decreased. The LC was increased in a rat brain

tumor model (Spence et al., 1990). Finally, a 17% decline in the LC in rats of ages 3–24 mo has been reported (Takei, Fredericks, and Rapoport, 1986). Because the calculated rCMRGlu is inversely proportional to the LC (Figure 5.8, bottom), the use of an incorrect value leads to a corresponding error in calculated rCMRGlu. Thus, in pathological conditions, it is necessary to redetermine both the LC and the rate constants to avoid errors in rCMRGlu calculation. These observations are relevant to the use of FDG in the neonatal period, when cerebral ischemia, seizure, and abnormal blood glucose levels may be found. FDG studies in neonates must therefore be interpreted with caution.

rCMRGlu can also be measured with ^{11}C-labeled glucose (Blomqvist et al., 1990). ^{11}C-glucose is transported and metabolized in the same fashion and at the same rate as natural glucose. Therefore, a correction factor such as the LC is not required to account for differences between radiotracer and glucose. A disadvantage is that the labeled metabolites of glucose, such as [11]CO_2, are not all trapped within the tissue. Thus, tracer models must account for the formation and loss of labeled metabolites. The use of ^{11}C-glucose is at a relatively early stage, but with further work it may become more widely applied, especially in pathological conditions.

PET IMAGE DISPLAY AND ANALYSIS

Although visual inspection of PET images may show abnormalities, quantitative data analysis is usually required to obtain scientifically useful information. In fact, the tasks of data reduction, analysis, and interpretation often are very demanding. After a PET study has been performed, the relevant tracer model is used to calculate the corresponding physiological variable. For the methods described earlier to measure CBF and metabolism, the model is applied to PET images on a point-by-point basis. In the resultant images, the intensity is proportional to the local value of the physiological variable. A bar scale indicates this correspondence (Figure 5.7). The analysis of PET images is greatly facilitated by interactive computer programs. Small regions of interest (ROIs) of arbitrary size and shape are placed over selected areas for which the average physiological variable is computed. The location of regions specified on one image (e.g., of CBF) can be stored and used with other physiological images (e.g., of $CMRO_2$) obtained in the same subject. Global measurements can be obtained by averaging over multiple contiguous PET slices. This approach, which has been used in neonatal PET studies, provides whole-brain CBF and metabolic measurements similar to those obtained with the Kety-Schmidt technique (Kety and Schmidt, 1948).

Regional PET measurements must be related to the corresponding anatomic brain regions. Early approaches used PET images obtained in standard planes, such as parallel to the canthomeatal line. The images were visually compared to corresponding anatomic sections in a brain atlas, and ROIs were manually drawn (Duara et al., 1984). That method, however, was subjective and liable to observer bias. Also, it cannot be assumed that PET images based on physiology delineate anatomy, especially if there is local abnormality. An alternative approach uses stereotactic localization (Fox, Perlmutter, and Raichle, 1985). A correspondence is established in three-dimensional space between anatomic regions in a stereotactic brain atlas and specific ROIs on the PET image. This provides objective and reproducible anatomic localization when brain anatomy is normal. Other methods are required when there are structural abnormalities, such as enlarged cerebrospinal fluid (CSF) spaces, or if there is a focal lesion from which PET measurements are desired. An approach being increasingly used in both normal brain and abnormal brain is to obtain anatomic images with computed tomography (CT) or magnetic-resonance imaging (MRI) in the same planes as the PET slices. Several methods have been described to achieve this (Evans et al., 1988; Pelizzari et al., 1989; Wilson and Mountz, 1989). Once coplanar anatomic and PET images are obtained, they can be accessed with an image-analysis program, and ROIs can be transferred between them. Use of these methods has not been reported in neonatal PET. Registration with anatomic images is feasible, however, and would help in the analysis of neonatal PET images, especially if there are focal brain lesions or enlarged CSF spaces.

RADIATION EXPOSURE AND TECHNICAL ISSUES IN NEONATAL PET

Radiation exposure

Although the short half-lives of PET radionuclides favorably affect the radiation exposure to subjects, this exposure is not negligible. Radiation exposure is an important consideration, because scan subjects typically are either normal adult volunteers or patients being studied for research purposes (Veatch, 1982; Huda and Scrimger, 1989). Limits on radiation exposure to research subjects are set by regulatory bodies such as the U.S. Food and Drug Administration and institutional radiation safety committees. The potential risks associated with low levels of radiation, such as those received from PET, are carcinogenesis and genetic effects in future generations (Hilton, 1984; Brill, 1987). Although the risk is very low, it is agreed that the least amount of radiotracer necessary to perform an adequate PET study should be administered. Methods have been developed to determine radiation exposure from internally administered radiopharmaceuticals (Cloutier and Watson, 1987; Loevinger, Budinger, and Watson, 1988; Kassis, 1992). One first determines the distribution of the radiotracer in the body as a function of time following its administration. This information can be calculated using physiological models of in vivo tracer behavior, extrapolated from measurements in animals, or can be measured in a small group of human subjects. Then the radiation exposure to each organ is calculated using a model of the body that simulates the size, shape, and properties of body organs. Appropriate models have been designed for the pediatric age group, including the neonate. Radiation exposures for typical PET studies in neonates, as well as for certain diagnostic procedures, are listed in Table 5.2.

Technical issues in neonatal PET

Clinical research with PET is more complex in neonates than in adults, for several reasons. In many centers, the PET facility is at a distance from the neonatal nursery. Therefore, care of the acutely ill neonate is an important consideration during transportation, as well as during scanning. Arterial blood sampling is required to perform truly quantitative studies. In the adult, arterial catheters can routinely be inserted purely for research purposes (Lockwood, 1985), but in infants, arterial samples have been obtained from catheters previously placed for intensive-care purposes (Volpe et al., 1983). One must limit the volume of blood sampled so as not to compromise the infant, while still obtaining satisfactory data. During a PET scan, it is necessary to prevent head movement. In cooperative adults, this is accomplished by means of a specially designed head holder affixed to the scanner couch. Some neonates studied are so ill that there is little, if any, spontaneous movement, whereas others have been studied while quietly resting or asleep. In one study, thiopental was administered (Shirane et al., 1991); this approach, however, may itself affect CBF and metabolism. Finally, although normal adults frequently are scanned to obtain control data for comparison with patient data, it is not possible to

Table 5.2. *Radiation dosimetry in neonates using PET radiotracers and selected diagnostic nuclear medicine procedures*

Agent/procedure	Dose (mCi)	Radiation exposure (rad)[a]		
		Critical organ	Bone marrow	Ovaries, testes
PET radiopharmaceuticals				
^{18}F-fluorodeoxyglucose (intravenous)[b]	0.24	1.02 (urinary bladder)	0.15	0.19, 0.15
$H_2^{15}O$ (intravenous)[c]	2.5	0.20 (lung, spleen)	0.084	0.12, 0.13
$C^{15}O$ (inhalation)[c]	3.5	0.77 (lung)	0.098	0.16, 0.17
$O^{15}O$ (inhalation)[c]	3.5	0.67 (lung)	0.098	0.15, 0.16
Nuclear-medicine procedures[d]				
Bone, ^{99m}Tc-MDP	0.7	1.5 (large intestine)	—	0.05, 0.04
Lung scan, ^{99m}Tc-MAA	0.2	0.74 (lung)	—	0.015, 0.012
Liver-spleen scan, ^{99m}Tc-sulfur colloid	0.3	0.96 (liver)	0.174	0.043, 0.012

[a]Data for a 3.5-kg newborn, except for ^{18}F-fluorodeoxyglucose, 3.4 kg. The administered dose of radioactivity for a given radiopharmaceutical may vary. The "critical organ" is the organ that receives the greatest radiation exposure. It is not necessarily the organ of physiological interest in the study.
[b]"^{18}FDG Internal Radiation Dosimetry for Use in Research Protocols," L. Coronado, Radiation Safety Branch, National Institutes of Health, Bethesda, MD, October 1991; assumes uniform voiding frequency of 1.5 h.
[c]From Powers et al. (1988).
[d]From Treves (1985).

scan normal neonates. Therefore, careful study design is required to obtain meaningful information from neonatal scans. This has been accomplished in some cases by testing hypotheses that do not require control data (e.g., Altman et al., 1989; Perlman and Altman, 1992). Alternatively, one can retrospectively select subjects scanned for appropriate clinical research indications, either those who had suffered only transient neurologic events not affecting brain development or those in whom neurologic disease was ultimately excluded (Chugani and Phelps, 1991). In spite of the increased complexity of PET in the neonate, several studies have been published, as described later.

PET STUDIES IN THE NEWBORN

Clinical research with PET in the newborn is considerably less well developed than in adults. Studies have been reported from a few medical centers with PET facilities. In general, there are only one or two publications for each clinical condition that has been investigated, so that findings have not been replicated. These studies, as reviewed later, have clearly demonstrated the feasibility and potential of PET in

this age group and also have yielded new insights into the pathophysiology of certain neonatal conditions.

rCBF in premature infants with intraventricular hemorrhage and hemorrhagic intracerebral involvement

Volpe and colleagues used PET to assess rCBF in six premature infants with periventricular-intraventricular hemorrhage (PVH-IVH) and hemorrhagic intracerebral involvement documented by cranial ultrasound (Volpe et al., 1983). Of all patients with PVH-IVH, this group exhibits the highest rates of neurologic morbidity and mortality. Birth weights ranged from 920 to 1,200 g. CBF was measured on postnatal days 5 to 17 with $H_2^{15}O$ and the PET/autoradiographic method. At the time of PET, all infants were stuporous and on ventilators. Although arterial time–activity curves were not always obtained, it was possible to determine relative flow differences because of the linear relationship between image counts and CBF. As would be expected, the scans showed markedly reduced CBF in the region of intracerebral hemorrhage. More interesting, however, were flow decreases more extensive than could be accounted for by the intracerebral blood. These involved cortical and subcortical areas in the affected hemisphere (Figure 5.9; color plate, following page 121).

That report demonstrated the feasibility of PET measurements of rCBF in critically ill neonates. The findings indicate that the hemorrhagic intracerebral involvement was a component of a larger ischemic lesion. Other factors contributing to this observation should be considered, however. Because of limited spatial resolution, the region of very low flow associated with the hemorrhagic parenchymal lesion would appear larger. Also, decreases in cortical flow do not necessarily represent impaired circulation to that region. With a subcortical lesion, rCBF may be depressed in an overlying cortical region because its afferent projections are interrupted, even though it is structurally normal. It is unlikely that these effects would be sufficient to explain all the rCBF findings, however, because the observation of decreased flow in the involved hemisphere was corroborated by postmortem findings of extensive non-hemorrhagic infarction in three infants. That study did not, however, demonstrate the cause and timing of the ischemia. There may have been a primary ischemic injury, possibly due to prior systemic hypotension, with secondary hemorrhagic intracerebral lesions. It is also possible that the ischemic lesion was due to the effects of blood in the lateral ventricle and cerebral parenchyma. It would require a prospective study in premature infants at high risk for developing these lesions to determine if cerebral ischemia occurs first.

rCBF in the term newborn with perinatal asphyxia

In a study by Volpe et al. (1985), scans were obtained with $H_2^{15}O$ and the PET/autoradiographic method in 17 asphyxiated term infants with hypoxic-ischemic encephalopathy (HIE). PET was performed on postnatal days 3 to 5 in 15 infants, on day 7 in 1 infant, and on day 20 in 1 infant. The consistent and apparently unifying abnormality was a relative decrease in rCBF in parasagittal regions, generally symmetrical but more marked posteriorly (Figure 5.10; color plate, following page 121). The affected parasagittal areas showed loss or even reversal of the expected cortical gray-matter-to-white-matter gradient of flow. The ratio of parasagittal to sylvian rCBF, a measure of the relatively lower rCBF in the parasagittal region, was calculated from either absolute rCBF or tissue radioactivity values.

The 8 infants with apparently normal neurologic outcomes had higher values for this ratio than did those with poor outcomes. The severity of these flow defects could not be quantitated precisely, however, because of the lack of normal values for rCBF in this age group and the small number of patients with absolute rCBF measurements. Further indication that these parasagittal deficits represented acute tissue injury, however, was provided by technetium brain scans in 3 patients. These showed increased uptake in parasagittal regions more prominent posteriorly, and they correlated closely with the PET scans. Also, neuropathologic study in 1 infant showed injury to the parasagittal cerebral cortex and subcortical white matter, especially posteriorly. As the authors noted, that study did not demonstrate the pathogenesis of the parasagittal brain injury. They hypothesized, however, that this brain region, the "watershed" between the major cerebral arteries, may be more susceptible to cerebral ischemia that may occur with systemic hypotension.

CBF requirements for brain viability in newborn infants

A study by Altman et al. (1988) provided data on the level of CBF compatible with neuronal viability in newborn infants and also examined the relationship between CBF and neurologic outcome. Measurements of rCBF in adults with cerebrovascular disease have demonstrated that values below 10 ml per 100 g per minute occur only in areas of cerebral infarction, and experimental data from adult animals indicate a similar threshold for neuronal death (Powers et al., 1986; Powers, 1988). The threshold of reversible ischemic neuronal dysfunction is approximately 20 ml per 100 g per minute. The investigators obtained quantitative rCBF measurements with $H_2^{15}O$ and the autoradiographic method in 16 preterm and 14 term infants with a variety of conditions, including PVH-IVH, HIE, and previous extracorporeal membrane oxygenation. Mean whole-brain CBF was measured by averaging PET slices through the cerebral hemispheres. The major observation was that very low whole-brain flow, less than 10 ml per 100 g per minute, was compatible with subsequent normal development. There were 3 preterm infants with normal neurologic examinations and cognitive testing at ages 6 to 24 mo who had mean brain blood flows of 4.9, 5.2, and 9.3, and there was 1 term infant with a mean flow of 9.0 who was developing normally until he died at age 5 mo from septicemia. Three infants with mean CBF values less than 10 had normal neurologic examinations at the time of PET. No significant relationship was observed between mean CBF and neurologic outcome.

That important study demonstrated that mean hemispheric CBF values below 10 and as low as 4.9 ml per 100 g per minute in newborn infants can be associated with a normal neurologic examination and normal neurologic outcome. The infants did not undergo follow-up neuroimaging procedures, so it was possible that some brain injury occurred. However, the low mean CBF values that were observed would, in adults, invariably be associated with destruction of all neuronal tissue. That clearly is not compatible with the normal developmental outcome observed in these infants. The findings were consistent with those of Greisen and Trojaberg (1987), who reported normal visual evoked responses in preterm infants with mean CBF values below 10, an observation suggesting that neuronal viability is preserved at low CBF levels. Another important conclusion of that study was that a single CBF measurement in the newborn does not indicate the degree of brain injury. A low CBF measurement did not predict a poor outcome, but higher values did not assure normal neurologic development. This lack of correlation between CBF and the apparent degree of brain injury is not surprising, however, given the impairment of the control mechanisms for CBF in acute brain injury.

rCBF in newborns after successful extracorporeal membrane oxygenation (ECMO)

Perlman and Altman (1992) studied 23 newborn infants after ECMO to determine whether or not there were reductions in CBF ipsilateral to the ligated common carotid artery. In 14 patients, the carotid remained ligated, but in 9 others it was reanastomosed after ECMO. None of the patients had clinical features of HIE, although 4 had subependymal germinal-matrix hemorrhage, and 2 had cerebellar hemorrhage. The PET studies were performed at a mean of 6 d after decannulation with intravenous $H_2{}^{15}O$ and the autoradiographic method. Right- and left-hemisphere CBF values were determined from PET slices through the cerebral hemispheres, and the right/left hemispheric CBF ratio was then calculated. Although some patients did not have absolute CBF values measured, because of the absence of an arterial line, the autoradiographic technique still permitted accurate right/left comparisons. The right/left CBF ratio was

0.98 in both infant groups, those with permanent carotid ligation and those with reanastomosis. A maximum asymmetry of 8% was observed in 2 infants. The authors concluded that hemispheric CBF is most likely to be symmetric in newborns who have been treated with ECMO if there is no evidence of brain injury. Therefore, the indications for reanastomosis should not include short-term improvement in ipsilateral CBF.

rCBF in an asphyxiated infant during a seizure

rCBF was fortuitously measured during a focal seizure in an infant with HIE and intermittent seizures after intrauterine asphyxia (Perlman et al., 1985). Just before injection of $H_2{}^{15}O$, a seizure began and persisted until after the scan. It consisted of eye deviation to the right, eye jerking, and clonic jerking of the right arm. An electroencephalogram 30 min after PET showed marked suppression of activity and bursts of multifocal sharp activity, particularly in the left-temporal–central-occipital leads. CBF was 40% higher in the left sylvian cortex (80 vs. 57 ml per 100 g per minute) (Figure 5.11; color plate, following page 121). In addition, there was decreased flow in parasagittal cortical regions, especially posteriorly, as has been observed in other asphyxiated term infants (discussed earlier). Therefore, there was an ictal CBF increase in the hemisphere clinically identified to be the site of origin of a focal seizure, similar to observations reported in adults. The authors did note that the interhemispheric difference in CBF could have resulted from increased CBF on the left (due to focal infarction and luxury perfusion) or decreased CBF on the right (due to focal infarction and impaired perfusion). Neither of these possibilities, however, was supported by cranial ultrasound scans. In addition, this degree of CBF asymmetry was not observed in 13 other asphyxiated term infants (Volpe et al., 1985).

Measurement of cerebral oxygen metabolism in newborn infants

Altman et al. (1989, 1993) reported measurements of $CMRO_2$, OEF, CBF, and CBV in 5 preterm and 6 term intubated neonates. They used ^{15}O-radiotracers and the brief-inhalation technique. Whole-brain $CMRO_2$ was calculated by averaging measurements over contiguous PET slices. In 5 of the term infants, mean $CMRO_2$ ranged from 0.4 to 1.3 ml per 100 g per minute; the sixth term infant was brain-dead, and no intracranial radioactivity was detected. Two of the term infants, with $CMRO_2$ of 0.4 and 0.7 ml per 100 g per minute, had no evidence of brain injury in the neonatal period and were developing normally at age 6 mo. In the preterm infants, with gestational ages 26–32 wk, $CMRO_2$ was even lower, 0.54 ml per 100 g per minute or less. $CMRO_2$ was virtually nil, 0.06, in 2 preterm infants who had minimal or no evidence of brain injury in the newborn period.

The demonstration of very low $CMRO_2$ (0.4, 0.7 ml per 100 g per minute) in 2 term infants and a virtual absence of $CMRO_2$ in 2 preterm infants, all with minimal or no evidence of brain injury, is in striking contrast to observations in adults. $CMRO_2$ is normally 3.0–3.5 ml per 100 g per minute in the adult human brain; values below 1.3 have been recorded only in nonviable tissue (Powers, 1988). The authors suggested that cerebral energy requirements in both premature and term newborns may be minimal or that they may be met by nonoxidative mechanisms such as glycolysis. The low OEF values that were also observed may indicate an extensive physiological reserve that could compensate for reductions in cerebral oxygen delivery. They noted that if further studies showed their findings to be common, the importance of hypoxemia in the pathogenesis of perinatal brain injury in preterm infants would need reexamination.

CBF and oxygen metabolism in infants with hydrocephalus

There has been a preliminary report of measurements of CBF, CBV, and $CMRO_2$ with the steady-state inhalation technique in 7 infants under age 2 yr with hydrocephalus (Shirane et al., 1990; 1991). Subjects received intravenous thiopental prior to the scans. The 2 infants studied in the first postnatal month had lower values for both rCBF and $rCMRO_2$ than did the older infants. One, with a Chiari malformation, had cortical $CMRO_2$ less than 0.8 ml per 100 g per minute and OEF values less than 0.20. Although a relatively high resolution scanner was used (7–8 mm), these results should be interpreted with caution because of the potential for partial-volume averaging with enlarged ventricles to have artifactually lowered the PET measurements.

FDG imaging in the term newborn with perinatal asphyxia and/or seizure

FDG imaging in infants was first reported in 5 patients aged 5 to 103 d with structural brain abnormalities seen on CT (Doyle et al., 1983). In the 2 neonates, one with HIE and the other with recurrent seizures, there was decreased FDG uptake in areas of decreased attenuation on CT. That study demonstrated the feasibility of FDG imaging in this population. The same group (Thorp et al., 1988) subsequently reported a study of 20 term infants, 2 with severe hypotonia, and 18 who had had one or more major motor seizures, 11 of whom had also experienced birth asphyxia. The babies were studied at ages ranging from 6 to 17 d. There was no blood sampling, so quantitative rCMRGlu was not calculated. Two patterns, a symmetrical pattern of FDG accumulation, or a loss of "metabolic architecture," with poor differentiation between gray and white matter, correlated with a history of perinatal asphyxia and HIE and an absence of focal echoes on cranial ultrasound. Marked hemispheric asymmetry or localized hypermetabolism or hypometabolism was seen in babies who had suffered mild or no birth asphyxia. No neuropathological studies or long-term follow-up were reported, and the prognostic significance of the various patterns of FDG uptake is unknown. Other investigators, in a preliminary report of FDG imaging in 3 infants with severe perinatal asphyxia, have also noted heterogeneous patterns of FDG accumulation (Suhonen-Polvi et al., 1991). FDG uptake in areas with structural abnormality seen on either CT or ultrasound should be interpreted with caution, however. This is because in abnormal brain regions, relative radioactivity measurements may not reflect relative differences in glucose metabolism, because of possible changes in the rate constants and lumped constant, as discussed earlier.

rCMRGlu during human brain development

Chugani and colleagues reported measurements of rCMRGlu during human brain development (Chugani and Phelps, 1986; Chugani, Phelps, and Mazziotta, 1987). Out of over 100 children with a variety of neurologic syndromes who had undergone PET, they selected 29 who had suffered only transient events that did not affect development or in whom neurologic disease was ultimately excluded. The subjects, ranging from age 5 d to 15 yr, were believed to be reasonably normal, given the impossibility of studying truly normal children. rCMRGlu was measured with FDG using venous blood sampling and values for the rate and lumped constants derived in normal adults. rCMRGlu in gray matter was low at birth (13–25 μmol per 100 g per minute), but rose to adult values (19–33) by 2 yr and subsequently continued to rise to approximately twice adult values. After age 9, there was a decline to

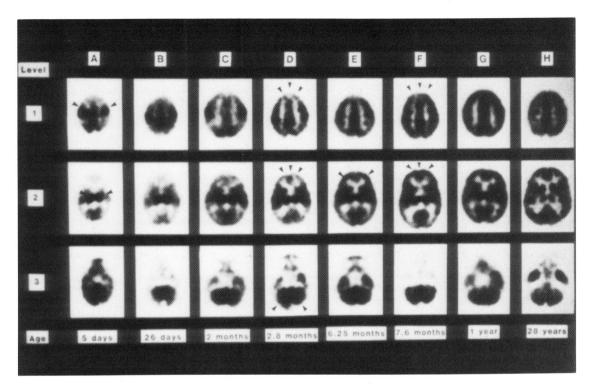

Figure 5.12. Images obtained with FDG that illustrate the developmental changes in rCMRGlu with increasing age. Level 1 is a superior section at the level of the cingulate gyrus, level 2 is at the level of the basal ganglia, and level 3 is at the level of the cerebellum. In the newborn, rCMRGlu is highest in sensorimotor cortex, thalamus, and cerebellar vermis. There

is subsequently a maturation of the metabolic pattern until a pattern similar to that in the adult is seen by age 1 yr. Note that image sizes are not on the same scale, and also images are not shown on the same absolute gray scale of rCMRGlu. (From Chugani et al., 1987. Courtesy of Dr. H. T. Chugani and by permission of Little, Brown and Company.)

adult values by about age 15. Those findings paralleled the pioneering observations of Kennedy and Sokoloff (1957), who, using the Kety-Schmidt technique, found that whole-brain CBF and oxygen metabolism in children aged 3–11 yr were respectively 76% and 23% greater than in young adults. In addition, Chugani observed that the pattern of rCMRGlu in the neonate was different from that in the adult, with rCMRGlu highest in sensorimotor cortex, thalamus, brain stem, and cerebellas vermis (Figure 5.12). By 3 mo, rCMRGlu became more prominent in parietal, temporal, and occipital cortices, basal ganglia, and cerebellar cortex. Subsequently, rCMRGlu increased in frontal cortex, and by age 1 yr the pattern resembled that in adults. Chugani noted that this maturation of the rCMRGlu pattern generally agreed with the behavioral, neurophysiological, and anatomic changes that accompany development in infants. Similar maturation patterns of rCBF and rCMRGlu in relation to development have been demonstrated in the rat, cat,

dog, and monkey (Kennedy et al., 1972, 1982; Nehlig, Pereira de Vasconcelos, and Boyet, 1988, 1989; Chugani et al., 1991).

CONCLUSIONS

This chapter has reviewed the principles of PET, with emphasis on the radiotracer techniques that have been used in the neonate to measure rCBF and metabolism of oxygen and glucose. In spite of the increased complexities involved, this technology has been successfully applied in several clinical research studies in the neonate. Such studies not only have demonstrated the feasibility of PET in the neonate but also have yielded new insights in several important areas. The studies of brain development, CBF and oxygen metabolism levels that are compatible with brain viability, and patterns of blood flow in infants with perinatal injury are particularly noteworthy. These early findings should stimulate further research with PET in the neonatal period.

REFERENCES

Alpert, N. M., Eriksson, L., Chang, J. Y., Bergstrom, M., Litton, J. E., Correia, J. A., Bohm, C., Ackerman, R. H., and Taveras, J. M. (1984). Strategy for the measurement of regional cerebral blood flow using short-lived tracers and emission tomography. *Journal of Cerebral Blood Flow and Metabolism* 4:28–34.

Altman, D. I., Lich, L. L., and Powers, W. J. (1991). Brief inhalation method to measure cerebral oxygen extraction with PET: accuracy determination under pathologic conditions. *Journal of Nuclear Medicine* 32:1738–41.

Altman, D. I., Perlman, J. M., Volpe, J. J., and Powers, W. J. (1989). Cerebral oxygen metabolism in newborn infants measured with positron emission tomography. *Journal of Cerebral Blood Flow and Metabolism* [*Suppl. 1*] 9:25.

—— (1993). Cerebral oxygen metabolism in newborn infants. *Pediatrics* 92:99–104.

Altman, D. I., Powers, W. J., Perlman, J. M., Herscovitch, P., Volpe, S. L., and Volpe, J. J. (1988). Cerebral blood flow requirement for brain viability in newborn infants is lower than in adults. *Annals of Neurology* 24:218–26.

Baron, J. C., Frackowiak, R. S. J., Herholz, K., Jones, T., Lammertsma, A. A., Mazoyer, B., and Weinhard, K. (1989). Use of PET methods for measurement of cerebral energy metabolism and hemodynamics in cerebrovascular disease. *Journal of Cerebral Blood Flow and Metabolism* 9:723–42.

Baron, J. C., Steinling, M., Tanaka, T., Cavalheiro, E., Soussaline, F., and Collard, P. (1981). Quantitative measurement of CBF, oxygen extraction fraction (OEF) and CMRO$_2$ with the ^{15}O continuous inhalation technique and positron emission tomography (PET): experimental evidence and normal values in man. *Journal of Cerebral Blood Flow and Metabolism* [*Suppl. 1*] 1:5–6.

Barrio, J. R. (1991). Approaches to the design of biochemical probes for positron emission tomography. *Neurochemical Research* 16:1047–54.

Bergmann, S. R. (1991). Positron emission tomography of the heart. In *Cardiac Nuclear Medicine*, 2nd ed., ed. M. C. Gerson (pp. 299–335). New York: McGraw-Hill.

Bergstrom, M., Eriksson, L., Bohm, C., Blomqvist, G., and Litton, J. (1983). Correction for scattered radiation in a ring detector positron camera by integral transformation of the projections. *Journal of Computer Assisted Tomography* 7:42–50.

Berridge, M. S., Adler, L. P., Nelson, A. D., Cassidy, E. H., Muzic, R. F., Bednarczyk, E. M., and Miraldi, F. (1991). Measurement of human cerebral blood flow with [^{15}O]butanol and positron emission tomography. *Journal of Cerebral Blood Flow and Metabolism* 11:707–15.

Berridge, M. S., Cassidy, E. H., and Terris, A. H. (1990). A routine, automated synthesis of oxygen-15-labeled butanol for positron tomography. *Journal of Nuclear Medicine* 31:1727–31.

Blomqvist, G., Stone-Elander, S., Halldin, C., Roland, P. E., Widén, L., Lindqvist, M., Swahn, C.-G., Långström, B., and Wiesel, F. A. (1990). Positron emission tomographic measurements of cerebral glu-

cose utilization using [1 – ^{11}C]ᴅ-glucose. *Journal of Cerebral Blood Flow and Metabolism* 11:467–83.

Brill, A. B. (1987). Biological effects of ionizing radiation. In *Nuclear Medical Physics*, ed. L. E. Williams (pp. 163–83). Boca Raton: CRC Press.

Brooks, R. A. (1982). Alternative formula for glucose utilization using labeled deoxyglucose. *Journal of Nuclear Medicine* 23:538–9.

Brooks, R. A., and Di Chiro, G. (1976). Principles of computer assisted tomography (CAT) in radiographic and radioisotopic imaging. *Physics in Medicine and Biology* 21:689–732.

Brooks, R. A., Sank, V. J., Friauf, W. S., Leighton, S. B., Cascio, H. E., and Di Chiro, G. (1981). Design considerations for positron emission tomography. *IEEE Transactions on Biomedical Engineering* 28:158–77.

Budinger, T. F., Derenzo, S. E., Greenberg, W. L., Gullberg, G. T., and Huesman, R. H. (1978). Quantitative potentials of dynamic emission computed tomography. *Journal of Nuclear Medicine* 19:309–15.

Carson, R. E. (1986). Parameter estimation in positron emission tomography. In *Positron Emission Tomography and Autoradiography*, ed. M. E. Phelps, J. C. Mazziotta, and H. R. Schelbert (pp. 347–90). New York: Raven Press.

Carson, R. E., Huang, S.-C., and Green, M. V. (1986). Weighted integration method for local cerebral blood flow measurements with positron emission tomography. *Journal of Cerebral Blood Flow and Metabolism* 6:245–58.

Chugani, H. T., Hovda, D. A., Villablanca, J. R., Phelps, M. E., and Wei-Fang, X. (1991) Metabolic maturation of the brain: a study of local cerebral glucose utilization in the developing cat. *Journal of Cerebral Blood Flow and Metabolism* 11:35–47.

Chugani, H. T., and Phelps, M. E. (1986). Maturational changes in cerebral function in infants determined by ^{18}FDG positron emission tomography. *Science* 231:840–3.

—— (1991). Imaging human brain development with positron emission tomography. *Journal of Nuclear Medicine* 32:23–6.

Chugani, H. T., Phelps, M. E., and Mazziotta, J. C. (1987). Positron emission tomography study of human brain functional development. *Annals of Neurology* 22:487–97.

Cloutier, R. J., and Watson, E. E. (1987). Internal dosimetry – an introduction to the ICRP technique. In *Nuclear Medical Physics*, ed. L. E. Williams (p. 143). Boca Raton: CRC Press.

Correia, J. A., Alpert, N. M., Buxton, R. B., and Ackerman, R. H. (1985). Analysis of some errors in the measurement of oxygen extraction and oxygen consumption by the equilibrium inhalation method. *Journal of Cerebral Blood Flow and Metabolism* 5:591–9.

Council on Scientific Affairs (1988a). Cyclotrons and radiopharmaceuticals in positron emission tomography. *Journal of the American Medical Association* 259:1854–60.

—— (1988b). Instrumentation in positron emission tomography. *Journal of the American Medical Association* 259:1351–6.

—— (1988c). Positron emission tomography in oncology. *Journal of the American Medical Association* 259:2126–31.

Cunningham, V., and Cremer, J. E. (1985). Current assumptions behind the use of PET scanning for measuring glucose utilization in brain. *Trends in Neurosciences* 8:96–9.

Cutler, P. D., Cherry, S. R., Hoffman, E. J., Digby, W. M., and Phelps, M. E. (1992). Design features and performance of a PET system for animal research. *Journal of Nuclear Medicine* 33:595–604.

Dannals, R. F., Ravert, H. T., and Wilson, A. A. (1990). Radiochemistry of tracers for neurotransmitter receptor studies. In *Quantitative Imaging: Neuroreceptors, Neurotransmitters, and Enzymes,* ed. J. J. Frost and H. N. Wagner (pp. 19–35). New York: Raven Press.

Daube-Witherspoon, M. E., and Carson, R. E. (1991). Unified deadtime correction model for PET. *IEEE Transactions on Medical Imaging* 10:267–75.

DeGrado, T. R., Turkington, T., Williams, J. J., Stearns, C. W., Hoffman, J. M., and Coleman, R. E. (1994). Performance characteristics of a whole-body PET scanner. *Journal of Nuclear Medicine* 35:1398–1406.

Derenzo, S. E., Huesman, R. H., Cahoon, J. L., Geyer, A. B., Moses, W. W., Uber, D., Vuletich, T., and Budinger, T. F. (1988). A positron tomograph with 600 BGO crystals and 2.6 mm resolution. *IEEE Transactions on Nuclear Science* 35:659–64.

Doyle, L. W., Nahmias, C., Firnau, G., Kenyon, D. B., Garnett, E. S., and Sinclair, J. C. (1983). Regional cerebral glucose metabolism of newborn infants measured by positron emission tomography. *Developmental Medicine and Child Neurology* 25:143–51.

Duara, R., Grady, C., Haxby, J., Ingvar, D., Sokoloff, L., Margolin, R. A., Manning, R. G., Cutler, N. R., and Rapoport, S. I. (1984). Human brain glucose utilization and cognitive function in relation to age. *Annals of Neurology* 16:702–13.

Eichling, J. O. Raichle, M. E., Grubb, R. J., Jr., and Ter-Pogrossian, M. M. (1974). Evidence of the limitations of water as a freely diffusible tracer in the brain of the rhesus monkey. *Circulation Research* 35: 358–64.

Evans, A. C., Thompson, C. J., Marrett, S., Meyer, E., and Mazza, M. (1991). Performance evaluation of the PC-2048: a new 15-slice encoded-crystal PET scanner for neurological studies. *IEEE Transactions on Medical Imaging* 10:90–8.

Fowler, J. S., and Wolf, A. P. (1991). Recent advances in radiotracers for PET studies of the brain. In *Radiopharmaceuticals and Brain Pathology Studied with PET and SPECT,* ed. M. Diksic and R. C. Reba (pp. 11–34). Boca Raton: CRC Press.

Fox, P. T., Perlmutter, J. S., and Raichle, M. E. (1985). A stereotactic method of anatomical localization for positron emission tomography. *Journal of Computer Assisted Tomography* 9:141–53.

Frackowiak, R. S. J., Lenzi, G.-L., Jones, T., and Heather, J. D. (1980). Quantitative measurement of regional cerebral blood flow and oxygen metabolism in man using ^{15}O and positron emission tomography: theory, procedure and normal values. *Journal of Computer Assisted Tomography* 4:727–36.

Gjedde, A., Wienhard, K., Heiss, W.-D., Kloster, G., Diemer, N. H., Herholz, K., and Pawlik, G. (1985). Comparative regional analysis of 2-fluorodeoxyglucose and methylglucose uptake in brain of four stroke patients. With special reference to the regional estimation of the lumped constant. *Journal of Cerebral Blood Flow and Metabolism* 5:163–78.

Gjedde, A., and Wong, D. F. (1990). Modelling neuro-

receptor binding of radioligands in vivo. In *Quantitative Imaging: Neuroreceptors, Neurotransmitters, and Enzymes,* ed. J. J. Frost and H. N. Wagner (pp. 51–79). New York: Raven Press.

Grafton, S. T., and Mazziotta, J. C. (1992). Cerebral pathophysiology evaluated with positron emission tomography. In *Diseases of the Nervous System: Clinical Neurobiology,* 2nd ed., ed. A. K. Asbury, C. M. McKhann, and W. I. McDonald (pp. 1573–88). Philadelphia: W. B. Saunders.

Graham, M. M., Spence, A. M., Muzi, M., and Abbott, G. L. (1989). Deoxyglucose kinetics in a rat brain tumor. *Journal of Cerebral Blood Flow and Metabolism* 9:315–22.

Greenberg, J. H., Hamar, J., Welsh, F. A., Harris, V., and Reivich, M. (1992). Effect of ischemia and reperfusion on λ of the lumped constant of the $[^{14}C]$ deoxyglucose technique. *Journal of Cerebral Blood Flow and Metabolism* 12:70–7.

Greisen, G., and Trojaberg, W. (1987). Cerebral blood flow, $Paco_2$ changes, and visual evoked potentials in mechanically ventilated, preterm infants. *Acta Pediatrica Scandinavica* 76:394–400.

Grubb, R. L., Jr., Raichle, M. E., Higgins, C. S., and Eichling, J. O. (1978). Measurement of regional cerebral blood volume by emission tomography. *Annals of Neurology* 4:322–8.

Hawkins, R. A., Phelps, M. E., and Huang, S.-C. (1986). Effects of temporal sampling, glucose metabolic rates, and disruptions of the blood-barrier on the FDG model with and without a vascular compartment: studies in human brain tumors with PET. *Journal of Cerebral Blood Flow and Metabolism* 6:170–83.

Herscovitch, P., Auchus, A., Gado, M., Chi, D., and Raichle, M. E. (1986). Correction of positron emission tomography data for cerebral atrophy. *Journal of Cerebral Blood Flow and Metabolism* 6:120–4.

Herscovitch, P., Markham, J., and Raichle, M. E. (1983). Brain blood flow measured with intravenous $H_2{}^{15}O$. I. Theory and error analysis. *Journal of Nuclear Medicine* 24:782–9.

Herscovitch, P., Mintun, M. A., and Raichle, M. E. (1985). Brain oxygen utilization measured with oxygen-15 radiotracers and positron emission tomography: generation of metabolic images. *Journal of Nuclear Medicine* 26:416–17.

Herscovitch, P., and Raichle, M. E. (1983). Effect of tissue heterogeneity on the measurement of cerebral blood flow with the equilibrium $C^{15}O_2$ inhalation technique. *Journal of Cerebral Blood Flow and Metabolism* 3:407–15.

(1985a). Effect of tissue heterogeneity on the measurement of regional cerebral oxygen extraction and metabolic rate with positron emission tomography. *Journal of Cerebral Blood Flow and Metabolism* [Suppl. 1] 5:671–2.

(1985b). What is the correct value for the brain-blood partition coefficient of water? *Journal of Cerebral Blood Flow and Metabolism* 5:65–9.

Herscovitch, P., Raichle, M. E., Kilbourn, M. R., and Welch, M. J. (1987). Positron emission tomographic measurements of cerebral blood flow and permeability–surface area product of water using $[^{15}O]$ water and $[^{11}C]$butanol. *Journal of Cerebral Blood Flow and Metabolism* 7:527–42.

Hilton, J. W. (1984). Radiation effects and protection in children. In *Practical Pediatric Radiology,* ed. S. v. H.

Hilton, D. K. Edwards, and J. Hilton (pp. 575–603). Philadelphia: W. B. Saunders.

Hoffman, E. J., Huang, S.-C., and Phelps, M. E. (1979). Quantitation in positron emission computed tomography: 1. Effect of object size. *Journal of Computer Assisted Tomography* 3:299–308.

Hoffman, E. J., Huang, S.-C., Phelps, M. E., and Kuhl, D. E. (1981). Quantitation in positron emission computed tomography: 4. Effect of accidental coincidences. *Journal of Computer Assisted Tomography* 5:491–500.

Hoffman, E. J., and Phelps, M. E. (1986). Positron emission tomography: principles and quantitation. In *Positron Emission Tomography and Autoradiography*, ed. M. E. Phelps, J. C. Mazziotta, and H. R. Schelbert (pp. 237–86). New York: Raven Press.

Huang, S.-C., Carson, R. E., Hoffman, E. J., Carson, J., MacDonald, N., Barrio, J. R., & Phelps, M. E. (1983). Quantitative measurement of local cerebral blood flow in humans by positron computed tomography and ^{15}O-water. *Journal of Cerebral Blood Flow and Metabolism* 3:141–53.

Huang, S.-C., Phelps, M. E., Hoffman, E. J., Sideris, K., Selin, C. J., and Kuhl, D. E. (1980). Non-invasive determination of local cerebral metabolic rate of glucose in man. *American Journal of Physiology* 238:E69–E82.

Huda, W., and Scrimger, J. W. (1989). Irradiation of volunteers in nuclear medicine. *Journal of Nuclear Medicine* 30:260–4.

Hutchins, G. D., Hichwa, R. D., and Koeppe, R. A. (1986). A continuous flow input function detector for O-15 H$_2$O blood flow studies in positron emission tomography. *IEEE Transactions on Nuclear Science* 33:546–9.

Hutchins, G. D., Holden, J. E., Koeppe, R. A., Halama, J. R., Gatley, S. J., and Nickles, R. J. (1984). Alternative approach to single-scan estimation of cerebral glucose metabolic rate using glucose analogs, with particular application to ischemia. *Journal of Cerebral Blood Flow and Metabolism* 4:35–40.

Iida, H., Kanno, I., Miura, S., Murakami, M., Takahashi, K., and Uemura, K. (1986). Error analysis of a quantitative cerebral blood flow measurement using H$_2$^{15}O autoradiography and positron emission tomography, with respect to the dispersion of the input function. *Journal of Cerebral Blood Flow and Metabolism* 6:536–45.

(1988). Evaluation of regional differences of tracer appearance time in cerebral tissues using [^{15}O] water and dynamic positron emission tomography. *Journal of Cerebral Blood Flow and Metabolism* 8:285–8.

Ingvar, M., and Siesjö, B. K. (1985). Measurements of brain glucose utilization in pathological states: problems and pitfalls. In *The Metabolism of the Human Brain Studied with Positron Emission Tomography*, ed. T. Greitz, D. H. Ingvar, and L. Widén (pp. 195–205). New York: Raven Press.

Jamieson, D. G., and Greenberg, J. H. (1989). Positron emission tomography of the brain. *Computerized Medical Imaging and Graphics* 13:61–79.

Jones, S. C., Greenberg, J. H., and Reivich, M. (1982). Error analysis for the determination of cerebral blood flow with the continuous inhalation of ^{15}O-labeled carbon dioxide and positron emission tomography. *Journal of Computer Assisted Tomography* 6:116–24.

Jones, T., Chesler, D. A., and Ter-Pogossian, M. M. (1976). The continuous inhalation of oxygen-15 for assessing regional oxygen extraction in the brain of man. *British Journal of Radiology* 49:339–43.

Karp, J. S., Daube-Witherspoon, M. E., Hoffman, E. J., Lewellen, T. K., Links, J. M., Wong, W.-H., Hichwa, R. D., Casey, M. E., Colsher, J. G., Hitchens, R. E., Muehllehner, G., and Stoub, E. (1991). Performance standards in positron emission tomography. *Journal of Nuclear Medicine* 32:2342–50.

Kassis, A. I. (1992). The MIRD approach: remembering the limitations. *Journal of Nuclear Medicine* 33:781–2.

Kearfott, K. J. (1982). Absorbed dose estimates for positron emission tomography (PET): C^{15}O, ^{11}CO, and CO^{15}O. *Journal of Nuclear Medicine* 23:1031–7.

Kennedy, C., Grave, G. D., Jehle, J. W., and Sokoloff, L. (1972). Changes in blood flow in the component structures of the dog brain during postnatal maturation. *Journal of Neurochemistry* 19:2423–33.

Kennedy, C., Sakurada, O., Shinohara, M., and Miyaoka, M. (1982). Local cerebral glucose utilization in the newborn macaque monkey. *Annals of Neurology* 12:333–40.

Kennedy, C., and Sokoloff, L. (1957). An adaptation of the nitrous oxide method to the study of the cerebral circulation in children; normal values for cerebral blood flow and cerebral metabolic rate in childhood. *Journal of Clinical Investigation* 36:1130–7.

Kessler, R. M., Ellis, J. R., Jr., and Eden, M. (1984). Analysis of emission tomographic scan data: limitations imposed by resolution and background. *Journal of Computer Assisted Tomography* 8:514–22.

Kety, S. S. (1951). The theory and applications of the exchange of inert gas at the lungs and tissues. *Pharmacological Reviews* 3:1–41.

(1960). Measurement of local blood flow by the exchange of an inert diffusible substance. *Methods in Medical Research* 8:228–36.

Kety, S. S., and Schmidt, C. F. (1948). The nitrous oxide method for the quantitative determination of cerebral blood flow in man: theory, procedure, and normal values. *Journal of Clinical Investigation* 27:476–83.

Kilbourn, M. (1991). Radiotracers for PET studies of neurotransmitter binding sites: design considerations. In *In Vivo Imaging of Neurotransmitter Functions in Brain, Heart and Tumors*, ed. D. E. Kuhl (pp. 47–65). Washington, DC: American College of Nuclear Physicians.

Kilbourn, M. R. (1990). *Fluorine-18 Labeling of Radiopharmaceuticals*. Washington, DC: National Academy Press.

Koeppe, R. A., Holden, J. E., and Ip, W. R. (1985). Performance comparison of parameter estimation techniques for the quantitation of local cerebral blood flow by dynamic positron computed tomography. *Journal of Cerebral Blood Flow and Metabolism* 5:224–34.

Lammertsma, A. A., Brooks, D. J., Beaney, R. P., Turton, D. R., Kensett, M. J., Heather, J. D., Marshall, J., and Jones, T. (1984). In vivo measurement of regional cerebral haematocrit using positron emission tomography. *Journal of Cerebral Blood Flow and Metabolism* 4:317–22.

Lammertsma, A. A., Brooks, D. J., Frackowiak, R. S. J., Beany, R. P., Herold, S., Heather, J. D., Palmer, A. J., and Jones, T. (1987). Measurement of glucose utilization with [^{18}F]2-fluoro-2-deoxy-D-glucose: a comparison of different analytical methods. *Journal of Cerebral Blood Flow and Metabolism* 7:161–72.

Lammertsma, A. A., Heather, J. D., Jones, T.,

Frackowiak, R. S. J., and Lenzi, G.-L. (1982). A statistical study of the steady-state technique for measuring regional cerebral blood flow and oxygen utilization using ^{15}O. *Journal of Computer Assisted Tomography* 6:566–73.

Lammertsma, A. A., and Jones, T. (1983). Correction for the presence of intravascular oxygen-15 in the steady-state technique for measuring regional oxygen extraction ratio in the brain. 1. Description of the method. *Journal of Cerebral Blood Flow and Metabolism* 13:416–24.

Lammertsma, A. A., Jones, T., Frackowiak, R. S. J., and Lenzi, G.-L. (1981). A theoretical study of the steady-state model for measuring regional cerebral blood flow and oxygen utilization using oxygen-15. *Journal of Computer Assisted Tomography* 5:544–50.

Lammertsma, A. A., and Mazoyer, B. M. (1990). EEC concerted action on cellular degeneration and regeneration studies with PET: modelling expert meeting, blood flow measurement with PET. *European Journal of Nuclear Medicine* 16:807–12.

Lammertsma, A. A., Wise, R. J. S., Heather, J. D., Gibbs, J. M., Leenders, K. L., Frackowiak, R. S. J., Rhodes, C. G., and Jones, T. (1983). Correction for the presence of intravascular oxygen-15 in the steady-state technique for measuring regional oxygen extraction ratio in the brain. 2. Results in normal subjects and brain tumor and stroke patients. *Journal of Cerebral Blood Flow and Metabolism* 3:425–31.

Landau, W. M., Freygang, W. H., Jr., Rowland, L. P., Sokoloff, L., and Kety, S. (1955). The local circulation of the living brain; values in the unanesthetized and anesthetized cat. *Transactions of the American Neurological Association* 80:125–9.

Lassen, N. A., and Ingvar, D. H. (1972). Radioisotopic assessment of regional cerebral blood flow. *Progress in Nuclear Medicine* 1:376–409.

Lassen, N. A., and Perl, W. (1979). *Tracer Kinetic Methods in Medical Physiology*. New York: Raven Press.

Lockwood, A. H. (1985). Invasiveness in studies of brain function by positron emission tomography. *Journal of Cerebral Blood Flow and Metabolism* 5:487–9.

Loevinger, R., Budinger, T. F., and Watson, E. E. (1988). *MIRD Primer for Absorbed Dose Calculations*. New York: Society of Nuclear Medicine.

Martin, W. R. W., Powers, W. J., and Raichle, M. E. (1987). Cerebral blood volume measured with inhaled $C^{15}O$ and positron emission tomography. *Journal of Cerebral Blood Flow and Metabolism* 7:421–6.

Mazziotta, J. C., Phelps, M. E., Plummer, D., and Kuhl, D. E. (1981). Quantitation in positron computed tomography. 5. Physical-anatomical effects. *Journal of Computer Assisted Tomography* 5:734–43.

Meyer, E. (1989). Simultaneous correction for tracer arrival delay and dispersion in CBF measurements by the $H_2^{15}O$ autoradiographic method and dynamic PET. *Journal of Nuclear Medicine* 30:1069–78.

Meyer, E., Tyler, J. L., Thompson, C. J., Redies, C., Diksic, M., and Hakim, A. M. (1987). Estimation of cerebral oxygen utilization rate by single-bolus $^{15}O_2$ inhalation and dynamic positron emission tomography. *Journal of Cerebral Blood Flow and Metabolism* 7:403–14.

Meyer, E., and Yamamoto, Y. L. (1984). The requirement for constant arterial radioactivity in the $C^{15}O_2$ steady-state blood-flow model. *Journal of Nuclear Medicine* 25:455–560.

Mintun, M. A., Raichle, M. E., Martin, W. R. W., and

Herscovitch, P. (1984). Brain oxygen utilization measured with O-15 radiotracers and positron emission tomography. *Journal of Nuclear Medicine* 25:177–87.

Muehllehner, G., and Karp, J. S. (1986). Positron emission tomography imaging – technical consideration. *Seminars in Nuclear Medicine* 16:35–50.

Nakai, H., Yamamoto, Y. L., Diksic, M., Matsuda, H., Takara, E., Meyer, E., and Redies, C. (1987). Time-dependent changes of lumped and rate constants in the deoxyglucose method in experimental cerebral ischemia. *Journal of Cerebral Blood Flow and Metabolism* 7:640–8.

Nehlig, A., Pereira de Vasconcelos, A., and Boyet, S. (1988). Quantitative autoradiographic measurement of local cerebral glucose utilization in freely moving rats during postnatal development. *Journal of Neuroscience* 8:2321–3.

(1989). Postnatal changes in local cerebral blood flow measured by the quantitative autoradiographic [^{14}C]iodoantipyrine technique in freely moving rats. *Journal of Cerebral Blood Flow and Metabolism* 9:579–88.

Nelson, A. D., Muzic, R. F., Miraldi, F., Muswick, G. J., Leisure, G. P., and Voelker, W. (1990). Continuous arterial positron monitor for quantitation in PET imaging. *American Journal of Physiological Imaging* 5:84–8.

Obrist, W. D., Thompson, H. K., King, C. H., and Wang, H. S. (1967). Determination of regional cerebral blood flow by inhalation of xenon-133. *Circulation Research* 20:124–35.

Ohta, S., Meyer, E., Thompson, C. J., and Gjedde, A. (1992). Oxygen consumption of the living human brain measured after a single inhalation of positron emitting oxygen. *Journal of Cerebral Blood Flow and Metabolism* 12:179–92.

Pelizzari, C. A., Chen, G. T. Y., Spelbring, D. R., Weichselbaum, R. R., and Chen, C.-T. (1989). Accurate three-dimensional registration of CT, PET, and/or MR images of the brain. *Journal of Computer Assisted Tomography* 13:20–6.

Perlman, J. M., and Altman, D. I. (1992). Symmetric cerebral blood flow in newborns who have undergone successful extracorporeal membrane oxygenation. *Pediatrics* 89:235–9.

Perlman, J. M., Herscovitch, P., Kreusser, K. L., Raichle, M. E., and Volpe, J. J. (1985). Positron emission tomography in the newborn: effect of seizure on regional cerebral blood flow in an asphyxiated infant. *Neurology* 35:244–7.

Phelps, M. E., and Hoffman, E. J. (1976). Resolution limit of positron cameras. *Journal of Nuclear Medicine* 17:757–8.

Phelps, M. E., Hoffman, E. J., Huang, S.-C., and Kuhl, D. E. (1979). Design considerations in positron computed tomography. *IEEE Transactions on Nuclear Science* NS-26:2746–51.

Phelps, M. E., Hoffman, E. J., Huang, S.-C., and Ter-Pogossian, M. M. (1975a). Effect of positron range on spatial resolution. *Journal of Nuclear Medicine* 16:649–52.

Phelps, M. E., Hoffman, E. J., Mullani, N. A., and Ter-Pogossian, M. M. (1975b). Application of annihilation coincidence detection to transaxial reconstruction tomography. *Journal of Nuclear Medicine* 16:210–24.

Phelps, M. E., Huang, S. C., Hoffman, E. J., and Kuhl, D. E. (1979a). Validation of tomographic measurement of cerebral blood volume with C-11-labeled car-boxyhemoglobin. *Journal of Nuclear Medicine* 20:328–34.

Phelps, M. E., Huang, S. C., Hoffman, E. J., Selin, C., Sokoloff, L., and Kuhl, D. E. (1979b). Tomographic measurement of local cerebral glucose metabolic rate in humans with (F-18)2-fluoro-2-deoxy-D-glucose: validation of method. *Annals of Neurology* 6:371–88.

Powers, W. J. (1988). Positron emission tomography in the evaluation of cerebrovascular disease: clinical applications? In *Clinical Neuroimaging*, ed. W. H. Theodore (pp. 49–74). New York: Alan R. Liss. (1991). Cerebral hemodynamics in ischemic cerebrovascular disease. *Annals of Neurology* 29:231–40.

Powers, W. J., Grubb, R. L., Jr., Darriet, D., and Raichle, M. E. (1986). CBF and CMRO$_2$ requirements for cerebral function and viability in humans. *Journal of Cerebral Blood Flow and Metabolism* 5:600–8.

Powers, W. J., Stabin, M., Howse, D., Eichling, J. O., and Herscovitch, P. (1988). Radiation absorbed dose estimates for oxygen-15 radiopharmaceuticals (H$_2^{15}$O, C^{15}O, O^{15}O) in newborn infants. *Journal of Nuclear Medicine* 29:1961–70.

Raichle, M. E., Martin, W. R. W., Herscovitch, P., Mintun, M. A., and Markham, J. (1983). Brain blood flow measured with intravenous H$_2^{15}$O. II. Implementation and validation. *Journal of Nuclear Medicine* 24:790–8.

Reivich, M., Alavi, A., Wolf, A., Fowler, J., Russell, J., Arnett, C., MacGregor, R. R., Shiue, C. Y., Atkins, H., Anand, A., Dann, R., and Greenberg, J. H. (1985). Glucose metabolic rate kinetic model parameter determination in humans: the lumped constants and rate constants for [^{18}F]fluorodeoxyglucose and [^{11}C]deoxyglucose. *Journal of Cerebral Blood Flow and Metabolism* 5:179–92.

Reivich, M., Kuhl, D., Wolf, A., Greenberg, J., Phelps, M., Ido, T., Casella, V., Fowler, J., Hoffman, E., Alavi, A., Som, P., and Sokoloff, L. (1979). The (^{18}F)-fluorodeoxy-glucose method for the measurement of local cerebral glucose utilization in man. *Circulation Research* 44:127–37.

Rhodes, C. G., Lenzi, G. L., Frackowiak, R. S. J., Jones, T., and Pozzilli, C. (1981). Measurement of CBF and CMRO$_2$ using continuous inhalation of C^{15}O$_2$ and ^{15}O$_2$: experimental validation using CO$_2$ reactivity in the anesthetised dog. *Journal of the Neurological Sciences* 50:381–9.

Sakai, F., Nakazawa, K., Tazaki, Y., Ishii, K., Hino, H., Igarushi, H., and Kanda, T. (1985). Regional cerebral blood volume and hematocrit measured in normal human volunteers by single-photon emission computed tomography. *Journal of Cerebral Blood Flow and Metabolism* 5:207–13.

Sakurada, O., Kennedy, C., Jehle, J., Brown, J. D., Carbon, G. L., and Sokoloff, L. (1978). Measurement of local cerebral blood flow with iodo[^{14}C]antipyrine. *American Journal of Physiology* 234:H59–H66.

Senda, M., Buxton, R. B., Alpert, N. M., Correia, J. A., Mackay, B. C., Weise, S. B., and Ackerman, R. H. (1988). The ^{15}O steady-state method: correction for variation in arterial concentration. *Journal of Cerebral Blood Flow and Metabolism* 8:681–90.

Shipley, R. A., and Clark, R. E. (1972). *Tracer Methods for In Vivo Kinetics*. New York: Academic Press.

Shirane, R., Sato, S., Kameyama, M., Ogawa, A.,

Yoshimoto, T., Hatazawa, J., and Ito, M. (1991). Cerebral blood flow and oxygen metabolism in infants with hydrocephalus measured with positron emission tomography. *Journal of Cerebral Blood Flow and Metabolism [Suppl. 2]* 11:199.

Shirane, R., Sato, S., Sato, K., Kameyama, M., Yoshimoto, T., Hatazawa, J., and Ito, M. (1990). Cerebral blood flow and oxygen metabolism in children with hydrocephalus. In *CYRIC Annual Report*, ed. H. Orihara, M. Fujioka, T. Ido, T. Nakamura, and M. Itoh (pp. 191–9). Sendai: Tohoku University.

Shuster, D. P. (1989). Positron emission tomography: theory and its application to the study of lung disease. *American Review of Respiratory Disease* 139:818–40.

Sokoloff, L. (1985). Basic principles in imaging of cerebral metabolic rates. In *Brain Imaging and Brain Function*, ed. L. Sokoloff (pp. 21–49). New York: Raven Press.

Sokoloff, L., Reivich, M., Kennedy, C., Des Rosiers, M. H., Patlak, C. S., Pettigrew, K. D., Sakurada, O., and Shinohara, M. (1977). The [^{14}C]deoxyglucose method for the measurement of local cerebral glucose utilization; theory, procedure, and normal values in the conscious and anesthetized albino rat. *Journal of Neurochemistry* 28:897–916.

Sorenson, J. A., and Phelps, M. E. (1987). Tracer kinetic modeling. In *Physics in Nuclear Medicine*, 2nd ed. (pp. 465–517). Orlando: Grune & Stratton.

Spence, A. M., Graham, M. M., Muzi, M., Abbott, G. L., Krohn, K. A., Kapoor, R., and Woods, S. D. (1990). Deoxyglucose lumped constant estimated in a transplanted rat astrocytic glioma by the hexose utilization index. *Journal of Cerebral Blood Flow and Metabolism* 10:190–8.

Steinling, M., Baron, J. C., Maziere, B., Lasjaunias, P., Loc'h, C., Cabanis, E. A., and Guillon, B. (1985). Tomographic measurement of cerebral blood flow by the ^{68}Ga-labelled-microsphere and continuous-C^{15}O$_2$-inhalation methods. *European Journal of Nuclear Medicine* 11:29–32.

Strauss, L. G., and Conti, P. S. (1991). The applications of PET in clinical oncology. *Journal of Nuclear Medicine* 32:623–48.

Subramanyam, R., Alpert, N. M., Hoop, B., Jr., Brownell, G. L., and Taveras, J. M. (1978). A model for regional cerebral oxygen distribution during continuous inhalation of ^{15}O$_2$, C^{15}O, and C^{15}O$_2$. *Journal of Nuclear Medicine* 19:13–53.

Suda, S., Shinohara, M., Miyaoka, M., Lucignani, G., Kennedy, C., and Sokoloff, L. (1990). The lumped constant of the deoxyglucose method in hypoglycemia: effects of moderate hypoglycemia on local cerebral glucose utilization in the rat. *Journal of Cerebral Blood Flow and Metabolism* 10:499–509.

Suhonen-Polvi, H., Ruotsalainen, U., Ahonen, A., Haaparanta, M., Aho, K., Riikonen, R., Kero, P., Korvenranta, H., Simell, O., and Wegelius, U. (1991). Positron emission tomography in asphyxiated infants. Preliminary studies of regional cerebral glucose metabolism using ^{18}F-FDG. *Acta Radiologica. Supplementum (Stockholm)* 376:173.

Takei, H., Fredericks, W. R., and Rapoport, S. I. (1986).The lumped constant in the deoxyglucose procedure declines with age in Fischer-344 rats. *Journal of Neurochemistry* 46:931–8.

Ter-Pogossian, M. M., Ficke, D. C., Hood, J. T., Sr., Yamamoto, M., and Mullani, N. A. (1982). PETT VI:

a positron emission tomography utilizing cesium fluoride scintillation detectors. *Journal of Computer Assisted Tomography* 6:125–33.

Ter-Pogossian, M. M., Phelps, M. E., Hoffman, E. J., and Mullani, N. A. (1975). A positron-emission transaxial tomograph for nuclear imaging (PETT). *Radiology* 114:89–98.

Ter-Pogossian, M. M., Raichle, M. E., and Sobel, B. E. (1980). Positron-emission tomography. *Scientific American* 243:170–81.

Thorp, P. S., Levin, S. D., Garnett, E. S., Nahmias, C., Firnau, G., Toi, A., Upton, A. R. M., Nobbs, P. T., and Sinclair, J. C. (1988). Patterns of cerebral glucose metabolism using [18]FDG and positron tomography in the neurologic investigation of the full term newborn infant. *Neuropediatrics* 19:146–53.

Townsend, D. W., Geissbuhler, A., Defrise, M., Hoffman, E. J., Spinks, T., Bailey, D. L., Gilardi, M. C., and Jones, T. (1991). Fully three-dimensional reconstruction for a PET camera with retractable septa. *IEEE Transactions on Medical Imaging* 10:505–12.

Treves, S. T. (1985). *Pediatric Nuclear Medicine.* New York: Springer-Verlag.

Veatch, R. M. (1982). The ethics of research involving radiation. *IRB: A Review of Human Subjects Research* 4:3–5.

Videen, T. O., Perlmutter, J. S., Herscovitch, P., and Raichle, M. E. (1987). Brain blood volume, flow, and oxygen utilization measured with [15]O radiotracers and positron emission tomography: revised metabolic computations. *Journal of Cerebral Blood Flow and Metabolism* 7:513–16.

Videen, T. O., Perlmutter, J. S., Mintun, M. A., and Raichle, M. E. (1988). Regional correction of positron emission tomography data for the effects of cerebral atrophy. *Journal of Cerebral Blood Flow and Metabolism* 8:662–70.

Volpe, J. J., Herscovitch, P., Perlman, J. M., Kreusser, K. L., and Raichle, M. E. (1985). Positron emission tomography in the asphyxiated term newborn: parasagittal impairment of cerebral blood flow. *Annals of Neurology* 17:287–96.

Volpe, J. J., Herscovitch, P., Perlman, J. M., and Raichle, M. E. (1983). Positron emission tomography in the newborn: extensive impairment of regional cerebral blood flow with intraventricular hemorrhage and hemorrhagic intracerebral involvement. *Pediatrics* 72:589–601.

Welch, M. J., Eichling, J. O., Straatman, M. G., Raichle, M. E., and Ter-Pogossian, M. M. (1975). New short-lived radiopharmaceuticals for CNS studies. In *Noninvasive Brain Imaging: Computed Tomography and Radionuclides,* ed. H. J. De Blanc, Jr., and J. A. Sorenson (pp. 25–44). New York: The Society of Nuclear Medicine.

Welch, M. J., and Kilbourn, M. R. (1985). A remote system for the routine production of oxygen-15 radiopharmaceuticals. *Journal of Labeled Compounds* 22:1193–200.

Wienhard, K., Dahlbom, M., Eriksson, L., Michel, C., Bruckbauer, T., Pietrzyk, U., and Heiss, W.-D. (1994). The ECAT EXACT HR: performance of a new high resolution positron scanner. *Journal of Computer Assisted Tomography* 18, 110–18.

Wienhard, K., Pawlik, G., Herholz, K., Wagner, R., and Heiss, W.-D. (1985). Estimation of local cerebral glucose utilization by positron emission tomography of [^{18}F]2-fluoro-2-deoxy-D-glucose: a critical appraisal of optimization procedures. *Journal of Cerebral Blood Flow and Metabolism* 5:115–25.

Wilson, M. W., and Mountz, J. M. (1989). A reference system for neuroanatomical localization on functional reconstructed cerebral images. *Journal of Computer Assisted Tomography* 13:174–8.

Yokoi, T., Kanno, I., Iida, H., Miura, S., and Uemura, K. (1991). A new approach of weighted integration technique based on accumulated images using dynamic PET and H_2[15]O. *Journal of Cerebral Blood Flow and Metabolism* 11:492–501.

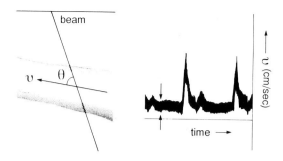

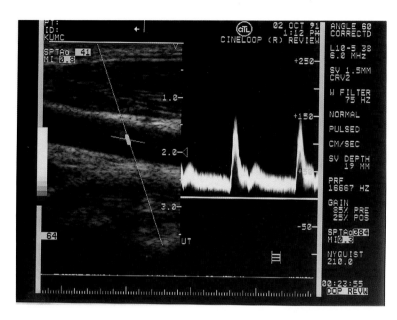

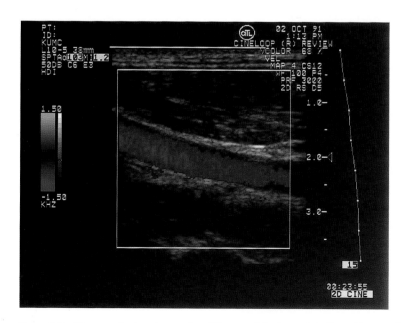

Figure 1.8. Diagrams (top) and examples of the use of duplex Doppler (middle) and color-flow Doppler (bottom) are illustrated for a normal carotid artery. The direction of blood flow is indicated by v, and the Doppler angle is θ. The variability of Doppler velocities is indicated by the width of the spectral trace (arrows).

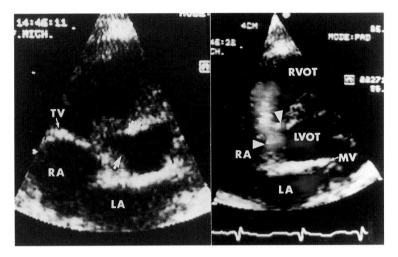

Figure 2.13. In this example of a parasternal short-axis view at the base of the heart, an area of dropout of echoes (arrows) is seen on the 2-D image (left). Use of color-flow Doppler clearly demonstrates a jet of flow toward the transducer in systole (arrowheads), representing a perimembranous ventricular septal defect.

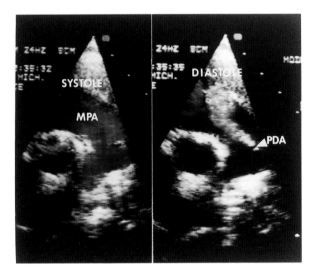

Figure 2.14. In this example of a high parasternal short-axis view at the base of the heart, the main pulmonary artery (MPA) is seen, with normal flow during systole (left). During diastole (right), a small jet of flow is seen in the proximal MPA, consistent with a patent ductus arteriosus (PDA).

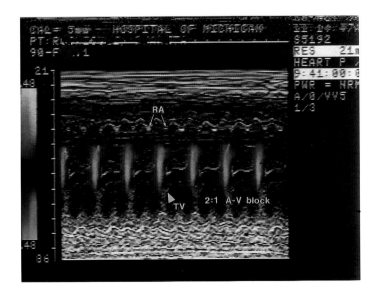

Figure 2.18. Combined M-mode and color-flow Doppler can be used to demonstrate a rhythm abnormality. Right atrial (RA) contraction at a rate of 400 bpm is shown by M-mode recording (arrows). The opening of the tricuspid valve (TV) is shown with a red-orange inflow signal occurring half as frequently (200 bpm) in this example of fetal atrial flutter with 2 : 1 AV block.

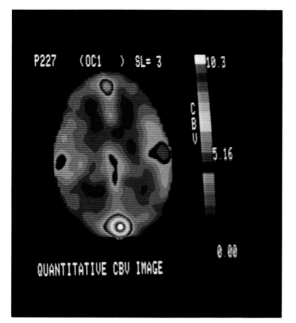

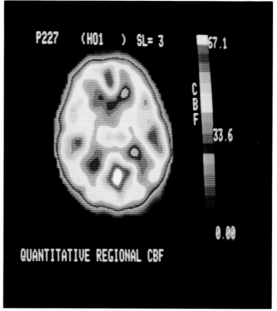

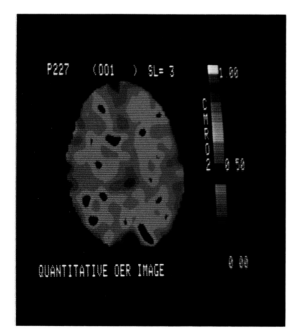

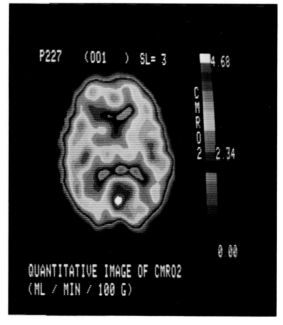

Figure 5.7. Quantitative PET images obtained with ^{15}O-labeled tracers and the PETT VI tomograph (transverse resolution 18 mm FWHM) (Ter-Pogossian et al., 1982) in a normal adult. These are horizontal slices at the level of the thalamus, oriented such that anterior is up and left is to the reader's left. *Top left:* Cerebral blood volume measured following C^{15}O inhalation. The superior saggital sinus is seen anteriorly and posteriorly, and the differences in vascular density between gray and white matter are delineated. *Top right:* Image of rCBF obtained with the PET/autoradiographic method and bo-

lus intravenous injection of H$_2$^{15}O. *Bottom left:* Image of cerebral oxygen extraction fraction (OEF) calculated from scan data obtained following the brief inhalation of ^{15}O$_2$ as well as from the CBV and CBF images. The image is relatively uniform throughout the brain because oxygen metabolism and blood flow are matched throughout the brain in the resting state. *Bottom right:* Image of the cerebral metabolic rate for oxygen. This image is obtained by multiplying data from the CBF and OEF images and the arterial oxygen content.

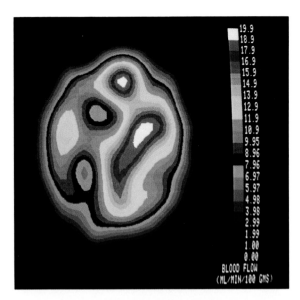

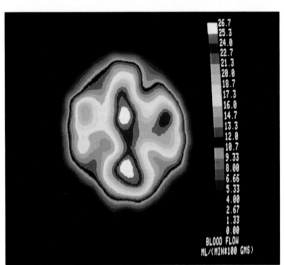

Figure 5.9. rCBF in a premature infant with PVH-IVH and marked hemorrhagic intracerebral involvement confined to the left frontal white matter demonstrated on cranial ultrasound. In the left frontal region of intracerebral hemorrhage there is a marked reduction in rCBF. In addition, there is a more extensive decrease in rCBF in the involved hemisphere laterally and posteriorly. The observation of widespread ischemia in this infant was confirmed by postmortem findings of extensive nonhemorrhagic infarction in frontal, temporal, and parietal cortices. (From Volpe et al., 1983. By permission of the American Academy of Pediatrics.)

Figure 5.10. rCBF in an asphyxiated term newborn with hypoxic-ischemic encephalopathy. There is a relative decrease in rCBF in the parasagittal regions. (From Volpe et al., 1985. By permission of Little, Brown and Company.)

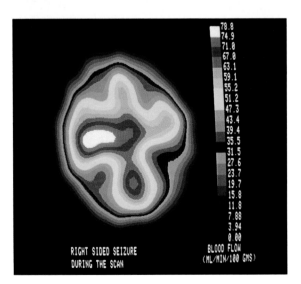

Figure 5.11. rCBF image obtained in an asphyxiated infant during a focal seizure clinically identified to be of left-hemisphere origin. rCBF is 40% higher in the left sylvian region. (From Perlman et al., 1985. By permission of Advanstar Communications, Inc.)

PART II

Oxygenation

Presumably because oxygen is the most vital substance provided to critically ill patients, technical means to measure its concentration in blood have been among the most important and useful of modern medical developments. In neonatal-perinatal medicine, oxygen monitors for newborn infants have led the way, but still it is surprising that measurement of maternal oxygenation has remained so far behind in application as well as in technology, given the direct dependence of fetal oxygenation on the maternal blood oxygen concentration and partial pressure. At least during cesarean-section delivery, maternal pulse oximetry now is standard – and if only it could be combined with some measure of uterine and/or placental blood flow, as well as fetal oxygenation, it would be powerful. A measure of maternal P_{CO_2} also would be helpful; older studies clearly documented delayed respiratory effort with neonatal hypocapnia that could be induced by maternal hyperventilation, and hypocapnia also shifts the oxygen–hemoglobin affinity curve to the left (increased affinity), thereby lowering the maternal uterine venous P_{O_2} and in turn the fetal umbilical venous P_{O_2} and oxygen supply to the fetus (although the effect of the latter is partially counterbalanced by the relative increase in fetal hemoglobin saturation with oxygen, because the fetus also develops hypocapnia and an increase in hemoglobin–oxygen affinity).

In-line monitoring of P_{O_2} and oxygen saturation has never gained widespread use. Although both are useful for moment-to-moment measurement of blood oxygenation, they require an indwelling catheter, and catheter failures for such monitors were frequent, though often unexplained, complications. Thus, it was easy to replace these monitoring devices, along with blood sampling through catheters, with noninvasive transcutaneous P_{O_2} instruments that provided the same sort of moment-to-moment measurement of blood oxygenation, but without the many risks of catheters. In turn, there were many problems associated with transcutaneous P_{O_2} instruments: atmospheric leak under the skin probe, thermal burns, the need for frequent checks on accuracy and proper functioning with painful percutaneous sticks and further bloodletting, relative inaccuracy in infants with chronic lung disease, and so forth. Admittedly, many of those problems were more or less frequent in one or another intensive-care unit, depending on the dedication of the staff working with them. Nevertheless, it was very easy to move on to pulse oximetry, which has become nearly universal in neonatal medicine. Pulse oximetry is accurate and sensitive and provides nearly instantaneous and continuous measurements; it also is noninvasive and relatively risk-free, and except for a relatively high false-alarm rate due to movement artifacts, it is very user-friendly.

Next in line is niroscopy, which essentially takes pulse oximetry to the tissue level and attempts to assess the adequacy of oxygen supply, blood flow, and oxygen utilization. Although more research is needed to develop clinical pathophysiological and outcome correlations, niroscopy is an exciting new development that gets us even closer to assessing cellular oxygenation.

The outcast among the procedures in this group is the measurement of fetal scalp pH. Though widely used, it is simply too variable and too poorly correlated with fetal condition and neonatal outcome to be reliably accurate or predictive. It is unfortunate that because of such limitations, it has played a more prominent role in litigation than in successful medical care.

The fetus needs a pulse oximeter or niroscope or both – they are on the horizon, and prototypes are under study. We may yet learn what is actually going on in the fetus, not what "perhaps" happened at some time, somehow.

6

Continuous (in-line) monitoring of blood gases

MICHAEL WEINDLING, B.Sc., M.D.

INTRODUCTION

The argument for continuous monitoring of arterial blood gases (O_2, PCO_2, and pH) is that careful intermittent sampling and subsequent analysis by a blood gas analyzer can provide accurate measurements, but only at a single point in time. The proponents of continuous monitoring argue that levels of PO_2 can fluctuate rapidly, particularly following suctioning, during handling of the baby, and during treatment for hyaline membrane disease, especially if there is pulmonary hypertension with right-to-left atrial and ductal shunting. In practice, continuous monitoring of only arterial PO_2 is possible at present. For completeness, however, intraarterial PCO_2 and pH monitoring will be considered briefly.

TECHNICAL CONSIDERATIONS

Oxygen monitoring

Sensor characteristics

The shape, size, and form of any sensor are determined by the measurement site (Rolfe, 1990). Measurements within tissues are made with relatively large needles, with diameters of around 0.8 mm, whereas intracellular measurements are made with microelectrodes a few microns thick. If direct intravascular measurements are to be made, the electrodes have to be built into flexible catheters, which can range between 0.5 and 2.0 mm in diameter. In the case of a neonate, the external diameter of a French 5-gauge umbilical arterial catheter is 1.7 mm,

and that of a French 3.5-gauge catheter is 1.32 mm. All sensors need to be calibrated, and in the case of intraarterial catheters, this needs to be done in vitro.

Sensor principles

The principles of measuring oxygen are the same whether one is determining the inspired oxygen concentration or the arterial PO_2. The standard method uses an electrode developed by Clark (1956) and an electrochemical cell. A potential of approximately -600 mV is applied between a cathode, consisting of a noble metal (gold, silver, platinum), and a silver/silver chloride reference electrode. This cathode potential is generally derived from an external power source. However, in 1962 a method was developed (Mancy, Okun, and Reilly, 1962) for its generation internally by a galvanic cell; a silver cathode was combined with a lead anode, and that couple was sufficient to generate the appropriate polarizing voltage.

The effect of applying a potential at the cathode is to reduce oxygen and produce a current proportional to the oxygen partial pressure (PO_2). The cathode, reference electrode, and electrolyte are all contained within a thin gas-permeable membrane, and this ensures that oxygen will diffuse in a controlled manner toward the cathode surface.

Sensor design

In the newborn baby, the basic membrane-covered oxygen electrode (Figure 6.1) needs to be incorporated into a suitable catheter. The selection of mate-

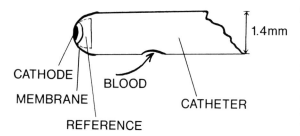

Figure 6.1. A catheter-tip oxygen sensor based on the Clark principle. Blood is sampled via a side-hold through one lumen. Electrical connections to the cathode pass separately.

rials and mechanical design is of the utmost importance to ensure safe and reliable operation. Since Clark's original invention, developments have been concerned with the problem of attaching the sensor and the membrane safely and securely to the tip. Various approaches have been reviewed by Rolfe (1976).

Biocompatibility

One problem with intravascular sensors is their interaction with the biological fluids with which they are in contact. This can take two forms. First, there may be reactions to the sensor, such as blood coagulation, complement activation, or an inflammatory response. Second, sensor performance may be impaired because of its becoming coated with protein and cells. Both situations are undesirable.

Both physical and chemical factors affect the tendency for reactions to occur around the sensor. The main physical problem is surface roughness. A smooth external surface is important to avoid blood clotting on the catheter and around the sensor. One method that has been employed in the most widely used sensor is to attach the membrane by "dip coating" (Soutter, Conway, and Parker, 1975). When the diffusion membrane is dip-coated onto the cathode and reference electrode, the membrane material is first dissolved in a suitable solvent. The advantages of the technique are that (1) it is faster than the previously used method of attaching the performed membrane to the catheter with an adhesive, and (2) the diffusion membrane can be made integral with the catheter wall, resulting in a safer design. The catheter can then be stored dry, and it will activate within a short time of being placed in the bloodstream. The thickness of the membrane can be varied by altering the viscosity of the polymer solution and the number of coats applied, and so the sensor response time can be changed. Different polymers,

such as polyurethanes, polystyrene, and the polyvinyl chlorides can be used (Rolfe, 1990).

Chemical factors that influence reactions around the sensor are wettability and surface charge (Sharma, 1981; Rolfe, 1990). This relates to the zeta potential, which results from the extent to which certain charged groups are exposed or concealed at the surface. Platelets, erythrocytes, and vascular endothelium exhibit a negative surface charge of around -12 to -15 mV, and the effect of this is for these objects to repel each other. But there is also a distribution of charge over the surfaces of biological materials, and this can vary in both polarity and magnitude. To minimize the risk of clotting around the catheter tip, some catheters have incorporated heparin bound to their surfaces (Nilsson et al., 1981).

Response time

Most electrochemical sensors for inspired gas monitoring of Po_2 have 95% response times between 20 and 60 s (Rolfe, 1990). The response time for intravascular monitoring of Po_2 is given in the technical literature as 30–90 s (Neocath 1000, Biomedical Sensors, Malvern, PA). The system developed by Soutter et al. (1975) was reported to have a 95% response time of about 50 s. Their transducer output was unaffected by changes in blood pH.

Other methods

Although these other methods are mentioned here for completeness, only the Clark-type electrode driven by an external voltage source has achieved general use.

Blood oxygen monitoring can also be carried out with fiber-optic oximeter catheters (Wilkinson, Phibbs, and Gregory, 1978). By this method (Oximetrix, Mountain View, CA), it is possible to measure the oxygen saturation of hemoglobin continuously in the arterial blood of newborn infants. The 4-FG polyurethane catheter has a dual lumen. One lumen is for infusing fluids, sampling blood, and measuring blood pressure; the other contains two optical fibers. One fiber transmits three wavelengths of red and near-infrared light between 600 and 1,000 nm; the light is transmitted in 1 ms pulses to the blood. The second fiber transmits the light reflected by the blood to a light detector, and the average Sao_2 is computed. The Sao_2 measured by this system correlated closely with the Sao_2 measured on a blood sample by co-oximetry ($r = 0.976$, $n = 139$). The accuracy was unaffected by hyper-

Table 6.1. *Advantages and disadvantages of different methods of arterial oxygen monitoring*

Method	Advantages	Disadvantages
Intermittent sampling	Accurate if indwelling catheter; cheap	Intermittent
Intraarterial PaO_2 sensor	Accurate, continuous	Disposable, single-use catheters are expensive; damping of blood pressure trace
PtcO_2	Noninvasive, continuous	Inaccurate if poor skin perfusion; rather tedious to apply
SaO_2	Noninvasive, easy to apply, continuous	Variable relation with PaO_2

bilirubinemia, hyperviscosity, acidosis, hypercarbia, or varying amounts of HbF. Complications were no more frequent with this system than with a conventional catheter. However, the convenience and noninvasive nature of pulse oximetry has superseded this technique. A combined fiber-optic oximeter and PO_2 sensor has also been reported (Parker, 1981).

Rolfe (1988) has described the measurement of oxygen in blood with a sensor based on fluorescence. A fluorescent dye, such as parlene butyrate, is adsorbed to organic beads contained within a hydrophobic, gas-permeable membrane. The dye is excited with blue light (468 nm), and it emits radiation in the green band of the spectrum (514 nm). The PO_2 can be calculated. The choice of dye is important to optimize sensitivity and brightness (Peterson, Fitzgerald, and Buckhold, 1984).

Mass spectroscopy measures the components of a complex gas by separating them according to their charge and mass. A small sample of the gas to be analyzed is drawn into a measurement chamber that is maintained at a very high vacuum (about 10^{-5} mm Hg). The gas mixture is bombarded by electrons that ionize the gas molecules; these charged particles are then accelerated through a magnetic field which separates them according to their charge : mass ratio. Because most ions have just a single charge, the most important factor that affects their separation is their mass. The lightest ions are deflected more than the heaviest and travel the least distance. Metal receivers are placed in such a way as to collect ions of each species. Each detector emits a small current in proportion to the rate at which ions impinge on it, so that a measure of the partial pressure of the gas is obtained.

There are two types of mass spectrometers: magnetic-sector and quadrupole. The latter is smaller and lighter and can be tuned to a specific gas. This is achieved by passing the ions through a quadrupole mass filter that comprises four rods, set in two parallel pairs at right angles to one another. A steady voltage is applied to all the rods, with a radio-frequency alternating component to the opposite pairs. By adjusting this frequency it is possible to filter out all the ions except those with a particular mass : charge ratio.

Mass spectrometers have a fast response time (about 100 ms for a 95% response) and require very small sample flow rates (Sykes, Vickers, and Hull, 1981). Mass spectrometry has been used for measuring intravascular gases by means of a gas-collection cannula with a supported membrane at its tip (Woldring, Owens, and Woolford, 1966; Owens, Belmusto, and Woldring, 1969; Brantigan, Dunn, and Albo, 1976; Rolfe, 1976). The tubing must be strong enough to withstand the vacuum at the inlet to the mass spectrometer and must be relatively impermeable to gas diffusion (Rolfe, 1990). Stainless steel (Pinard, Seylaz, and Mamo, 1978; Lundsgaard, Gronlund, and Einer-Jensen, 1978; Lundsgaard, Jensen, and Gronlund, 1980), for the connecting cannula, and a nylon catheter coated on the inside with polyurethane have been used (Parker and Delpy, 1983). The main disadvantages of mass spectrometry are the size of the machines and their high capital and servicing costs. They are not used for routine clinical monitoring.

pH and Pco$_2$ measurements

Measurement of pH is generally regarded as essential for measuring Pco$_2$, but the necessary apparatus has been dogged by manufacturing problems (Rolfe, 1990). The most popular approach to the monitoring of Pco$_2$ has been to use an electrochemical potentiometric sensor for pH, surrounded by a CO_2-permeable membrane, the Stow-Severinghaus electrode (Stow and Randall, 1957). Even metal/metal oxide pH sensors, using antimony, iridium, or palladium, have been tried instead of the traditional glass electrode, as discussed later (Coon,

Lai, and Kampine, 1976; Parker, Delpy, and Lewis, 1978). It is impossible to measure CO_2 with an amperometric sensor in which the electrolyte is nonaqueous (e.g., dimethyl sulfoxide), but such electrodes are difficult to build because of the aggressive nature of the solvent (Rolfe, 1990).

Glass membranes have been used for measuring various cations and anions, and a glass pH electrode that can be inserted into an artery through a modified needle has been reported (Band and Semple, 1967). But because of the obvious disadvantage of a glass electrode (namely, its fragility), the technique has never achieved widespread clinical use, and others (e.g., Le Blanc et al., 1976; Cobbe and Poole-Wilson, 1980; Ammann et al., 1981) have investigated polymer membranes. Most often a reference electrode is connected by a salt bridge to the intravascular space, although skin-surface-mounted silver/silver chloride electrodes have also been used (Rolfe, 1990).

A polymer pH membrane was used in a combined pH and Pco_2 sensor (Biochem International, Malvern, PA). This tiny sensor was made of an outer polymer membrane (Le Blanc et al., 1976), with a palladium/palladium oxide pH sensor for pH measurement, and a bicarbonate solution and silver/silver chloride reference electrode within the polymer membrane for Pco_2 measurement (Coon et al., 1976; Sugioka, 1981).

Another approach has involved the ion-selective field-effect transistor (ISFET), as first described by Bergveld (1970). This is a low-cost micro-miniature sensor. The principle is that of a device for measuring an electrical potential with high-input impedance. It is made by removing the metal gate region normally present in a field-effect transistor. The potential applied at the gate is derived by an ion-selective process and modulates the current between the source and the drain. ISFETs are made in the form of needles by anisotropic etching of the silica substrate (Esahi and Matsuo, 1978). An ISFET device for pH and Pco_2 has been described (Shimada et al., 1980). The catheter pH ISFET is 0.5 mm in diameter, and the chip is embedded in silicon resin at the tip of a nylon tube, with a hydrogel coating over the surface to improve biocompatibility. This device has been converted for CO_2 monitoring by expert miniaturization. A silver/silver chloride reference is incorporated on the chip, with a deposit of polyvinyl alcohol gel containing NaCl and $NaHCO_3$ over the ISFET and reference electrode, with both regions coated with a thin silicon resin. Unfortunately, one problem has been to encapsulate ISFETs sufficiently well to prevent damage by water vapor, and gener-

ally it has not been possible to operate them for more than 24 h.

An optical approach, like that for oximetry, has been tried for pH sensors (Saari and Seitz, 1982). A pH sensor was made in which the fluorescence intensity of immobilized fluorescein amine at 520 nm was measured following excitation at 480 nm. A single device containing optical sensors for pH, Pco_2, and Po_2, together with a thermocouple for temperature compensation, has been described (Gehreich et al., 1986). This device has not yet been manufactured commercially.

Manufacturing difficulties

Some manufacturing difficulties have already been mentioned. It must be asked why only the Po_2 continuous-monitoring electrode has achieved general clinical acceptability. It is not simply a matter of the cost of such sensors, which must be discarded after a single use, but rather of inadequate overall performance. The problem has been addressed by Rolfe (1990): "It is clear to anyone who has observed the rigours of a busy intensive care unit that instrumentation must first, be straightforward to use, secondly must provide reliable information . . . and thirdly must be safe." All these criteria have not yet been met.

End-tidal CO₂

This measurement is mentioned in this context because of claims that it might be as useful for monitoring sick neonates as it is for anesthetized patients. End-tidal CO_2 ($Petco_2$) is considered to be a reflection of intraalveolar Pco_2. The argument is that because of the very rapid equilibration between intraalveolar Pco_2 and pulmonary arterial Pco_2 ($Paco_2$), the former will sufficiently closely mirror the latter. In practice, because of the pulmonary parenchymal abnormalities that invariably occur in hyaline membrane disease, $Paco_2$ and $Petco_2$ correlate very poorly during the acute phases of this disease (Watkins and Weindling, 1987). The technique may be useful for monitoring the chronically ventilated patient who has normal lungs, but in practice this situation hardly arises in the neonatal nursery. In any case, continuous monitoring of Pco_2 is of doubtful clinical relevance in such situations. The only conceivable situation where this technique may be useful is in the physiology laboratory.

The most widely used technique for respiratory CO_2 analysis is based on the infrared absorption properties of carbon dioxide. The gas for analysis is

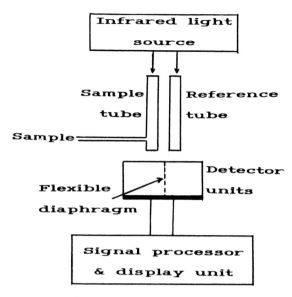

Figure 6.2. Schematic diagram of an infrared gas analyzer.

drawn into a sample tube, and a differential optical absorption measurement is made between this and a reference tube. The absorption measurement is carried out by allowing the infrared light transmitted through the sample and reference tubes to be absorbed by two gas-filled detector units positioned on either side of a flexible diaphragm (Rolfe, 1990). Earlier Pco_2 monitors relied on the absorption of light on the detector unit causing a rise in temperature (Figure 6.2). The consequent expansion resulted in a pressure difference across the diaphragm, the difference being proportional to the CO_2 concentration. More recent CO_2 monitors simply use infrared detectors to measure the absorption by the sample gas. Because other gases and vapors also absorb infrared radiation, a specific absorption band of 4.26 μm is used for CO_2 measurements.

CLINICAL CONSIDERATIONS

Relative value of continuous intraarterial monitoring of Po_2 compared with other methods

One of the cardinal prerequisites for successful neonatal intensive support is the ability to maintain sick infants in a stable condition. Such babies are, however, likely to experience sudden disturbances in their conditions. These changes must be promptly recognized so that appropriate restorative measures can be implemented as quickly as possible. For this reason, several physiological parameters must be continuously measured and assessed. One of these is blood gas status, although not all neonatologists would agree that Po_2 needs to be recorded continuously.

The problem with Po_2 monitoring is that, like other physiological variables, the Po_2 must be kept within a fairly narrow range. Generally accepted values are 60–90 mm Hg (8.0–12.0 kPa). Every cell depends on a sufficient supply of oxygen; there is no evidence to support a view that the cells of more premature babies are better able to withstand hypoxia than are those of term infants. Too little oxygen, and the cell is injured; too much, and arteriolar constriction occurs. One of the best-known consequences of hyperoxia is retinopathy of prematurity. A detailed consideration of the evidence that pertains to the causation of this problem is beyond the scope of this review, but in spite of recent speculation about the multifactorial causes of this problem, there is general agreement that hyperoxia is one significant factor (e.g., Ng et al., 1988).

Oxygen is driven into cells by the partial pressure of oxygen (Po_2) in the capillaries, and its availability is determined by the arterial Po_2 (Pao_2). Several strategies are available for assessing Pao_2: first, by sensors on the skin surface that measure the Po_2 *at that site*. This caveat is important: although so-called transcutaneous Po_2 ($Ptco_2$) generally correlates well with Pao_2, the method depends on the blood supply to the skin and on the skin's own metabolism and utilization of oxygen. (The same arguments apply to skin-surface Pco_2 measurements, but here the production of CO_2 by the skin is even more important.) $Ptco_2$ therefore correlates well with Pao_2 only in the hemodynamically stable infant. The accuracy of the method, which depends on dilatation of the cutaneous capillaries, is seriously reduced in the face of peripheral vasoconstriction and cardiogenic or hypovolemic shock. These are conditions that affect the most seriously ill patients, precisely the group to benefit most from intensive support. It is also necessary to reposition the skin sensor every 3–4 h to avoid skin burns, and this interrupts the continuous recording of data.

In practice, the relative difficulties of recording reliable data from skin-surface sensors, the necessity to reposition the sensor, the cost of replacing the sensor when its cable becomes damaged by being trapped in an incubator door, and, most important, the development of pulse oximetry have resulted in this method being less popular than it was 5 yr ago. Neonatal nurses generally prefer the much greater convenience of pulse oximetry.

The main problem with pulse oximetry – which is

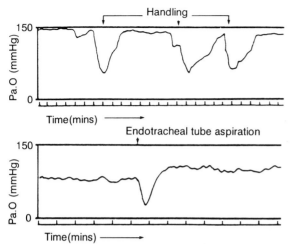

Figure 6.3. Traces from a ventilated neonate, showing re-duced oxygenation during handling and endotracheal-tube aspiration. (From Rolfe, 1988.)

easy to apply, requires no calibration, and gives continuous information – is that it provides a mea-sure of arterial oxygen saturation (Sao_2) rather than Pao_2. It cannot be stressed too strongly that there is not a constant relationship between these two phys-iological variables. Their relationship changes ac-cording to pH, fetal hemoglobin content, and tem-perature. This point is fundamental, but often ignored. Although pulse oximetry cannot indicate hyperoxia, small changes in Pao_2 below the "knee" of the Po_2–oxygen saturation curve result in large changes in Sao_2. For this reason, pulse oximetry is an excellent monitor, but, as with every monitor, it is important that users be aware of the precise phys-iological variable that is being measured.

Any system to monitor patients should give clini-cally relevant information accurately. It should be easy to apply, and it should not interfere with other information systems. The continuous intraarterial Pao_2 monitor fulfills most of these criteria. It is cer-tainly very accurate. Several independent studies have shown excellent correlations between Pao_2 values measured intermittently and by intraarterial sensor. Overall correlation coefficients were better than 0.97 (Bratanow et al., 1985; Rithalia, Edwards, and Doran, 1992), although Kettler and Hentze (1979) observed a lower correlation ($r = 0.773$, $n = 14$) at lower oxygen tensions ($Pao_2 = 4$–9.3 kPa) than at a higher range ($r = 0.93$, $n = 64$ at $Pao_2 = 9.3$–20).

There are, however, two main concerns about the usefulness of this method. One is that the side-hole

of the catheter may cause damping of the blood pressure waveform. In a recent series of 11 adults in whom a sensor was introduced into the radial ar-tery, damping of the arterial pressure trace was a recurrent problem in 2 patients (Rithalia et al., 1992). This is of particular importance, because in-creasing emphasis is placed on the correction of hypotension in these very sick infants (Weindling, 1989). At our neonatal intensive-care unit, intermit-tent monitoring of blood gases is used in conjunc-tion with pulse oximetry and invasive blood pres-sure monitoring. The other drawback is the high cost of the single-use, disposable catheter with its integral oxygen sensor.

Continuous monitoring of intraarterial oxygen tension

Continuous monitoring of intraarterial oxygen ten-sion has been available for a long time. One report described 282 instances of umbilical artery catheters with oxygen electrodes on their tips passed into the aortas of 268 newborn infants between 1974 and 1977 (Pollitzer et al., 1980); 90% of the electrodes re-corded Pao_2 satisfactorily for a mean of 66 h; 75% of the electrodes were still functioning when removed after a mean of 87 h, even though they were no longer needed. In that study, 10% of electrodes failed to function after initial insertion; manufac-turers' representatives claim that such figures are now considerably less. Problems with clot forma-tion over the tip of the catheter were recorded in 51 cases. The overall incidence of clots forming was be-lieved by the authors to be no greater than with or-dinary umbilical arterial catheters.

There is no doubt that the continuous availability of Pao_2 data has raised the awareness of medical and nursing attendants regarding the major distur-bances that can be caused by handling a sick neo-nate and by fairly straightforward nursing pro-cedures (Figure 6.3). This has resulted in the development of a minimal-handling policy toward sick and unstable infants. The main strength of con-tinuous in-line measurement of Pao_2 is its ability to provide a continuous readout. However, this has now been largely superseded by pulse oximetry, a technique that is both cheaper and easier to apply.

Invasive on-line measurements of biochemicals in the blood would provide a direct and rapid indica-tion of a patient's clinical condition. Although con-tinuous arterial O_2, CO_2, and pH measurements would be invaluable guides to a patient's cardio-respiratory status, only oxygen sensors are available for routine clinical use at present.

CONCLUSIONS

Laboratory blood gas analyzers have been developed and refined over the past few years and are now commonplace in the neonatal intensive-care nursery. They provide reliable and rapid analysis of very small blood samples. It is already possible with the current generation of machines to measure potassium, calcium, and sodium ions with built-in ion-selective electrodes. It is probable (Rolfe, 1990) that the next step will be to include sensors for glucose measurement. A further development may be for these variables to be monitored within the patient continuously. The next important advance is likely to be the ability to measure blood glucose concentrations continuously in the sick newborn infant, who is so vulnerable to hypoglycemia.

REFERENCES

Ammann, D., Lanter, F., Steiner, R. A., Schulthess, P., Shijo, Y., and Simon, W. (1981). Neutral carrier based hydrogen ion selective microelectrode for extra- and intracellular studies. *Analytical Chemistry* 53:2267–9.

Band, D. M., and Semple, S. J. G. (1967). Continuous measurement of blood pH with an indwelling glass electrode. *Journal of Applied Physiology* 22:854–7.

Bergveld, P. (1970). Development of an ion-sensitive solid-state device for neurophysiological measurements. *IEEE Transactions* BME-17:70–1.

Brantigan, J. W., Dunn, K. L., and Albo, D. (1976). A clinical catheter for continuous blood gas measurement by mass spectrometry. *Journal of Applied Physiology* 40:443–6.

Bratanow, N., Pol, K., Bland, R., Krom, H., and Taishon, L. (1985). Continuous polarographic monitoring of intra-arterial oxygen in the perioperative period. *Critical Care Medicine* 13:859–60.

Clark, L. C. (1956). Monitor and control of blood and tissue oxygen tension. *Transactions of American Society of Artificial Organs* 2:41–6.

Cobbe, S. M., and Poole-Wilson, P. A. (1980). Catheter tip pH electrodes for continuous intravascular recording. *Journal of Medical Engineering and Technology* 4:122–4.

Coon, R. I., Lai, N. J. C., and Kampine, J. P. (1976). Evaluation of dual-function P_t and P_{CO_2} *in vivo* sensor. *Journal of Applied Physiology* 40:625–9.

Esahi, M., and Matsuo, T. (1978). Integrated micro multi-ion sensor using field effect of semiconductor. *IEEE Transactions* BME-25:184–92.

Gehreich, J. L., Lubbers, D. W., Opitz, N., Hansmann, D. R., Miller, W. W., Tusa, J. K., and Yasufo, M. (1986). Optical fluorescence and its application to an intravascular blood gas monitoring system. *IEEE Transactions* BME-33:1117–32.

Kettler, D., and Hentze, G. (1979). Clinical suitability and accuracy of a new combined system for the transcutaneous and intravascular determination of P_{O_2}. *Biotelemetry Patient Monitoring* 1–2:66–74.

Le Blanc, O. H., Brown, J. F., Klebe, J. F., Niedrach, L. W., Slusarczuk, G. M. J., and Stoddard, W. H. (1976). Polymer membrane sensors for continuous intravascular monitoring of blood pH. *Journal of Applied Physiology* 40:644–7.

Lundsgaard, J. S., Gronlund, J., and Einer-Jensen, N. (1978). *In-vivo* calibration of flow-dependent blood gas catheters. *Journal of Applied Physiology and Respiration* 44:124–8.

Lundsgaard, J. S., Jensen, B., and Gronlund, J. (1980). Fast responding flow-independent blood gas catheter for oxygen measurement. *Journal of Applied Physiology and Respiration* 48:376–81.

Mancy, K. H., Okun, D. A., and Reilly, C. N. (1962). A galvanic cell oxygen analyser. *Journal of Electroanalytical Chemistry* 4:65–92.

Ng, Y. K., Shaw, D. E., Fielder, A. R., and Levene, M. I. (1988). Epidemiology of retinopathy of prematurity. *Lancet* 2:1235–8.

Nilsson, E., Alme, B., Edwall, G., Larsson, R., and Olsson, P. (1981). Continuous intra-arterial P_{O_2} registrations with conventional and surface heparinized electrodes. In *Monitoring of Vital Parameters during Extracorporeal Circulation*, ed. H. P. Kimmich (pp. 127–33).

Owens, G., Belmusto, L., and Woldring, S. (1969). Experimental intracerebral p_{O_2} and p_{CO_2} monitoring by mass spectrometry. *Journal of Neurosurgery* 30:110–15.

Parker, D. (1981). Continuous measurement of blood oxygen tension and saturation. In *Monitoring of Vital Parameters during Extracorporeal Circulation*, ed. H. P. Kimmich (pp. 23–8). Basel: Karger.

Parker, D., and Delpy, D. T. (1983). Blood gas analysis by invasive and non-invasive techniques. In *Measurement in Clinical Respiratory Physiology*, ed. G. Laszlo and M. F. Sudlow (pp. 75–111). London: Academic Press.

Parker, D., Delpy, D., and Lewis, M. (1978). Catheter tip electrode for continuous measurement of P_{O_2} and P_{CO_2}. *Medical and Biological Engineering and Computing* 16:599–600.

Peterson, J. L., Fitzgerald, R. V., and Buckhold, D. K. (1984). Fibre-optic probe for *in vivo* measurement of oxygen partial pressure. *Journal of Analytical Chemistry* 52:864–9.

Pinard, E., Seylaz, J., and Mamo, H. (1978). Quantitative continuous measurement of p_{O_2} and p_{CO_2} in artery and vein. *Medical and Biological Engineering and Computing* 16:59–64.

Pollitzer, M. J., Soutter, L. P., Reynolds, E. O. R., and Whitehead, M. D. (1980). Continuous monitoring of arterial oxygen tension in infants: four years of experience with an intravascular oxygen electrode. *Pediatrics* 66:31–6.

Rithalia, S. V. S., Edwards, D., and Doran, B. R. H. (1992). Intra-arterial O_2 electrode. *British Journal of Intensive Care* January/February:29–33.

Rolfe, P. (1976). Arterial oxygen measurement in the newborn with intra-vascular transducer. In *Medical Electronics Monographs 18–22*, ed. D. W. Hill and B. W. Watson. Stevenage: Peter Peregrinus.

(1988). Review of chemical sensors for physiological measurement. *Journal of Biomedical Engineering* 10:138–45.

(1990). *In vivo* chemical sensors for intensive-care monitoring. *Medical and Biological Engineering and Computing* 28:B34–47.

Saari, L. A., and Seitz, W. R. (1982). pH sensor based on immobilized fluorescein amine. *Analytical Chemistry* 54:821–3.

Sharma, C. P. (1981). Possible contributions of surface energy and interfacial parameters of synthetic polymers to blood compatibility. *Biomaterials* 2:57–64.

Shimada, K., Yano, M., Shibatani, K., Komoto, Y., Esahi, M., and Matsuo, T. (1980). Application of catheter-tip i.s.f.e.t. for continuous *in vivo* measurement. *Medical and Biological Engineering and Computing* 18:741–5.

Soutter, L. P., Conway, M. J., and Parker, D. (1975). A system for monitoring arterial oxygen tension in sick newborn babies. *Biomedical Engineering* 1:257–60.

Stow, R. W., and Randall, B. E. (1957). Rapid measurement of the tension of carbon dioxide in the blood. *Archives of Physical Medicine and Rehabilitation* 38:646–50.

Sugioka, K. (1981). Continuous measurement of $Paco_2$, pH and bicarbonate in humans. In *Monitoring of Vital Parameters during Extracorporeal Circulation*, ed. H. P. Kimmich (pp. 138–42). Basel: Karger.

Sykes, M. K., Vickers, M. D., and Hull, J. C. (1981). *Principles of Clinical Measurement*. Oxford: Blackwell.

Watkins, A. M. C., and Weindling, A. M. (1987). Monitoring of end tidal CO_2 in neonatal intensive care. *Archives of Disease in Childhood* 62:837–9.

Weindling, A. M. (1989). Blood pressure monitoring in the newborn. *Archives of Disease in Childhood* 64:444–447.

Wilkinson, A. R., Phibbs, R. H., and Gregory, G. A. (1978). Continuous measurement of oxygen saturation in sick newborn infants. *Journal of Pediatrics* 93:1016–19.

Woldring, S., Owens, G., and Woolford, D. C. (1966). Blood gases: continuous *in vivo* recording of partial pressure by mass spectrometry. *Science* 155:885–8.

7

Transcutaneous monitoring of blood gases

WILLEM P. F. FETTER, M.D., Ph.D.
HARRY N. LAFEBER, M.D., Ph.D.

INTRODUCTION

Over the past two decades, skin sensors have been developed to allow continuous measurements of oxygen tension (Po_2) and carbon dioxide tension (Pco_2). The use of transcutaneous sensors has become a standard of care, especially in the treatment of neonates with respiratory problems, where invasive techniques are to be avoided as much as possible. In this chapter, the methodology, reliability, and clinical applications of transcutaneous blood gas sensors are described.

TRANSCUTANEOUS Po_2 MEASUREMENT

History

Measurement of Po_2 has been possible since 1923, when Heyrovský and Shikata published their report on a dropping mercury electrode (Heyrovský and Shikata, 1923). For technical reasons, however, it was impossible to measure Po_2 in tissue. Measurement of Po_2 in blood samples and tissues has been made possible by Clark, who described the membrane-covered electrode (Clark et al., 1953; Clark, 1956).

It was shown in 1851 by Gerlach, at the Royal Veterinary School in Berlin, that both oxygen and carbon dioxide can diffuse through intact skin. One hundred years later the observations of Gerlach were confirmed by Baumberger and Goodfriend. In their experiment, Po_2 was measured in a phosphate buffer solution after immersion of a subject's finger in the solution for 15 min (Baumberger and Goodfriend, 1951). By using platinum needles, Montgomery and Horwitz (1950) could measure Po_2 intracutaneously. Because they used bare needles, the electrode turned out to be very unstable, making calibration difficult and measurements unreliable.

In 1966, a membrane-covered electrode for intracutaneous measurement was described (Evans and Naylor, 1966). The measured Po_2 was half the intra-arterial Po_2 (Pao_2). One year later the same authors described a membrane-covered platinum electrode for Po_2 measurement on the skin surface (Evans and Naylor, 1967). The measurement was improved by local application of a nicotinic acid derivative that induced hyperemia of the skin.

The same principle was applied by Huch and co-workers in their first description of a transcutaneous Po_2 sensor (Huch, Huch, and Lübbers, 1969). Four years later, the first transcutaneous Po_2 sensor was described, with a heating system to produce skin hyperemia (Huch et al., 1973a). The first results with this device in newborn infants were published in the same year (Huch et al., 1973c). The heating system for the sensor was set at 45°C, which provided a temperature at the skin surface of 43°C. Other kinds of transcutaneous oxygen sensors were described in the years thereafter (Eberhard et al., 1973; Vesterager, 1977). The prototypes were soon followed by commercially available sensors.

Principles of transcutaneous P_{O_2} measurement

All transcutaneous P_{O_2} sensors are modified Clark-cell electrodes. Clark and co-workers described the polarographic techniques of oxygen measurement in 1953 (Clark et al., 1953). Oxygen is reduced at an electrode made of a noble metal, such as gold or platinum, after a polarization current of 600–700 mV has been applied between this electrode (the cathode) and usually a silver reference electrode (the anode). The reduction reaction generates an electric current that is proportional to the number of oxygen molecules presented to the cathode, and therefore proportional to the P_{O_2}. The sensor is covered with a semipermeable membrane (polystyrene, polypropylene, or Teflon), making diffusion of oxygen molecules to the cathode possible. The cathode is glass-coated to prevent a change in the surface area during the measurement.

An electrolyte solution is applied between sensor and membrane for the electrochemical reactions at the cathode and anode. For further information on polarography, the reader is referred to the monograph by Fatt (1976).

Transcutaneous P_{O_2} sensors use a built-in heating system to induce skin hyperemia. A heating temperature of 44–45°C is sufficient for maximal vasodilatation (Al-Siaidy and Hill, 1979). The skin consists of three functional layers: one oxygen-consuming layer with blood vessels, a second oxygen-consuming layer without blood vessels, and a third non-oxygen-consuming layer (the stratum corneum). Living cells in the skin receive just enough P_{O_2}. The P_{O_2} drops from arterial values at the end of the capillary loops to very low values in the non-living stratum corneum. Normally, very low P_{O_2} values (0–3 mm Hg) are measured at the skin surface (Evans and Naylor, 1967).

The skin serves as a regulator of body temperature by increasing its blood flow with rising body temperature. This principle is used when local heating is applied to the skin by a heated sensor. In this way the oxygen supply is increased far above local oxygen consumption. On their route from capillary vessels to the cathode, oxygen molecules pass through several layers: the three skin layers, the sensor membrane, and the electrolyte solution. With an unheated sensor, P_{O_2} falls rapidly as a result of countercurrent shunting from the arteriolar to the venous limbs in the capillary loops and as a result of oxygen consumption by the living skin cells. Consequently, P_{O_2} measured at the sensor membrane is far below Pa_{O_2}. Oxygen consumption can be blocked by topical application of cyanide, but this compound is not suitable for clinical use (Engel, Delpy, and Parker, 1979).

Heating increases the oxygen supply to the skin layers by arterialization of the capillary loops. Moreover, P_{O_2} is increased with rising temperature because of the shift to the right in the oxygen dissociation curve; in this way, hemoglobin-oxygen binding is reduced, and oxygen release to the tissues is increased. Another effect of heating is an alteration of fat that makes it more permeable to oxygen (Van Dussee, 1975).

The effect of temperature on P_{O_2} values varies from 1.3% per 1°C to 7.2% per 1°C when arterial saturation is less than 90% (Palmisano and Severinghaus, 1990). Humidification of the skin using a droplet of water will decrease the skin's oxygen-diffusion resistance 20-fold (Vaupel, 1976).

Transcutaneous P_{O_2} sensor and monitor

A cross section of a transcutaneous P_{O_2} sensor is shown in Figure 7.1. The sensor consists of a glass-coated wire serving as cathode. In most sensors, very small cathodes are used (diameters 15–50 μm). Therefore, dependence on an influx of oxygen molecules is low, and thus oxygen consumption is limited. A silver ring serves as the reference anode. The membrane and electrolyte solution are fixed by a fixation ring.

The heating system is regulated by thermistors and an integrated circuit. The monitor includes circuitry for P_{O_2} measurement, heating and temperature controls covering the range 37–45°C, digital display and outputs for recorder and printer, and controls for calibration adjustments. Furthermore, alarms can be set for P_{O_2} values outside certain limits and for temperature values that deviate more than 0.3°C from the selected temperature (Wimberley et al., 1990).

The in vitro response times (time necessary to reach 90% or 95% of the ultimate Ptc_{O_2}) vary among the different sensors and depend on the type and thickness of the sensor membrane and on the cathode diameter.

Drift is defined as the percentage of change in the Ptc_{O_2} value measured at a constant P_{O_2} value. Drift should be less than ±5% over a period of 4 h (Wimberley et al., 1990). Because oxygen sensors are linear over a wide range of P_{O_2}, a two-point calibration is sufficient. Calibration can be performed with an oxygen-free solution (sodium bisulfate) au-

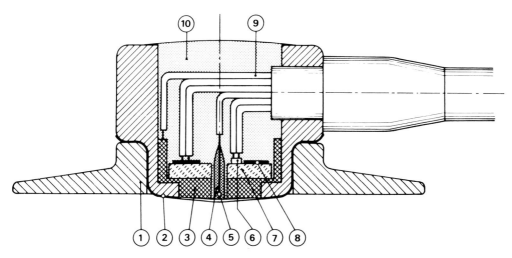

Figure 7.1. Cross section of a transcutaneous oxygen sensor: 1, fixation ring; 2, membrane (polypropylene); 3, anode (silver/silver chloride); 4, glass coating; 5, cathode (platinum); 6, integrated circuit; 7, ceramic plate; 8, heating element; 9, insulated connection wires; 10, casting (epoxy resin). (From Fetter, 1983.)

tomatically to set a $Ptco_2$ of 0 mm Hg, and in atmospheric air to set a $Ptco_2$ of 150–160 mm Hg (at sea level). The Po_2 in air can be calculated from the following equation:

$$Po_2 = (P_B - P_{H_2O}) \cdot F_{IO_2}$$

where P_B is ambient barometric pressure, P_{H_2O} is the partial H_2O pressure in air, and F_{IO_2} is the oxygen fraction in air.

Some types of equipment have facilities to measure the amount of energy necessary to keep the sensor at a constant temperature. It was thought that such a heating-energy system could serve as an indicator of skin blood flow and therefore as an indicator of circulation (Huch, Lübbers, and Huch, 1974; Huch, Huch, and Lübbers, 1981b). However, when skin blood flow was blocked completely, a maximum decrease in heating energy of 30% was reached (Severinghaus, Stafford, and Thunstrom, 1978b). Furthermore, no relationship could be found between heating energy and skin blood flow beneath the sensor when skin blood flow was measured by means of a laser Doppler flow technique (Enkema et al., 1981).

Fixation on the skin is facilitated by a self-adhesive ring. Optimal measuring conditions are found in skin areas with high densities of capillaries, ample capillary blood flow, thin epidermis, and small or no fat depositions. Optimal places are the abdomen and chest. Extremities are best avoided, because vasoconstriction is induced at an earlier stage

if the circulation is compromised. Preferably, sensors in a newborn must be placed on the right part of the chest, in case of a right-to-left shunt through a patent ductus arteriosus. Hair should be removed.

The $Ptco_2$ is usually measured at a sensor temperature of 44°C. Higher temperatures are to be avoided to prevent skin burns. After a preheating period at 44°C, $Ptco_2$ can be measured accurately at 42°C; $Ptco_2$ measured at 42°C is lower than $Ptco_2$ measured at 44°C, but quite similar to the latter value when corrected for the temperature difference (Friis-Hansen et al., 1987). The maximum measuring time is 4 h. Even at a shorter period, skin erythema may develop, disappearing after 1–2 d (Peabody et al., 1978). Permanent skin damages were reported by Golden (1981). After removal from the skin, the sensor should be checked in a calibration gas to document drift. The membrane and electrolyte solution should be changed weekly (Wimberley et al., 1990).

Reliability of transcutaneous oxygen sensors

Under ideal conditions, $Ptco_2$ values are approximately equal to Pao_2 values. To ensure a correct interpretation of $Ptco_2$, a comparison is advised with Po_2 values determined in arterial blood. Capillary blood samples are not suitable because of the poor correlation between capillary and arterial Po_2 values (Banister, 1969; Lewis and Haslan, 1984; Mclain, Evans, and Dear, 1988). Any change in $Ptco_2$ may be caused by a change in Pao_2 or by a change in skin blood perfusion, provided the sensor is working correctly. The quality of correlation between $Ptco_2$ and Pao_2 can be expressed by a coefficient of correlation, as shown in many publications. For a review, the reader is referred to a monograph by Huch, Huch, and Lübbers (1981a,b).

However, in many circumstances $Ptco_2$ is not a good indicator of Pao_2. $Ptco_2$ is far below Pao_2 when the sensor temperature is set inappropriately, causing insufficient skin blood flow (Bossi et al., 1975; Duc, Bucher, and Micheli, 1975). In vivo calibration improves accuracy (Pollitzer et al., 1980). Pressure on the sensor can diminish blood flow, leading to artifactual hypoxia (Whitehead, Pollitzer, and Reynolds, 1979). The risk for compression of the capillaries is increased when the sensor is placed over bony structures.

Poor clinical conditions, as indicated by acidosis, low blood pressure, or anemia, make $Ptco_2$ measurement unreliable (Versmold et al., 1979). In infants with hyperoxemia, $Ptco_2$ may underestimate Pao_2 (Löfgren et al., 1978; Duc et al., 1979; Martin, Robertson, and Hopple, 1982). Drugs that influence circulation may disturb skin blood perfusion, leading to underestimation of Pao_2 (Peabody et al., 1978). $Ptco_2$ may underestimate Pao_2 beyond the neonatal period (Versmold et al., 1978; Hamilton, Whitehead, and Reynolds, 1985; Mok et al., 1988). In infants with bronchopulmonary dysplasia, $Ptco_2$ may also underestimate Pao_2 (Rome et al., 1984; Lafeber et al., 1987).

$Ptco_2$ measurements can be influenced by interference from anesthetic gases like halothane and nitrous dioxide (Severinghaus et al., 1971; Eberhard and Mindt, 1979). Halothane interference can be prevented by using a Teflon membrane, and nitrous dioxide interference can be prevented by an altered polarization voltage (Tremper, 1984).

Clinical applications of transcutaneous Po_2 sensors

Continuous measurements of Po_2 have made nursing staff and neonatologists aware of the fact that many procedures (e.g., chest x-rays, endotracheal intubation, endotracheal suctioning, heel puncture, infusion puncture) can have tremendously negative influences on the oxygenation of infants (Dangman et al., 1976; Emmrich, 1976; Simbruner et al., 1981; Danford et al. 1983; Murdoch and Darlow, 1984).

Periods of hypoxia due to excessive handling can be shortened by continuous Po_2 measurement (Long, Philip, and Lucey, 1980; Kilbride and Mer-

enstein, 1984). Continuous Po_2 measurement can decrease the number of arterial blood samples needed, which can have a beneficial effect on the financial burden (Peevy and Hall, 1985). A reduced incidence of retinopathy of prematurity among infants whose birth weights were less than 1,000 g was reported as a consequence of continuous $Ptco_2$ monitoring (Bancalari et al., 1987). Apneic attacks are detected more frequently by continuous $Ptco_2$ measurement (Peabody et al., 1977). By using two sensors (one on the abdomen and one on the right chest), pathological right-to-left ductal shunts can be found (DeGeeter et al., 1979; Heinonen and Hakulinen, 1986).

$Ptco_2$ measurement has proved to be beneficial in the treatment of neonates with respiratory distress (Emmrich, 1976; Löfgren et al., 1978; Okken, Rubin, and Martin, 1978).

Summary

$Ptco_2$ measurement can be used as a trend parameter for continuous noninvasive Po_2 monitoring. As an adjunct to intermittent Pao_2 measurement, $Ptco_2$ measurement can detect hypoxemia and hyperoxemia in infants with respiratory distress, persistent fetal circulation, apneic attacks of prematurity, and cardiac anomalies.

The major limitation of $Ptco_2$ measurement is its dependence on skin blood flow. $Ptco_2$ can never be used as a complete replacement for Pao_2. Because of the necessity for sensor maintenance, calibration procedures, and frequent application-site changes, the technique of $Ptco_2$ measurement requires extensive staff training in the neonatal intensive-care unit (NICU). For this reason, many NICUs have abandoned transcutaneous measurements in favor of pulse oximetry. This latter technique does not require any calibration or extensive maintenance techniques, but it also suffers from some limitations in practice, as discussed elsewhere in this volume.

TRANSCUTANEOUS Pco_2 MEASUREMENTS

History

The first publications on transcutaneous Pco_2 measurements date to 1973–8 (Huch, Lübbers, and Huch, 1973b, 1977; Severinghaus, Stafford, and Bradley, 1978a). As was the case with transcutaneous Po_2 measurements, the first sensors were based on equipment developed for blood gas analysis. Those first developments have been described by Severinghaus et al. (1978a), comparing a large, modified electrode for blood gases (Stow-Severinghaus glass, pH-sensitive) mounted in a circulated, thermostated copper jacket with a prototype of a miniaturized electrode. The first electrodes were still too large, causing measurement disturbances, but many experiments proved that glass pH electrodes could detect the CO_2 diffused through the skin if the skin was heated to a stable temperature. Earlier attempts had been made to measure CO_2 diffused through the skin in infrared analysis, similar to the method applied for respiratory gases (Eletr et al., 1978). That technique proved to be rather impractical, because the upper layer of the skin (stratum corneum) had to be stripped before application of the sensor. Another technique to measure skin CO_2 was mass spectrometry (Delpy and Parker, 1975, McIlroy, Simbruner, and Sonoda, 1978; Parker, Delpy, and Reynolds, 1978). Although that technique proved to be effective, its technology turned out to be too complicated and costly, and it has never seen general use in clinical medicine.

The most successful improvements were achieved using miniaturized pH-sensitive glass or metal/metal oxide electrodes. The technique of liquid-filled pH-sensitive glass electrodes to measure CO_2 has been known for more than 80 yr and has proved to be very reliable regarding sensitivity and stability. For transcutaneous use, these electrodes experienced problems because of the heating of the skin, causing air bubbles in the electrolyte solution, followed by drifting and a "noisy" response. Use of ethylene glycol reduced those problems (Severinghaus et al., 1978a). The use of the glass electrode led to other problems, such as high resistance, necessitating high-input impedance and requiring high-quality shielding of the electrodes. Its use in practice was also limited because of the fragile nature of glass. Therefore, alternative techniques were tested using metal/metal oxide electrodes, such as antimony/antimony oxide, palladium/palladium oxide, or iridium/iridium oxide (Yeung, Beran, and Huxtable 1978; Beran et al., 1978), or reduction–oxidation electrodes, such as the quinhydrone electrode (Van Kempen, Deurenberg, and Kreuzer 1971; Yeung et al., 1978). Eventually, over the past 10 yr, iridium/iridium oxide and pH-sensitive glass electrodes, combined with thick-film technology, have proved to be most successful for mass production and practical clinical use. Because both Po_2 and Pco_2 sensors use silver/silver chloride (Ag/AgCl) as cathode/reference electrodes, the idea of combining the two electrodes in one sensor was introduced a few years after the initial introduction of the separate sensors (Halsall et al., 1980; Severinghaus,

1981). Ag/AgCl was also used as a heating element (Severinghaus, Bradley, and Stafford, 1979), and the combination of Clark and Stow-Severinghaus electrodes became possible by using HCO_3 as an electrochemical stabilizing reagent in the electrolyte solution under the membrane covering the combined electrodes (Severinghaus, 1981). The performance of the transcutaneous sensors was further improved by determining the best skin temperature settings and correction algorithms for comparison with arterial Pco_2.

Measurement principles for pH-sensitive glass or metal/metal oxide electrodes

The Pco_2 measurement is in fact a pH measurement. As CO_2 is released from the skin, it diffuses through the membrane into the electrolyte solution, where it reacts with water, forming carbonic acid, which immediately dissociates into HCO_3^- and H^+, according to the following equation:

$$H_2O + CO_2 \leftrightarrow H_2CO_3 \leftrightarrow H^+ + HCO_3^-$$

The changes in H^+ in the electrolyte solution imply changes in pH, as the HCO_3^- content of the electrolyte is kept fixed. As the pH in the electrolyte changes, the voltage between the glass or metal/metal oxide electrode and the reference electrode changes. The pH change is converted to a Pco_2 reading on the basis of the linear relationship between pH and log Pco_2, as expressed by the Henderson-Hasselbalch equation:

$$pH = pK + \log \frac{[HCO_3^-]}{a \cdot Pco_2}$$

where pK is the dissociation constant for carbonic acid, $[HCO_3^-]$ is the concentration of HCO_3^-, a is the solubility coefficient for CO_2 in electrolyte solution, and Pco_2 is the partial pressure of CO_2. As no charged molecules can penetrate the membrane, the change in pH is due strictly to carbon dioxide diffusion in the electrolyte. The potential, measured across the combined electrode chain, is fed into the Pco_2 channel, where it is digitized. This digitized signal is then passed on to a microcomputer, where it is converted to display the Pco_2 value in millimeters of mercury or kilopascals. A diagram and illustration of one of the most advanced combined $Ptco_2$/$Ptcco_2$ sensors are shown in Figures 7.2 and 7.3.

This is a combined-electrode sensor using a solid-state pH-sensitive glass electrode. This electrode, with thermistor-servocontrolled heating element,

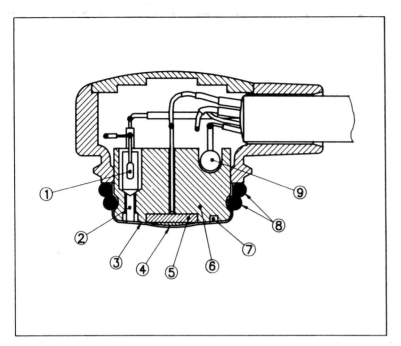

Figure 7.2. Cross section of a modern combined Po_2/Pco_2 sensor using a pH-sensitive glass electrode manufactured using thick-film technology: 1, high-precision negative-temperature-coefficient (NTC) resistors–temperature sensors; 2, platinum cathode (Po_2 electrode); 3, electrolyte covering the electrode surface; 4, O_2/CO_2-permeable membranes; 5, reinforced solid-state pH-sensitive electrode (Pco_2 electrode); 6, Ag/AgCl reference electrode; 7, electrolyte reservoir; 8, O-rings for securing membranes; 9, heating element. (From Larsen and Linnet, 1990, with permission.)

combines the advantages of the stability and sensitivity of a glass electrode with a low rate of breakage by using a special thick-film manufacturing technique on a basis of ceramic material (Larsen and Linnet, 1990) (Figure 7.4).

Before each application to the skin, the sensor is calibrated by one or two calibration gases (usually containing 5% or 10% CO_2), preferably at the measuring temperature. The site of application to the skin must be changed every 3–4 h, thus preventing edema and other skin damage that could make the measurement unreliable.

Reliability of transcutaneous Pco_2 measurement

As discussed later, close correlations between Ptcco$_2$ and arterial Pco_2 have been demonstrated in neonates as well as in adults. Owing to the elevated temperature at which the transcutaneous electrode operates, the measured values will be significantly higher than arterial values at 37°C. The Ptcco$_2$ readout, however, can be temperature-correlated to 37°C, thus enabling a readout comparable to 37°C values as obtained by means of invasive blood gas analysis (Bradley, Stupfel, and Severinghaus, 1956). However, a small deviation is caused by a metabolic contribution of the epidermis. Hence, arterial Pco_2 estimation by means of Ptcco$_2$ measurement depends mainly on the electrode temperature, the skin perfusion, and the amount of metabolic CO_2 contribution. Evaluation of the temperature setting can be performed in vitro, but ultimately a correct comparison can be made only in vivo in various groups of patients (Severinghaus et al., 1978b; Eberhard, 1980; Eberhard and Schäfer, 1980; Herrell et al., 1980; Eberhard, Mindt, and Schäfer, 1981a,b; Frey, Ruh, and Ruh, 1981; Hazinski and Severinghaus, 1982; Vesterager, 1982; Melberg and Vesterager, 1983; Mindt, Eberhard, and Schäfer, 1983; Monaco, McQuitty, and Nickerson, 1983; Severinghaus, 1983; Friis-Hansen et al., 1987; Martin et al., 1987).

In general, the relation between arterial Pco_2 and

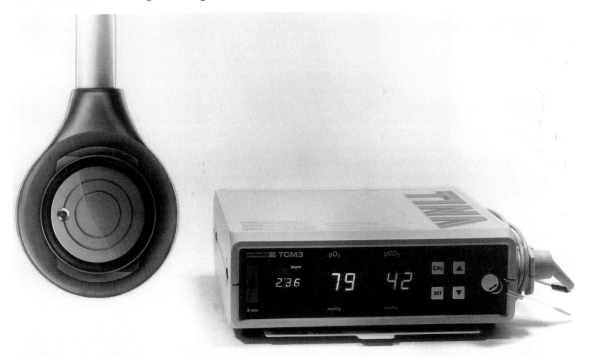

Figure 7.3. Modern combined P_{O_2}/P_{CO_2} sensor with monitor. (Radiometer A/S, Copenhagen, Denmark.)

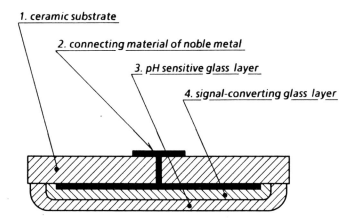

Figure 7.4. Cross section of pH-sensitive glass electrode produced by thick-film technique on a basis of ceramic material. (From Larsen and Linnet, 1990, with permission.)

transcutaneous P_{CO_2} is determined mainly by the three parameters discussed next (Baumbach, 1986).

Capillary blood temperature

From in vitro studies of blood gas analysis (Bradley et al., 1956), the exact expression for P_{CO_2} at a higher temperature $T°C$ is known (according to Siggaard Anderson):

$$P_{CO_2}(T) = P_{CO_2}(37°C)^{10^{0.021(T-37°C)}}$$

According to this formula, P_{CO_2} at 42°C is 1.27 times the P_{CO_2} at 37°C, and at 43°C the P_{CO_2} is approximately 1.34 times the P_{CO_2} at 37°C.

Metabolic carbon dioxide contribution

The living cells of the epidermis produce CO_2, which is added to the CO_2 from the capillary blood. This metabolic skin production is highly variable, depending on age, thickness, and clinical condition. This phenomenon is still physiologically poorly understood, but it appears to be independent of skin temperature. It is not suprising that in various validation studies, as described later, variable values for this metabolic contribution have been found. On average, it may amount to 4 mm Hg (0.5 kPa).

Blood flow

The effect of local blood flow on $Ptcco_2$ readings is not as pronounced as it is for oxygen measurements. This is mainly due to the fact that the difference between arterial and venous Pco_2 normally amounts to only a few millimeters of mercury, whereas CO_2 diffuses much faster than O_2 in tissue (Severinghaus, Stafford, and Thurnstrom, 1978b; Eberhard et al., 1981b). Consequently, a reduction in local blood flow will increase $Ptcco_2$ readings by only a few millimeters of mercury. The blood flow, however, is responsible for CO_2 washout/washin in the skin. Thus, a reduced blood flow will lower the $Ptcco_2$ response time, and in severe cases (e.g., shock) $Ptcco_2$ will not reflect arterial Pco_2, but will merely be an indicator of the shock condition (Tremper, Mentelos, and Shoemaker, 1980a; Tremper et al., 1980b; Versmold et al., 1981)

Clinical use of $Ptcco_2$ monitoring

General use

Over the past decade, the clinical use of $Ptcco_2$ has been investigated in all patient categories, as reviewed by several authors (Severinghaus, 1982; Cassady, 1983; Avery et al., 1989; Wimberley et al., 1990; Rennie, 1990; Schultz, De Kleine, and Koppe, 1991).

In general, it can be concluded that transcutaneous Pco_2 measurements, like those of $Ptco_2$, have been most successfully applied in neonatology. This is mainly due to the fact that under normal circumstances, transcutaneous readings in these infants are more closely related to arterial values than are those in adults. The most important factor influencing the clinical success of transcutaneous Pco_2 monitoring, however, is the clinician's understanding of the concept of "skin CO_2" being physiologically different from arterial CO_2. As in the case of $Ptco_2$,

other factors limiting the clinical success of transcutaneous Pco_2 monitoring are the necessity for calibration, frequent skin-site changes, sensor maintenance, and choice of heating temperature.

The latter depends to a large extent on the philosophy of the user: Higher temperatures may cause more arterialization of the skin, creating a closer relationship with arterial values. Higher temperatures, however, may also cause increases in the Pco_2 readings. High temperatures limit the time during which the sensor can be fixed to one position on the skin. Lower temperatures can be used, allowing measurements for 24 h, especially for trend monitoring purposes (Bucher et al., 1986).

In practice, $Ptcco_2$ has been validated in many clinical studies and has proved to be useful for monitoring of several clinical conditions: the progress of labor, neonatal intensive-care treatment, and intensive-care treatment of older infants and children (Bompard et al., 1981; Hazinski et al., 1981; Vyas, Helms, and Cheriyan, 1988; Fanconi et al., 1990) and adults (Eberhard et al., 1981a; Mahutte et al., 1984; Palmisano and Severinghaus, 1984, 1990; Rithalia, Clutton-Brock, and Tinker, 1984; Wimberley et al., 1985). For the latter patient groups, its use in the operating room has been validated in regard to interference by narcotic gases, such as halothane, enflurane, and nitrous oxide. In contrast with $Ptco_2$ measurements, the use of narcotic gases shows hardly any interference with $Ptcco_2$ measurements (Eberhard and Mindt, 1981; Rafferty et al., 1981; Tremper et al., 1981; Nolan and Shoemaker, 1982). $Ptcco_2$ measurement has also proved to be an important tool in exercise monitoring (Ewald, Tuvemo, and Rooth, 1985; Rooth, Ewald, and Caligara, 1985; Nickerson et al., 1986).

Perinatal use of $Ptcco_2$

Following the reports of success in transcutaneous measurements during the neonatal period, several attempts were made to apply $Ptcco_2$ sensors to the head of the fetus during birth. Usually, standard sensors were used, sometimes with special fixation techniques (Hansen, 1984; Schmidt and Saling, 1987; Nickelsen, 1989; Van den Berg et al., 1991). Most fetal scalp measurements show strong interference due to poor skin blood perfusion caused by local pressure exerted on the skull by the birth canal. Thus, although fetal $Ptco_2$ measurement often is impossible, $Ptcco_2$ measurements show high CO_2 readings, with slow response times. The higher $Ptcco_2$ values do not allow an easy interpretation regarding fetal surveillance, and Pco_2

measurement seems to be useful only for trend detection in between fetal scalp measurements of blood gases and acid–base balance (Van den Berg et al., 1991).

Neonatal use of Pco_2 measurements has been very successful for management of respiratory failure and application of surfactant in respiratory distress syndrome. Most often, $Ptcco_2$ is used for continuous CO_2 monitoring in between samplings of arterial blood gases. Most validation studies have shown good correlation between arterial and transcutaneous Pco_2 values under normal conditions, with a wide variety of suggested "correction factors," depending on the type of electrode and the temperature setting (Hansen and Tooley, 1979; Versmold et al., 1980; Whitehead, Halsall, and Pollitzer, 1980; Bhat et al., 1981; Cabal et al., 1981; Erny, Messer, and Willard, 1981; Laptook and Oh, 1981; Meritt, 1981; Monaco and McQuitty, 1981; Whitehead, 1981; Löfgren and Anderson, 1982; Vesterager, 1982; Kost, Chow, and Kenny, 1983a,b; Epstein et al., 1985; Marsden et al., 1985; Whitehead et al., 1985; Wimberley et al., 1985; Bucher et al., 1986; Cheriyan et al., 1986; Friis-Hansen et al., 1987; Martin et al., 1987; Lee, Broadhurst, and Helms, 1989; Schultz et al., 1991). Several of the validation studies described situations in which $Ptcco_2$ seemed less reliable, most of the time because of poor clinical conditions, with diminished skin perfusion (Versmold et al., 1981), poor calibration procedures, and improper tenures of application of the skin (Avery et al., 1989). Reports on the selection of the best electrode temperature have been in conflict, for reasons described earlier, and often different types of equipment show different absolute $Ptcco_2$ values. In most cases, the $Ptcco_2$ values obtained with iridium/iridium oxide electrodes are somewhat higher than those with the new solid-state glass electrodes (Schultz et al., 1991), which in part may be due to the temperature-correction algorithms used by the manufacturers. Use of $Ptcco_2$ seems to be most effective for trend monitoring, such as in the development of pneumothorax, detection of sleep states, and detection of obstructive apnea (Rowe et al., 1980; Martin, Herrell, and Pultusher, 1981). Measurements in older newborn infants with chronic lung disease often show poor correlation with arterial Pco_2 (Rome et al., 1984). Like $Ptco_2$ measurements, most $Ptcco_2$ measurements used as a day-to-day routine are hampered by poor instrument management, and strict guidelines have been suggested to manufacturers and users (Avery et al., 1989; Wimberley et al., 1990).

Mainly because of all the technical handling involved in using transcutaneous sensors (calibration, changing the membrane, site changes), alternative monitoring techniques such as capnography (end-tidal CO_2 measurement) have been validated for neonatal use (Phan et al., 1987; McEvedy, McLeod, and Mulera, 1988). Measurement in small neonates became possible because of the introduction of low-flow side-stream systems that could be connected to the ventilator. Newborns with normal pulmonary function show good correlation among arterial Pco_2, end-tidal CO_2, and transcutaneous Pco_2. But, as can be predicted on the basis of pathophysiological reasoning, neonates with poor pulmonary function due to respiratory distress syndrome show variable end-tidal CO_2 values, depending on vascular shunting in the lungs (McEvedy et al., 1988). For this reason, for most patients in neonatal intensive care, end-tidal CO_2 measurement is of only limited clinical value.

Summary

$Ptcco_2$ measurements are nowadays usually combined with $Ptco_2$ measurements, and both have proved to be useful for continuous estimation of arterial blood gases in neonates. Transcutaneous measurements on the fetal scalp during labor are of limited value regarding surveillance of the fetus, because of diminished perfusion in the presenting part of the fetal head. The requirements for proper sensor maintenance and calibration procedures have limited the use of transcutaneous sensors in practice. Many neonatal intensive-care units currently favor the use of pulse oximetry instead of $Ptco_2$, and $Ptcco_2$ is no longer used. Modern solid-state $Ptco_2/Ptcco_2$ sensors, applied by trained personnel, may add tremendously to our ability to monitor high-risk situations in neonatology (i.e., hyperoxemia during surfactant replacement therapy or hypercarbia during mechanical ventilation).

REFERENCES

Al-Siaidy, W., and Hill, D. W. (1979). The importance of an elevated skin temperature in transcutaneous oxygen tension measurement. In *Continuous Transcutaneous Blood Gas Monitoring*, ed. A. Huch, R. Huch, and J. F. Lucey (pp. 149–65). New York: Alan R. Liss.

Avery, G. B., Bancalari, E. H., Engler, A., Guilfoile, T. D., Hodgson, A. J., Hodson, W. A., Huch, A., Huch, R., Jay, A. W. L., Lucey, J. F., Martin, R. J., Caffey, C., and Lochhart, J. D. (1989). Task force on transcutaneous oxygen monitors. *Pediatrics* 83:122–6.

Bancalari, E., Flynn, J., Goldberg, R. N., Bawol, R., Cassady, J., Schiffman, J., Feuer, W., Roberts, J., Gillings, D., and Sim, E. (1987). Influence of transcutaneous monitoring on the incidence of retinopathy of prematurity. *Pediatrics* 79:663–9.

Banister, A. (1969). Comparisons of arterial and arterialized capillary blood in infants with respiratory distress. *Archives of Disease in Childhood* 44:726–8.

Baumbach, P. (1986). *Understanding Transcutaneous pO$_2$ and pCO$_2$ Measurements.* TC 100. Copenhagen: Radiometer A/S.

Baumberger, D. M., and Goodfriend, R. B. (1951). Determination of arterial oxygen tension in man by equilibration through intact skin. *Federation Proceedings* 15:3–6.

Beran, A. V., Huxtable, R. F., and Sperling, D. R. (1976). Electrochemical sensor for continuous transcutaneous Pco$_2$ measurement. *Journal of Applied Physiology* 41:442–7.

Beran, V., Shigezawa, G. Y., Yeung, H. N., and Huxtable, R. F. (1978). An improved sensor and a method for transcutaneous CO$_2$ monitoring. *Acta Anaesthesiologica Scandinavica [Suppl. 68]*, pp. 111–17.

Bhat, R., Shukla, A., Kins, W. D., and Vidyasagar, D. (1981). Simultaneous tissue pH and transcutaneous carbon dioxide monitoring in critically ill neonates. *Critical Care Medicine* 9:744–9.

Bompard, Y., Aufront, C., Mercier, J. C., and Beaufils, P. (1981). Cutaneous pCO$_2$ monitoring in respiratory distress in infants and children. *Intensive Care Medicine* 7:255–6.

Bossi, E., Breitenstein, M., Lenzin, B., and Pfenninger, J. (1975). Percutane Messung des Sauerstoffpartialdruckes beim kranken Neugeborenen. *Helvetica Paediatrica Acta [Suppl. 35]*, pp. 22–3.

Bradley, A. F., Stupfel, M., and Severinghaus, J. W. (1956). Effect of temperature on Pco$_2$ and Po$_2$ of blood in vitro. *Journal of Applied Physiology* 9:201–4.

Brünstler, I., Enders, A., and Versmold, H. T. (1982). Skin surface pCO$_2$ monitoring in newborn infants in shock: effect of hypotension and electrode temperature. *Journal of Pediatrics* 100:454–7.

Bucher, H. U., Fanconi, S., Fallenstein, F., and Duc, G. (1986). Transcutaneous carbon dioxide tension in newborn infants: reliability and safety of continuous 24 hour measurements at 42°C. *Pediatrics* 78:631–5.

Cabal, L., Hodgman, J., Siassi, B., and Playstek, C. (1981). Factors affecting heated transcutaneous Po$_2$ and unheated transcutaneous Pco$_2$ in preterm infants. *Critical Care Medicine* 9:298–301.

Cassady, G. (1983). Transcutaneous monitoring in the newborn infant. *Journal of Pediatrics* 103:837–48.

Cheriyan, G., Helms, P., Paky, F., Marsden, G., and Chiu, M. C. (1986). Transcutaneous estimation of arterial carbon dioxide in intensive care. *Archives of Disease in Childhood* 61:652–6.

Clark, L. C., Jr. (1956). Monitor and control of blood and tissue oxygen tensions. *Transactions of the American Society for Artificial Internal Organs* 2:41–6.

Clark, L. C., Jr., Wolf, R., Granger, D., and Taylor, Z. (1953). Continuous monitoring of blood oxygen tensions by polarography. *Journal of Applied Physiology* 6:189–93.

Danford, D. A., Miske, S., Headley, J., and Nelson, R. M. (1983). Effects of routine care procedures on transcutaneous oxygen in neonates; a quantitative approach. *Archives of Disease in Childhood* 58:20–3.

Dangman, B. C., Heygi, T., Hiatt, M., Indyk, L., and

James, L. S. (1976). The variability of Po$_2$ in newborn infants in response to routine care. *Pediatric Research* 10:422A.

DeGeeter, B., Messer, J., Benoit, M., and Willard, D. (1979). Right-to-left ductal shunt and transcutaneous Po$_2$. In *Continuous Transcutaneous Blood Gas Monitoring*, ed. A. Huch, R. Huch, and J. F. Lucey (pp. 387–92). New York: Alan R. Liss.

Delpy, D., and Parker, D. (1975). Transcutaneous measurement of arterial blood-gas tensions by mass-spectrometry. *Lancet* 1:1076–7.

Duc, G., Bucher, H. U., and Micheli, J. L. (1975). Is transcutaneous pO$_2$ reliable for arterial oxygen monitoring in newborn infants? *Pediatrics* 55:566–7.

Duc, G., Frei, H., Klar, H., and Tuchschmid, P. (1979). Reliability of continuous transcutaneous Po$_2$ (Hellige) in respiratory distress syndrome in the newborn. In *Continuous Transcutaneous Blood Gas Monitoring*, ed. A. Huch, R. Huch, and J. F. Lucey (pp. 305–13). New York: Alan R. Liss.

Eberhard, P. (1980). Skin sensor for continuous monitoring of pCO$_2$ measuring principle. In *Fetal and Neonatal Physiological Measurements*, ed. P. Rolfe (pp. 413–17). London: Pitman Medical.

Eberhard, P., and Mindt, W. (1979). Interference of anesthetic gases at oxygen sensors. In *Continuous Transcutaneous Blood Gas Monitoring*, ed. A. Huch, R. Huch, and J. F. Lucey (pp. 65–74). New York: Alan R. Liss.

(1981). Interference of anesthetic gases at skin surface sensors for oxygen and carbon dioxide. *Critical Care Medicine* 9:717–20.

Eberhard, P., Mindt, W., Jann, F., and Hammacher, K. (1973). Oxygen monitoring of newborns by skin electrodes. Correlation between arterial and cutaneously determined pO$_2$. *Advances in Experimental Medicine and Biology* 37b:1097–101.

Eberhard, P., Mindt, W., and Schäfer, R. (1981a). Cutaneous blood gas monitoring in the adult. *Critical Care Medicine* 9:702–5.

(1981b). Methodologic aspects of cutaneous Pco$_2$ monitoring. *Intensive Care Medicine* 7:249–50.

Eberhard, P., and Schäfer, R. (1980). A sensor for noninvasive monitoring of carbon dioxide. *British Journal of Clinical Equipment* 5:224–7.

Eletr, S., Jimison, H., Ream, A. K., Polan, W. H., and Rosenthal, H. H. (1978). Cutaneous monitoring of systematic Pco$_2$ on patients in the respiratory intensive care unit being weaned from the ventilator. *Acta Anaesthesiologica Scandinavica [Suppl. 68]*, pp. 123–7.

Emmrich, P. (1976). Die transkutane Sauerstoffpartialdruckmessung in der Paediatrie. *Monatsschrift für Kinderheilkunde* 124:504–10.

Engel, R. F., Delpy, D. T., and Parker, D. (1979). The effect of topical potassium cyanide on transcutaneous gas measurement. In *Continuous Transcutaneous Blood Gas Monitoring*, ed. A. Huch, R. Huch, and J. F. Lucey (pp. 117–21). New York: Alan R. Liss.

Enkema, L., Jr., Holloway, G. A., Jr., Piraino, D. W., Harry, D., Zick, G. L., and Kenny, M. A. (1981). Laser Doppler velocimetry vs heater power as indicators of skin perfusion during transcutaneous O$_2$ monitoring. *Clinical Chemistry* 27:391–6.

Epstein, M. F., Cohen, A. R., Feldman, H. A., and Raemer, D. B. (1985). Estimation of Paco$_2$ by two noninvasive methods in the critically ill newborn infant. *Journal of Pediatrics* 106:282–6.

Erny, P., Messer, J., and Willard, D. (1981). Cutaneous pCO_2 monitoring and artificial ventilation in the newborn. *Intensive Care Medicine* 7:252–3.

Evans, N. T. S., and Naylor, P. F. D. (1966). Steady states of oxygen tension in human dermis. *Respiration Physiology* 2:46–50.

(1967). The systemic oxygen supply to the surface of human skin. *Respiration Physiology* 3:21–37.

Ewald, U., Tuvemo, T., and Rooth, G. (1985). Detection of exercise induced lactic acidoses using transcutaneous carbon dioxide. *Critical Care Medicine* 13:630–1.

Fanconi, S., Burger, R., Maurer, H., Uehlinger, J., Ghelfi, D., and Mühleman, C. (1990). Transcutaneous carbon dioxide pressure for monitoring patients with severe croup. *Journal of Pediatrics* 117:701–5.

Fatt, I. (1976). *Polarographic Oxygen Sensor.* Cleveland: C.R.C. Press.

Fetter, W. P. F. (1983). Transcutane meting van de zuurstofspanning in de Neonatologie. Thesis, Erasmus University, Rotterdam.

Frey, P., Ruh, H., and Ruh, P. (1981). Continuous pCO_2 monitoring by means of skin surface sensors: the influences of various sensor temperatures and first clinical experiences. *Intensive Care Medicine* 7:260.

Friis-Hansen, B., Voldsgaard, P., Witt, J., Pedersen, K. G., and Frederiksen, P. S. (1987). The measurement of $tcpCO_2$ and $tcpO_2$ in newborn infants at 44°, 42° and 37°C. after initial heating to 44°C. *Advances in Experimental Medicine and Biology* 220:35–40.

Gerlach, P. (1851). Ueber das Hautatmen. *Archiven der Anatomie und Physiologie,* pp. 431–79.

Golden, S. M. (1981). Skin craters – a complication of transcutaneous oxygen monitoring. *Pediatrics* 67:514–16.

Halsall, D., Delpy, D., Parker, D., Whitehead, M. D., Pollitzer, M. J., and Reynolds, E. O. R. (1980). Transcutaneous pO_2 and pCO_2 measured by a combined electrochemical sensor. In *Fetal and Neonatal Physiological Measurements,* ed. P. Rolfe (pp. 424–9). London: Pitman Medical.

Hamilton, P. A., Whitehead, M. D., and Reynolds, E. O. R. (1985). Underestimation of arterial oxygen tension by transcutaneous electrode with increasing age in infants. *Archives of Disease in Childhood* 60: 1162–5.

Hansen, P. (1984). Transcutaneous carbon dioxide measurements during labor. *American Journal of Obstetrics and Gynecology* 150:47–50.

Hansen, T. N., and Tooley, W. H. (1979). Skin surface carbon dioxide tension in sick infants. *Pediatrics* 64:942–5.

Hazinski, T. A., Hansen, T. N., Simon, J. A., and Tooley, V. H. (1981). Effect of oxygen administration during sleep on skin surface oxygen and carbon dioxide tensions in patients with chronic lung disease. *Pediatrics* 67:626–30.

Hazinski, T. A., and Severinghaus, J. W. (1982). Transcutaneous analysis of arterial Pco_2. *Medical Instrumentation* 16:150–3.

Heinonen, K., and Hakulinen, A. (1986). Transcutaneous pO_2 recording using two sensors in a neonate with preductal coarctation of the aorta. *Critical Care Medicine* 14:298–9.

Herrell, N., Martin, R. J., Pultusher, M., Lough, M., and

Fanaroff, A. (1980). Optimal temperature for the measurement of transcutaneous carbon dioxide tension in the neonate. *Journal of Pediatrics* 97:114–17.

Heyrovský, J., and Shikata, M. (1923). Researches with the dropping mercury cathode. Part 2. The polarograph. *Recoltes Traveaux Chimiques des Pays-Bas* 44:496–502.

Huch, A., Huch, R., Arner, B., and Rooth, G. (1973a). Continuous transcutaneous oxygen tension measured with a heated electrode. *Scandinavian Journal of Clinical and Laboratory Investigations* 31:269–75.

Huch, A., Huch, R., and Lübbers, D. W. (1969). Quantitative polarographische Sauerstoffdruckmessung auf der Kopfhaut des Neugeborenen. *Archiven der Gynäkologie* 207:443–51.

Huch, A., Lübbers, D. W., and Huch, R. (1973b). Patienten Uberwachung durch transcutane Pco_2 Messung bei gleichzeitige Kontrolle der relativen Perfusion. *Anaesthetist* 22:379–80.

(1977). Transcutaneous pCO_2 measurement with a miniaturized electrode. *Lancet* 1:982–8.

Huch, R., Huch, A., and Lübbers, D. W. (1973c). Transcutaneous measurement of blood $Po_2(tcPo_2)$. Method and application in perinatal medicine. *Journal of Perinatal Medicine* 1:183–91.

(1981a). Principle and technique of transcutaneous Po_2 measurement. In *Transcutaneous pO_2,* ed. R. Huch, A. Huch, and D. W. Lübbers (pp. 71–107). New York: Thieme-Stratton.

(1981b). Results of clinical and physiologic investigations with the transcutaneous pO_2 technique. In *Transcutaneous pO_2,* ed. R. Huch. A. Huch, and D. W. Lübbers (pp. 108–51). New York: Thieme-Stratton.

Huch, R., Lübbers, D. W., and Huch, A. (1974). Reliability of transcutaneous monitoring of arterial Po_2 in newborn infants. *Archives of Disease in Childhood* 49:213–18.

Kilbride, H. W., and Merenstein, G. B. (1984). Continuous transcutaneous oxygen monitoring in acutely ill preterm infants. *Critical Care Medicine* 12:121–4.

Kost, G. J., Chow, J. L., and Kenny, M. A. (1983a). Monitoring of transcutaneous carbon dioxide tension. *American Journal of Clinical Pathology* 80:832–8.

(1983b). Transcutaneous carbon dioxide for short term monitoring of neonates. *Clinical Chemistry* 29:1534–6.

Lafeber, H. N., Fetter, W. P. F., Van der Wiel, A. R., and Jansen, T. C. (1987). Pulse oximetry and transcutaneous oxygen tension in hypoxemic neonates and infants with bronchopulmonary dysplasia. *Advances in Experimental Medicine and Biology* 220: 181–6.

Laptook, A., and Oh, W. (1981). Continuous transcutaneous carbon dioxide monitoring in the newborn period. *Critical Care Medicine* 9:759–60.

Larsen, J., and Linnet, N. (1990). *Solid State Transcutaneous Combined pO_2/pCO_2 Electrode.* TC 110. Copenhagen: Radiometer A/S.

Lee, H. K., Broadhurst, E., and Helms, P. (1989). Evaluation of two-combined oxygen and carbon dioxide transcutaneous sensors. *Archives of Disease in Childhood* 64:279–82.

Lewis, I. G., and Haslan, R. R. (1984). A comparison of pO_2 monitoring techniques in newborn infants. *Australian Paediatric Journal* 20:309–11.

Löfgren, O., and Anderson, D. (1982). Continuous transcutaneous carbon dioxide monitoring in the newborn period. *Critical Care Medicine* 9:750–1.

Löfgren, O., Henriksson, P., Jacobson, L., and Johansson, O. (1978). Trancutaneous pO_2 monitoring in neonatal intensive care. *Acta Paediatrica Scandinavica* 67:693–7.

Long, J. G., Philip, A. G. S., and Lucey, J. F. (1980). Excessive handling as a cause of hypoxemia. *Pediatrics* 65:203–7.

McEvedy, B. A. B., McLeod, M. C., and Mulera, M. (1988). End tidal transcutaneous and arterial Pco_2 measurements in critically ill neonates: a comparative study. *Anaesthesiology* 69:112–16.

McIlroy, H. B., Simbruner, G., and Sonoda, Y. (1978). Transcutaneous blood gas measurements using a mass spectrometer. *Acta Anaesthesiologica Scandinavica [Suppl. 68]*, pp. 128–30.

Mclain, B. I., Evans, J., and Dear, P. R. F. (1988). Comparison of capillary and arterial blood gas measurement in neonates. *Archives of Disease in Childhood* 63: 743–7.

Mahutte, C. K., Michiels, T. M., Hassell, K. T., and Trueblood, D. M. (1984). Evaluation of a single transcutaneous pO_2/pCO_2 sensor in adult patients. *Critical Care Medicine* 12:1063–6.

Marsden, D., Chiu, M. C., Paky, F., and Helms, P. (1985). Transcutaneous oxygen and carbon dioxide monitoring in intensive care. *Archives of Disease in Childhood* 60:1158–61.

Martin, R. J., Beoglos, A., Miller, M. J., DiFiore, J. M., and Carlo, W. A. (1987). Current correction factors inadequately predict the relationship between transcutaneous and arterial pCO_2 in sick neonates. *Advances in Experimental Medicine and Biology* 220:51–3.

Martin, R. J., Herrell, N., and Pultusher, M. (1981). Transcutaneous measurement of carbon dioxide tension: effect of sleep state in term infants. *Pediatrics* 67:622–5.

Martin, R. J., Robertson, S. S., and Hopple, M. M. (1982). Relationship between transcutaneous and arterial oxygen tension in sick neonates during mild hyperoxemia. *Critical Care Medicine* 10:671–2.

Melberg, S. G., and Vesterager, P. (1983). Temperature effects in transcutaneous carbon dioxide monitoring. In *Continuous Transcutaneous Blood Gas Monitoring*, ed. R. Huch & A. Huch (pp. 217–31). New York: Marcel Dekker.

Meritt, T. (1981). Skin surface CO_2 measurement in sick preterm and term infants. *Journal of Pediatrics* 99:782–6.

Mindt, W., Eberhard, P., and Schäfer, R. (1983). Methodologic factors affecting the relationship between transcutaneous and arterial pCO_2. In *Continuous Transcutaneous Blood Gas Monitoring*, ed. R. Huch & A. Huch (pp. 199–215). New York: Marcel Dekker.

Mok, J. Y., Hak, H., McLaughlin, F. J., Pintar, M., Casnny, G. J., and Levison, H. (1988). Effect of age and state of wakefulness on transcutaneous oxygen values in preterm infants; a longitudinal study. *Journal of Pediatrics* 113:706–9.

Monaco, F., and McQuitty, J. C. (1981). Transcutaneous measurements of carbon dioxide partial pressures in sick neonates. *Critical Care Medicine* 9:756–8.

Monaco, F., McQuitty, J. C., and Nickerson, B. G. (1983). Calibration of a heated transcutaneous CO_2 electrode

to reflect arterial CO_2. *American Review of Respiratory Diseases* 127:322–4.

Monaco, F., Nickerson, B. G., and McQuitty, J. C. (1982). Continuous transcutaneous oxygen and carbon dioxide monitoring in the pediatric ICU. *Critical Care Medicine* 10:765–6.

Montgomery, H., and Horwitz, O. (1950). Oxygen tension of tissues by the polarographic method. 1. Introduction: Oxygen tension and blood flow of the skin of human extremities. *Journal of Clinical Investigation* 29:1120–30.

Murdoch, D. R., and Darlow, B. A. (1984). Handling during neonatal intensive care. *Archives of Disease in Childhood* 59:957–61.

Nickelsen, C. (1989). Monitoring of fetal carbon dioxide tension during labour. *Danish Medical Bulletin* 36:537–50.

Nickerson, B. G., Patterson, C., McCrea, R., and Monaco, F. (1986). In vivo response times for a heated skin surface CO_2 electrode during rest and exercise. *Pediatric Pulmonology* 2:135–40.

Nolan, L. S., and Shoemaker, W. C. (1982). Transcutaneous O_2 and CO_2 monitoring of high risk surgical patients during the perioperative period. *Critical Care Medicine* 10:762–6.

Okken, A., Rubin, I. L., and Martin, R. J. (1978). Intermittent bag ventilation of preterm infants on continuous positive airway pressure: the effect on transcutaneous Po_2. *Journal of Pediatrics* 93:279–82.

Palmisano, B. W., and Severinghaus, J. W. (1984). Clinical accuracy of a combined transcutaneous pO_2/pCO_2 electrode. *Critical Care Medicine* 12:276–80.

(1990). Transcutaneous pCO_2 and pO_2: a multicenter study of accuracy. *Journal of Clinical Monitoring* 6:189–95.

Parker, D., Delpy, D., and Reynolds, E. O. R. (1978). Transcutaneous blood gas measurements by mass spectrometry. *Acta Anaesthesiologica Scandinavica [Suppl. 68]*, pp. 131–6.

Peabody, J. L., and Emery, J. R. (1985). Noninvasive monitoring of blood gases in the newborn. *Clinics in Perinatology* 12:147–60.

Peabody, J. L., Gregory, G. A., Willis, M. M., Lucey, J. F., and Tooley, W. H. (1977). Failure of conventional respiratory monitoring to detect hypoxia. *Clinical Research* 25:190A.

Peabody, J. L., Willes, M. M., Gregory, G. A., Tooley, W. H., and Lucey, J. F. (1978). Clinical limitations and advantages of transcutaneous oxygen electrodes. *Acta Anaesthesiologica Scandinavica [Suppl. 68]*, pp. 76–82.

Peevy, K. J., and Hall, M. W. (1985). Trancutaneous oxygen monitoring: economic impact on neonatal care. *Pediatrics* 75:1065–7.

Phan, C. Q., Tremper, K. K., Lee, S. E., and Barker, S. J. (1987). Noninvasive monitoring of carbon dioxide: a comparison of the partial pressure of transcutaneous and end tidal carbon dioxide with the partial pressure of arterial carbon dioxide. *Journal of Clinical Monitoring* 3:149–54.

Pollitzer, M. J., Whitehead, M. D., Reynolds, E. O. R., and Delpy, D. (1980). Effect of electrode temperature and in vivo calibration on accuracy of transcutaneous estimation of arterial oxygen tension on infants. *Pediatrics* 65:515–22.

Rafferty, T. D., Schachter, E., Mentelos, R. A., and Yoker, R. E. (1981). In vitro evaluation of a transcutaneous CO_2 and O_2 monitor: the effects of nitrous oxide, enflurane and halothane. *Medical Instrumentation* 15:316–18.

Rennie, J. M. (1990). Transcutaneous carbon dioxide monitoring. *Archives of Disease in Childhood* 65:345–6.

Rithalia, S. V. S., Clutton-Brock, T. H., and Tinker, J. (1984). Characteristics of transcutaneous carbon dioxide tension monitors in normal adults and critically ill patients. *Intensive Care Medicine* 10:149–53.

Rome, E. S., Stork, E. K., Carlo, W. A., and Martin, R. J. (1984). Limitations of transcutaneous pO_2 and pCO_2 monitoring in infants with bronchopulmonary dysplasia. *Pediatrics* 74:217–20.

Rooth, G., Ewald, U., and Caligara, F. (1985). Anaerobic skin metabolism in healthy men estimated with transcutaneous pCO_2 electrode. *Scandinavian Journal of Clinical and Laboratory Investigation* 45:393–6.

Rowe, L. D., Hansen, T. S., Neilson, D., and Tooley, W. H. (1980). Continuous measurements of skin surface oxygen and CO_2 tensions in obstructive sleep apnea. *Laryngoscope* 90:1797–803.

Schmidt, S. C., and Saling, E. Z. (1987). The continuous measurement of transcutaneous carbon dioxide tension: an atraumatic tool to verify fetal acidosis? *British Journal of Obstetrics and Gynaecology* 94:963–6.

Schultz, M. J., De Kleine, M. J. K., and Koppe, J. G. (1991). Transcutane pCO_2 meting in de neonatologie. *Tijdschrift voor Kindergeneeskunde* 59:44–50.

Severinghaus, J. W. (1981). A combined transcutaneous pO_2/pCO_2 electrode with electrochemical HCO_3 stabilisation. *Journal of Applied Physiology* 15:1027–32.

(1982). Transcutaneous blood gas analysis. *Respiratory Care* 27:152–9.

(1983). Skin CO_2 electrode design and function. In *Continuous Blood Gas Monitoring*, ed. R. Huch & A. Huch (pp. 177–84). New York: Marcel Dekker.

Severinghaus, J. W., Bradley, A. F., and Stafford, M. J. (1979). Transcutaneous pCO_2 electrode design with internal silver heath path. In *Continuous Transcutaneous Blood Gas Monitoring*, ed. A. Huch, R. Huch, and J. F. Lucey (pp. 265–70). New York: Alan R. Liss.

Severinghaus, J. W., Stafford, M., and Bradley, A. F. (1978a). TcpCO_2 electrode design, calibration and temperature gradient problems. *Acta Anaesthesiologica Scandinavica* [Suppl. 68], pp. 118–22.

Severinghaus, J. W., Stafford, M., and Thurnstrom, A. (1978b). Estimation of skin metabolism and blood flow with tcPo_2 and tcpco_2 electrodes by cuff occlusion of the circulation. *Acta Anaesthesiologica Scandinavica* [Suppl. 68], pp. 9–15.

Severinghaus, J. W., Weiskopf, R. B., Nishimura, M., and Bradley, A. F. (1971). Oxygen electrode errors due to polarographic reduction of halothane. *Journal of Applied Physiology* 31:640–4.

Simbruner, G., Coradello, H., Fodor, M., Havelec, L., Lubec, G., and Pollak, A. (1981). Effect of tracheal suctioning on oxygenation, circulation, and lung mechanics in newborn infants. *Archives of Disease in Childhood* 56:326–30.

Tremper, K. K. (1984). Transcutaneous pO_2 measurement. *Canadian Anaesthetists' Society Journal* 31:664–77.

Tremper, K., Mentelos, R. A., and Shoemaker, W. C. (1980a). Effect of hypercarbic and shock on transcutaneous carbon dioxide at different electrode temperatures. *Critical Care Medicine* 8:608–12.

Tremper, K., Shoemaker, W. C., Shippy, C. R., and Nolan, L. S. (1981). Transcutaneous pCO_2 monitoring on adult patients in the ICU and the operating room. *Critical Care Medicine* 9:752–5.

Tremper, K. K., Waxman, K., Bowman, R., and Shoemaker, W. C. (1980b). Continuous transcutaneous oxygen monitoring during respiratory failure, cardiac decompensation, cardiac arrest. *Critical Care Medicine* 8:377–81.

Van den Berg, P., Gembruch, V., Schmidt, S., Hansmann, M., and Krebs, D. (1991). Continuous intrapartum transcutaneous carbon dioxide measurement during fetal arrythmia. *Journal of Perinatal Medicine* 19:81–5.

Van Dussee, B. F. (1975). Thermal analysis of human stratum corneum. *Journal of Investigations in Dermatology* 65:404–8.

Van Kempen, L. H. J., Deurenberg, H., and Kreuzer, F. (1971). The CO_2–quinhydrone electrode. A new method to measure partial CO_2 pressure in gases and liquids. *Respiration Physiology* 14:366–70.

Vaupel, P. (1976). Effect of percental water content in tissue and liquids on the diffusion coefficient of O_2, CO_2, N_2, H_2. *Pflügers Archiv* 361:201–4.

Versmold, H. T., Brünstler, I., Grauber, V., Kopecky, M., Schultess, J., Sengespeik, C., Wittermann, C., and Zimmer, V. (1981). Transcutaneous pCO_2 monitoring of newborn infants in shock at electrode temperatures of 41–44°C. *Intensive Care Medicine* 7:251–2.

Versmold, H. T., Holzmann, M., Linderkamp, O., and Riegel, K. (1978). Skin oxygen permeability in premature infants. *Pediatrics* 62:488–91.

Versmold, H. T., Linderkamp, O., Holzman, M., Strohhacker, I., and Riegel, K. (1979). Trancutaneous monitoring of pO_2 in newborn infants: where are the limits? Influence of blood pressure, blood volume, blood flow, viscosity, and acid base state. In *Continuous Transcutaneous Blood Gas Monitoring*, ed. A. Huch, R. Huch, and J. F. Lucey (pp. 285–94). New York: Alan R. Liss.

Versmold, H. T., Severinghaus, J. W., Müller, C., Paikert, I., and Riegel, K. P. (1980). Transcutaneous monitoring of pCO_2 in newborn infants. *Pediatric Research* 13:170A.

Vesterager, P. (1977). Transcutaneous pO_2 electrode. *Scandinavian Journal of Clinical and Laboratory Investigations* [Suppl. 146] 37:27–30.

(1982). Effect of electrode temperatures on monitoring of transcutaneous carbon dioxide (tcpCO_2) in prematures. *Biotelemetry Patient Monitoring* 9:18–27.

Vyas, H., Helms, P., and Cheriyan, G. (1988). Transcutaneous oxygen monitoring beyond the neonatal period. *Critical Care Medicine* 16:844–7.

Whitehead, M. D. (1981). Transcutaneous pO_2 and pCO_2 monitoring with a single electrochemical sensor: its clinical use and advantages in neonatal intensive care. *Intensive Care Medicine* 7:256–7.

Whitehead, M. D., Halsall, D., and Pollitzer, M. J. (1980). Transcutaneous estimation of arterial pCO_2 in newborn infants with a single electrochemical sensor. *Lancet* 1:1111–14.

Whitehead, M. D., Lee, B. V. W., Pagdins, T. M., and Reynolds, E. O. R. (1985). Estimation of arterial oxygen and carbon dioxide tension by a single transcutaneous sensor. *Archives of Disease in Childhood* 60:356–9.

Whitehead, M. D., Pollitzer, M. J., and Reynolds, E. O. R. (1979). Artefactual hypoxemia during estimation of p_aO_2 by skin electrode. *Lancet* 2:157.

Wimberley, P. D., Burnett, R. W., Covington, A. K., Maas, A. H. J., Müller-Plathe, O., Siggaard-Andersen, O., Weisberg, H. F., and Zijlstra, W. G. (1990). Guidelines for transcutaneous pO_2 and pCO_2 measurement. *Clinica Chimica Acta [Suppl. 190]*, pp. 41–50.

Wimberley, P. D., Frederikson, P. S., Witt-Hansen, J.,

Melberg, S. G., and Friis-Hansen, B. (1985). Evaluation of a transcutaneous oxygen and carbon dioxide monitor in a neonatal intensive care department. *Acta Paediatrica Scandinavica* 74:352–9.

Wimberley, P. D., Grönlund Pedersen, K., Olsson, J., and Siggaard-Andersen, O. (1985). Transcutaneous carbon dioxide and oxygen at different temperatures in healthy adults. *Clinical Chemistry* 31:1611–15.

Yeung, H. N., Beran, A. V., and Huxtable, R. F. (1978). Low impedance pH sensitive electrochemical devices that are potentially applicable to transcutaneous pCO_2 measurements. *Acta Anaesthesiologica Scandinavica [Suppl. 68]*, pp. 137–41.

8

Pulse oximetry

ELIZABETH H. THILO, M.D.
JULIA BROCKWAY CURLANDER, M.D.
WILLIAM W. HAY, JR., M.D.

INTRODUCTION

Pulse oximetry, following its development in Japan in the mid-1970s and its commercial availability in the United States since the early 1980s, has become the most widely used method for monitoring blood oxygenation in neonates. Its ease of application and accuracy, combined with the fact that it needs no calibration and produces no side effects, all make it attractive for use in the neonatal intensive-care unit (NICU). Despite its apparent simplicity, however, pulse oximetry involves sophisticated technology, and there are clear limitations to its usefulness. The purpose of this chapter is to review the principles behind the technology of pulse oximetry, the principles of oxygen transport important in applying the technology, and common clinical applications of pulse oximetry in the NICU.

HISTORY OF OXIMETRY

A detailed and personalized history of the development of oximetry has been published by Severinghaus (1986). Briefly, the use of spectrophotometry to analyze oxygen saturation in tissue was introduced by Nicolai in 1932, and the first instruments for measuring oxygen saturation in vivo were developed independently by Matthes and Kramer in 1935. Millikan introduced the name "oximeter" for these devices in 1942. The initial devices were large and cumbersome, but were soon scaled down for use in the unpressurized military aircraft available during World War II. Millikan's ear oximeter was later refined by Wood and Geraci to include an inflatable balloon that would render the pinna of the ear bloodless for a time, so that the "absolute" degree of saturation could be measured as the ear was reperfused. They even devised an electronic means of displaying the degree of saturation continuously.

Unfortunately, classic oximetry (nonpulsatile) could not discriminate between the arterial blood to be measured and the other light absorbers in the tissue, and the optical components available to those early workers were too unreliable to achieve reproducible results. Consequently, classic in vivo oximetry was never widely applied, and progress in that area ground to a halt in the 1950s.

In 1956, Clark developed his polyethylene-covered oxygen cathode, now known as the Clark electrode. That was a true turning point in blood gas analysis and respiratory physiology allowing easy, accurate measurement of the partial pressure of oxygen (Pao_2) in blood. For the next 30 yr, clinicians learned to think in terms of Pao_2 as the measure of oxygenation, rather than saturation.

Two technological advances, light-emitting diodes (LEDs) and microprocessors, plus the ingenious idea of analyzing the change in light absorption produced by arterial pulsations, resulted in the development of a new generation of oximeters: the pulse oximeter (Tremper and Barker, 1986). Now, clinicians are again thinking of oxygenation as a function of the degree of saturation and oxygen content, as the pulse oximeter becomes the preferred monitoring device. As we shall discuss, however, there are situations in which measurement of Pao_2 will continue to be necessary.

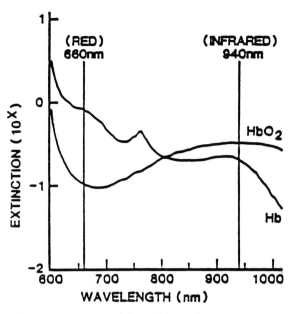

Figure 8.1. Oxygenated hemoglobin (HbO_2) and reduced hemoglobin (Hb) exhibit markedly different absorption (extinction) characteristics to red light at 660 nm and infrared light at 940 nm. (Courtesy of Ohmeda, 1986.)

PRINCIPLES OF MEASURING BLOOD OXYGEN SATURATION

The basic principle underlying all of oximetry is quite simple: The color change of blood as it becomes saturated with oxygen is a function of the optical properties of the hemoglobin (and specifically the heme) molecule. As the blood deoxygenates, it becomes less permeable to red light, and therefore becomes less red and more "blue" in appearance. An oximeter, then, needs to measure the "blueness" of the arterial blood, without interference from the patient's pigmentation, from the venous blood, or from other absorbers light that may be present in the tissue being studied, and display this "blueness" in terms of the degree of saturation.

If light of a specific wavelength is passed through a substance, and only a negligible amount passes through, the substance is considered opaque to (has a high extinction or absorbance for) that wavelength of light. As can be seen in Figure 8.1, hemoglobin's absorbance at wavelengths above 600 nm decreases rapidly; that is, it becomes more transparent. The predominant color of light above 600 nm is red; thus, hemoglobin transmits red light. An example may be helpful: When the light from a flashlight passes through one's hand in a darkened room, the

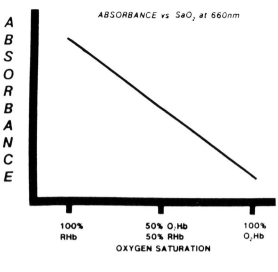

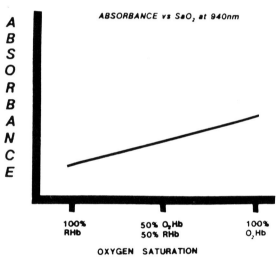

Figure 8.2. Comparison of absorbance and oxygen saturation (SaO_2) values at 660 and 940 nm. (From Pologe, 1987a, with permission.)

light transmitted appears red, even though the incident light is white. This is because hemoglobin absorbs the shorter wavelengths of light, allowing only the longer, red wavelengths to pass through. Between 600 and 800 nm, oxygenated hemoglobin (HbO_2 or oxyhemoglobin) has a lower extinction, compared with reduced hemoglobin (Hb), and appears more red.

The opposite relationship between Hb and HbO_2 extinctions occurs at higher wavelengths (above 800 nm). Thus, as shown in Figure 8.2, as the degree of oxygen saturation (percentage oxyhemoglobin) in-

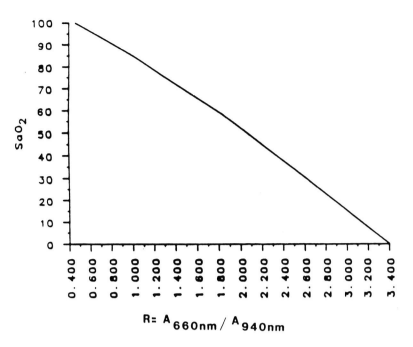

$$R = \frac{A_{660nm}}{A_{940nm}}$$

Figure 8.3. Calibration curve used by the oximeter to calculate arterial oxygen saturation (SaO_2) from the ratio (R) of the light absorbed (A) by the tissue being monitored. (Courtesy of Ohmeda, 1987)

creases (and, reciprocally, as the percentage of Hb decreases), absorption at 660 nm decreases in a linear relationship, whereas absorption at 940 nm, in the near-infrared spectrum, increases. If both wavelengths of light are used, their opposite changes in the amount of light absorbed by oxyhemoglobin (or Hb) will produce a sensitive index of blood oxygen saturation, calculated as $R = A_{660nm}/A_{940nm}$ (Figure 8.3). This ratio is unique for any given degree of oxygen saturation.

The path length that light travels through the blood or tissue affects the amount absorbed or transmitted. Using a ratio of two different absorbances (A_{660nm}/A_{940nm}) over the same path length will eliminate the path length as a variable.

The curve defining the relationship between the degree of oxygen saturation and the absorbance ratio (Figure 8.3) is called the calibration curve. Although this curve could be derived entirely theoretically, accuracy is improved by deriving it empirically using healthy subjects with arterial catheters in place under conditions of controlled hypoxemia. The data points that are gathered, down to approximately 65% saturation, are plotted against the absorbance ratio, yielding the calibration curve for the particular oximeter in question. The low end of the calibration curve, below 65% saturation, is derived theoretically or is extrapolated, with some sacrifice in accuracy at these low levels.

Because oximetry is based only on the extinction curves for hemoglobin, it is unaffected by pH, unlike the hemoglobin–oxygen dissociation curve. Although variations in hematocrit will affect light absorption, use of the ratio of absorbances at two wavelengths eliminates this problem, just as it eliminates differences in path length. Because the calibration curve for a specified wavelength of light is unchanging, it can be committed to software in the pulse oximeter and used to determine the degree of saturation for any input absorbance ratio.

Because the extinction curves for fetal hemoglobin are not significantly different from those for adult hemoglobin, in either oxygenated or reduced states (Pologe and Raley, 1987), the saturation by pulse oximetry (SpO_2) is not significantly affected by the amount of fetal hemoglobin present. Theoretically, this makes sense, because the extinction curves are dependent almost exclusively on the heme molecule, not the globin chains, and only the chains differ in fetal versus adult hemoglobin.

Other light absorbers may be present, however, and may interfere with the oximeter's reading. Both methemoglobin (MetHb) and carboxyhemoglobin (COHb) have significant extinction values at both 660 nm and 940 nm (Figure 8.4). It can be seen that at 660 nm, MetHb has roughly the same extinction coefficient as Hb, and COHb roughly the same as HbO_2. If only two wavelengths of light are used, as in the pulse oximeter, the effect essentially is to "lump" or combine absorbance due to MetHb with

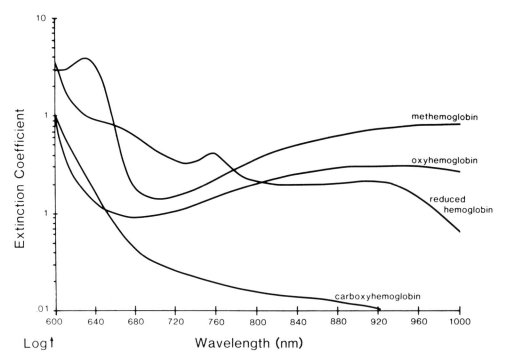

Log↑

Wavelength (nm)

Figure 8.4. Hemoglobin extinction curves showing relationships of reduced hemoglobin, oxyhemoglobin, carboxyhemoglobin, and methemoglobin to light absorption. (From
Wukitsch et al., 1988, with permission.)

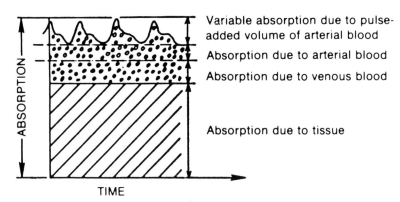

Variable absorption due to pulse-
added volume of arterial blood

Absorption due to arterial blood

Absorption due to venous blood

Absorption due to tissue

Figure 8.5. Tissue composite shows
dynamic and static components affecting light absorption. (From Wukitsch
et al., 1988, with permission.)

that due to Hb, and absorbance due to COHb with
that due to HbO₂. Multiwavelength oximeters have
been developed to measure these fractions separately in the blood; examples are the IL-282 CO-
oximeter and the Radiometer OSM3 CO-oximeter.
The effects of abnormal amounts of these other absorbers on Spo₂ will be discussed later.

PRINCIPLES OF PULSE OXIMETRY

As described for classic oximetry, two wavelengths
of light are passed through the tissue, the amount of

light transmitted at each wavelength is detected and
subtracted from the incident light (to calculate absorbance), and the degree of saturation is derived
from the ratio of the amounts of light absorbed at
the two wavelengths. The difference from the classic oximeter is that only the added volume of arterial
blood as it pulses through the tissue is analyzed,
with the constant baseline of transmitted light due
to the tissue and the venous and capillary blood being "ignored" (actually, electronically and computationally filtered out) (Figure 8.5). In other words,
the pulse oximeter measures the change in absor-

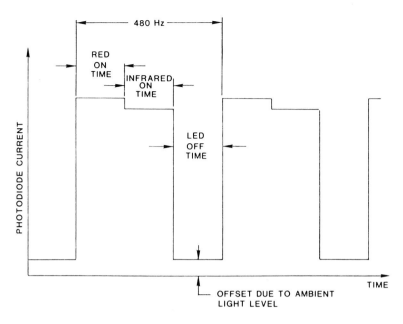

Figure 8.6. Output of the photodetector on the Ohmeda 3700 pulse oximeter (LED, light-emitting diode). (From Wukitsch et al., 1988, with permission.)

bance at 660 nm divided by the change in absorbance at 940 nm as the blood pulsates. In this way, constant absorbers such as pigmentation are canceled out, and a closer approximation of the degree of arterial saturation can be made.

The oximeter probe consists of the light sources, a photodetector (photodiode), and a means of identifying itself to the microprocessor. The light sources are LEDs, which are tiny, lightweight, and cheap and yet emit a tremendous amount of light over an extremely narrow portion of the electromagnetic-energy spectrum. They also require very little power and generate very little heat. By a fortunate coincidence, 660 nm, one of the wavelengths at which LEDs are available, is also the best wavelength for use in oximetry, because at this wavelength the oxyhemoglobin extinction curve is fairly flat (so that small variations in LED wavelength cause minimal error), and the separation between the extinction curves for oxyhemoglobin and reduced hemoglobin is large (yielding detectable changes in absorbance with small changes in saturation). In the selection of the second wavelength, one criterion is essential: The extinction curve should be as different as possible from that for the first wavelength, preferably even inverted, giving a large change in the absorption ratio (R) for any change in saturation. At 940 nm, for which an LED also happens to be available, the curves are inverted and separated, fulfilling this criterion.

The detector, a silicon photodiode, is also lightweight and small and responds to light through the visible region up to 1,100 nm. In a two-wavelength oximeter, there is only one detector to measure three different light levels: red (660 nm), infrared (940 nm), and ambient or background light. This is accomplished by sequencing the red and infrared light sources on and off, allowing an interval when both are off to detect (and then "subtract out") the transmittance of ambient light. An example of such sequencing for the Ohmeda 3700 pulse oximeter is shown in Figure 8.6. Sequencing the red and infrared LEDs at a frequency that is an integer multiple of the power-line frequency allows the system to operate synchronously with flickering room lights. For example, fluorescent lights generate a 120-Hz flicker on 60-Hz power. The sequencing avoids potential interference from light flickers on the photodiode that would distort or disguise the tiny pulse signals of arterial pulse flow. The light-timing sequence shown in Figure 8.6 cycles 480 times per second at 60-Hz power; 16 of the red–infrared–off sequences are used to calculate SpO_2 every 0.033 s. These signals are used differently by different pulse-oximeter manufacturers; for example, one calculates the peak SaO_2 of each pulse of arterial blood, maximizing the differences between minimum and maximum transmitted light intensities (for both the red and the infrared wavelengths), whereas another calculates the red and infrared transmissions 30 times per second and calculates a weighted average SaO_2 (Figure 8.7). Such frequent determinations allegedly allow a more stable calculation and more rapid response time, while being independent of heart rate.

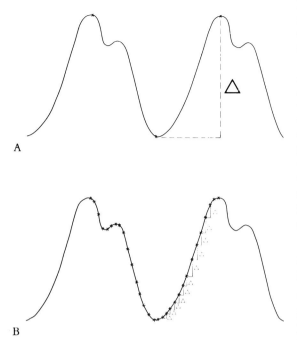

Figure 8.7. Changes in light intensity for both red and infrared wavelengths can be measured at the minimum and maximum points of the pulse wave, or many times along the wave. (A) Change in light intensity from the minimum to the maximum point on the arterial pressure waveform, from which saturation can be calculated once per heartbeat. (B) The multiple measurements depicted allow many sample points that can be subjected to validation schemes, such as the running weighted average. (From Wukitsch et al., 1988, with permission.)

Because the pulsatile fraction of the total light transmitted is quite small, perhaps only 1–3% of the total under ideal circumstances, and as low as 0.1–0.2% of the total at times (Wukitsch et al., 1988), pulse oximeters have a large amount of automatic gain built in, so that the signal can be amplified. The problem, of course, is that as the gain is increased, sometimes by as much as 4 billion times (Pologe, 1987a), interference by background noise is also heightened. The noise can then be run through the calibration curve, and a degree of saturation can be calculated, even when no pulse or no patient exists. This problem is addressed in two ways. First, the oximeter can display the strength of the signal pulsation either as a column of pulsating light or as a plethysmographic waveform. The latter can let the clinician know at a glance whether or not a true arterial pulsation is being "seen" by the oximeter, thus greatly enhancing the trust placed in the saturation reading (Pologe, 1987a; Kopotic et al., 1987; Hay, Thilo, and Curlander, 1991). Second, the devices

have a "low-quality signal" warning to indicate that inadequate pulsations are being detected, either because of probe misalignment or because of inadequate perfusion.

Interestingly, any motion artifact that is consistent and of significant duration will make the degree of saturation determined by the pulse oximeter tend toward 85%. This occurs because the motion will introduce a large signal of similar magnitude into both the red and infrared channels. R will become close to 1.0, and converting an R of 1.0 to the degree of saturation using the calibration curve will yield a value of 85% (Pologe, 1987b). This is a somewhat unfortunate consequence of the physics involved, and it can lead the untrained observer to false conclusions about the patient's condition.

PRINCIPLES OF OXYGEN TRANSPORT AND RELEVANCE TO PULSE OXIMETRY

Oxygen is carried in the blood both bound to hemoglobin ($\approx$98%) and dissolved in plasma ($\approx$2% in the physiological Pao_2 range) (Figure 8.8), and the amount carried can be calculated as

$$Cao_2 = (1.34 \times [Hb] \times Sao_2) + (0.003 \times Pao_2)$$

where Cao_2 is the arterial oxygen content (volume percent), [Hb] is the hemoglobin concentration (grams per 100 ml), Sao_2 is the fraction of hemoglobin saturated with oxygen (percent), 1.34 equals the milliliters of oxygen bound to 1 g of Hb at 100% saturation (milliliters per gram), 0.003 is the solubility of oxygen in plasma (volume percent per millimeter of mercury), and Pao_2 is the arterial partial pressure of oxygen (millimeters of mercury). Both bound oxygen and dissolved oxygen are directly dependent on Pao_2, because Pao_2, together with the type of hemoglobin, the pH, the Pco_2, the temperature, and the amount of 2,3-diphosphoglycerate (2,3-DPG) present, will determine the Sao_2. This relationship is commonly expressed as the oxygen–hemoglobin affinity curve, or the oxyhemoglobin dissociation curve, shown in Figure 8.9. HbO_2 affinity is modified primarily by four factors: hydrogen-ion concentration ($[H^+]$), Pco_2, temperature, and 2,3-DPG concentration. Increased values for these factors will act to decrease HbO_2 affinity. For example, increased values for $[H^+]$, Pco_2, and temperature will occur in tissues at sites of active metabolism and thus will aid in releasing oxygen from hemoglobin, raising the local Po_2 and making oxygen more available for tissue uptake. These conditions are reversed in the lungs, where hemoglobin uptake of oxygen is more important.

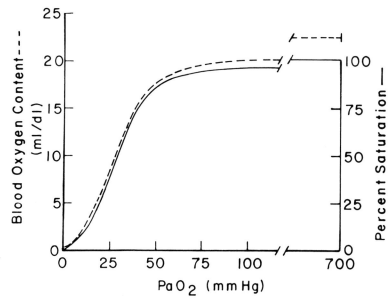

Figure 8.8. Blood oxygen content (dash curve) is shown to be a function of the blood partial pressure of oxygen (Pao$_2$). Blood oxygen content consists primarily of oxygen bound to hemoglobin (reflected in the figure by the solid line in relation to percent saturation) and a much smaller portion of oxygen dissolved in the plasma (reflected in the figure by the difference between the curve for oxygen content and the curve for percent saturation).

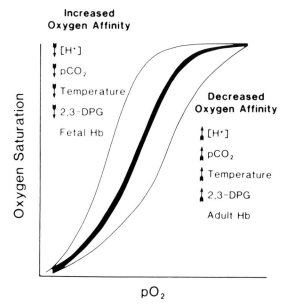

Figure 8.9. Factors affecting hemoglobin–oxygen affinity. (From Hay, 1987a, with permission.)

The position of the oxyhemoglobin dissociation curve under a specific set of circumstances may shift to the right (lower affinity) or to the left (higher affinity) and is described by the P$_{50}$, (the Pao$_2$ at which the hemoglobin is 50% saturated). Adult hemoglobin has a P$_{50}$ of about 30 mm Hg under standard conditions, and fetal hemoglobin has a P$_{50}$ of approximately 20 mm Hg under the same conditions (Figure 8.10). Under the relatively hypoxic conditions of intrauterine life, where the best-oxygenated umbilical venous blood has a Po$_2$ of only about 30 mm Hg, the increased affinity of fetal hemoglobin for oxygen (lower P$_{50}$) is an advantage that favors oxygen uptake by fetal blood as it passes through the placenta. This same property, however, makes judging the adequacy of oxygenation on the basis of skin color more difficult in the newborn. Because of high levels of fetal hemoglobin and a low P$_{50}$, the newborn may have a high degree of saturation and appear "pink" even with a suboptimal Pao$_2$ (Hay, 1987a).

Over the first weeks following birth, production of adult hemoglobin supersedes that of fetal hemoglobin, and 2,3-DPG levels rise, both serving to shift the oxyhemoglobin curve to the right. This decreases the affinity of hemoglobin for oxygen and increases unloading of oxygen to the tissues. This occurs as the hemoglobin concentration is falling to its postnatal nadir and allows continued adequate supply of oxygen to the tissues despite a developing physiological anemia.

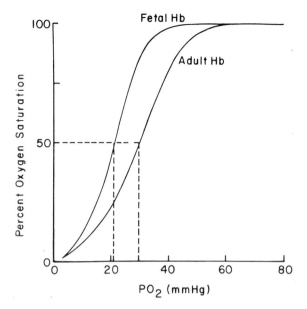

Figure 8.10. Fetal hemoglobin has greater affinity for oxygen; thus, the fetal oxyhemoglobin affinity curve is "left-shifted" relative to that for adult hemoglobin. As a measure of this left shift, the P_{50} (PO_2 at 50% saturation) for fetal hemoglobin is about 20–22 mm Hg, and the P_{50} for adult hemoglobin is about 27–30 mm Hg.

DEGREE OF SATURATION OR Pao_2: WHICH IS BETTER?

On the basis of the preceding discussion of oxygen transport, it is apparent that both Sao_2 (Spo_2) and Pao_2 are useful measurements. The degree of saturation is useful in that it provides a physiological measurement of tissue oxygen supply and allows calculation of Cao_2. Saturations above 80–85% probably will be adequate for tissue needs, even with a low Pao_2. Second, at a constant Hb concentration, blood flow to the "vital" organs (brain and heart) is related inversely to blood flow to other tissues (muscle, skin, gut) as the degree of blood oxygen saturation (and thus Cao_2) changes (Figure 8.11) (Peeters et al., 1979; Sheldon et al., 1979). Thus, the degree of saturation can be used to estimate organ blood flow and to predict changes in organ perfusion.

Measurement of Pao_2 also is important, however. The pulmonary circulation and the ductus arteriosus are responsive to Pao_2 rather than to oxygen content (Fishman, 1961), with a high Pao_2 causing pulmonary vascular dilation and ductal constriction (Figure 8.12). Neonates, during the transition from intrauterine life to extrauterine life, often are prone to pulmonary hypertension and seem to have very

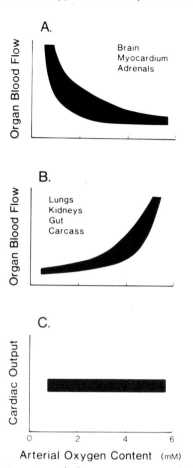

Figure 8.11. Redistribution of organ blood flow as blood O_2 content changes, adapted from studies in late-gestation fetal lambs. (From Hay, 1987a, with permission.)

reactive pulmonary vascular beds (Geggel and Reid, 1986). It is certainly feasible that the degree of saturation might be "adequate" for tissue needs (i.e., 80–85% or more), but with a Pao_2 low enough to cause pulmonary vasoconstriction. On the other hand, hyperoxia is not well detected by oximetry either, because at the upper end of the dissociation curve, the degree of saturation changes little, despite large changes in Pao_2. Hyperoxia also can be damaging to the neonate and is to be avoided, necessitating measurement of Pao_2 if the degree of saturation is at the upper limit for any prolonged time (probably more than 20–30 min).

If Pao_2 measurements are to be accurate reflections of baseline conditions in the newborn, they require the presence of indwelling arterial catheters, to eliminate the effects of crying or breath-holding that occur almost universally when a needle punc-

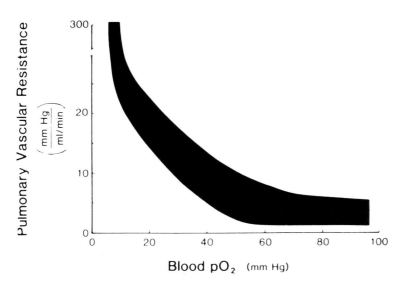

Figure 8.12. In contrast to the situation in other organs, pulmonary vascular resistance (and thus pulmonary blood flow) is Po_2-dependent. (From Hay, 1987a, with permission.)

tures the skin. Such catheters certainly are not without risks, such as thrombosis and infection, and cannot be maintained in place indefinitely. Also, intermittent measurements are only that: They cannot continuously reveal trends in the infant's progress. Transcutaneous oxygen/carbon dioxide monitors are available and are helpful in certain situations, but require rigorous calibration and application techniques to achieve useful correlation with Pao_2 (Peabody and Emery, 1985; Rooth, Huch, and Huch, 1987; AAP, 1989). Additionally, they commonly cause thermal burns at the site of application, necessitating frequent changes of the electrode site. In vivo correlation with an arterial sample is recommended with each change in electrode site (AAP, 1989), but this only compounds the problems described earlier, including skin (and, potentially, nerve) damage, pain, breath-holding, and vasoconstriction. These monitors are greatly affected by conditions that decrease skin perfusion, such as hypotension, edema, acidosis, and hypothermia, all of which are common in sick neonates. Finally, transcutaneous Po_2 monitors correlate less well with Pao_2 as the infant ages, making them less useful in infants with chronic lung disease (Rome et al., 1984; Solimano et al., 1986; Durand and Ramanatham, 1986; Ramanathan, Durand, and Larrazabal, 1987). Nevertheless, transcutaneous Po_2 and Pco_2 measurements are helpful, particularly in acutely ill, newly born infants who may be prone to pulmonary hypertension, in whom hypoxemia is to be strictly avoided, and trends in Pco_2 are helpful in monitoring the hyperventilation used to manage this disease.

The accuracy of transcutaneous Po_2 versus Pao_2 depends on the technique employed in calibration and probe application, on local factors affecting skin perfusion, and on the age of the patient. Correlation coefficients greater than 0.95 are obtained under the best of circumstances in the immediate newborn period, with correlations of only 0.78–0.81 in older infants with bronchopulmonary dysplasia (Durand and Ramanathan, 1986; Solimano et al., 1986; Ramanathan et al., 1987). Under these circumstances, Pao_2 may be underestimated by as much as 29% (Solimano et al., 1986).

Pulse oximetry is a much easier technique to apply in that it requires no calibration, no membrane changes, and no in vivo correlation with arterial samples (Dziedzic and Vidyasagar, 1989). It is less sensitive to local tissue perfusion than is the transcutaneous oxygen monitor, and it functions well even during severe hypotension (Severinghaus and Spellman, 1990). In the physiological range of saturations, Spo_2 is generally reported to be within 1.5% of measured Sao_2 for saturations of 85% or greater, and within 3–5% for saturations of 60–70% or greater (Dziedzic and Vidyasagar, 1989). Below 60% saturation, its accuracy is less predictable (Fanconi, 1988), but because this level is dangerously low and requires therapeutic intervention regardless of the absolute figure, this is not clinically important. Correlation coefficients for Spo_2 versus Sao_2 are generally 0.86–0.95 (Dziedzic and Vidyasagar, 1989), with values as high as 0.98–0.99 having been reported (Hay, Brockway, and Eyzaguirre, 1989). Unlike the situation for the transcutaneous oxygen monitor, the pulse oximeter's accuracy is not decreased by increasing skin thickness or age of the patient, and it has proved to be very useful in infants with bronchopulmonary dysplasia.

It should be remembered that the *calculated* Sao_2 that is included in the clinical laboratory's report of blood gases is not the same as Sao_2 *measured* by a CO-oximeter and should not be compared or "correlated" with Spo_2. The calculated Sao_2 assumes adult hemoglobin, P_{50} of 27 mm Hg, pH 7.40, and temperature 37° C, assumptions that bear little connection to the typical newborn intensive-care patient. It should also be noted, however, that a "correlation" of Spo_2 with Pao_2 should be performed for each patient at the lower ($Spo_2 < 88$–90%) and higher ($Spo_2 > 96\%$) saturation levels before relying entirely on Spo_2 determinations for oxygen management (Hay et al., 1991). This will help assure, for each patient, that hypoxemia and hyperoxemia are avoided, and it is best done early in postnatal life when an arterial catheter is in place.

LIMITATIONS OF PULSE OXIMETRY

Pulse oximeters are exquisitely sensitive to movement of the extremity to which the probe is applied. Because pulse oximetry is based on the principle of detecting a tiny pulsatile change in absorbance, motion disturbances are always likely to pose problems. Because of the large amplitude of any such movement compared with the tiny pulse amplitude normally sought, R (A_{660nm}/A_{940nm}) will approach unity, and the Spo_2 reading will trend toward 85%. Additionally, the pulse rate will deviate markedly from the electronically determined heart rate, and the pulse waveform will be lost on those instruments that feature a plethysmographic display, making it immediately obvious that the problem is movement-related. As a general rule, for those instruments without a plethysmographic display, if the pulse rate displayed on the oximeter is within 1–2 beats per minute of the electronically determined heart rate that is simultaneously and independently monitored, the Spo_2 value will be believable. The presence of a plethysmographic display of the pulse waveform is, in our opinion and that of others (Kopotic et al., 1987), a major advantage, because one can tell at a glance whether or not a good pulse is being detected and the Spo_2 reading is credible.

Probe application is a minor problem at times, with the geometry of the probe and the intensity of the light limiting the size of the body part that can be selected for application. It is important that the LED be directly opposite the photodiode and that not too much ambient light strike the photodiode. If the light levels reaching the photodiode are too high, the oximeter will signal "Probe Off Patient." If the light levels reaching the photodiode are too small to be "seen," despite maximum gain, the oximeter will display "Insufficient Light." In either case, adjusting the probe position, and possibly shielding it from ambient light with an opaque cover, such as a diaper or drape, should rectify the situation. One needs to be cautious about excessive pressure in applying the probe; rare instances of pressure necrosis, especially in edematous patients, have been described (Hay et al., 1991).

The presence of other absorbers, such as skin pigment and bilirubin, usually is inconsequential, because pulse oximetry looks only at substances that are pulsatile (in the blood), and bilirubin's extinction curve for light is out of the wavelength range used (Anderson, 1987). Dyes such as methylene blue can interfere with Spo_2 readings, the relationship being inversely proportional: The greater the amount of methylene blue, the lower the Spo_2 (Sidi et al., 1987). Fortunately, use of this substance is rare, but the clinician should be aware that there is an effect. Likewise, dark red shades of fingernail polish may interfere with accurate reading (Bowes, Corke, and Hulka, 1989); such polish should be removed before applying the probe (obviously this problem is more germane to the mothers than to their babies).

The issue of fetal hemoglobin arises frequently as a possible source of error in pulse oximetry. In fact, the extinction curves for fetal and adult hemoglobins are very similar (Pologe and Raley, 1987), so that HbF has little effect on Spo_2 readings. Large amounts of HbF will, however, give falsely elevated carboxyhemoglobin readings with CO-oximetry unless appropriate corrections are made (Ryan et al., 1986; Hodgson, 1987; Thilo et al., 1993). Methemoglobin levels are unaffected even by very large amounts of HbF (Figure 8.13). As mentioned previously, HbF does have a left-shifted oxygen dissociation curve compared with adult hemoglobin, so that the relationship between Spo_2 and Pao_2 will be affected by changes in the relative proportion of HbF in the blood (e.g., following exchange transfusions or massive direct transfusions).

Elevated amounts of carboxyhemoglobin (COHb) and methemoglobin (MetHb) do interfere with the accuracy of pulse oximetry. Both tend to elevate the Spo_2 value relative to actual Sao_2–COHb more so than MetHb (Hay, 1987b; Wukitsch et al., 1988). The reason for this is that the extinction curves for COHb and MetHb are sufficiently similar to those for HbO_2 and Hb that the pulse oximeter, using

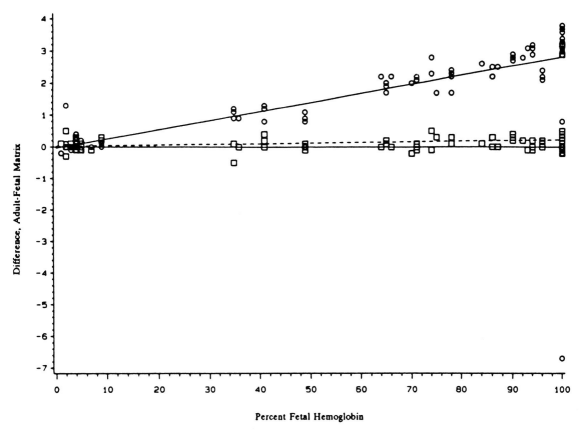

Figure 8.13. COHb (circles) determination by co-oximetry is falsely elevated by large amounts of HbF ($y = 0.029x - 0.04$, $r = 0.70$, $p < 0.001$), whereas MetHb (squares) deter-mination is not ($y = 0.002$ $x + 0.02$, $r = 0.17$, $p < 0.05$). (Data from Thilo et al., 1993, with permission.)

only two wavelengths of light, cannot distinguish them (Figure 8.4). Consequently, if large amounts of either are present, a falsely elevated Spo_2 will result. For example, if the true Sao_2 is 90%, and COHb is 10%, the Spo_2 value will be 97–98%; approximately 80% of the COHb added to the Sao_2 will give the Spo_2. For MetHb, the effect is smaller, such that for an actual Sao_2 of 90% and a MetHb of 10%, the Spo_2 will be on the order of 91–92%. The lower the actual Sao_2, however, the greater the error. MetHb absorbs more light at both 660 nm and 940 nm than does either HbO_2 or Hb, but proportionately more at 660 nm. This serves to increase R (A_{660}/A_{940}), lowering the Spo_2 reading (Figure 8.3). When 65% or more of the total hemoglobin is MetHb, R approaches 1.27, which yields an Spo_2 of 75–80%, even though the maximum possible HbO_2 is 35%. Therefore the pulse oximeter progressively overestimates saturation with increasing MetHb (Watcha, Connor, and Hing, 1989). Fortunately,

large amounts of COHb and MetHb are rare. Furthermore, as long as their concentrations remain relatively stable and unchanging, Spo_2 can still be used to follow trends in oxygenation.

Interinstrument variability is another issue that should be addressed. Each brand of oximeter has its own calibration curve, arrived at independently. There are both variable and systematic differences between these curves, although most clinicians mistakenly view the saturation values as interchangeable from one brand to another. For example, Bucher et al. (1989) have shown that the Nellcor N-100 pulse oximeter (Nellcor, Hayward, CA) consistently overestimates the measured Sao_2, and Thilo et al. (1992) have shown that the Ohmeda 3700 pulse oximeter (Ohmeda, Louisville, CO) consistently reads lower than the Nellcor N-100. Russell and Helms (1990) have shown similar systematic differences in readings in older children as well. Thilo et al. (1993) found that the Nellcor reading for Spo_2 was 1.61 ±

Table 8.1. *Correlation of* SpO_2 *with fractional and functional* SaO_2 *(corrected for amount of fetal hemoglobin) by linear-regression analysis and paired t test*

Parameter	SpO_2 (Ohmeda 3700)	SpO_2 (Nellcor N-100)
Fractional SaO_2 fetal matrix		
Slope	1.01	0.97
95% confidence interval	0.95–1.08	0.90–1.04
r value	0.94	0.93
Functional SaO_2 fetal matrix		
Slope	0.98	0.94
95% confidence interval	0.91–1.04	0.87–1.00
r value	0.94	0.93
Mean difference $SpO_2 - SaO_2$ fetal matrix ($\pm SD$)		
Fractional SaO_2	0.00 ± 3.23 ($p = 1.00$)	1.66 ± 3.45 ($p < 0.001$)
Functional SaO_2	− 1.25 ± 3.22 ($p < 0.001$)	0.41 ± 3.44 ($p = 0.20$)

Source: Data from Thilo et al. (1993).

2.69% higher than that for the Ohmeda, nearly identical with the difference between these two instruments of 1.63 ± 2.65% as reported by Russell and Helms (1990). The basis for these differences is in the calibration algorithm built into the pulse oximeter's software, where either the functional oxygen saturation $(HbO_2/HbO_2 + Hb) \times 100$ or the fractional oxygen saturation $(HbO_2/HbO_2 + Hb + COHb + MetHb) \times 100$ is chosen as the standard (Table 8.1). Unfortunately, often the consumer is not well versed in these details, and many believe that all machines measure or approximate SaO_2 (itself not a particularly exact measurement) (Nickerson, Sarkisian, and Tremper, 1988) in the same way. Although this is not important in some clinical circumstances (e.g., an SpO_2 of 75% vs. 78%, where both are significantly low), it can be important for newborns at borderline low and high SpO_2 values, because both hypoxemia and hyperoxemia are to be avoided, and prediction of PaO_2 from SpO_2 is more variable than later in life because of fetal hemoglobin.

CLINICAL APPLICATION

What is the desired range of SpO_2, and what is appropriate oxygenation? Answers to these questions have not been determined using conventional experimental methods. Instead, SpO_2 values have been arbitrarily declared as acceptable, based on fairly obvious but definitely crude criteria, such as absence of metabolic acidosis, success in weaning infants from oxygen or in lowering ventilator settings, demonstration of sustained growth (in chronically O_2-dependent infants), and even "pink" coloration of the skin. More reliably, indirect

association of SpO_2 values with transcutaneous PO_2 and PaO_2 values has allowed prediction of appropriate oxygenation based on "normal" or "acceptable" PaO_2 levels. Though controversy remains regarding the actual (or potential) risks (or benefits) of moderately low (45–60 mm Hg) or high (90–110 mm Hg) PaO_2 values, most clinicians would accept the PaO_2 range of 60–90 mm Hg as appropriate and safe for preterm and term newborn infants and those infants with sustained oxygen requirements owing to respiratory system diseases. To date, however, determination of PaO_2 by controlling and measuring SpO_2 has not been accomplished. Instead, clinically determined PaO_2 values have been compared with simultaneously recorded SpO_2 values, allowing, at best, a reverse, indirect assumption of PaO_2 for an observed SpO_2. For example, Hay et al. (1989) reported 117 simultaneous correlations of SpO_2 (Ohmeda, Louisville, CO) with PaO_2 (via indwelling catheter) in 58 preterm infants less than 1 wk of age (Figure 8.14), wherein SpO_2 values of 92% or greater were associated with PaO_2 values as low as 46 mm Hg, and SpO_2 values of 97% or greater were associated with PaO_2 values as high as 122 mm Hg. A sensitivity-specificity analysis showed that the SpO_2 range of 94 ± 3% (>90% to <98%) indicated a PaO_2 range of 45–100 mm Hg with 100% sensitivity and 100% specificity. To restrict PaO_2 values to 60–90 mm Hg with more than 95% confidence, SpO_2 would have to be greater than 94% and less than 98%, a very narrow range that would be difficult to achieve and maintain.

In more recent research not yet published, Brockway and Hay studied a group of infants recovering from respiratory distress syndrome who had umbilical arterial catheters placed on clinical grounds.

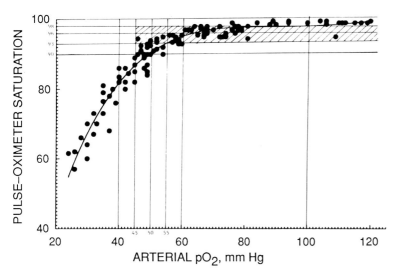

Figure 8.14. Comparison of pulse-oximeter saturation (SpO$_2$) with PaO$_2$ (catheter) in infants in first week of life. OSM-2 is the Radiometer hemoximeter. The hatched area represents the SpO$_2$–PaO$_2$ correlations from 93% to 97% SpO$_2$. (Data from Hay et al., 1989.)

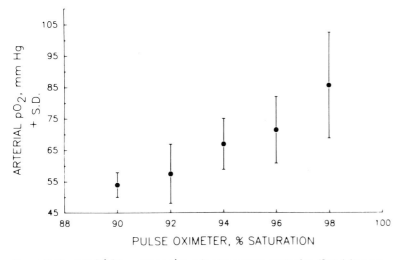

Figure 8.15. Arterial PO$_2$ versus pulse-oximeter percent saturation (SpO$_2$) in near-term newborn infants in whom pulse saturation was fixed by adjusting FIO$_2$ first, and then PaO$_2$ was measured. Values are mean ± SD. (J. M. Brockway and W. W. Hay, Jr., unpublished data.)

They first adjusted the fractional concentration of inspired oxygen (FIO$_2$) to achieve and maintain SpO$_2$ values of 90%, 92%, 94%, 96%, and 98% at five sampling times and then measured PaO$_2$ at each SpO$_2$ value. Figure 8.15 shows that with 10 infants studied at each of the selected SpO$_2$ values, SpO$_2$ values of 94–96% included the "acceptable" PaO$_2$ range of 60–90 mm Hg. Thilo et al. (1993) showed that the SpO$_2$ range "desired" should be adjusted based on

the brand of instrument used: a range of 90–96% for SpO$_2$ using the Ohmeda 3700, and a range of 92–98% of SpO$_2$ using the Nellcor N-100, giving a positive predictive value of 0.94 and 0.95, respectively, for PO$_2$ between 50 and 100 mm Hg (Table 8.2). Clearly, more investigation is needed to verify these ranges, to determine if the previously noted systematic difference between instruments is clinically important, and to define the potential for clinically un-

Table 8.2. *Results from predictive-value analysis for Spo$_2$ vs. Pao$_2$ of 50–100 mm Hg*

Spo$_2$ range	Sensitivity	Specificity	PPV[a]	Accuracy
90%–95%				
Spo$_2$ (Ohmeda)	0.40	0.91	0.92	.55
Spo$_2$ (Nellcor)	0.35	0.80	0.68	.36
90%–96%				
Spo$_2$ (Ohmeda)	0.56	0.91	0.94	0.67
92%–98%				
Spo$_2$ (Nellcor)	0.70	0.91	0.95	0.77

[a]PPV, positive predictive value.
Source: Data from Thilo et al. (1993).

satisfactory consequences of Spo$_2$ values outside of these ranges. Furthermore, in babies that are especially susceptible to the dangers of high or low Po$_2$ values, pulse oximetry should not be used exclusive of direct Pao$_2$ measurements to manage blood oxygenation.

CONCLUSIONS

Pulse oximetry, because of its ease of application, accuracy, and truly noninvasive nature, has become the standard means for continuous assessment of oxygenation in neonatal medicine. Although there are limitations to its use, and situations where knowledge of Pao$_2$ is essential, no instrument in recent years has gained such rapid and widespread acceptance. Clinicians need to be aware of the principles involved in its design and use so that they can make intelligent decisions based on the information it provides.

REFERENCES

AAP (1989). AAP Task Force on Transcutaneous Oxygen Monitors: Report of consensus meeting, December 5–6, 1986. *Pediatrics* 83:122–6.

Anderson, J. V. (1987). The accuracy of pulse oximetry in neonates: effects of fetal hemoglobin and bilirubin. *Journal of Perinatology* 7:323.

Bowes, W. A., Corke, B. C., and Hulka, J. (1989). Pulse oximetry: a review of the theory, accuracy and clinical applications. *Obstetrics and Gynecology* 74:541–6.

Bucher, H. U., Fanconi, S., Baeckert, P., and Duc, G. (1989). Hyperoxemia in newborn infants: detection by pulse oximetry. *Pediatrics* 84:226–30.

Durand, M., and Ramanathan, R. (1986). Pulse oximetry for continuous oxygen monitoring in sick newborn infants. *Journal of Pediatrics* 109:1052–6.

Dziedzic, K., and Vidyasagar, D. (1989). Pulse oximetry in neonatal intensive care. *Clinics in Perinatology* 16:177–97.

Fanconi, S. (1988). Reliability of pulse oximetry in hypoxic infants. *Journal of Pediatrics* 112:424–7.

Fishman, A. P. (1961). Respiratory gases in the regulation of the pulmonary circulation. *Physiological Reviews* 41:214–80.

Geggel, R. L., and Reid, L. M. (1986). The structural basis of PPHN. *Clinics in Perinatology* 11:525–49.

Hay, W. W. (1987a). Physiology of oxygenation and its relation to pulse oximetry in neonates. *Journal of Perinatology* 7:309–19.

(1987b). The uses, benefits and limitations of pulse oximetry in neonatal medicine; consensus on key issues. *Journal of Perinatology* 7:347–9.

Hay, W. W., Brockway, J. M., and Eyzaguirre, M. (1989). Neonatal pulse oximetry: accuracy and reliability. *Pediatrics* 83:717–22.

Hay, W. W., Thilo, E., and Curlander, J. B. (1991). Pulse oximetry in neonatal medicine. *Clinics in Perinatology* 18:441–72.

Hodgson, A. J. (1987). CO-oximetry is reliable standard for pulse oximetry in the neonate? *Journal of Perinatology* 7:327–8.

Kopotic, R. J., Mannino, F. L. Colley, C. D., and Horning, N. (1987). Display variability, false alarms, probe cautions, and recorder use in neonatal pulse oximetry. *Journal of Perinatology* 7:340–2.

Nickerson, B. G., Sarkisian, C., and Tremper, K. (1988). Bias and precision of pulse oximeters and arterial oximeters. *Chest* 93:515–17.

Peabody, J. L., and Emery, J. R. (1985). Noninvasive monitoring of blood gases in the newborn. *Clinics in Perinatology* 12:147–60.

Peeters, L. L. H., Sheldon, R. E., Jones, M. D., Jr., Makowskie, L., and Meschia, G. (1979). Blood flow to fetal organs as a function of arterial content. *American Journal of Obstetrics and Gynecology* 135:637–46.

Pologe, J. A. (1987a). Pulse oximetry: technical aspects of machine design. *International Anesthesiology Clinics* 25:137–58.

(1987b). The theory and principles of pulse oximetry. *Journal of Perinatology* 7:320–2.

Pologe, J. A., and Raley, D. M. (1987). Effects of fetal hemoglobin on pulse oximetry. *Journal of Perinatology* 7:324–6.

Ramanathan, R., Durand, M., and Larrazabal, C. (1987). Pulse oximetry in very low birth weight infants with acute and chronic lung disease. *Pediatrics* 79:612–17.

Rome, E. S., Stork, E. K., Carlo, W. A., and Martin, R. J. (1984). Limitations and transcutaneous Po$_2$ and Pco$_2$

monitoring in infants with bronchopulmonary dysplasia. *Pediatrics* 74:217–20

Rooth, G., Huch, A., and Huch, R. (1987). Transcutaneous oxygen monitors are reliable indicators of arterial oxygen tension (if used correctly). *Pediatrics* 79:283–6.

Russell, R. I. R., and Helms, P. J. (1990). Comparative accuracy of pulse oximetry and transcutaneous oxygen in assessing arterial saturation in pediatric intensive care. *Critical Care Medicine* 18:725–7.

Ryan, C. A., Barrington, K. J., Vaughan, D., and Diner, N. N. (1986). Directly measured arterial oxygen saturation in the newborn infant. *Journal of Pediatrics* 109:526–9.

Severinghaus, J. W. (1986). Historical development of oxygenation monitoring. In *Pulse Oximetry*, ed. J. P. Payne and J. W. Severinghaus (pp. 1–18). Berlin: Springer-Verlag.

Severinghaus, J. W., and Spellman, M. J. (1990). Pulse oximeter failure thresholds in hypotersions and vasoconstriction. *Anesthesiology* 73:532–7.

Sheldon, R., Peeters, L. L. H., Jones, M. D., Jr., Makowskie, L., and Meschia, G. (1979). Redistribution of cardiac output and oxygen delivery in the hypoxemic fetal lamb. *American Journal of Obstetrics and Gynecology* 135:1071–8.

Sidi, A., Paulus, D. A., Rush, W., Gravenstein, N., and Davis, R. F. (1987). Methylene blue and indocyanine green artifactually lower pulse oximetry readings of oxygen saturation. Studies in dogs. *Journal of Clinical Monitoring* 3:249–56.

Solimano, A. J., Smyth, J. A., Mann, T. K., Albersheim, S. G., and Lockitch, G. (1986). Pulse oximetry advantage in infants with bronchopulmonary dysplasia. *Pediatrics* 78:844–9.

Thilo, E. H., Andersen, D., Wasserstein, M. L., Schmidt, J., and Luckey, D. (1993). Saturation by pulse oximetry: comparison of the results obtained by instruments of different brands. *Journal of Pediatrics* 122:620–6.

Thilo, E. H., Schmidt, J., Andersen, D., and Luckey, D. (1992). Saturation by pulse oximetry: are different brands' results interchangeable? *Clinical Research* 40:133A.

Tremper, K. K., and Barker, S. J. (1986). Pulse oximetry and oxygen transport. In *Pulse Oximetry*, ed. J. P. Payne and J. W. Severinghaus (pp. 19–27). Berlin: Springer-Verlag.

Watcha, M. F., Connor, M. T., and Hing, A. V. (1989). Pulse oximetry in methemoglobinemia. *American Journal of Diseases of Children* 143:845–7.

Wukitsch, M. W. Petterson, M. T., Tobler, D. R. and Pologe, J. A. (1988). Pulse oximetry: analysis of theory, technology, and practice. *Journal of Clinical Monitoring* 4:290–301.

9

Near-infrared monitoring of cerebral metabolic signals

FRANS F. JÖBSIS VAN DER VLIET, Ph.D.
JANE E. BRAZY, M.D.

INTRODUCTION

Noninvasive optical monitoring of cerebral oxidative metabolic status, specifically of intraneuronal availability of oxygen, is a new bedside method to provide direct information on the organ most at risk in a large number of intensive-care situations. It closes the information gap between more peripheral signals, such as pulmonary and circulatory parameters from pulse oximetry and blood-pressure monitoring, and our need to know whether or not the neurons are actually receiving adequate levels of oxygen. Within the past 15 yr, much effort has been expended to develop methods for supplying information by means of optical monitoring utilizing wavelengths in the near infrared (NIR), now referred to as near-infrared spectroscopy (NIRS). The primary signal in this method pertains to the oxidation state of the intraneuronal enzyme that catalyzes the use of oxygen in the process of oxidative phosphorylation. Ancillary signals can be obtained regarding regional oxygenated and deoxygenated hemoglobin. In contrast to the optical technique of pulse oximetry to determine arterial blood oxygenation, NIR monitoring of oxygen sufficiency (niroscopy) presents information on the actual delivery of oxygen in the tissues, most importantly in the brain. In addition, regional cerebral blood flow (rCBF) can be determined intermittently, such as by administration of a dye bolus or other means of contrast. These signals are available "on line," that is, continuously in real time. Although this monitoring

technique as yet does not provide all the information desired by the neonatologist, it does appear that clinical applications can now be made in a more or less routine manner to ascertain pathophysiology trends and the efficacy of treatment.

The idea of using the NIR range of the spectrum to monitor physiological oxygen sufficiency arose in 1977 when it was discovered that NIR photons could penetrate relatively dense tissues, including skin and bone (Jöbsis, 1977).* It was soon shown that this property makes it possible to monitor metabolic conditions in intact tissues and body parts in a nontraumatic, noninvasive way (Kariman, Jöbsis, and Saltzman, 1982; Proctor et al., 1983; Mook et al., 1984; Seeds et al., 1984; Ferrari et al., 1985; Jöbsis van der Vliet, 1985; Brazy et al., 1985a; Fox, Jöbsis van der Vliet, and Mitnick, 1985). NIRS has been and continues to be used primarily for cerebral monitoring in the operating room during anesthesia (Jöbsis van der Vliet, Fox, and Sugioka, 1987) and in the neonatal intensive-care unit (NICU) (Brazy, 1990). More recently, the technique has been applied toward the crucially important detection of fetal hypoxia during the birth process (Schmidt et al., 1989; Rolfe, Thorniley, and Wickramasinghe, 1991). NIRS has also been used for in vivo monitoring of skeletal muscle (Piantadosi and Jöbsis van der Vliet, 1985; Piantadosi, Hemstreet, and Jöbsis van der Vliet, 1986; Hampson, Jöbsis van der Vliet, and Pi-

---

* Prior to 1984, the first author of this chapter published under this abbreviated name.

antadosi, 1987) and the heart after surgical exposure (Jöbsis, 1977; Parsons et al., 1990).

In the first report on biomedical NIR applications it was realized that it might be possible to obtain NIR images similar to those produced by computed tomography (CT) and magnetic-resonance imaging (MRI). They would provide a metabolic topography of the organ or tissue, rather than a morphological map. Much effort has been and is being expended to achieve a useful level of clarity (Chance et al., 1993; Benaron and Stevenson, 1993; Benaron, van Houten, and Stevenson, 1994), and success may soon be achieved.

Monitoring of metabolic conditions over time with NIRS is now gaining acceptance in critical-care medicine, with neonatal care in the NICU leading the way. Monitoring of cerebral oxygen sufficiency in neonates received some of the earliest attention (Brazy et al., 1985b; Brazy and Lewis, 1986; cf. Brazy, 1990), and this is still the most active area of application, with new research and clinical articles appearing each month. A workshop organized by the National Institutes of Health concluded that NIR applications in neonatology constitute a promising field of basic and clinical research and should be stimulated. (Hirtz, 1993).

This review is limited to spectrophotometric monitoring of signals pertaining to cerebral oxidative metabolism. It is not so much the purpose to review the clinical observations, but rather to describe the derivation and interpretation of the signals. Nevertheless, a brief introduction to clinical experience is included, with special emphasis on applications to low birth-weight infants.

PRINCIPLES OF IN VIVO SPECTROPHOTOMETRY

In the NIR range, spectrophotometric signals are generated by only a very limited number of commonly occurring biological molecules. This number is further reduced when one considers only those molecules that respond to changing metabolic conditions by changes in their NIR absorption spectra. They are hemoglobin, myoglobin, and cytochrome c oxidase, the enzyme that catalyzes 90% or more of oxygen consumption in the cell. These are the molecules of interest for monitoring oxygen sufficiency in intact tissues and organs.

The "metabolic signals" that can be monitored are the amount of oxidized cytochrome c oxidase (a.k.a. cytochrome aa_3 and abbreviated cyt-aa_3) and the amounts of deoxygenated hemoglobin (Hb) and oxygenated hemoglobin (HbO_2 or HbO). (In muscle

tissue, myoglobin can also be monitored, but in the NICU, applications have been limited to cerebral monitoring.) The signals pertain to conditions in the *tissue* or in the *region* under optical observation, and to emphasize this point the abbreviations are usually preceded by the letter t or letter r.

The instrumentation generally employs laser diodes to generate the required NIR "light" at low, safe levels. The intensity needed to monitor cerebral oxygen sufficiency is many times less than the amount of NIR the brain would receive during an outdoor walk on a sunny winter's day in North Carolina. But the NIR light generated by the laser diodes (abbreviated LADs), a special form of light-emitting diodes (LEDs), is limited to a small number of distinct, monochromatic wavelengths. Safety is enhanced by the fact that photon energy decreases with increasing wavelength, and photochemical reactions induced by NIR photons are not known to occur in mammalian tissues. The NIR light from the input bundle is not a coherent or collimated beam and poses no significant risk. In addition, because the electrical voltage and current for the solid-state detectors are minimal, and the latter can be insulated electrically from the subject by an NIR-translucent plastic covering, this aspect also provides no significant risk.

Nevertheless, when working with an NIR monitoring instrument, it is advisable not to look at close range into the optical module that delivers the NIR. Because the retina does not register NIR light, no pupillary adaptation can take place to adjust the eye to the intensity, and the lens might concentrate a beam to an image small enough that theoretically it might injure the retina by local heating. For this reason the output of the fiber-optic cable is dispersed to spoil its beam characteristics. Nevertheless, patients can wear opaque eye shields to guard against the slim chance of inadvertent long-time exposure. Phototherapy eye patches do very well for the purpose. It is generally advisable that the upper part of the neonate's head, including the areas of NIR input and pickup, be covered with an opaque bonnet to exclude ambient room light from being sensed by the detector.

Physical principles

The "biological" or "metabolic" signals of NIRS are mostly presented in terms of deviations from the baseline, in units similar to the standard spectrophotometric units of absorbance (A) or optical density (OD), defined as A or $OD = \log I_0/I$ (discussed later). The earliest and still the most prevalent NIRS monitor (the Niroscope®) reports the data in terms of variations in density (abbreviated as v/d units). In order to explain NIRS and the implications of the v/d units, we must refer to the principles of spectrophotometry and the differences among single-wavelength, dual-wavelength, and multiwavelength differential modes of operation.

Spectrophotometry is a technique within the larger field of spectroscopy and commonly is used to determine the amount or concentration of a material. In the simplest case, light absorption is measured while a single monochromatic beam is transmitted through a cuvette. The Beer-Lambert equation is used to determine the concentration of the absorbing component. It states that the ratio of the light intensity *without* the absorber to that *with* the absorber is logarithmically related to the concentration of the absorbing molecules, their ability to absorb the light, and the distance that the light travels through the solution. Thus,

$$\log_{10}(I_0/I) = c \times e \times d$$

where I_0 is the light intensity observed without the absorber present (in terms of solution chemistry: pure solvent without the solute), I is the light intensity observed in the presence of the absorber, c is the concentration of the absorber, in moles per liter, e is the molar extinction coefficient of the absorber (i.e., light loss, at the wavelength employed, incurred per centimeter of travel through a 1-molar solution, with dimension of $cm^{-1} \cdot$ concentration^{-1}), and d is the optical path length through the solution, in centimeters.

To determine the concentration of a solute, the equation is rewritten as

$$c = \log_{10}(I_0/I) \times d^{-1} \times e^{-1}$$

The term log I_0/I is dimensionless and is called the absorbance (A) or optical density (OD). An A or OD unit equals 1.00 when the light has been attenuated 10-fold. Most spectrophotometry for quantitative chemical analysis is performed in the range of 0.1–1.0 OD unit. NIR determinations on tissues and organs usually are performed in the 6.0–10.0 OD range.

Spectrophotometry of turbid samples has long been a problem for bench-top measurements. In most instruments, light that is lost from the collimated beam cannot be distinguished from light losses caused by absorption. The well-known dual-wavelength differential method, introduced by Britton Chance in the early 1950s for the visible and near-ultraviolet ranges, utilizes subtraction of the signal at one wavelength (the reference) from that at the primary one (the measuring wavelength) to cor-

rect for light losses due to scattering in turbid samples (Chance, 1951). Standardly, the latter is chosen at the peak of the absorption spectrum of the molecule to be determined. A nearby reference wavelength is selected at which the molecule absorbs much less strongly. The requirement for success is that a narrow, strong absorption band of the molecule to be measured dominate the spectrum. The implicit assumption is that the degrees of light scattering at the two wavelengths will be so similar that any difference will be negligible compared with the difference in strength of absorption by the targeted molecule at those wavelengths. Studies employing this technique must also fulfill the requirement that the turbid biological samples (suspensions of red cells, mitochondria, etc., or excised tissue slices) be clear or thin enough so that most of the detected light will have traveled only once through the sample (i.e., that multiple scattering and its effect on path length will be negligible). Excised muscle slices 1–2 mm thick, for example, can be transilluminated successfully in a bench-top approach.

Dual- and triple-wavelength reflectance techniques using visible-range light were applied successfully to solid tissues such as the cerebral cortex (Jöbsis et al., 1977). However, because of the limited depth of penetration of photons in that range, the cortex had to be exposed for those studies. For clinical monitoring, a new, noninvasive, atraumatic approach was indicated.

Spectrophotometry of normally perfused solid tissues

Spectrophotometry of solid tissues and organs in vivo differs from the standard bench-top technique in five important respects. It must deal with (1) light losses by processes other than absorption, (2) inability to determine I_0 in the absence of the absorber, (3) an unknown optical path length caused by multiple scattering, (4) heterogeneity of tissues in the body part under observation, and (5) light absorption by several absorbers.

In addition, in the NIR range we also must cope with the following:

1. weak absorption coefficients, necessitating relatively large tissue samples (preferably several centimeters in diameter for transillumination, and 4 cm or more in lateral dimension for the reflectance mode of monitoring)
2. the fact that none of the three molecules of interest has a narrow, strong absorption band in the NIR

3. the fact that absorption by cytochrome c oxidase is about eightfold weaker than that by the hemoglobin in the cerebral circulation
4. the fact that absorption spectra determined in vivo differ sufficiently from those of purified material measured in vitro that it complicates separation of the cyt-aa$_3$ signal from the hemoglobin signals.

The operating principle of NIR tissue monitors is called multiwavelength differential spectrophotometry (MWDS). It employs several (four or five, rather than three) monochromatic light sources, for two purposes: (1) to monitor the three absorbing molecules separately and (2) to distinguish between scattering losses and loss of NIR light due to molecular absorption. The latter are caused by intracellular inclusions (such as mitochondria, nuclei, and microsomes), by cell membranes and myelination, by tissue structures (such as bone and connective tissue), and by any other nonhomogeneous tissue elements (such as red cells in the microvasculature).

Overlapping NIR absorption spectra of similar intensities necessitated a new and different approach that normalizes the intensities of absorption of the three molecules at one "reference" wavelength (usually in the range of 810 ± 8 nm), according to experimentally measured spectrophotometric absorption in situ. It then scales the absorption intensities at the other wavelengths according to the in situ absorption spectrum of the molecule to be monitored (Jöbsis van der Vliet, 1985; Jöbsis van der Vliet et al., 1988).

The algorithms to accomplish separate monitoring of the three components in the NIR utilize all wavelengths and take the form of multiple simultaneous equations. These are continuously solved for the three unknowns (Hb, HbO, and Cyt-aa$_3$) by a microprocessor program in the monitoring instrument. The MWDS technique can distinguish between scattering losses and loss of light due to molecular absorption.

At first it was deemed possible to monitor only changes from a baseline taken from the patient at the start of a monitoring session, and most of the published studies have been limited to that mode. That limitation arose because of two factors: Multiple scattering of photons lengthens their path through the tissue to an unknown extent, and skull geometry and thickness and scalp color can vary considerably. That made it impossible to arrive at absolute concentration indices and prevented a diagnosis of status. More recently, however, two

techniques have been suggested that may overcome some or all of these hurdles, though proof of that contention has not yet been established, and their reproducibility is questionable from patient to patient, or in a given patient under different metabolic conditions. In this review, primary emphasis will be placed on the results from trend-recording studies. Later, in discussing the outlook for the future, we shall return briefly to this issue.

APPLICATION TO CEREBRAL MONITORING

NIR monitoring of oxidative metabolism has been applied to a number of tissues. Some of these, such as muscle, have other reactive molecules (i.e., myoglobin) that contribute NIR signals. However, we shall limit this discussion to cerebral monitoring, with emphasis on applications to neonates.

Five factors contribute to concentration- and oxygen-related optical changes when monitoring the intact brain:

1. Changes in the oxidized copper complement in cytochrome c oxidase, designated Δcyt-aa$_3$
2. Changes in oxygenated hemoglobin, usually designated ΔrHbO or ΔtHbO
3. Changes in deoxygenated hemoglobin, designated ΔrHb or ΔtHb

[The sum of the rHbO and rHb changes is representative of the regional blood volume (BV) changes, commonly designated ΔrBV or ΔtBV, although it might more correctly have been called "Δr (total hemoglobin)."]

4. In addition, following changes in tissue oxygenation, an absorption is found to occur in the form of a minor band of mitochondrial origin with a peak at approximately 870 nm (as yet unconfirmed regarding its nature).
5. There is also a mild wavelength dependence of the scattering-function changes.

(These last two are lumped together in the algorithm treatment and are not shown among the reported parameters.)

Each of these five parameters contributes at most of the wavelengths in the NIR region of interest (i.e., 750–920 nm). It would seem to follow that a minimum of five wavelengths must be employed to construct five simultaneous absorption equations to be solved for the contribution of each of these five parameters. However, combination of the last two parameters reduces the requirements to four wavelengths and four algorithms. A number of instruments employ only three wavelengths. They provide satisfactory results except during the major light-scattering changes that occur at or close to death, when large shifts between intracellular and extracellular water occur. Thus, a complement of three is the absolute minimum number of wavelengths required to solve for the three unknowns. Four will provide an extra degree of confidence during major challenges to the tissue, by correcting for the influences of items 4 and 5.

In addition to the three direct signals due to cytochrome c oxidase, Hb, and HbO_2, and their sum BV, it was recognized early that measurements of regional cerebral blood flow (rCBF) could be made available on-line by niroscopy. The first attempt relied on the transit time of a bolus of indocyanine green, a dye that is clinically well accepted, with intensive light absorption in the NIR range. The first animal study established a satisfactory correlation between the NIR signal and standard xenon-133 measurements of CBF (Colacino, Grub, and Jöbsis, 1981). Neonatal studies of rCBF signals were first performed with NIR signals in Copenhagen: Vasodilations or contractions, signaled by the BV parameter, were found to be positively and closely correlated with the ^{133}Xe signals of rCBF (Pryds et al., 1990).

One of the drawbacks of NIR monitoring as currently practiced is the inability to provide an absolute number, such as a concentration, for each of the parameters measured. All monitoring is started by tuning the output intensity of the lasers to provide signals of appropiate strength at the site of detection. After this "baselining" routine, which takes about half a minute, the strength of the laser output is locked in and is maintained during the monitoring period, which may last for many hours. All results are recorded as deviations from the original baseline. In other words, there is no opportunity to make a diagnostic statement in terms of the concentrations of the components in the region being monitored optically. This inability and the possible ways to remedy it will be addressed in a later section.

What should be emphasized here is the fact that the signals are nevertheless quantitative in the sense that they are directly related to the amount of the absorber in the field of observation. Even though we cannot use expressions in terms of *concentration* (because the length of the path taken by the photons is not known), the changes in the metabolic NIR signals are directly related to changes in the *content* of the absorber. In other words, if one kind of manipulation produces twice the increase in the rHbO signal produced by a second manipula-

tion, then the first produced twice the increase in the regional oxygenated hemoglobin content compared with the second. The measured parameters concerning tissue content are expressed in terms of variation in density units (v/d) similar to absorbance (*A*) or optical density (OD) units of the concentration parameter.

The physiological signals

A cerebral monitoring trace is presented in Figure 9.1 for the purpose of illustrating the behavior of the so-called biological or physiological signals. It was obtained from a 4-kg female New Zealand white (NZW) rabbit, anesthetized with intramuscular ketamine, supplied with a femoral venous catheter for further drug administration, and intubated for positive-pressure ventilation. After local shaving, the input "optrode" was placed on the caudal aspect of the head, and the detector on the midline between the eyes. Before exposure to severe hypoxia, the animal was treated with an additional dose of anesthetic and was relaxed by administration of gallamine triethiodide.

Figure 9.1 shows the effects of a hypoxic/anoxic episode on the four signals. This part of the experiment followed exposures to a number of ventilatory gas mixtures, ending with a period of apnea produced by turning the ventilator off for approximately 90 s. Afterward, the traces were displaced from their original baseline values, showing a mild hypervolemia resulting from the anoxic episode 15 min earlier. That increased cerebral vasodilation was of arterial origin, as witnessed by the higher level of oxygenated hemoglobin (HbO). In fact, the deoxygenated hemoglobin (Hb) had fallen slightly from baseline conditions. The record shows that the previous manipulations had produced a net increase in the regional blood volume (BV), calculated as the sum of the Hb and HbO traces.

After the hypoxic gas mixture has traversed the dead space, and blood with a lower PaO_2 arrives in the cerebral circulation, we see, almost simultaneously, an increase in the Hb trace and decreases in the HbO and cyt-aa_3 traces. It can be shown, at faster rates of display, that the beginning of the reduction in cyt-aa_3 lags anywhere from 1 s to 3 s behind the hemoglobin traces. This delay tends to increase after repeated hypoxic/anoxic insults, possibly because of hyperemia. Conversely, following reoxygenation, the onsets of the responses of HbO, Hb, and cyt-aa_3 are almost simultaneous, with the latter sometimes leading the way by a few seconds. These observations on the kinetics agree with the

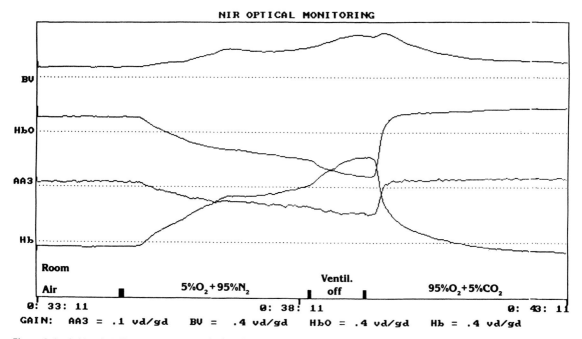

Figure 9.1. A 10-min NIR monitoring record of a rabbit's cerebral responses to ventilatory manipulations. The traces were smoothed by a 5-s running-average routine. The dotted lines represent the starting levels for the four physiological traces. They also represent the grid referred to in the notations at the bottom. The expression vd/gd stands for vander units per distance between two grid lines. This record was transcribed from a floppy disc that captured the data during the experiment. The time designation at the bottom refers to time from the beginning of a new file.

fact that the blood is the source of the oxygen, and cytochrome c oxidase is the sink of the oxygen, and that little or no O_2 reserve or excess exists in the brain under normal circumstances.

It can be noted from the rBV trace that an initial vasodilatory stage was followed by an interim period of trading HbO_2 for Hb, with a subsequent faster rise in the Hb. At that point the ventilator was switched off, and in the subsequent minute of apnea the traces rapidly attained their final levels. It is important to note that a downturn in the rBV trace occurred before ventilation was restored. This signifies a decrease in cardiac output and is a telltale sign of the end of the cardiovascular system's ability to compensate for the falling oxygen delivery.

Following renewed administration of oxygen, in the form of a hyperoxic and hypercarbic gas mixture, the traces reversed and overshot their points of departure. It is of interest that rabbits are much better able to maintain viability at low FIO_2 and also do not react strongly to an elevated $Paco_2$. In cats and in domestic swine, an FIO_2 or an $FICO_2$ of 0.05 will have immediate and dramatic effects on cardiac output and on cerebral vasodilation. In those species, the hypoxic period would have shown a greater early increase in cerebral blood volume, to be followed by a severe decrease in cardiac output and inability to maintain cerebral viability. Hypercarbia would have had about twice the effect on the regional cerebral blood volume. It could be speculated that the differences between species are related to the rabbit's evolutionary adaptation to life in an underground warren with limited ventilation–similar to the reactions of rats, but the opposite of the special ability of birds to be unresponsive to extreme hypocarbia because of hyperventilation during flight at high altitudes. However, surveys of the NIR responses of subterranean dwellers have not yet been made.

Interpretation of the signals

Because of the novel nature of optically monitoring cerebral metabolism, many questions arise concerning the biological signals. Some of these can usefully be addressed here as a means toward elucidating various aspects of the information obtained by NIR monitoring. Other questions are addressed in the later section on limitations.

The anatomic and histologic origins of the signals

are among the most frequently questioned aspects. Four or five different tissues are traversed by the photons between the input and detection points, and they may contribute to the signals. Of these, the meninges can be dismissed out of hand, because they are optically clear and metabolically inert for all practical purposes. The scalp and the skull do not contain sufficient amounts of cytochrome c oxidase to be measured in the NIR range. This is in keeping with their very low rates of oxidative metabolism. Red blood cells are totally devoid of the enzyme, and white cells are sparse compared with the nerve cells supplied by the blood. Thus, the cyt-aa$_3$ signal can confidently be assigned a neuronal origin.

Blood flow in bone is low, negligible compared with that in the brain. Blood flow and blood content in the scalp might not be negligible were it not for the fact that pressure from the optrodes eliminates most blood at the places of entry and exit of the photons. This is certainly the case when the devices are applied firmly against the adult cranium. In the case of the softer neonate skull, pressure should remain moderate, and a larger fraction of the so-called blood signals might be contributed by the scalp vasculature. Nevertheless, we should recognize that, in contrast to the situation of the radioactive xenon used for cerebral blood-flow determinations, only the thicknesses of the tissues and their relative blood contents (not their morphology or relative location) count in neonatal NIR monitoring. In the adult cat, for example, less than 5% of the blood signals are found to be derived from the scalp circulation (F. F. Jöbsis van der Vliet, unpublished observations). Thus, we can state that the blood signals derive primarily, almost exclusively, from the regional cerebral circulation.

Therefore, questions about signal derivation essentially boil down to gray versus white matter. In the adult brain, the gray matter forms a relatively thin but highly convoluted layer overlying the white, which pokes wispy fingers toward the calvarium. The thin columns supporting the gyri are likely to be the only part of the white matter traversed by the NIR photons when using reflectance monitoring; the more solid body of this tissue is optically almost impenetrable.

There are two reasons that white matter appears white to our eyes. First, a strong diffuse reflectance is produced by the many layers of myelin. It scatters light so efficiently that most of the light is turned back at or near the surface. Second, the white matter is only poorly supplied with mitochondria, whose flavoproteins impart most of the beige color

to the gray matter. In fact, by far most of the mitochondria dwell in the neuronal cell bodies, rather than in the dendrites, in the more distal axons, or in the glia (O'Connor, 1977). Thus, the cerebral signals are primarily derived from the neurons in the gray matter.

The cerebral region of signal derivation varies considerably between adult and neonatal applications. In the reflectance mode, used in the former case, the optrodes are applied 4 cm or more apart on the forehead. This leads to an elliptically shaped field of observation, with the optrodes at the two foci. The field is almost totally confined to the more glazy gray matter through which the photons travel on their helter-skelter paths as time and again they are deflected by myelin, by other membranes, and by intracellular inclusions.

In the neonatal brain, transillumination is the preferred mode of observation. This can be accomplished in either a temple-to-temple or a frontal-to-occipital configuration. The ease of transmitting an adequate optical signal is doubtless related to the incomplete myelination at this stage of development: An adult cat's head of considerably smaller diameter produces a much greater attenuation of the optical signal. Nevertheless, considerable scattering does take place, and it is best to adopt the point of view that most of the photons have roamed through most of the brain before being detected at the exit point. Thus, the physiological NIR signals provide a global representation of oxygen sufficiency in the neonatal brain.

Interpretation of the physiological signals is straight forward in a trend-monitoring sense, but difficult in a quantitative diagnostic sense. In addition, because of the interspecific differences noted earlier, it is highly relevant to stress that the reactions seen in human subjects and patients must be interpreted from a solid base of experience. An extensive data base must be accumulated for the purpose, and separately for newborns and adults. The first observations on neonates in the intensive-care nursery showed unexpected differences from the findings in adults. The very close relationship between the HbO trace and the cyt-aa$_3$ redox trace was not found in the neonates, especially the low-birth-weight babies (Brazy et al., 1985b). In other words, autoregulation between oxygen consumption and supply is not nearly as firm and seamless in neonates as in adults. Similarly, it was observed that newborn piglets quite unexpectedly adapted to life-threatening hypoxic/anoxic challenges by an apparent increase in the oxygen affinity of cytochrome oxidase. After several minutes of ventilation with pure nitrogen, the enzyme was found to be at a much higher oxidation state at the same normoxic and hypoxic conditions than before the anoxic episode (Jöbsis van der Vliet, 1991). Thus, it would appear that the cytochrome signal provides more telling information than does the state of the regional cerebral blood oxygenation. When cytochrome oxidase trends to a more reduced state, intraneuronal oxygenation is decreasing. However, given the current state of our technology, we are not yet able to state the danger limits for incurring cellular damage. Clinical research and experience must provide the answers, as was required in the past for arterial blood gas data, for end-tidal CO_2, for glucose, for blood pressure, for temperature, and for a host of other data.

CLINICAL OBSERVATIONS

The technique of NIRS was first applied to neonates in the early 1980s (Brazy et al., 1985a,b). Those early observations demonstrated the ability of the technique to detect changes in hemoglobin oxygenation, cerebral blood volume, and the cytochrome c oxidase redox state (Brazy and Lewis, 1986; Brazy, 1990). In addition, they showed the potential usefulness of the technique for continuous real-time, noninvasive monitoring of cerebral oxygenation in sick preterm neonates.

However, early NIRS provided information only on trends or patterns of change in the monitored parameters. Using an estimation of path length and an inhalation technique to provide blood-borne markers, recent studies have attempted to quantitate the changes in the signals to provide information that will be familiar to the clinician and will allow comparison between the NIRS technique and other assessments. The first studies were performed by Reynold's group in London, using a variation of the niroscope instrument constructed by Delpy after consultation at Duke University. Most of the findings obtained with those two instruments can therefore be compared, allowing extrapolations between the two with some confidence. The same holds for the work of Rolfe and Wickramasinghe in Keele, England, who independently produced their own instruments early on (Crowe et al., 1984). The Copenhagen instruments used by the groups of Greisen and Schmidt produce acceptable Hb, HbO, and BV signals, but fail to measure cyt-aa_3 because of an incorrect set of wavelengths.

Edwards and associates of the London group measured cerebral blood flow in sick but stable infants, using an inhalation technique, and found a range of 7–33 ml per 100 g per minute, which is consistent with the ranges obtained using other techniques (Edwards et al., 1988). Mean cerebral blood volume in term and preterm infants who were believed to have normal brains was 2.2 ± 0.4 ml per 100 g (Wyatt et al., 1990). Cerebral blood-flow reactivity was also studied. The normal range for reactivity was 0.1–0.7 ml per 100 g per 1 kPa (Wyatt et al., 1991). There was a close linear correlation between gestational age and blood-flow reactivity to changing $Paco_2$, with more mature infants demonstrating greater reactivity.

In addition to defining normal neonatal physiology, NIRS is helpful in understanding the pathophysiology of disease states. Brazy and associates demonstrated decreases in cerebral oxygen delivery during hypertensive peaks and during episodes of crying in unstable sick preterm infants (Brazy and Lewis, 1986; Brazy, 1988). Two groups have studied term infants after asphyxia. Cerebral blood volume and blood flow were both significantly elevated post asphyxia, and cerebral vascular reactivity was reduced. The degree of disturbance correlated with the severity of the encephalopathy (McCormick et al., 1991). Van Bel et al. (1993) compared severely asphyxiated infants to normal infants and to moderately asphyxiated infants. From 2 to 12 h after birth, cerebral blood volume decreased in the severely asphyxiated, but remained stable in the others. Those decreases were associated with declines in both oxyhemoglobin and deoxyhemoglobin and, in two infants, decreases in cytochrome oxidation. Those observations suggest that postasphyxic hypoperfusion of the brain during the first few hours of life may extend cerebral tissue damage. Both studies noted a correlation between mean arterial pressure and cerebral blood volume, suggesting a pressure-passive circulation after asphyxia.

NIR monitoring permits continuous observation of cerebral responses to administration of drugs and reactions to procedures. Intravenous infusions of indomethacin, aminophylline, and phenobarbital all cause decreases in cerebral blood flow or blood volume that can persist for several hours (Edwards et al., 1990; McDonald, Ives, and Hope, 1992; Fahnenstich et al., 1992). Cerebral responses to procedures such as suctioning, surfactant administration, extracorporeal membrane oxygenation, and deep hypothermia have been investigated (Shah et al., 1992; Edwards et al., 1992; Liem et al., 1992; Kurth et al., 1992).

Little is known about the development of the cytochrome system throughout gestation and the adaptive changes that occur after delivery. But it is known that there are significant differences between the neonatal and adult systems, specifically in cytochrome c oxidase (Mela, Goodwin, and Miller, 1976; cf. Mela, 1979). During NIR monitoring of low-birth-weight babies, it became clear that the close relationship between the cyt-aa$_3$ redox state and cerebral oxyhemoglobin content seen in adults was not present or was easily disturbed, as noted in sick preterms (Brazy et al., 1985b; cf. Jöbsis van der Vliet, 1991). In other words, the feedback loop between the metabolic demand for oxygen and its local supply system is not as closely implemented, not as sturdy, in the neonate as in the adult. Currently, therefore, it is not possible to provide an accurate, fine-tuned interpretation of the cytochrome signals noted during hypoxic events and hemodynamic fluctuations in neonates. Nevertheless, decreases in cyt-aa$_3$ oxidation are sure signals that the mitochondria are suffering a decrease in oxygen availability for oxidative metabolism. Coupled with further research in this area, NIRS offers the potential to identify more closely and quantitatively cellular oxygen insufficiency before it progresses to cell death. Until that can be achieved, whenever trend monitoring of cyt-aa$_3$ shows a decreased oxidation of the enzyme, steps should be considered to reverse that trend, because the ancillary blood signals may be inconclusive.

LIMITATIONS

It might be useful to summarize the status of NIR monitoring of tissue oxygen sufficiency (niroscopy) in the form of a review of its current limitations. At present, the three major shortcomings of spectrophotometric NIR monitoring are the lack of a diagnostic mode, the absence of a gold standard for calibrating the new signals, and the need to perfect the art and craft of easier routine application. In addition, as with any novel measurement, we lack sufficient clinical experience for precise evaluation of the results obtained with an individual patient.

An ability to provide diagnostic information regarding the metabolic status of a tissue would greatly improve the trend-monitoring value. Neither the concentration of the target molecules in standard terms (i.e., moles per liter or grams per kilogram wet weight) nor the relative concentrations of the two forms, oxidized and reduced, can currently be calculated. This inability stems from lack of reliable measurements of path length and of I_0, the light intensity in the absence of the absorber. However, it appears that this diagnostic deficiency may well be resolved in the near future.*

As noted earlier, the optical path is unknown because of multiple scattering. Two approaches are being used in efforts to provide an index to path length: (1) assessment of photon absorption by water at adjacent NIR wavelengths, as a determination of the amount of solvent encountered by the photon stream, and (2) measurement of the time of flight (TOF) of photons through the tissue.

1. At somewhat longer NIR wavelengths, water features an increasingly intense absorption spectrum. Gradually starting at about 900 nm this leads to peaks at 1,000 and 1,300 nm, followed by a large number of increasingly intense bands. In the late 1980s it was realized that the first water bands might serve the purpose of measuring the amount of water encountered by the photon stream, with that number being used to calculate the concentrations of other absorbers (i.e., amount of solute per amount of solvent) (Cope et al., 1989). That approach has not yet been implemented for routine observations, partially because of a lack of reliable lasers of sufficient power at these wavelengths, but also because of the need for much spectroscopic research in this neglected region of the spectrum. Efforts to overcome these problems, however, appear to be on their way toward a solution.

2. The second technique focuses on the fact that the average path length can be judged from the time required for passage of the photons. This approach is called time-of-flight (TOF) analysis or time-resolved spectroscopy (TRS). The geometric distance between input and detection points would lead us to anticipate a certain time of arrival for a very short train of photons – say a laser pulse lasting only a few picoseconds (1 ps = 10^{-12} s). However, the pulse that emerges is delayed and no longer has its original rectangular shape. Very few photons are detected at the expected time of arrival. Instead, after a threefold to sixfold delay, a muted peak is finally observed, followed by a protracted "tail"

---

* Recently (August/September 1994), we have succeeded in determining that percentage of the blood in the region being monitored that is saturated with O_2 (P. D. Jöbsis and F. F. Jöbsis van der Vliet, unpublished data). When applied to the brain, it has been designated regional cerebral blood oxygen saturation (rCBOS). Testing of this new quantitative parameter and development of a data base for on-line diagnostic purposes in the clinical setting should be achieved in 1995. Industrial sources predict that it can be incorporated into commercial, clinical models that could become available in early 1996, depending on success in testing and the speed of FDA approval.

stretching out many fold farther. The last photons to arrive have traveled the longest path and may have skittered around in the farthest reaches of the brain. (The tales they will tell once we are better versed in their dialect!) From the ratio between the average TOF and the expected TOF, and from the decay curve, an estimated average path length and absorber concentration can be calculated, respectively (Wyatt et al., 1990; Sevick et al., 1991). It has been shown that multiple scatterings increase the average path length through a newborn baby's head to three to six times the geometric distance. Similar numbers and variabilities are found in other body parts, such as the adult arm, for example. Large variations are observed between individuals regarding the factor by which the geometric path length is multiplied by multiple scatterings. Differences in metabolic states also contribute to the variability, although they may do so to a lesser extent. However, we have no quantitative or even relative assessment of the latter. It appears that an individual path-length determination with continuous updating will be required, though the current picosecond technology does not lend itself to bedside measurements.

An alternative way to determine the optical path length by TOF analysis is to apply phase-shift techniques to the delay in the moment of occurrence of the peak photon flux, sometimes referred to as time-resolved spectroscopy (TRS). This has been accomplished by rapid modulation of the intensity of a light source and measurement of the phase shift in the detected signal (Sevick et al., 1991). It is a frequency-modulation (FM) technique, for which sensitive and inexpensive FM detection has been perfected. It has the advantages that the peak is somewhat less influenced by the intensity of absorption than the decay and that the equipment and technical support are much simpler than for picosecond pulse analysis. However, phase-shift techniques are relatively insensitive for concentration determinations, because slight differences in the small extinction coefficients of the absolute absorption spectra must be employed. Situations of small differences between large signals typically generate unfavorable signal-to-noise ratios. Good solutions to these problems inherent in TOF and TRS analysis have not yet been found.

In conclusion it can be stated that thus far we have failed to find acceptable solutions to the problems of determining absolute concentrations because of lack of a reliable on-line means to determine optical path length. However, research efforts are under way in several laboratories working on various means to provide continuous, real-time information that can allow quantitative assessments of the concentrations of the absorbers.

The absence of a gold standard (i.e., an ability to extrapolate the NIR data to a proven and accepted parameter) is a consequence of the truly novel nature of these signals. Currently, there is no information on intracerebral blood content and its oxygenation state averaged over arteries, capillaries, and veins. No other method exists to provide a cross-reference for these NIR signals. In animal experimentation, certain limits can be set, such as the onset of total anoxia or total hyperoxia at 4–5 atm of oxygen pressure in a hyperbaric chamber. But normoxic values for the intracerebral blood are not available. It will therefore be necessary to derive a quantitative number at the extremes of oxygenation and deoxygenation. Then we must generate experimental data by trend-monitoring the limits of hypoxic effects compatible with survival and the NIR signal changes observed. Transfer to the clinical setting will then follow.

A number of technical problems must yet be solved to make the use of this instrumentation routine in the nursery. The suppression of motion artifacts could still be improved, as could the procedures for applying the optrodes to the neonate's head. These and other improvements, which are not trivial, can be expected to be achieved by a combination of engineering and experience in the field.

CONCLUSIONS

In summary, it can be stated with confidence that NIR monitoring is sufficiently advanced that it can be recommended for routine monitoring of trends in patients at risk for cerebral oxygen insufficiency. The technique is rapidly gaining acceptance in Europe, Japan, and other Pacific countries. In the United States, we are waiting on the accumulation of sufficient clinical experience to win approval by the Food and Drug Administration. Once that is achieved, the NIR technique will rapidly find its niche in the armamentarium of the neonatologist.

REFERENCES

Benaron, D. A., and Stevenson, D. K. (1993). Optical time-of- flight and absorbance imaging of biologic media. *Science* 259:1463–6.

Benaron, D. A., van Houten, J., and Stevenson, D. K. S. (1994). Imaging cerebral pathology and function using time-of-flight optical scanning. *Lancet.*

Brazy, J. E. (1988). Effects of crying on cerebral blood volume and cytochrome aa₃. *Journal of Pediatrics* 112:457–61.

(1990). Near infrared spectrophotometry. In *Current Therapy in Neonatal-Perinatal Medicine*, 2nd ed., ed. N. M. Nelson (pp. 139–44). Toronto: B. C. Decker.

Brazy, J. E., and Lewis, D. V. (1986). Changes in cerebral blood volume and cytochrome aa$_3$ during hypertensive peaks in preterm infants. *Journal of Pediatrics* 108:983–7.

Brazy, J. E., Lewis, D. V., Mitnick, M. H., and Jöbsis van der Vliet, F. F. (1985a). Monitoring of cerebral oxygenation in the intensive care nursery. *Advances in Experimental Medicine and Biology* 191:843–8.

(1985b). Noninvasive monitoring of cerebral oxygenation in preterm infants: preliminary observations. *Pediatrics* 75:217–5.

Chance, B. (1951). Rapid and sensitive spectrophotometry. III: A double beam apparatus. *Review of Scientific Instruments* 22:634–8.

(1991). Optical method. *Annual Review of Biophysics and Chemistry* 20:1–28.

Chance, B., Kang, K., He, L., Weng, J, and Sevick, E. (1993). Highly sensitive object location in tissue models with linear in-phase and anti-phase multi-element optical arrays in one and two dimensions. *Proceedings of the National Academy of Sciences USA* 90:3423–7.

Colacino, J. M., Grubb, B., and Jöbsis, F. F. (1981). Infrared technique for cerebral bloodflow. Comparison with ^{133}xenon clearance. *Neurological Research* 3:17–31.

Cope, M., Delpy, D. T., Wray, S., Wyatt, J. S., and Reynolds, E. O. R. (1989). A CCD spectrophotometer to quantitate the concentration of chromophores in living tissue utilizing the absorption peak of water at 975 nm. *Advances in Experimental Medicine and Biology* 248:33–40.

Crowe, J., Rea, P. A., Wickramasinghe, Y. A. B. D., and Rolfe, P. (1984). Towards non-invasive monitoring of cerebral metabolism. In *Proceedings of the 2nd International Conference on Fetal and Neonatal Physiological Measurements*, ed. P. Rolfe (pp. N5–6). Oxford University Press.

Edwards, A. D., McCormick, D. C., Roth, S. C., Elwell, C. E., Peebles, D. M., Cope, M., Wyatt, J. S., Delpy, D. T., and Reynolds, E. O. R. (1992). Cerebral hemodynamic effects of treatment with modified natural surfactant investigated by near infrared spectroscopy. *Pediatric Research* 32:532–6.

Edwards, A. D., Wyatt, J. S., Richardson, C., Delpy, D. T., Cope, M. and Reynolds, E. O. R. (1988). Cotside measurement of cerebral blood flow in ill newborn infants by near infrared spectroscopy. *Lancet* 2:770–1.

Edwards, A. D., Wyatt, J. S., Richardson, C., Potter, A., Cope, M., Delpy, D. T., and Reynolds, E. O. R. (1990). Effects of indomethacin on cerebral haemodynamics and oxygen delivery investigated by near infrared spectroscopy in very preterm infants. *Lancet* 335:1491–5.

Fahnenstich, H., Schmidt, S., Krebs, D., and Kowaleski, S. (1992). Intrakranielle Hämodynamik unter Phenobarbitalmedikation. *Zeitschrift für Geburtshilfe und Perinatolgie* 196:74–7.

Ferrari, M., Giannini, F., Sideri, G, and Zanette, E. (1985). Continuous non invasive monitoring of human brain by near infrared spectroscopy. *Advances in Experimental Medicine and Biology* 191:873–82.

Fox, E., Jöbsis van der Vliet, F. F., and Mitnick, M. H. (1985). Monitoring of cerebral oxygen sufficiency in anesthesia and surgery. *Advances in Experimental Medicine and Biology* 191:849–54.

Greeley, W. J., Bracey, V. A., Ungerleider, R. M., Griebel, J. A., Kern, F. H., Boyd, J. L., Reves, J. G., and Piantadosi, C. A. (1991). Recovery of cerebral metabolism and mitochondrial oxidation state are delayed after hypothermic circulation arrest. *Circulation* 84:400–6.

Hampson, N. B., Jöbsis van der Vliet, F. F., and Piantadosi, C. A. (1987). Skeletal muscle oxygen availability during respiratory acid–base disturbances in cats. *Respiration Physiology* 70:143–58.

Hirtz, D. G. (1993). Report of the National Institute of Neurological Diseases and Stroke workshop on near infrared spectroscopy. *Pediatrics* 91:414–7.

Jöbsis, F. F. (1977). Non-invasive, infra-red monitoring of cerebral and myocardial oxygen sufficiency and circulatory parameters. *Science* 198:1264–7.

Jöbsis, F. F., Keizer, J. H., LaManna, J. C., and Rosenthal, M. (1977). Reflectance spectrophotometry of cytochrome a,a$_3$ in vivo. *Journal of Applied Physiology* 43:858–72.

Jöbsis van der Vliet, F. F. (1985). Non-invasive, near infrared monitoring of cellular oxygen sufficiency in vivo. *Advances in Experimental Midicine and Biology* 191:833–42.

(1991). Near infrared monitoring of cerebral cytochrome c oxidase: past and present (and future?). In *Fetal and Neonatal Physiological Measurements*, ed. H. N. Lafeber (pp. 41–55). Amsterdam: Excerpta Medica.

Jöbsis van der Vliet, F. F., Fox, E., and Sugioka, K. (1987). Monitoring of cerebral oxygenation and cytochrome a,a$_3$ redox site. In *Advances in Oxygen Monitoring: International Anesthesiology Clinics*, ed. K. K. Tremper (pp. 209–30). Boston: Little, Brown.

Jöbsis van der Vliet, F. F., Piantadosi, C. A., Sylvia, A. L., Lucas, S. K., and Keizer, H. H. (1988). Near infra red monitoring of cerebral oxygen sufficiency I: Spectra of cytochrome c oxidase in situ. *Neurological Research* 10:7–17.

Kariman, K., Jöbsis, F. F., and Saltzman, H. A. (1982). "Cytochrome a,a$_3$ reoxidation: early indicator of metabolic recovery from hemorrhagic shock. *Journal of Clinical Investigation* 72:180–91.

Kurth, C. D., Steven, J. M., Nicolson, S. C., Chance, B., and Delivoria-Papadopoulos, M. (1992). Kinetic of cerebral deoxygenation during deep hypothermic circulatory arrest in neonates. *Anesthesiology* 77:656–61.

Liem, K. D., Hopman, J. C., Koll, L. A., Kollee, L. A., and Oeseburg, B. (1992). Assessment of cerebral oxygenation and hemodynamics by near infrared spectrophotometry during induction of ECMO: preliminary results. *Advances in Experimental Medicine and Biology* 317:841–6.

McCormick, D. C., Edwards, A. D., Roth, S. C., Wyatt, J. S., Elwell, C. E., Cope, M., Delpy, D. T., and Reynolds, E. O. R. (1991). Relation between cerebral haemodynamics and outcome in birth asphyxiated newborn infants studied by near infrared spectroscopy. *Pediatric Research* (abstract).

McDonald, M., Ives, N. K., and Hope, P. L. (1992). Intravenous aminophylline and cerebral blood flow in preterm infants. *Archives of Disease in Childhood* 67:416–18.

Mela, L. (1979). Mitochondrial function in cerebral ischemia and hypoxia: Comparison of inhibitory and adaptive responses. *Neurological Research* 1:51–64.

Mela, L., Goodwin, C. W., and Miller, L. D. (1976). In vivo control of mitochondrial enzyme concentrations and activity by oxygen. *American Journal of Physiology* 231:1811–16.

Mook, P. H., Proctor, H. J., Jöbsis, F. F. and Wildevuur, C. R. H. (1984). Assessment of brain oxygenation: a comparison between an oxygen electrode and near-infrared spectrophotometry. *Advances in Experimental Medicine and Biology* 169:841–7.

O'Connor, M. J. (1977). Origin of labile NADH tissue fluorescence. In *Oxygen and Physiological Function*, ed. F. F. Jöbsis (pp. 79–89). Dallas: Professional Information Library.

Parsons, W. J., Reinbert, J. C., Bauman, R. P., Greenfield, J. C., Jr., and Piantadosi, C. A. (1990). Dynamic mechanisms of cardiac oxygenation during brief ischemia and reperfusion. *American Journal of Physiology* 259:477–85.

Piantadosi, C. A., Hemstreet, T. M., and Jöbsis van der Vliet, F. F. (1986). Near infrared spectrophotometric monitoring of oxygen distribution to intact brain and skeletal muscle tissues. *Critical Care Medicine* 14:698–706.

Piantadosi, C. A., and Jöbsis van der Vliet, F. F. (1985). Near infrared optical monitoring of intact skeletal muscle during hypoxic and hemorhagic hypotension in cats. *Advances in Experimental Medicine and Biology* 191:855–62.

Proctor, H. J., Palladino, G. W., Cairns, C., and Jöbsis, F. F. (1983). An evaluation of perfluorochemical resuscitation after hypoxic hypotension. *Trauma* 23:79–83.

Pryds, O., Greisen, G., Skov, L. L., and Friis-Hansen, B. (1990). Carbon dioxide-related changes in cerebral blood volume and cerebral blood flow in mechanically ventilated preterm neonates: comparison of near infrared spectrophotometry and [113]xenon clearance. *Pediatric Research* 27:445–9.

Rolfe, P., Thorniley, M., and Wickramasinghe, Y. A. B. D. (1991). The potential of near infra-red spectroscopy for detection of fetal cerebral hypoxia. *European Journal of Gynaecology and Obstetrics* 42: S24–8.

Schmidt, S., Eilers, H., Lenz, A., Helledie, N., and Krebs, D. (1989). Laserspectroscopy in the fetus. *Journal of Perinatal Medicine* 17:57–62.

Seeds, J. W., Cefalo, R. C., Proctor, H. J., and Jöbsis van der Vliet, F. F. (1984). The relationship of intracranial infrared light absorbance to fetal oxygenation. I: Methodology. *American Journal of Obstetrics and Gynecology* 149:679–84.

Sevick, E. M., Chance, B., Leigh, J., Nioka, S. and Maris, M. (1991). Quantitation of time- and frequency-resolved optical spectra for the determination of tissue oxygenation. *Analytical Biochemistry* 195:330–51.

Shah, A. R., Kurth, C. D., Gwiazdowski, S. G., Chance, B., and Delivoria-Papadopoulos, M. (1992). Fluctuations in cerebral oxygenation and blood volume during endotracheal suctioning in preterm infants. *Journal of Pediatrics* 120:769–74.

Tamura, M. (1991). Non-invasive monitoring of brain oxygen metabolism during cardiopulmonary bypass by near infra-red spectrophotometry. *Japanese Circulation Journal* 55:330–5.

van Bel, F., Dorrepaal, C. A., Benders, M. J. N. L., Zeeuwe, P. E. M., van der Bol, M., and Berger, H. M. (1993). Changes in cerebral hemodynamics and oxygenation in the first 24 hours following birth asphyxia. *Pediatrics* 92:365–72.

Wyatt, J. S., Cope, M., Delpy, D. T., Richardon, C. E., Edwards, A. D., Wary, S., and Reynolds, E. O. R. (1990). Quantitation of cerebral blood volume in newborn human infants by near infrared spectroscopy. *Journal of Applied Physiology* 68:1086–91.

Wyatt, J. S., Edwards, A. D., Cope, M., Delpy, D. T., McCormick, D. C., Potter, A., and Reynolds, E. O. R. (1991). Response of cerebral blood volume to changes in arterial carbon dioxide tension in preterm and term infants. *Pediatric Research* 29:553–7.

10

Fetal scalp pH and heat flux

GEORGE SIMBRUNER, M.D.
OSMAN IPSIROGLU, M.D.
RUDOLF RUDELSTORFER, M.D.

INTRODUCTION

The concentrations of hydrogen ions (H^+) in body fluids and the heat flowing from the body are all end products of metabolism. They are measured to determine whether or not energy is supplied to the fetus in sufficient amounts, and waste products are removed in sufficient amounts from the fetus, to maintain a thermodynamic force for life. Large amounts of H^+ are produced by metabolism and re-used in metabolic reactions (e.g., H^+ unites with O_2 to form H_2O). In a healthy adult, 13,000 mmol of H^+ would accumulate daily from metabolic CO_2 production if CO_2 were not breathed out, and more than 200 mmol of organic acids, produced by metabolic breakdown of amino acids and lipids, would accumulate if not excreted by the kidney. Under pathological conditions, either H^+ cannot be excreted or, when there is a lack of oxygen, metabolic reactions that normally consume H^+ are stopped, and H^+ accumulates in the form of lactate or other organic acids.

All of the free energy of nutrients, whether aerobically or anaerobically metabolized, finally appears in the form of the waste product heat. The amount of heat stored in a tissue depends on the amount of heat produced by metabolism and the amount removed by conductive and convective heat-transfer mechanisms, the convective heat transfer being mainly a function of blood flow. Under pathological conditions, the pathways for heat removal can be altered, or if there is a lack of oxygen, heat production may drop to 5% of its normal aerobic level.

pH MEASUREMENTS

The concentrations of H^+ to be measured in water or body fluids are very small. Water at 15°C contains only 0.0000001 mol of H^+ per liter; therefore, H^+ concentrations (cH^+) are expressed in nanomoles (1 nmol = 10^{-9} mol) per liter, or on a logarithmic scale, so that the *potentia hydrogenii* (pH) = $-\log_{10}$ (cH^+). When electrometric methods are used to determine pH, the activity of H^+, not its concentration, is measured. The concentration and the activity of H^+ are identical only if the activity coefficient is unity. In view of the difficulty of assigning values for the activity coefficient for single ions, the concentrations of H^+, even when derived from reliable pH measurements, are all to some degree uncertain (Robins, 1975).

Such small concentrations can be measured by chemical, electrometric, and other methods. Among the chemically based methods are (1) indirect assessment from measurements of P_{CO_2} and bicarbonate, using the Henderson-Hasselbalch equation, and (2) colorimetric methods, using either colored indicator dyes or light-absorption techniques. With the light-absorption techniques, the absorption of either white (polychromatic) or monochromatic light in the visible or the ultraviolet range of the spectrum is utilized. Among the electrometric methods, use of a glass pH-sensitive electrode is the best-known. Alternative methods use polymer membranes, noble-metal oxides, hydrated palladium, and ion-sensitive field-effect transistors (ISFETs) (Mindt, Maurer, and Möller, 1978). In this chapter we shall

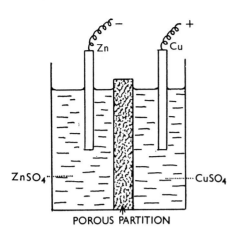

Figure 10.1. The Daniel cell. (From Sykes, 1974, with permission.)

focus on the pH-sensitive glass electrode and on a method based on light absorption by fluorescent dyes.

ELECTROMETRIC METHODS

The most accurate measurements of pH have been and still are made by means of pH-sensitive electrode. Among the various forms of electrodes (hydrogen or quinhydrone electrode), the glass electrode is extremely versatile, does not affect the solution to be measured, and can be used with oxidizing, reducing, and colloidal solutions.

Principle of the measuring method

The principle of measuring pH with a glass electrode has been described by Sykes (1974). When a metal is placed into a solution of one of its salts, there is a tendency for the metal ions to go into solution, leaving the metal with an excess negative charge. If two different metals and their salts are separated by a porous partition, an electromotive force is produced, because there is a greater tendency for one metal ion than for the other to go into solution (Figure 10.1). The electromotive force of the whole cell can be regarded as the difference between the separate electromotive forces produced by the two half cells. This electromotive force remains constant as long as the temperature and concentrations of the solutions remain constant (saturated).

In the measurement of pH, one also uses two half cells that are connected by the solution being tested and by a "salt bridge" of saturated potassium chloride solution (Figure 10.2). One half cell, the reference electrode, is made of mercury and of a saturated solution of mercury chloride (Hg_2Cl_2 or calomel). The other half cell, the glass electrode, is made of a glass tube, with a bulb of pH-sensitive glass (permeable to H^+) filled with a 0.1-N HCl solution into which a silver wire dips to effect an electrical connection and to provide, together with HCl, a silver/silver chloride solution (in analogy to the mercury/mercury chloride solution). Within the pH cell, four potentials can be distinguished. Two are the fixed potentials of the two half cells. A third potential develops at the pH-sensitive part of the glass, between the glass and test solution, depending on the H^+ concentration in the test solution. A fourth potential is generated between the test solution and the salt bridge at the so-called liquid junction. This kind of potential always develops at the interface between two solutions of different compositions or concentrations, because of differences in ionic transport across the boundary layer. The magnitude of this potential depends on a number of factors related to compositions or concentrations (the presence of red cells, leakage of KCl solution and intrusion of body fluids, dissimilar solute concentrations adjacent to different parts of the junction) and to the geometry of the junction of any individual electrode system (Sykes, 1974; Redstone, 1978). For this reason, the electrode manufacturer must exercise great care in designing a liquid junction that will be accurately reproduced each time a measurement is made.

According to the principles of thermodynamics, the variable electromotive force at the surface of the glass electrode should indicate the difference in pH between the test solution and the other solution, provided that all other potentials remain constant. Various pH electrodes for use in laboratory with point-to-point samples, and for tissue and intracellular (cytosol) measurements, have been constructed according to this principle (Figures 10.3 and 10.4) The scalp pH can be determined from blood samples collected from a wound in the scalp skin at various times (Saling, 1962) or can be monitored continuously in the scalp tissue by a tissue pH electrode during delivery (Stamm et al., 1974). Among the tissue pH electrodes used in perinatology, the Roche (Basel, Switzerland) electrode has been studied most thoroughly and is used as an example, although this type of glass electrode for use in tissue is no longer produced. In practice, numerous technical problems can limit the accuracy of

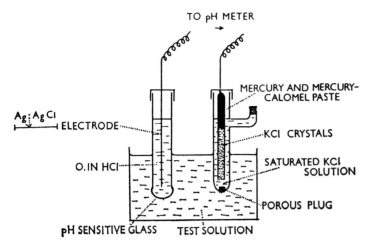

Figure 10.2. The glass–calomel electrode system. The liquid junction is between the test solution and the saturated KCl solution. (From Sykes, 1974, with permission.)

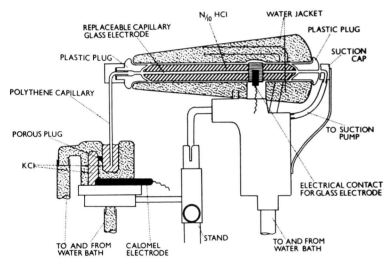

Figure 10.3. The Radiometer (Copenhagen, Denmark) microelectrode system to measure pH in blood samples. (From Sykes, 1974, with permission.)

pH measurements, as well as the application of tissue pH electrodes to the scalp site during delivery.

Technical problems

The thermodynamic activities of H^+ in the test solution and in the chloride salt-bridge solution, creating the potentials, are not related to the concentrations of this ion. Thus, inaccurate estimation of the thermodynamic activity (e.g., of the chloride ion) may limit the accuracy of pH determination to ± 0.02 (Sykes, 1974). The temperature of the pH electrode (especially of a mercury/mercury chloride solution, as it adjusts extremely slowly to changes in temperature) must be stable and therefore should be controlled accurately to $37.0 \pm 0.1°C$. Temperature increases from 20°C to 40°C, and the drift over time (e.g., over 6 h), can decrease pH by 0.02–0.03 unit in the electrode, according to in vitro tests (Mindt et al., 1978). An in vivo drift of ± 0.05 pH unit occurs in 20% of all applications (Rüttgers et al., 1978). Chemical and gas sterilizations apparently do not alter the reliability of the tissue pH electrode. The varying impedance across liquid and glass-membrane junctions and the high internal impedance of the pH cell itself can affect the accuracy of

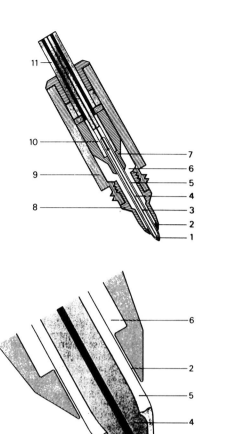

Cross section of pH probe. *1* pH sensitive tip; *2* liquid junction; *3* Ag/AgCl; *4* internal reference solution; *5* glass shaft; *6* reference solution; *7* reference electrode Ag/AgCl; *8* removable reference junction part; *9* electrode body; *10* electrical insolation (10^{12} Ω); *11* coaxial cable

pH sensitive tip and liquid junction. *1* pH sensitive glass membrane; *2* liquid junction; *3* Ag/AgCl; *4* internal reference solution; *5* glass shaft; *6* reference solution

Figure 10.4. The Roche (Basle, Switzerland) glass pH electrode for continuous measurement of scalp pH. (From Mindt et al., 1978, with permission.)

measurement of the true electromotive force. For example, with a current flowing, the potential measured will be lower than the true electromotive force. A liquid junction with a geometric design, which can provide a constant potential, is difficult to produce. In the Roche tissue pH electrode, the impedance at the liquid junction can vary between 0.8 and 3kΩ initially and may increase during measurements in body fluids up to 10 kΩ because of deposition of protein and red blood cells. Also, impedance can vary at the glass membrane with time and deposition of contaminants. Therefore, the glass capillary of a laboratory pH meter should be flushed frequently with saline or butter after blood samples have been introduced into the capillary and then should be cleaned with 1% pepsin in 0.1-N HCl solution. Fibrin deposits on the glass-membrane tip of the tissue pH electrode (Roche) will pro-

long the time required for stabilization, but will not actually influence the pH level (Löfgren, 1978).

Problems with application

A primary problem is preventing contamination of the test solution. A blood sample must not be contaminated by air, because gaseous CO_2 can diffuse out of blood and alter the pH, and tissue fluids must not be contaminated by amniotic fluid or air. The tissue electrode should be sealed off from the environment. The electrode tip must be placed into the scalp tissue at the correct depth. Therefore, the scalp skin must be incised by means of an incision blade 2–3 mm in length. Fixation and stabilization of the electrode have been improved by using a wide, double-helix screw electrode (Hochberg, 1978a), but these problems still limit its application.

The rate for obtaining records is about 80% (Uzan et al., 1978; Nickelsen and Weber, 1991), and the rate for recordings of good quality is around 50% (Flynn and Kelly, 1978), ranging from 35% (Weber and Hahn-Pedersen, 1978) to 80% (Laursen, Miller, and Paul, 1978; Young et al., 1978; Zacutti and Ciuffi, 1978). Electrodes break in 2% of applications (Hochberg, 1978b), and the mean lifetime for electrodes is less than 25 uses in experienced hands (Nickelsen and Weber, 1991). The electrodes become detached in 20% of cases, mainly because of the mechanical effects of labor and vaginal examination. A comprehensive review of measurements with tissue pH electrodes has been published (Hirsch et al., 1978).

Validity of the method

The correlation between pH measured by a tissue electrode and in a scalp blood sample, described by the correlation coefficient, was less than 0.7 in half of the studies examined ($r_2 = 0.5$). However, within the frequency distribution of correlation coefficients there is a peak of excellent correlations, with correlation coefficients of 0.8 or 0.9, which were obtained with an improved type of electrode applied by expert groups. However, only a few studies have reported data for a pH range below 7.2 (Henner, Ehrsam, and Haller, 1978; Rüttgers et al., 1978; Zacutti and Ciuffi, 1978), and none have reported the standard deviation of the error (in pH units of H^+ concentration). Animal and clinical studies indicate that the correlation in the acidotic range seems to be distinctly worse than in the physiological pH range (Boos et al., 1978).

pH MEASUREMENTS WITH OPTICAL FLUORESCENCE SYSTEMS

Optical fluorescence systems for continuous measurements of pH and blood gases have been made available for use in extracorporeal circuits during cardiopulmonary bypass (Clark, O'Brien, and McCulloch, 1984), in blood vessels (Shapiro et al., 1989) and in fetal scalp tissue (Small et al., 1989). These systems are based on the following principle: When light strikes a photoluminescent dye, specific wavelengths are absorbed, and electrons in the dye are excited to higher energy status. Each of these excited electrons can decay to a lower energy level by emitting a photon of a wavelength different from that of the incident absorbed light. In some specific photoluminescent dyes, the emission of photons is competitively inhibited by molecules like H^+, CO_2,

and O_2. Because the energy from the excited electrons is absorbed by these molecules, the photoluminescent dye emits fewer photons when the concentrations of these molecules rise (Opitz and Lübbers, 1987). When this method is applied to pH measurements, H^+ will diffuse either through a semipermeable membrane or freely into a dye bound to a gel matrix. This dye is a nontoxic, reversibly pH-sensitive fluorescent chemical (e.g., phenol red polyacrylamide). The dye made fluorescent by light changes its emitted light (i.e., its color) according to the concentration of H^+. For example, red and green light pass through a fiber-optic cable to the fluorescence-based sensor. Because the absorbance of green light is affected by H^+ concentration, its reflectance is used to indicate ("reflect") pH, whereas the red light is unaffected by pH and serves as a reference signal and as a test for probe integrity.

Such a system consists of a sensor, an optical-fiber system, a patient-interface module, the microprocessor-based analyzer, and the display module. The technical design of the fiber-optic pH probe includes a hollow stainless-steel needle (22 gauge) with a window through which H^+ can diffuse into the dye, a mirror to reflect light, which then passes through the dye, and the hollow optical fibers to guide the light signal to the patient-interface module (Figure 10.5). The needle with the sensor, being spiral-shaped and mounted on the fiber-optic pH probe, penetrates 3–4 mm into the fetal scalp tissue. The fiber-optic probe is somewhat larger than the usual scalp electrode for fetal electronic monitoring (Figure 10.6), but can also be positioned with an applicator. The interface module provides for photodetection of the returned fluorescent signal and for conversion of the signal from analog to digital presentation. This interface module ensures minimal transmission distance of the light signal returning from the sensor. Sophisticated electronics are required for analysis and display. In one available fiber-optic system (Fetascan 1000, Obstetrical Data System, Biomedics International, Bothell, WA), the pH range accessible for measurements is limited to values greater than 7.09, and the time lag between a change in capillary blood pH and the corresponding tissue change has been reported not to be constant (varying between 6 and 13 min).

Technical and applications problems with the method

Sufficient data on the rates of successful applications and recordings, on the problems of calibration

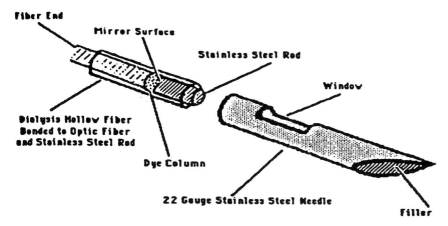

Figure 10.5. Principle of construction of the fiber-optic pH probe. (From Hochberg et al., 1987, with permission.)

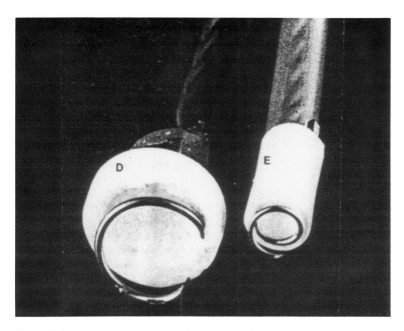

Figure 10.6. Comparison of tissue pH fiber-optic probe (D) to electronic scalp electrode (E) for fetal monitoring; original magnification ×9. (From Small et al., 1989, with permission.)

and drift, and on the incidence of clinical complications (tissue wounds, bleeding) are not yet available to allow comparison with other methods, such as the glass pH electrode (Nickelsen and Weber, 1991). In one study, application of this new technique was reported to be successful in 39 of 59 cases (66%), but for final analysis, 40(!) of 59 cases (68%) were excluded. Quoting those authors, "user related problems included a probe that became loose or fell off,

broken cables, recalibration of the machine by mistake, dislodgment of the probe by the fetal scalp sampling cone for capillary pH measurements, unplugging of the machine, which causes loss of calibration, repeated gain sets required during a study, leakage of fluid at the cable joint, migration of the probe application site posterior under the edge of the cervix, slow stabilization of the probe, bent probe, unstable heat block, necessity to recalibrate the probe, and refusal of the machine to display fetal echocardiogram or tissue pH" (Small et al., 1989).

Validation of the method

In one recent report, the correlation between tissue pH and scalp blood pH was poor ($r = 0.188$, or $r^2 = 0.035$, $n = 93$ measurements in 39 successfully monitored out of 59 attempted cases) and was improved only by selecting 19 data pairs after excluding less reliable measurements ($r = 0.487$, or $r^2 = 0.237$, $n = 19$) (Small et al., 1989). In another recent report, acidotic tissue pH was found to be more frequently associated with fetal, neonatal, and maternal problems than was acidotic capillary pH, but no relationship between tissue pH and capillary blood pH was presented (Chatterjee and Hochberg, 1991).

Risks of scalp tissue pH electrodes

The risks from both the electrometric and light-absorption techniques for pH measurement stem from skin invasiveness and injury, as well as the introduction of foreign material into the birth canal. Application of the glass pH electrode for use in tissue resulted in distinct skin wounds in 20% of cases and required sutures in 1%.

Costs and commercial availability

The tissue pH electrode has been manufactured in some laboratories and was produced in larger numbers by Roche in the 1970s, but commercial products are not available at present. The fluorescence light-absorption pH electrode developed in the 1980s by Biomedics International (Bothell, WA) appears to be technically more feasible, but at the cost of accuracy and reliability. Because of their sophisticated technologies, both tissue pH electrodes have had high developmental costs, and if they become available commercially, prices in the range of $10,000 to $100,000 are to be expected.

Interpretation of pH values and their changes

When interpreting pH values, one should first remember that pH values are not on a linear scale: A pH of 7.0 is equal to 100 nanoequivalents of H^+ per liter (nEq/l), pH 7.2 equals 63 nEq/l, 7.4 equals 40 nEq/l, 7.6 equals 25 nEq/l, and 8.0 equals 10 nEq/l. Second, pH is determined by the amounts of CO_2-dissolved bicarbonate (as described by the Henderson-Hasselbalch equation) and nonbicarbo-

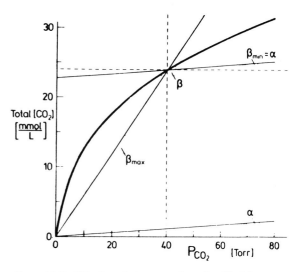

Figure 10.7. CO_2 dissociation curve for a simplified "homogenized blood" model. The thick line is the CO_2 dissociation curve corresponding to "homogenized" human arterial blood. The slope β_{min} is for the unbuffered solution, and β_{max} is for an infinitely buffered solution. (From Piiper et al., 1988, with permission.)

nate buffers. The significance of acid–base changes cannot be determined on the basis of pH measurements alone, but requires that P_{CO_2} or CO_2 content and nonbicarbonate buffer capacity be known. To illustrate this point, consider a condition with increasing amounts of CO_2, which results in a large amount of H^+. If a high concentration of nonbicarbonate buffer "mops up" the H^+ and allows HCO_3^- to be formed from CO_2, then P_{CO_2} will rise more slowly than in a system with a low concentration of nonbicarbonate buffer or no nonbicarbonate buffer at all (Figure 10.7). Hemoglobin is the main component of the nonbicarbonate buffer power. Hemoglobin changes its own buffering capacity in proportion to its O_2 saturation (Haldane effect). For example, if human blood is deoxygenated, the pH value will decrease from 7.41 to 7.25 with the Haldane effect, and to 7.17 without the Haldane effect. In the case of lactic acid formation in tissues, blood is acidified, P_{CO_2} rises, and pH falls. Consequently, pH and its changes cannot be correlated to the pathophysiological changes without determining P_{CO_2}, buffering capacity, and lactic acid formation. Additional problems in interpreting pH values arise as the H^+ concentrations and pH values differ in various compartments. A pH value measured at the scalp tissue or at the wound cavity caused by an electrode will differ significantly from the values in venous and arterial blood or in the extracellular and intracellular spaces of the fetus. The pH of the fetus, in turn, is affected by the acid–base balance of the mother (Bowen et al., 1986). Little is known about the dynamics of H^+ fluxes within these compartments and the compensatory changes in acid–base status in the fetal kidney or the placenta.

Usefulness of pH measurements for medical decisions

More than 90% of all fetuses are born as vigorous infants, if the tracings of their fetal heart rates and intrauterine pressures (FHR/IUP) are normal. In the remaining fetuses, even when FHR/IUP readings are suggestive of fetal distress, most fetuses still have normal Apgar scores at birth. The microchemical method of measuring pH intrapartum facilitates detection of the truly endangered fetus. Saling, who developed the method of fetal microlevel blood sampling (Saling, 1962), and many other investigators have demonstrated that a fetal scalp pH above 7.25 preceding birth is associated with a vigorous infant, with Apgar scores greater than 7 and pH values in umbilical arterial and venous blood greater than 7.25 in more than 80% of cases, whereas a fetal scalp pH below 7.20 indicates a depressed infant, with Apgar scores less than 6 and pH values in both umbilical vessels less than 7.2 in about 80% of cases (Saling, 1962; Tejani, Mann, and Bhakthavathsalan, 1976). The usefulness of scalp pH measurements for making medical decisions regarding various end points (vaginal vs. operative delivery; mortality and morbidity among infants at birth, at 1 mo, or at 1 yr) has not yet been evaluated by prospective, randomized studies. Previous publications have reported conflicting data, mainly because of variations in the FHR/IUP criteria used to determine fetal risk and in the policies followed in response to the risks. In term infants, pH has been found to be only slightly related to neonatal neurological morbidity (Dijxhoorn et al., 1985). Van den Berg et al. (1987) claimed a 60% reduction in the rate of cesarean section by employing fetal pH measurements in addition to a cardiotocogram (CTG) score. Nickelsen and Weber (1991) reported a significant reduction in forceps or vacuum deliveries from 26% to 9%.

SCALP HEAT-FLUX MEASUREMENTS

Heat is the end product of metabolism, and its production drops to about 5% of normal under anaerobic conditions. In the fetus, more than 75% of the total heat is estimated to be produced in the brain, and 25% in the rest of the body tissues. Hence the brain functions as a stove, whose heat is conducted to the cooler surroundings and is convected by circulation to the rest of the body and to the placenta. It is estimated that 75% of all heat produced is dissipated via the placenta, a superb heat exchanger, and 25% via the skin surface to the fetal environment (i.e., maternal structures such as amniotic fluid, uterus, and the mother's tissues). In monitoring fetal heat flux, the amount of heat per unit surface area and per unit time, flowing from the accessible fetal surface (i.e., the scalp or breech), is measured electronically by a heat-flux transducer.

Principles of heat-flux measurements

A heat-flux transducer or heat-flux meter consists of a sensitive thermopile, composed of many fineguage thermocouples connected in series on the opposite side of a flat core whose thermal resistance is known and stable. The thermopile and core are covered with a protective material. As heat flows normally through the flat matrix, a transient or steady-state temperature difference is established across the core. In practical systems, this temperature difference is rather small, about 0.005°C to 5°C. However, the signal is magnified approximately 100 to 1,000 times because of the multijunction sensor, the many thermocouples in series. When placed in contact with the subject, the heat-flux transducer generates a direct-current (dc) voltage directly proportional to the heat flux passing through it. That voltage then is amplified and recorded. Heat-flux transducers are linear over a wide range of voltage outputs. Output is exactly zero at exactly zero heat flux in the steady state. Application of a disc sensor 2.5 cm in diameter and less than 2 mm thick (Thermonetics, San Diego, CA) to the fetal scalp usually yields a voltage output of 0.15 mV, corresponding to 15 W $\cdot$ m^{-2}. Because of the low "noise" characteristics of the device, as little as 0.03 W $\cdot$ m^{-2} can be reliably resolved. The practical limits of calibration accuracy range from $\pm 1\%$ for a disc sensor of about 8 cm^2 to $\pm 10\%$ for the smaller sensors of 2 cm^2. The heat-flux transducer is insensitive to pressure and temperature changes (1.5% over 10°C). No drifts or changes in the calibration constant are found over periods of months. The calibration constant is provided by the manufacturer. Calibration by the user is not recommended, because it requires elaborate and precise apparatus (Ducharme, Frim, and Tikuisis, 1990). The accuracy of in vivo applications, however, will depend on the relationship between the thermal resistances to heat flux at the site with and without the heat-flux transducer in place.

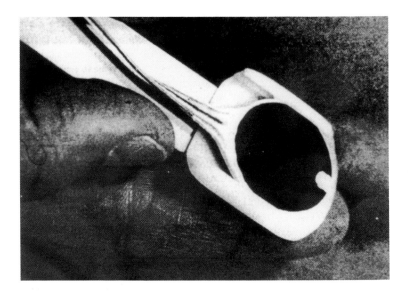

Figure 10.8. The heat-flux transducer (black-platelet) within its introducer; original size. (From Rudelstorfer, 1990, with permission.)

Heat flux can be underestimated if the conductance of the underlying tissue is high and tissue insulation by the overlying heat-flux transducer occurs (Ducharme et al., 1990). Heat-flux transducers are gas-sterilized.

The use of a heat-flux transducer before and after rupture of membranes is possible. Heat-flux measurements before rupture of membranes are possible if the heat-flux transducer is placed at the required site on the head and is kept in place by the pressure exerted on the fetal head by the surrounding tissues. When the amniotic membranes have been ruptured, the heat-flux transducer can be glued onto the head, and this is the most reliable way to measure scalp heat flux. Attachment of the heat-flux transducer by glue can be accomplished using either an amnioscope or a special introducing device. Using an amnioscope 40 mm in diameter, we dry the scalp with gauze, introduce the heat-flux transducer (with glue on its surface) into the vagina, attach it to the parieto-occipital region of the fetal scalp, and after removal of the amnioscope firmly press the transducer onto the scalp in order to ensure good contact. Because of the inconvenience of the amnioscope, the use of a special introducing device is preferred. This heat-flux introducer consists of a lid that covers the side of the heat-flux transducer with the glue on it, allowing unhindered insertion of the heat-flux transducer into the vagina and placement close to the head surface (Figure 10.8). At the site of attachment, usually the parieto-occipital region, the heat-flux transducer is then slid out of the protective lid onto the fetal scalp. The glue used is a water-resistant silicone adhesive, approved for use in humans (Dow Corning, Brussels, Belgium). The glue on the scalp and the heat-flux transducer can be easily removed with acetone.

Application of the method

The rate of successful measurements on the first attempt to place the heat-flux transducer is 93% with introducer and glue (Table 10.1). Once the transducer is applied, the rate of successful recordings is nearly 100%. Vaginal examinations do not detach the transducer. However, heat-flux measurements are affected for a period of 3–5 min because of the altered thermal environment.

Risks of the method

The intrapartum attachment and postnatal removal of the heat-flux transducer onto the scalp are not invasive and do not injure the skin. In contrast to other methods of pH monitoring, it can be applied to fetuses with coagulopathies. The main risk lies in introducing a foreign body into the birth canal and increasing the risk of infection.

Costs and commercial availability

The heat-flux transducer employed, model HA 15-15-13(C) (Thermonetics, San Diego, CA), can be purchased for about $200. Its use is limited by phys-

Table 10.1. *Frequency of attachment of heat-flux transducers necessary for successful recordings*

Technique of attachment	n	Frequency of attachment		
		Once	Twice	<Twice
Introducer and glue	54	50	4	0
Amnioscope and glue	147	124	19	4
Direct, no glue	7	3	2	2

ical damage. The heat-flux introducer is available from the author of this chapter (G. Simbruner). Any electronic equipment suitable to amplify and record the voltage output in the microvolt range can be used. No commercial device for monitoring fetal scalp heat flux is available at present.

Validity of the method

In experiments on lamb fetuses, Rudelstorfer et al. (1986) demonstrated a close correlation between the heat flux from and the oxygen uptake by the utero-placental unit under various conditions of uterine blood flow. Several investigators have employed measurements of fetal–maternal temperature gradients in humans, which are proportional to heat flux, to assess fetal conditions (Walker, Walker, and Wood, 1969; Rooth et al., 1977; Zilianti et al., 1983). Zilianti et al. (1983) found a close relationship between the fetal–maternal temperature gradient and the pH of the umbilical arterial blood, as well as the 1-min Apgar score. Monitoring of fetal scalp heat flux was introduced and investigated by Rudelstorfer and Simbruner in 1980 (Rudelstorfer et al., 1983; Simbruner, 1983). They demonstrated that fetal scalp heat fluxes in newborns with good outcomes, defined as a pH value of the arterial cord blood greater than 7.2, were significantly higher within the last 30 min before delivery than were the heat fluxes in newborns with bad outcomes (pH < 7.2); also, fetal scalp heat fluxes at delivery and 10 and 20 min before delivery were significantly correlated to the pH of arterial cord blood (Rudelstorfer et al., 1983). Furthermore, in 25 fetuses, fetal scalp heat flux was significantly related to scalp blood pH obtained according to the method of Saling ($r = 0.771$, $n = 25$, $p < 0.001$), and changes in scalp heat flux paralleled changes in scalp pH in 11 of 13 paired measurements (Rudelstorfer et al., 1987). A recent study demonstrated that the scalp heat fluxes of postmature and growth-retarded fetuses were higher and that their heat fluxes decreased significantly, compared with those of normal fetuses, dur-

ing delivery. Thus, measurements of scalp heat flux may be able to indicate not only abnormal oxygen transport and uptake by the fetus but also a disturbed placental exchange function (Rudelstorfer, Simbruner, and Nanz, 1991).

Interpretation of heat-flux values and their changes

Assessment of oxygen transport and uptake by the fetus, using measurements of heat flux from fetal head/scalp, is based on the following pathophysiological concept: The heat flux from the fetal head is a function of the temperature difference between the core of the head and the fetal surroundings (i.e., maternal structures) [$HF = k\ (T_{brain} - T_{envir})$]. If the thermal environment of the fetus (T_{envir}) is considered to be constant, then scalp heat flux will depend on the brain temperature (T_{brain}) or the core temperature of the head, which in turn will depend on cerebral heat production and removal. Heat removal from the head/brain is a function of cerebral circulation (cerebral blood flow, CBF) and the temperature difference between venous blood leaving and arterial blood entering the brain/head [heat removed $= CBF\ (T_{venous} - T_{arterial})$]. If the fetal heart rate, and thus cardiac output, decreases (stagnant hypoxia), CBF will also decrease and remove less heat from the head. Decreased CBF and decreased O_2 transport are usually compensated for by increased O_2 extraction, so that normal or slightly reduced O_2 uptake and heat production are maintained. Consequently, as long as cerebral heat removal decreases to a greater extent than cerebral heat production, the brain temperature will rise, and scalp heat flux will increase. Similarly, if placental heat removal is impaired, fetal scalp heat flux will be expected to increase. If the O_2 saturation of fetal blood falls (hypoxic hypoxia), and CO_2 and H^+ concentrations increase, CBF will increase to compensate. With increased CBF, more cerebral heat will be removed, and scalp heat flux will decrease. If the increase in CBF no longer compensates for the

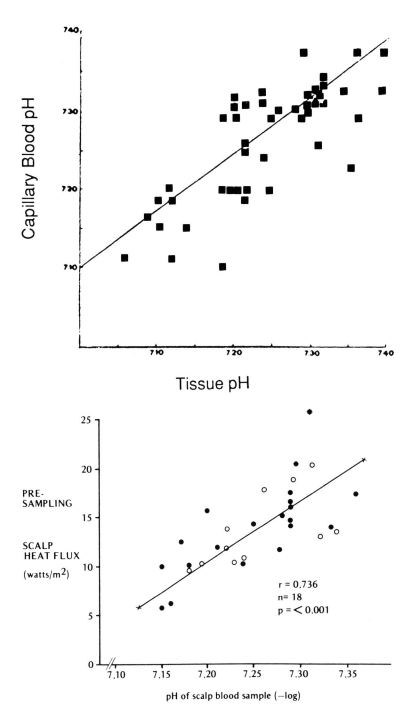

Figure 10.9. Relationship between the pH of capillary scalp blood and scalp tissue pH determined using the Roche glass pH electrode (above, top); the relationship between the pH of capillary scalp blood and scalp heat flux (above, bottom); and relationships between the pH of capillary scalp blood and scalp tissue pH determined using the fiber-optic pH electrode in unselected (opposite, top) and selected (opposite, bottom) cases. (From Zacutti and Ciuffi, 1978, Small et al., 1989, Rudelstorfer et al., 1987, with permission.)

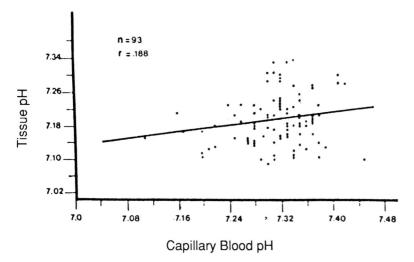

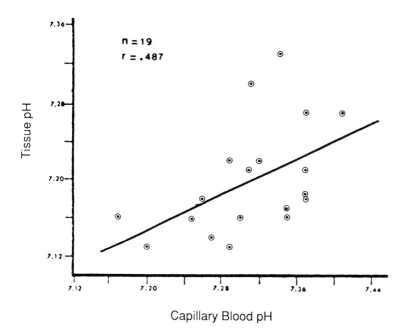

decrease in O_2 saturation, cerebral metabolism will also decrease. If less cerebral heat is being produced, and more heat is being removed, the result will be a decrease in brain temperature and consequently in scalp heat flux. In case of hemoglobin loss (anemic hypoxia), changes in oxygen and heat transport similar to those of hypoxic hypoxia will occur.

Simplifying the complex pathophysiology, we can state (1) that a decrease in CBF associated with maintenance of cerebral heat production must result in increased scalp heat flux and (2) that a decreased O_2 content of fetal blood associated with increased CBF and normal or decreased cerebral heat production must result in decreased scalp heat flux. This concept has been validated in a number of animal experiments and clinical investigations in newborn infants (Morishima et al., 1977; Simbruner et al., 1985a,b; Rudelstorfer et al., 1986), as well as by mathematical models (Simbruner, 1983; Simbruner et al., 1994). At present, scalp heat-flux values can be interpreted only in relation to fetal pH and outcome, not in terms of the pathophysiological events that cause the fetal distress.

Clinical usefulness for medical decisions

Little can be said about any useful comparison with other methods used for fetal surveillance. The one study available demonstrates that the overall accuracy for predicting fetal acidosis is 82% by monitoring fetal scalp heat flux, and 77% using cardiotocography (Rudelstorfer et al., 1990). An extensive review of a fetal heat flux has been published by Rudelstorfer (1990).

CONCLUSIONS

Enormous efforts have been made to measure the H^+ concentration in fetal tissue or blood during labor. The biotechnical devices developed allow continuous monitoring of fetal scalp pH, with various degrees of accuracy and precision (Figure 10.9). The correlations between fetal scalp pH or heat flux and scalp blood pH, determined according to the method of Saling, do not seem to differ significantly for the three methods described in this chapter. The rate of successful measurements undoubtedly is highest with the scalp heat-flux method, followed by the method of the glass electrode for use in tissue. From a viewpoint encompassing the invasiveness and risks, the technical construction and reliability, and the costs of production and maintenance, the monitoring of scalp heat flux appears to be superior to the use of either tissue pH electrode. In contrast to pH values measured directly by tissue electrodes, the scalp heat-flux values are related to only fetal blood pH and indicate its changes. However, monitoring scalp heat flux may provide more direct information on fetal metabolism, particularly in the fetal brain, especially if used in conjunction with ultrasonically determined fetal or placental blood flows. The monitoring of the end products of fetal metabolism in the form of either H^+ concentration or heat will remain an open field for physiological and biotechnological research, as clinically applicable and useful devices for this purpose are still needed.

REFERENCES

Boos, R., Heinrich, D., Muliawan, D., Rüttgers, H., Mittmann, U., and Kubli, F. (1978). In vivo performance of the pH tissue electrode during acute acid–base changes in the dog. *Archives of Gynecology* 226:45–50.

Bowen, L. W., Kochenour, N. K., Rehmn, N. E., and Woolley, F. R. (1986). Maternal–fetal pH difference and fetal scalp pH as predictors of neonatal outcome. *Obstetrics and Gynecology* 67:487–95.

Chatterjee, M. S., and Hochberg, H. M. (1991). Continuous intrapartum measurement of tissue pH of the human fetus using newly developed techniques. *Journal of Perinatal Medicine* 19:93–6.

Clark, C. L., O'Brien, J., and McCulloch, J. (1984). Early clinical experience with gas. *Journal of Extracorporeal Technology* 18:185.

Dijxhoorn, M. J., Visser, G. H., Huisjes, H. J., Fidler, V., and Touwen, B. C. (1985). The relationship of umbilical cord pH with the neonatal neurological morbidity in full term appropriate-for-dates infants. *Early Human Development* 11:33–42.

Ducharme, M. B., Frim, J., and Tikuisis, P. (1990). Errors in heat flux measurements due to thermal resistance of heat flux disks. *Journal of Applied Physiology* 69:776–84.

Flynn, A. M., and Kelly, J. (1978). An evaluation of the continuous tissue pH electrode (tpH) during labor in the human fetus. *Archives of Gynecology* 226:105–13.

Henner, H., Ehrsam, A., and Haller, U. (1978). Continuous tissue pH measurement on the fetus during delivery. *Archives of Gynecology* 226:129–32.

Hirsch, H. A., Kaufmann, C., Loeffler, F. E., and Ober, K. G. (eds.) (1978). *Archives of Gynecology* 226:1–216.

Hochberg, H. M. (1978a). New instrument developments for fetal pH monitoring. *Archives of Gynecology* 226:79–84.

(1978b). Multicenter clinical trials of fetal pH monitoring in the USA. *Archives of Gynecology* 226:93–8.

Hochberg, H. M., Roby, P. V., Snell, H. M., Smith, W. D., and Chatterjee, M. S. (1987). Continuous intrapartum fetal scalp tissue pH and ECG monitoring by a fiberoptic probe. *Journal of Perinatal Medicine* [Suppl. 1] 16:71–86.

Lauersen, N. M., Miller, F., and Paul, R. H. (1978). Evaluation of continuous fetal scalp pH during labor. *Archives of Gynecology* 226:141–8.

Löfgren, O. (1978). The effect of fibrin deposition on the sensitivity of the continuous monitoring pH electrode and the recorded pH value. An in vitro study. *Archives of Gynecology* 226:17–21.

Mindt, W., Mauer, H., and Möller, W. (1978). Principle and characteristics of the Roche tissue pH electrode. *Archives of Gynecology* 226:9–14.

Morishima, H., Yeh, M., Nieman, W., and James, L. (1977). Temperature gradient between fetus and mother as an index for assessing intrauterine fetal condition. *American Journal of Obstetrics and Gynecology* 129:443–8.

Nickelsen, C., and Weber, T. (1991). The current status of intrapartum continuous fetal tissue measurements. *Journal of Perinatal Medicine* 19:87–92.

Opitz, N., and Lübbers, D. W. (1987). Theory and development of fluorescent based optical sensors: oxygen optodes. *International Anesthesiology Clinics* 25:177–97.

Piiper, J., Gros, G., Forster, R. E., and Dodgson, S. J. (1988). CO_2/HCO_3 equilibria in the body. In *pH Homeostasis: Mechanisms and Control*, ed. D. Häussinger (pp. 203–32). London: Harcourt Brace Jovanovich.

Redstone, D. (1978). Fundamental basis of tissue pH measurements. *Archives of Gynecology* 226:1–5.

Robins, J. R. (1975). *Fundamentals of Acid–Base Regulation*, 5th ed. Oxford: Blackwell.

Rooth, G., Huch, A., Huch, R., and Peltonen, R. (1977). Fetal–maternal temperature differences during labor. *Contributions to Gynecology and Obstetrics* 3:54–62.

Rudelstorfer, R. (1990). *Fetal Heat Flux: Non Invasive Diagnosis of Fetal Distress*. Whitstable, Kent, UK: Smith-Gordon & Co.

Rudelstorfer, R., Simbruner, G., Bernaschek, G., Szalay, S., and Janisch, H. (1983). Heatflux from the fetus during delivery and fetal outcome. *Archives of Gynecology* 233:85–91.

Rudelstorfer, R., Simbruner, G., and Nanz, S. (1991). Scalp heat flux in postmature and in growth-retarded fetuses. *Archives of Gynecology and Obstetrics* 249:19–25.

Rudelstorfer, R., Simbruner, G., Neunteufel, W., and Nanz, S. (1990). Wärmeflussmessungen vom fetalen Skalp und Kardiotokographie zur Vorhersage von Azidosezuständen sub partu–ein Vergleich zweier Methoden. *Geburtshilfe und Frauenheilkunde* 50:278–85.

Rudelstorfer, R., Simbruner, G., Sharma, V., and Janisch, H. (1987). Scalp heat flux and its relationship to scalp blood pH. *American Journal of Obstetrics and Gynecology* 157:372–7.

Rudelstorfer, R., Tabsh, K., Khoury, A., Nywayhid, B., Brinkman, C., III, and Assali, N. S. (1986). Heat flux and oxygen consumption of the pregnant uterus. *American Journal of Obstetrics and Gynecology* 154:462–70.

Rüttgers, H., Muliawan, D., Boos, U., and Kubli, F. (1978). Influence of sterilization and temperature changes on the in vitro characteristics of the pH electrode. *Archives of Gynecology* 226:25–8.

Saling, E. (1962). A new method for examination of the child during labor. Introduction, technique and principles. *Archives of Gynecology* 197:108–22.

Shapiro, B. A., Cane, R. D., Chomka, C. M., Bandala, L. E., and Peruzzi, W. T. (1989). Preliminary evaluation of an intra-arterial blood gas system in dogs and humans. *Critical Care Medicine* 17:455–60.

Simbruner, G. (1983). *Thermodynamic Models for Diagnostic Purposes in the Newborn and Fetus*. Wein-Müchen: Facultas Verlag.

Simbruner, G., Nanz, S., Fleischhacker, E., and Derganc, M. (1994). Brain temperature discriminates between neonates with damaged, hypoperfused, and normal brains. *American Journal of Perinatology* 11:137–43.

Simbruner, G., Weninger, M., Popow, C., and Herholdt, W. (1985a). Regional heat loss in newborn infants. Part I. Heat loss in healthy newborns at various environmental temperatures. *South African Medical Journal* 68:940–4.

(1985b). Regional heat loss in newborn infants. Part II. Heat loss in newborns with various diseases – a method of assessing local metabolism and perfusion. *South African Medical Journal* 68:945–8.

Small, M. L., Beall, M., Platt, L. D., Dirks, D., and Hochberg, H. (1989). Continuous tissue pH monitoring in the term fetus. *American Journal of Obstetrics and Gynecology* 161:323–9.

Stamm, O., Latscha, U., Janecek, P., and Campana, A. (1974). Development of a special electrode for continuous subcutaneous pH measurement in the infant scalp. *American Journal of Obstetrics and Gynecology* 124:193–5.

Sykes, M. K. (1974). The determination of pH. In *Scientific Foundations of Anaesthesia*, ed. C. Scurr and S. Feldman (pp. 107–14). London: Heinemann.

Tejani, N., Mann, L. I., and Bhakthavathsalan, A. (1976). Correlation of fetal heart rate patterns and fetal pH with neonatal outcome. *Obstetrics and Gynecology* 48:460–3.

Uzan, S., Sturbois, G., Salat-Baroux, J., and Sureau, C. (1978). Application technique of tissue pH electrode on human fetuses. Clinical application of tissue pH monitoring during labor. Second series of 61 cases. *Archives of Gynecology* 226:61–7.

Van den Berg, P., Schmidt, S., Gesche, J. and Saling, E. (1987). Fetal distress and condition of the newborn using cardiotocography and fetal blood analysis during labor. *British Journal of Obstetrics and Gynaecology* 94:72–5.

Walker, D., Walker, A., and Wood, C. (1969). Temperature of the human fetus. *British Journal of Obstetrics and Gynaecology of the British Commonwealth* 76:503–11.

Walker, T., and Hahn-Pedersen, S. (1978). Analysis of sixty consecutive cases of continuous fetal pH-measurement. *Archives of Gynecology* 226:163–7.

Weber, T., and Hahn-Pedersen, S. (1978). Analysis of 60 consecutive cases of continuous fetal pH measurements. *Archives of Gynecology* 226:169–74.

Young, B. K., Hirschl, I. T., Klein, S. H., and Katz, M. (1978). Continuous fetal tissue pH monitoring in labor with high risk pregnancies. *Archives of Gynecology* 226:169–74.

Zacutti, A., and Ciuffi, F. G. (1978). Experience with continuous tissue pH electrode in the human fetus during labor. *Archives of Gynecology* 226:175–80.

Zilianti, M., Cabello, F., Chacon, N., Rincon, C. S., and Salazar, J. R. (1983). Fetal scalp temperature during labor and its reaction to acid–base balance and condition of the newborn. *Obstetrics and Gynecology* 61:474–9.

PART III

Electrical monitoring

One of the mainstays of modern biomedical technology is electrical monitoring. No neonatal patient lies in bed alone; each is constantly under surveillance for heart rate, respiratory rate, beat-to-beat variability in heart rate, blood pressure, or some combination of these or other parameters. The electrical impulses that chronicle these monitoring procedures act as the eyes and ears of the nursing staff when they are busy elsewhere and cannot see or hear. But they can also drive the unaccustomed to distraction, and they have been commandeered unnecessarily and far too often for litigation purposes. They are in desperate need of a computer whiz to figure out how to interpret them, accurately and meaningfully, for they signal inconsistently, even when monitoring the healthy. And they do not always predict with certainty the potential for serious illness. Think of the thousands of dollars in hospital and physician charges and hundreds of hours of hospital stay necessary simply for "feeding and growing" that so many preterm infants must accumulate before their ECG and respiratory-rate monitors show, "for a minimum of 5 days," *no* so-called apnea or bradycardia, before they can go home. And what neonatologist would not love a combination monitor that could provide on-line measurements of electrocortical activity, intracranial pressure, cerebral blood flow, and oxygenation as guides to brain function. Perhaps with such an instrument we could establish correlations with other aspects of the functioning of the central nervous system, including metabolic condition, neurotransmission or neuroexcitatory toxicity (normal versus pathological, e.g., seizures, hypoxic-ischemic injury, hypoglycemia, drug effects, cell death), nutrient and oxygen sufficiency, and edema. We have come to feel that we could not possibly perform adequately without these monitors, that we could not live without them, but we desperately need to come to a better understanding of how to live with them.

11

Cardiotocography

MICHAEL R. NEUMAN, Ph.D., M.D.

Unlike other patients, the fetus during gestation is, for the most part, inaccessible to the conventional methods of physical examination and diagnosis. It is not possible to directly observe, touch, or listen to the fetus in utero as one does with a patient on the examining table. As we have seen in preceding chapters, we can, to some extent, visualize the fetus and observe fetal behavior, as well as look inside at the functioning of the cardiovascular and other systems, but the devices that allow us to do so involve extensive use of complex technology. They do not allow clinicians to directly use their senses to assess and diagnose patients. Thus, clinicians must rely on technology to make biophysical measurements of the fetus during the antenatal and intrapartum periods. Most of these measurements are necessarily indirect measurements: Because of lack of accessibility to the fetus without performing invasive procedures on the mother, the sensor that is to make the biophysical measurement cannot be placed in contact with the fetus. Only during active labor, when membranes have ruptured, is it possible to have direct access to the fetus, and even then the access is indeed quite limited. Thus, most fetal measurements are necessarily indirect, and the mother serves as a conduit to connect the fetus to the measurement instrumentation.

These measurements, nevertheless, are very important in assessing fetuses, especially those who are believed to be at increased risk for various problems. Such problems can be identified only by observing the functioning of vital fetal systems, such as the central nervous system and the cardiovascular system. It is important to know that these vital tissues are receiving adequate perfusion, oxygenation, and nutrition for normal growth and development. Hemodynamic and metabolic variables are

important parameters for assessing these vital systems, and there is little that can be done toward assessing these systems without the assistance of technology. Measurements of hemodynamic variables such as blood pressure, blood flow, and tissue perfusion can be taken only with the assistance of electronic instrumentation. In an earlier chapter we saw how ultrasound instrumentation can assist in measuring flow velocity. Important metabolic variables for assessing the fetus include tissue and arterial blood pH values, oxygen tension, and carbon dioxide tension. These measurements can be made only by direct contact between chemical sensors and the tissue being studied. Thus, it is possible to consider making these measurements only during active labor, once membranes have been ruptured. In this chapter we shall consider those variables that can be measured in the fetus both antenatally and during active labor. We shall emphasize cardiovascular measurements; metabolic measurements were considered in previous chapters.

CARDIAC MEASUREMENTS

Assessment of the fetal heart has been one of the main aspects of antepartum care for many years. Long before the development of electronic technology for observing the fetal heart, simpler auscultatory instrumentation existed: the fetoscope, a short, straight tube with a bell on either end that was placed between the maternal abdomen and the ear of the examiner to serve as a sound conduit (Herbert et al., 1987). That instrument was later modified to look more like a stethoscope, but its basic principle of operation remained the same. It was necessary to exert pressure on the fetoscope bell against the maternal abdomen to better conduct the relatively weak fetal heart sounds through the uterine and abdominal walls to the fetoscope and the listener. Although that device allowed the clinician to examine the fetal heart, it was limited in that it allowed assessment of only the fetal heart rate, and only over a short time period. The heart rate that was determined was a mean rate, generally averaged over a sampling duration of 1 min or less, and the information obtained was of greatest value for reassurance that the heart was functioning properly. During labor, the fetoscope could also be used to detect fetal bradycardia, a hallmark of fetal distress. It is clear that such aural measurements are subjective and depend on the experience of the physician for their interpretation. As a result of such interpretations, more objective methods for evaluating the fetal heart have been developed.

Fetal electrocardiography

An early electrical technique that was used to evaluate the fetal heart was electrocardiography (Macrae, 1962; Shenker, 1966). The technique involved obtaining an electrocardiogram (ECG) from the fetus by placing electrodes on the maternal abdominal wall. The conduction pathway for electrical signals from the fetal heart to the maternal abdominal skin is not well understood, and so electrode placement must be empirical, seeking the optimal signals. Some investigators believe that the most likely signal pathways are through the umbilical cord and the fetal airway, which contains conductive amniotic fluid. Thus, electrodes placed over the placenta and fetal head should give the best results. There is, however, no convincing evidence that such is the case.

The fetal ECG usually is quite weak, having an amplitude of less than 50 μV. Thus, it is important that the least amount of "noise" be introduced by the measurement process, for noise can corrupt the signal. Low-noise silver/silver chloride electrodes should be used, and the skin should be carefully prepared, to minimize artifacts. Some clinicians recommend removing or at least interrupting the stratum corneum to minimize noise. This can be done by gently scraping the skin with sandpaper at the location where the electrodes are to be placed. It has been shown that the stratum corneum can introduce noise in low-level biopotential recordings, and by removing the stratum corneum or providing an electrical shunt path around it, it is possible to greatly diminish this source of noise (Tam and Webster, 1977). It is also important to have the subject relaxed when the measurement is made, be-

cause movement can introduce artifacts that will obliterate the signal. The major source of interference comes from the maternal ECG, as shown in Figure 11.1. This recording was made from a resting patient during active labor who also had a fetal scalp electrode (discussed later) placed to pick up the fetal ECG and electrodes on her chest to pick up the maternal ECG. It is seen from the abdominal ECG that the maternal signal, denoted by M, is much stronger than the fetal signal, denoted by F. In some cases the fetal signal will almost coincide with the maternal signal and will be obliterated by the latter. It can be seen from this recording, which is an example of an abdominal-fetal ECG of very good quality, that it is difficult to use this type of signal clinically. It certainly would not be possible to determine the instantaneous fetal heart rate for very long from this signal, unless some additional electronic processing of the signal were undertaken. It also would not be possible to look at the cardiac rhythm, because it is not possible to see any component of the ECG other than the fetal R wave on this recording.

By using various methods of electronic signal processing, one can enhance the fetal component of the abdominal ECG while greatly diminishing the maternal component. One such method is to collect the maternal ECG simultaneously with the abdominal ECG and subtract the maternal signal from the abdominal waveform, leaving just the fetal signal (Vanderschoot et al., 1987). It is then possible to process the remaining fetal signal to determine the heart rate, but usually it is not possible to determine the rhythm from this signal, because there is still enough noise to obliterate the fetal P and T waves. Although this method has, on occasion, been demonstrated to produce clinically useful signals of fetal heart rates, it is limited in that it is difficult to completely subtract the maternal ECG from the abdominal signal, and a great deal of signal manipulation is required to achieve a usable signal.

A second approach to improving the abdominal-fetal ECG is to average the signal using a computer. Computer averaging takes a strip of the abdominal-fetal ECG and identifies the fetal R waves. A large number of these, say 100, and a fraction of a second of the signal on each side of these, are rearranged so that the R waves appear to occur at the same instant of time. These signals are then added together in such a way that the fetal ECG is enhanced, and any other signals such as the maternal ECG or noise will appear to be random with respect to the fetal R wave. The contribution of these random signals to the sum signal is small with respect to the ECG, so this manipulation of the signal extracts a mean of

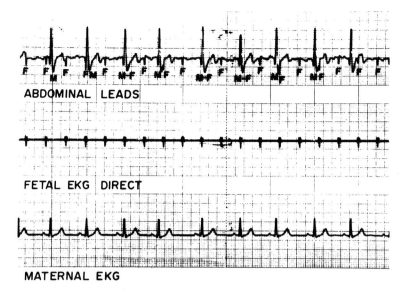

ABDOMINAL LEADS

FETAL EKG DIRECT

MATERNAL EKG

Figure 11.1. An abdominal-fetal ECG, with simultaneous direct fetal ECG and maternal ECG. *Top:* Signal taken from abdominal leads; F denotes a fetal R wave, and M denotes a maternal R wave. *Middle:* Filtered signal from a direct fetal scalp electrode. *Bottom:* Maternal ECG taken from chest leads. (From Roux et al., 1975, with permission.)

the ECG configurations that were added together, with a reduction in noise. When the average value of the sum is displayed on the computer screen, the enhanced fetal ECG can show the full P-QRS-T configuration (Bergveld, Koülling, and Peuscher, 1986). This technique has some limitations. In addition to the complexity of the computer analysis, an average signal has meaning only if the majority of the fetal cardiac cycles that are averaged are very similar to one another. If they are not, the differences will behave the same as the noise or the maternal ECG, and the averaging effect is diminished. Thus, this technique cannot be used to show a fetal arrhythmia unless that arrhythmia occurs quite frequently and is the same each time it occurs.

Continuous monitoring of fetal heart rate

Although the abdominal-fetal ECG is the only way to measure the electrical activity of the fetal heart antenatally, there are nonelectrical methods for detecting the fetal heart rate. During the intrapartum period, it may be possible to have direct access to the fetus, which allows the use of additional methods for determining the fetal heart rate. In general, there are two methods for obtaining information on fetal heart rate: direct and indirect. The indirect method, being noninvasive, offers advantages

in terms of convenience and can be used to study the fetal heart rate through the second and third trimesters of pregnancy. The direct method, on the other hand, provides a signal of higher quality and is the method of choice for patients in active labor who are believed to be at increased risk for complications.

Direct determination of fetal heart rate

Direct determinations of the fetal heart rate are derived from signals provided by a sensor placed on the fetal presenting part during active labor, once membranes have been ruptured. The sensor usually is a special fetal ECG electrode that makes possible a direct connection between the fetus and an electronic cardiac monitor. The ECG seen by the monitor is from a unipolar lead, whereby an electrode is placed on the fetus and the reference signal comes from a second electrode in the maternal vaginal fluids. These electrodes are connected to an electronic system that amplifies the weak signal and provides further processing to detect each fetal heartbeat and determine the fetal heart rate. Unlike the abdominal ECG signal, this signal is relatively strong and contains little, if any, interference from the maternal ECG.

Although several different types of electrodes

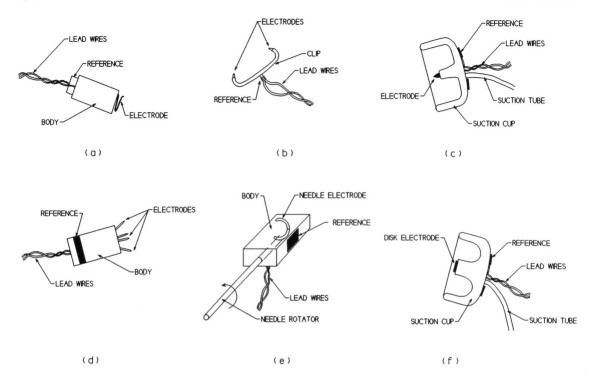

Figure 11.2. Examples of electrodes for direct fetal ECG: (a) spiral electrode, (b) clip, (c) suction cup with penetrating electrode (shown in cross section), (d) quadruped, (e) suture-needle electrode, (f) suction cup with nonpenetrating electrode.

have been used for obtaining a direct fetal ECG, they can be classified into two categories: those that penetrate the fetal skin, and those that do not. The fundamental principle of the penetrating electrodes is based on the fact that the fetus lies in a bath of amniotic fluid that is electrically conductive because of its electrolyte content. The amniotic fluid, bathing the entire skin, tends to connect all points on the fetal skin surface electrically. Even if it were physically possible to place conventional chest electrodes on the fetus to pick up the ECG signal, a poor-quality signal would be obtained because of this electrical shunting effect. On the other hand, this common connection of the amniotic fluid to all points on the skin surface makes the amniotic fluid a good reference electrode or central terminal for a unipolar ECG. Thus, the sensing electrode must be located at a position where it will not be in contact with the skin surface, and hence not in contact with the amniotic fluid, if a voltage difference representing the ECG signal is to be obtained. This can easily be achieved by having the unipolar electrode penetrate the outer layers of the fetal skin and make contact with the dermal or subcutaneous tissue. Because there is an electrical resistance associated with the

stratum corneum, by having the electrode make contact under the stratum corneum it is possible to measure the voltage drop across this resistance to obtain the fetal ECG. Penetration of the skin also helps to keep the electrode in place on the fetus during labor.

Various types of penetrating fetal electrodes have been developed over the years, but the most frequently applied sensor consists of a helical-spiral electrode first described by Hon (Hon, Paul, and Hon, 1972). This electrode (Figure 11.2a) consists of a short section of a helix of stainless-steel wire on an electrically insulating support. The tip of the wire is sharpened to a point that can penetrate the skin, and an applicator used with the electrode allows it to be "screwed" into the skin, such that almost one turn of the helix will be intracutaneous. A second stainless-steel electrode in the form of a metal strip is located on the opposite end of the insulator from the helix and contacts the vaginal pool, to serve as the reference connection. Lead wires connect the electrodes to the electronic monitor. The principal advantages of this electrode are the ease with which is can be applied and the fact that it can be applied with the cervix being dilated no more than 2 cm.

Although the penetration wound to the skin caused by the electrode is believed to be innocuous, there have been reports of local infection in the neonatal scalp following the use of this type of electrode for fetal monitoring (Hutchins, 1978).

Other types of penetrating electrodes have been described for obtaining a direct fetal ECG. The original electrode described by Hon (1963) consisted of a modified wound clip that could be attached to the fetal presenting part once the membranes had been ruptured. An example of such an electrode is illustrated in Figure 11.2b. The tines of the clip have a silver/silver chloride surface to minimize the effects of motion artifact, and these penetrate the fetal skin to make contact with the subcutaneous tissues. A silver wire with a silver chloride surface is located near the center of the clip and makes contact with the vaginal pool, to provide a reference. This sensor was kept in place because it was clipped to the skin in the same way that it would be used to close a wound.

The suction electrode is another variation of the same principle. A small suction cup, 10–15 mm in diameter, has a pointed silver/silver chloride, platinum, or stainless-steel electrode at its center, as illustrated in Figure 11.2c (Roux, Neuman, and Goodlin, 1975). For best results, this electrode should be insulated, with only 1 mm of the point exposed. It should also have a structure that will limit its penetration into the fetal skin to no more than 2 mm, so as to avoid serious trauma. In practice, the sensor is held against the fetal presenting part, and suction is applied. Thus draws the fetal skin into the suction cup, and the electrode penetrates the skin, making contact with the intracutaneous and/or subcutaneous tissue. The suction holds the electrode in place against the fetal skin.

A quadruped electrode that has been developed by Hoffman LaRoche has a plastic body similar to that of the spiral electrode. Four stainless-steel "legs" retracted in the body of this structure are released when it is pressed against the fetal skin. These legs extend 2–3 mm beyond the base of the sensor when released, and they enter the fetal skin obliquely, so that they hold the sensor firmly in place. A reference electrode on the opposite end of the plastic body of the sensor contacts the vaginal pool.

Another variation of the penetrating fetal scalp electrode is shown in Figure 11.2e. This electrode consists of a small, curved suture needle, with a lead wire replacing the suture. The needle is housed in a plastic structure, with an assembly for rotating the needle from the outside. With the needle retracted into the plastic housing, the housing is pressed against the fetal presenting part with a finger of one hand, while the needle is rotated with the other hand as if to place a suture in the fetal skin. Instead of completely rotating the needle through the skin, it is stopped once it enters the skin about a quarter of a turn, and this makes electrical contact to the intracutaneous tissue. A reference electrode on the side of the housing in which the needle is located contacts the vaginal pool.

Because all of these penetrating electrodes can produce local trauma to the fetal skin, with the remote possibility of infection, investigators have considered nonpenetrating electrodes for the same purpose. One of these is a variation of the penetrating suction electrode shown in Figure 11.2c. In this case, the sharp central electrode is replaced with a silver/silver chloride disc, as shown in Figure 11.2f (Goodlin and Fabricant, 1970). In this case, the electrode and suction cup are larger than those used for the penetrating electrode, and frequently they are made of an elastomer, so as to be somewhat flexible and able to conform to the shape of the fetal presenting part. When suction is applied, the region of skin under the suction cup becomes isolated from the amniotic fluid, and this portion is no longer in electrical contact with the fluid. Thus, a voltage can be measured on the surface of the skin under the suction cup that is different from the voltages at other points on the skin, and this is sensed by the central electrode. This signal, however, usually is weaker than the signal obtained by penetrating the skin, and the effects of artifacts often are more pronounced. Nevertheless, useful signals can be obtained with this method. The reference electrode in contact with the vaginal pool often is a larger silver/silver chloride disc on the back of the suction-cup assembly.

Another type of nonpenetrating electrode that has been reported need not even contact the fetus. This consists of a probe that is introduced into the uterine cavity in much the same way that a catheter or probe for making direct intrauterine pressure measurements is used. As a matter of fact, this can be the same probe that is used for the intrauterine pressure measurements. Several electrodes are positioned on the outside surface of this probe and make contact with the amniotic fluid. These usually are silver/silver chloride electrodes, to minimize electrical artifacts secondary to motion. As mentioned earlier, the amniotic fluid does not present a perfect short circuit for ECG signals appearing on the fetal skin, because the amniotic fluid is not a perfect electrical conductor. Thus, some of the ECG signal can be seen in the amniotic fluid and measured between pairs of electrodes on the probe. By trying different pairs of electrodes, it is possible to obtain an optimal signal. It is important to note that this method is different from other methods in that it is a bipolar rather than a unipolar measurement. It is similar to obtaining the abdominal ECG, but the fetal signal is stronger, and the maternal signal is weaker, than those seen when electrodes are placed on the abdomen. Nevertheless, the fetal signal is still quite weak as compared with the signal from electrodes in direct contact with the fetus, and significant interference from the maternal ECG signals can occur, depending on the electrode pairs being used. Although there have been some clinical demonstrations of this technique, it remains experimental (Strong et al., 1991).

Indirect methods for determining fetal heart rate

Signals related to the fetal heart often can be used for determination of the fetal heart rate. In some cases, such as the abdominal-fetal ECG mentioned earlier, these signals can be obtained from the maternal abdomen without any direct contact with the fetus. These methods for determining fetal heart rate are known as indirect sensing methods and will be described next.

Doppler ultrasound detection
of the fetal heartbeat

Anyone who has observed that the pitch of the sound of an automobile horn or the whine of the engines of a jet aircraft is higher when the vehicle is approaching the observer, and lower when it is speeding away, has experienced the Doppler effect. This basic principle of physics states that when an object emitting or reflecting sound is approaching the observer, the sound is heard at a higher pitch than if the sound source were stationary, and the opposite occurs as the object is moving away from the observer. This is the underlying principle of the most widely used indirect method for detecting the fetal heartbeat during the second and third trimesters of pregnancy and during parturition (Bernstine, 1968; Bishop, 1968). Instead of using audible waves, indirect fetal heart monitors use ultrasound energy, sound energy at a high frequency well beyond the range of hearing.

The fundamental operation of this instrument is illustrated in Figure 11.3. A source of continuous ultrasound energy, usually of a frequency in the range from 2 to 5 MHz and at a power level of less than 50 mW, is used to insonate the maternal pelvic region using an ultrasound transducer placed on the maternal abdomen. The sound waves are collimated into a beam that illuminates the fetal thorax within the amniotic cavity. It is well known by physicists that ultrasound energy is reflected by interfaces between different types of tissues and liquids in the beam path. Even cells in the fetal circulation reflect the ultrasound when they pass through the beam. If the reflector is moving, the Doppler effect tells us that the reflected ultrasound energy will be at a frequency different from that of the incident energy. This frequency difference will be proportional to the velocity of the reflecting surface in a direction along the beam axis. Thus, the faster the reflector moves, the greater the change in frequency of the reflected ultrasound waves with respect to the incident waves. The greatest frequency change usually is produced by the leaflets of the valves of the fetal heart as they open and close during the fetal cardiac cycle. The reflected ultrasound wave can be electronically processed so that only the frequency difference between the transmitted and reflected signals is shown as the output signal. The electronic circuits represented by the blocks in Figure 11.3 carry out this function and produce a signal such as that illustrated in Figure 11.4. This is the signal seen when the ultrasound beam illuminates the leaflets of the valves of the fetal heart. Note that for each heartbeat, there are two peaks in the signal – one resulting from the Doppler shift when the valve is opening, and the other from the Doppler shift as the valve is closing. One can further process this signal electronically to detect each fetal heartbeat, and this technique is used in indirect Doppler ultrasound monitors for the fetal heart, as well as in other devices for assessment of the fetal heart. In many cases, the signal revealing the frequency difference between the incident and reflected ultrasound waves is amplified in the instrument and played through a loudspeaker or earphones. The characteristic sounds of beating fetal hearts provide a familiar background in the labor and delivery and antenatal wards.

Doppler ultrasound techniques can be used to detect the fetal heartbeat as early as the 8–10 wk of gestation and are very useful clinically for evaluating intrauterine life throughout much of pregnancy. The characteristics of the ultrasound beam used to illuminate the fetal heart to monitor for optimal performance change as the fetus grows, and the reason for using ultrasound changes as gestation progresses. Early in pregnancy, Doppler ultrasound is

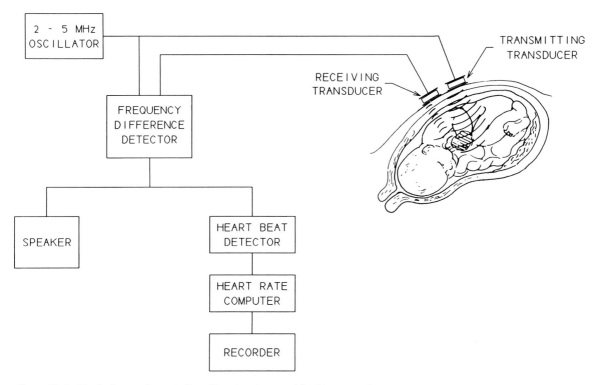

Figure 11.3. Block diagram for an indirect Doppler ultrasound fetal heart monitor.

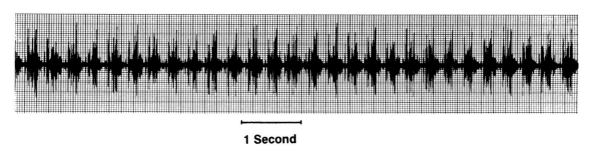

1 Second

Figure 11.4. Example of a Doppler ultrasound signal from the fetal heart for a fetus at term. (From Neuman, 1988, with permission.)

not used to monitor the fetal heart continuously, but rather is an instrument for detecting fetal life and sampling the heart rate over a short period of time, in much the way the fetoscope will be used later in gestation. To do this effectively, the beam from the ultrasound generator should be narrow, so that the weak reflections from the fetal heart will not be overpowered by stronger reflections from other tissue interfaces. The use of this narrow beam, however, means that the examining clinician must carefully aim the beam to pick up the signal from the fetal heart, and the beam position must be changed frequently throughout the examination, especially when the fetus moves. In later gestation, the clinician is concerned about a continuous record of the fetal heart rate over a longer period of time. The use of a narrow beam would be impractical for that purpose, because the beam would have to be repositioned every time the fetus moved. In that case, and in the case of monitoring the fetus during labor, it is better to have a transducer that produces a broad beam, so that the fetal heart will continue to be illuminated as the fetus moves. Of course, if the fetus and/or mother are moving, there will be many tissue interfaces that will be undergoing movement, and that will result in a Doppler-shifted ultrasound wave being reflected. These additional reflections will interfere with the reflection from the fetal heart or circulation and will result in artifacts, so that it will be difficult to detect the fetal heartbeat. Thus, Doppler ultrasound examinations should be carried out while the mother and fetus are resting quietly. This is one of the major limitations on the use of Doppler ultrasound in monitoring the fetal heart during active labor. Because the ultrasound beam needed for continuous fetal monitoring is broad, there will be more interference because of reflections from other parts of the mother and fetus, which can make the signal more noisy. Yet, because the fetal heart will be larger at later stages of gestation, the reflected signals from the fetal heart will also be stronger, and so the overall signal-to-noise ratio will not be changed by much and will still be favorable for detecting the fetal heartbeat.

The primary advantage of Doppler ultrasound for fetal heart monitoring is its simplicity. A transducer containing a means for producing the ultrasound beam and several sensors for detecting the reflected waves can be attached to the abdomen with an elastic strap or an adhesive pad. The transducer itself can be coupled to the tissue of the abdomen using a special gel formulated to transfer ultrasound energy efficiently from the transducer to the abdominal tissue. This is necessary because ultrasound signals at the frequencies used in fetal monitoring do not propagate well through air. If the transducer were placed in contact with the maternal abdomen without the use of the coupling agent, there would always be a thin layer of air between the transducer and the skin of the abdomen. Because ultrasound signals do not propagate well through air, that very small air gap could greatly decrease the sensitivity of the monitoring system.

Another advantage of this indirect method of detecting the fetal heartbeat is that it is entirely noninvasive. The procedure can easily be carried out in a physician's office, in a clinic, or in the labor and delivery suites, and the primary skill that is needed for use of this instrument is the ability to position the transducer in such a way that the fetal heart is imaged.

Whether or not the energy from Doppler ultrasound fetal heart monitors (or imaging equipment, for that matter) is safe has been an issue of great concern for many years (Mannor et al., 1972). Although the issue has not been definitively resolved, there have been no reports linking fetal or maternal morbidity to the use of ultrasound instrumentation.

Care has been taken in the design of these devices to use the smallest amount of energy required for the measurement task, and most clinicians take precautions not to expose their patients to any more ultrasound energy than is necessary for the examination, just in case there might yet be some risk discovered.

The major disadvantage of Doppler ultrasound for assessment of the fetal heart is that the technique is motion-sensitive, and movements by the mother and fetus can obliterate the fetal heart signal. Thus, the utility of the ultrasound technique during active labor is somewhat limited. Patients who do a lot of moving during labor will not be good subjects in whom to use ultrasound for continuous monitoring of the fetal heart; for those patients, a more reliable signal can be obtained using a direct fetal ECG sensor. The Doppler ultrasound signal also has major limitations when used to assess the beat-to-beat variability of the fetal heart rate. This will be discussed in more detail in a later section.

Phonocardiographic assessment of the fetal heart

An electronic device can be used to carry out the same function as the fetoscope, namely, to pick up fetal heart sounds from the maternal abdomen and process them in such a way as to enhance those sounds emanating from the fetal heart. An electronic circuit identifies each fetal heartbeat, and a cardiotachometer is used to determine the fetal heart rate from those beats. A contact microphone, instead of the bell of the fetoscope, is placed against the abdomen, and this sensor picks up the weak fetal heart tones, along with other sounds occurring in the maternal abdomen and its environment (Hammacher, 1962; Ginsburg, 1964). Because the fetal heart sounds are weak, the electrical impulses from the contact microphone are similarly weak and can be obliterated by other sound sources in and around the body. The electrical signal from the contact microphone is processed by an electronic filter system that reduces the effect of sounds outside the frequency range of the fetal heart and enhances the fetal heart sounds. Unfortunately, these systems are not entirely successful in their endeavors; artifacts and other sounds of biologic origin remain major problems with this acoustical method. This is especially true when it is used on patients who are moving a lot, are speaking or making other sounds, or are in a noisy environment. Thus, the technique generally is not suitable for use on patients in active labor. Today, this technique is not widely used, having been replaced by Doppler ultrasound methods.

Monitoring uterine activity

In monitoring the fetus during labor and antenatally it is important not only to look at the fetal physiological variables but also to look at maternal stressors that could affect those variables. The primary maternal function to be monitored to obtain such information is uterine or myometrial activity. This generally consists in monitoring the strength, frequency, and duration of uterine contractions. Measurements of uterine activity can be made by direct and indirect methods, as in the case of the fetal heart rate (Csapo, 1970). In the former case, it is necessary to have instrumentational access to the uterus itself, and so direct techniques are limited to use during the late latent phase and active phase of labor. The indirect method, on the other hand, can be used to assess uterine activity through the maternal abdomen and can be used antenatally as well as during labor.

Direct measurement of uterine activity

A truly direct method of measuring the contractions of the myometrium, the muscle of the uterine wall, would be able to reveal the tension and displacement of this muscle. Although it is possible to do that in the research laboratory, it is not practical to make such measurements during routine clinical monitoring. Thus, a secondary variable that is strongly affected by myometrial contraction must be measured. Such a variable is the hydrostatic pressure of the amniotic fluid within the pregnant uterus. If this fluid were homogeneous and were contained within a closed chamber made up of the uterine wall, pressure increases should be seen whenever uterine contractions occurred and should be related to the overall strength of the contraction. If one were to model the uterus as a spherical structure, with the tension in this idealized muscle the same no matter at what point on the spherical surface it was measured, then Pascal's law would give a direct relationship between the observed pressure in the fluid and the tension in the muscular wall. This simplified model, of course, is not an accurate picture of the uterus and its contents, and so the relationship between myometrial tension and intrauterine pressure is a qualitative one, as opposed to a generalizable quantitative relationship. Nevertheless, measurement of intrauterine pressure during labor can be a useful method for assessing the stresses experienced by the fetus during labor, as well as monitoring the uterus itself during this important time.

The pressure change in the amniotic fluid during a uterine contraction can be measured directly by coupling the amniotic fluid to an electrical manometer. This instrument consists of an electrical pressure sensor and the appropriate electronic circuitry for processing, displaying, and recording the measured pressure. The pressure sensor can be miniaturized and placed directly in the amniotic fluid, or the amniotic fluid can be coupled to an external pressure sensor by means of a fluid-filled catheter. It is possible to measure amniotic fluid pressure directly only after the membranes surrounding the fetus have been ruptured, and that can be done only when the patient is committed to labor. Even though membranes can rupture before a patient goes into labor, it is not a wise idea to place a catheter in the amniotic fluid at such a time, because the catheter could serve as a conduit for introducing infectious agents into the uterine cavity, leading to pathological results.

When a transcervical catheter is used to couple an external pressure transducer to the uterine cavity (Figure 11.5), it is important that the proximal end of the catheter be at the same elevation as the distal tip in the amniotic fluid. Otherwise, a hydrostatic-pressure difference would exist along the catheter, and the pressure baseline measured by the external transducer would be in error (Alvarez and Caldeyro-Barcia, 1950). This technique can be used to record high-quality signals indicating frequency, duration, shape, and relative strength of contractions, but some investigators have found that when more than one catheter and one external pressure transducer are used simultaneously to measure intrauterine pressure, errors are seen (Neuman et al., 1972a; Knoke et al., 1976). These errors are thought to be the results of nonideal catheter placement and limited communication between the amniotic fluid and fluid in the catheter lumen. Pressure differences between separate pockets of amniotic fluid in the uterine cavity can also introduce errors, especially when each pocket is coupled to a separate catheter and pressure transducer. There can also be obstruction or partial obstruction of the catheter by mucus or by the vernix caseosa, and this can lead to errors. Variations on the basic catheter design, such as placement of a small balloon at the distal tip of the catheter or an open-cell sponge over the distal tip of the catheter, are methods that have been reported in efforts to avoid these problems (Csapo, 1970).

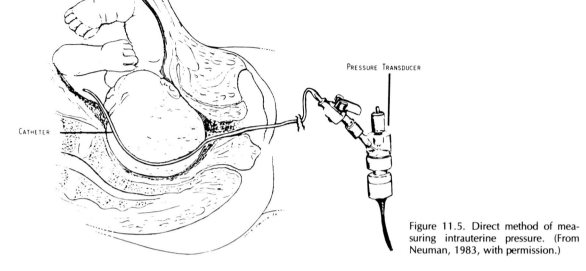

Figure 11.5. Direct method of measuring intrauterine pressure. (From Neuman, 1983, with permission.)

The catheter itself can be eliminated by placing a miniature solid-state pressure transducer into the amniotic cavity (Neuman, Picconnatto, and Roux, 1972b). Pressure sensors no larger than the catheters they replace have been reported (Neuman, 1977), and commercial products somewhat larger are readily available (Devoe et al., 1989). These intrauterine pressure sensors have been shown to be reliable, and a comparison of two sensors in one group of patients during labor has shown closer agreement than was seen in the earlier catheter work (Devoe, Smith, and Stoker, 1993). The advantage of a miniature intrauterine pressure sensor over the more traditional technique of catheter with external transducer is that most of the problems associated with the catheter are eliminated. Because the pressure sensor is within the amniotic cavity itself, there can be no hydrostatic-pressure errors. Most intrauterine pressure sensors have several orifices for communication between the sensor and the amniotic fluid, so the problem of full or partial obstruction is reduced. They also eliminate the possibility of artifacts associated with catheter movements internal and external to the patient, and because of the small size of the intrauterine pressure sensors and the absence of a catheter, they are better able to reproduce the structure of the intrauterine pressure waveform.

There are a few limitations on direct intrauterine pressure measurements. The placement of a transcervical catheter or pressure sensor is an invasive procedure that can be performed only after the chorioamniotic membranes have been ruptured and the patient is committed to labor. Skill is required in advancing and positioning the catheter, because one cannot observe the catheter's progress past the cervix and along the fetus. There is, therefore, a risk of uterine perforation or trauma to the fetus.

Indirect monitoring of uterine contractions

The clinician is able to determine when a patient in labor is having a uterine contraction by palpating the maternal abdomen. One of the earliest electrical sensors of uterine activity, the tocodynamometer, was developed by Reynolds to emulate this method of sensing uterine activity (Reynolds et al., 1948). This noninvasive method of measuring uterine activity has changed little since its original description, and it is widely applied today in fetal monitors and uterine activity monitors for use in the home. The basic principle of operation is identical with what the clinician does in palpating uterine contractions. A typical tocodynamometer (Figure 11.6) is made up of a movable probe attached to an electrical sensor to detect mechanical displacement. A spring gently presses the probe against the maternal abdomen, so that it indents the abdomen with respect to a guard ring around the periphery of the tocodynamometer. When there is no uterine contraction, the probe causes a slight indentation in the abdominal wall, just as an examiner's hand would be able to feel the increased compliance of the abdominal wall due to relaxation of the abdominal muscles and the myometrium. When a contraction of the myometrium occurs, the abdomen will feel less compliant to the examiner. Similarly, this will cause the spring-loaded probe to be pressed back into the

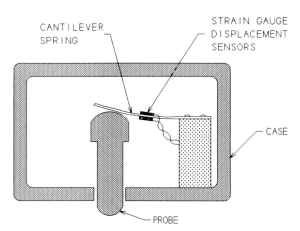

CANTILEVER SPRING

STRAIN GAUGE DISPLACEMENT SENSORS

CASE

PROBE

Figure 11.6. Cross-sectional view of a tocodynamometer.

tocodynamometer housing, thereby reducing the slight depression in the abdominal wall. This movement of the probe is sensed by the displacement sensor, and an electrical signal proportional to the displacement is provided at the output.

The principal advantage of the tocodynamometer is the noninvasive way in which it measures uterine activity. It is the only safe method that can be used before the patient is in active labor, but it obviously cannot offer quantitative assessment of uterine activity. Although it is capable of providing only a qualitative measure of the strength of contractions, it can be used to estimate the frequency and duration of the contractions. The quality of the signals obtained is strongly related to how well the sensor is placed on the abdomen, in terms of its position over the uterus and the tension in the belt holding it in place. The response seen is also dependent on the anatomy of the patient being studied. The closer the tocodynamometer is to the myometrium, the better it will perform. In a patient with a thick abdominal wall due to adipose tissue, the findings will be of poor quality as compared with the signals obtained from lean patients. The tocodynamometer is unable to differentiate between myometrial activity and that of the skeletal muscles of the abdominal wall. Thus, movement of the patient or poor relaxation of the muscles of the abdominal wall can generate many artifacts in this measurement. It has been found that this severely limits its usefulness in patients experiencing a great amount of discomfort during active labor.

THE CARDIOTOCOGRAPH

Electronic fetal monitoring of patients in labor was developed on the basis of the cardiac and uterine activity signals described in the preceding sections. Originally, electronic fetal monitors, or cardiotocographs, as they have come to be known, were capable of monitoring only direct signals, such as the fetal ECG and the intrauterine pressure (Paul and Hon, 1970). As the technology for indirect monitoring of fetal heart and uterine activity improved, cardiotocographs took on this noninvasive modality as well (Roux et al., 1975).

The functioning of the cardiotocograph can be understood using the block diagram in Figure 11.7. Most cardiotocographs have two possible inputs for assessing the fetal heart and two for assessing uterine activity. Thus, the operator can choose between using a direct or indirect method for sensing each of these functions. In determining the fetal heart rate, either Doppler ultrasound or the fetal ECG from a direct electrode on the fetus can be selected, but both of these signals are relatively weak and must be amplified before further processing can be carried out. Because the purpose of obtaining either of these signals is to determine when a fetal heartbeat occurs so that the fetal heart rate can be calculated, a special heartbeat detector circuit must be used to determine the point in time at which each heartbeat occurs. With the ECG signal, this is a relatively simple task, because the detector can identify the peak of the R wave as the time when the heartbeat occurred. It is not as easy to determine when a heartbeat has occurred when one is reading a fetal ultrasound signal, as can be seen from Figure 11.4. Each heartbeat has two major peaks, and each of these peaks is itself made up of individual peaks. Usually, heartbeat detector circuits in fetal monitors identify the heartbeat as occurring at some time during the first major peak, but the timing within that peak can vary, because of its complex nature. Thus, if a Doppler ultrasound signal is being used to determine beat-to-beat variability, there is a strong possibility that error can be introduced because of the lack of a well-defined marker to determine the exact time when the heartbeat occurs.

Once several heartbeats have been detected, a special computer circuit in the cardiotocograph determines the beat-to-beat fetal heart rate. This is done by precisely measuring the interval of time between successive heartbeats and taking the reciprocal of that value. A more detailed description of this process can be found in Chapter 12. The output of the cardiotachometer is a signal that shows the fetal heart rate as a function of time. This signal will be updated with each successive heartbeat and can be plotted on a strip chart and/or displayed on a computer screen on the monitor and at a central station.

Intrauterine pressure signals from either direct or

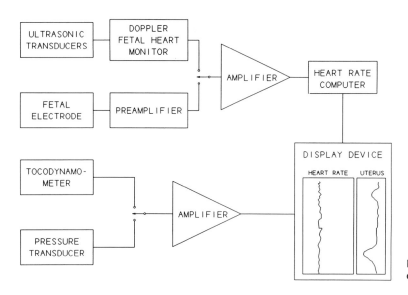

Figure 11.7. Block diagram for a cardiotocograph.

indirect sensors are weak and need to be amplified. The signal is also electronically filtered to reduce artifact. This signal is then plotted on a second channel of the strip-chart recorder and/or computer screen.

Clinicians interpret cardiotocograms to assess the health of the fetus and maternal uterine activity during labor. This interpretation involves examining the baseline value for each channel and the perturbations from that baseline. Clinicians have become familiar with the appearances of certain patterns and can rapidly recognize patterns that arouse concern by looking at the chart or the computer screen. For them to be able to do this, however, requires that the patterns be plotted in the same way on monitors made by different manufacturers. Otherwise, clinicians would have to learn the appearances of warning patterns for each type of monitor that is used. To avoid that problem, a de facto standard has been adopted in which the chart paper or its equivalent on the computer screen is 70 mm wide for the channel showing fetal heart rate, and the paper is linearly calibrated from a rate of 30 beats per minute (bpm) on one side of the chart to 240 bpm on the other. The channel showing uterine contractions is 40 mm wide and is calibrated with a linear scale (0–100). This scale is only qualitative when the tocodynamometer is used as the signal source, but it corresponds to the pressure in millimeters of mercury when direct intrauterine pressure sensors are used to monitor uterine contractions.

There are two standard speeds that are used for the chart paper or the display on the computer screen. The faster rate of 30 mm $\cdot$ min^{-1} is usually used, but a slow rate of 10 mm $\cdot$ min^{-1} can be used to conserve paper and compress the data for long-term or trend monitoring. An example of a cardiotocogram taken at 30 mm $\cdot$ min^{-1} is shown in Figure 11.8.

Cardiotocography can be used to monitor mother and fetus during labor and as an antenatal test of fetal condition. In the former case, both direct and indirect methods of sensing the two variables can be used, but antenatal monitoring requires that only noninvasive methods be used. In evaluating a cardiotocogram, a clinician considers the fetal heart rate and information on uterine contractions both independently and as variables that interact with one another. We have already indicated how the uterine-activity signal can be used to determine frequency, duration, and, in the case of direct monitoring, amplitude and baseline information. Similar types of information can be obtained from direct and indirect monitoring of fetal heart rate. One can determine the baseline heart rate and also estimate heart-rate variability from this channel of the monitor. Certain ominous heart-rate patterns such as sinusoidal variation can be identified from this channel (Manseau et al., 1972).

It is in assessing the interaction between uterine activity and fetal heart rate that cardiotocography is believed to be most useful. One can view a uterine contraction as a stress applied to the fetus, and the resulting changes in the fetal heart rate as the response to that stress. When the pattern of such changes bears a direct linear relationship to the pattern of uterine contractions, these are referred to as periodic changes in the fetal heart rate. The various

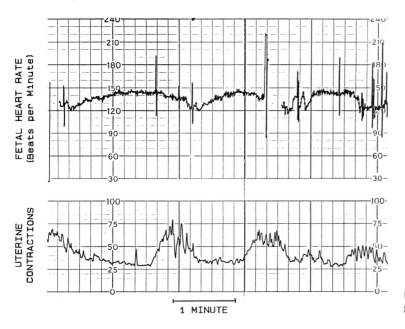

FETAL HEART RATE (Beats per Minute)

UTERINE CONTRACTIONS

1 MINUTE

Figure 11.8. Example of a cardiotocogram.

periodic changes seen in cardiotocography are well described in the research literature and textbooks and will not be considered in detail here (Hon, 1968; Aladjem and Vidyasagar, 1982; Fanaroff and Martin, 1992). It is interesting to note, however, that even though these patterns have been observed in fetal monitoring for almost 30 yr, it has taken clinicians nearly that long to realize that they are not highly specific for identifying fetal abnormalities. Recent clinical data are indicating that fetal cardiotocography may not in itself be as good a method of identifying fetal distress as was once thought (Haverkamp et al., 1979; Vintzileos et al., 1993).

Antepartum fetal cardiotocography is used to assess those fetuses believed to be at increased risk for fetal distress. In the nonstress test, a cardiotocograph is applied to a patient who is resting quietly. The patient is monitored for about an hour, and the data on uterine activity are examined to determine if there have been any spontaneously occurring uterine contractions. It is possible for the tocodynamometer to be used to identify fetal movements as well, and often the mother is instructed to indicate on the chart when she feels fetal movements. Fetal movements and uterine contractions can be considered stimuli that elicit a response in the fetal heart rate. This response usually is a brief acceleration in the heart rate, followed by a return to baseline; however, decelerations can occur, and these can be cause for concern (Paul, 1982).

One can also apply artificial stimuli and observe the responses of the fetal heart rate, rather than wait

for them to occur spontaneously. Contraction stress testing, as by administering oxytocin to the mother, will ensure that some uterine activity will be seen during the test period (Freeman, 1982). Another type of stimulation is to apply a vibroacoustic stimulus to the maternal abdomen for a brief period of time and observe the responses of the fetal heart and fetal movements (Gagnon et al., 1986). Monitors have been developed that include a vibroacoustic stimulator, making this process semiautomatic. Investigators have also considered other types of physical stimuli, such as flashes of light, sound bursts, and rapid positional changes of the mother, but these have been used only for research purposes thus far.

Complete cardiotocographic monitoring systems have been developed for labor and delivery suites. A block diagram for such a system is shown in Figure 11.9. A standard cardiotocographic monitor, such as that illustrated in Figure 11.7, is located at each bed in the labor unit and displays the cardiotocogram for the patient in that bed. Each of these monitors is also connected to a central system located at the nurse's station. Cardiotocograms from each patient site can be shown on this central system, but the display in this case is generally a series of computer screens that can be set to show a standard $30-\text{mm} \cdot \text{min}^{-1}$ cardiotocogram or show a longer sample of data with the sweep rate at 10 $\text{mm} \cdot \text{min}^{-1}$. This central station is also connected to a large computer memory that is used for archiving the cardiotocograms from all patients. The

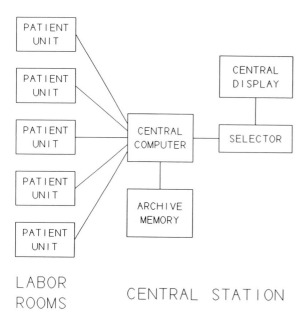

LABOR
ROOMS   CENTRAL STATION

Figure 11.9. Block diagram for a cardiotocographic system for labor and delivery suites, showing patient units and the central station.

memory usually is an optical disc that is capable of archiving and retrieving a large number of fetal cardiotocograms. Because it is required that the fetal cardiotocogram be stored as part of the patient's chart, storage of the paper charts produced by a cardiotocograph can occupy a considerable amount of space in a busy obstetrical unit, requiring a significant amount of clerical time to file and retrieve such data. The computer storage method, on the other hand, can be carried out as part of the monitoring procedure, occupying little additional space and requiring little additional staff time. Although a centralized monitoring system, such as that shown in Figure 11.9, cannot be considered an innovation from the standpoint of gaining more information about the patient, it does make the administration of care more convenient and perhaps even more cost-effective.

It is important to point out that whereas centralized monitoring may be more convenient for the clinical staff, this technical innovation does have the potential to diminish the quality of care. If clinicians begin to rely on the central-station monitors, they will not have as much contact with the patients as they would if they were to continue to check the monitor at each patient's bed, and that can deprive the clinician of important clinical information, in addition to the data on fetal heart rate and uterine ac-

tivity. Although the monitor provides objective data on two functions believed to be important in the management of patients at obstetrical risk, these functions represent only a small part of the overall status of the patient. By examining the patient, as well as the monitor, clinicians obtain important subjective information, as well as objective information, and they also have valuable opportunities to interact with the patient and provide reassurance. Thus, the central station should never replace the local monitor, but should be used only to augment it.

Wireless cardiotocography

Radiotelemetry is a method whereby a signal based on a measurement made at one location is transmitted to another location using radio waves instead of wires. This technique has been applied to transmit the fetal ECG and/or intrauterine pressure using a miniature radio transmitter worn by the patient. A nearby radio receiver picks up these signals and displays them on a conventional cardiotocograph (Neuman and O'Connor, 1980). Telemetry transmitters small enough to be placed in the vagina have been reported (Neuman, Critchfield, and Lin, 1970; Neuman et al., 1972b). In this case, once direct sensors are placed on the fetal presenting part and within the amniotic cavity, the patient has no external wires or catheters to add to her discomfort or limit mobility. Wireless cardiotocography can broadcast signals at distances up to 100 m, so it is possible for a subject to be monitored while ambulating, if so desired. This also is useful when it is necessary to transfer a patient from one location in the obstetrical suite to another, there being no need to disconnect the patient from the monitor and reconnect her at the new location. A continuous recording of the cardiotocogram can be obtained throughout the transfer process.

Variability in fetal heart rate

As mentioned earlier, instantaneous or beat-to-beat variability of the fetal heart rate has been of interest in fetal monitoring for almost as long as the monitor has been in existence. The functioning of the fetal heart follows a complex algorithm that involves nonlinear interactions of many physiological inputs. When these systems are operating properly, the result is a beat-by-beat variation in the cardiac period that makes the heart rate fluctuate around a central value, rather than being fixed at one value. An example of this variability is seen in the heart-rate recording in Figure 11.8. Numerous investigators have proposed means to measure this variability. There are many methods to calculate heart-rate variability (Roux et al., 1975). Most of these methods involve some sort of descriptive statistical means to measure variance. For example, a simple measure of variability would be the standard deviation of a series of R-R intervals from the fetal ECG. There are far more complicated ways of determining a measure of heart-rate variability, and many investigators like to differentiate between short-term variability and long-term variability. It is important to point out that an accurate measurement of the variability in fetal heart rate can be made only from the fetal ECG, where a sharp R wave can be used as the fiduciary mark from which to measure the interval precisely. As discussed earlier, the Doppler ultrasound signal has multiple peaks, and it is difficult to determine a fiduciary point that is the same from one cardiac cycle to the next.

One technique that has been shown to facilitate improved estimation of the beat-to-beat variability in fetal heart rate from an ultrasound signal is autocorrelation. Beat-to-beat variability determined from ultrasound signals using this technique can be very similar to that measured from a simultaneously recorded fetal ECG. This computer technique looks at the Doppler signal from one heartbeat and tries to superimpose it on the next heartbeat by shifting it in time until it comes as close to a perfect match to the next heartbeat as possible. The time over which the original heartbeat signal has to be shifted to match the subsequent heartbeat signal is then taken as the cardiac period. Then the computer determines the next cardiac period by trying to match the next heartbeat signal with the one that follows. This technique, of course, is based on the premise that the ultrasound signals from a string of heartbeats will look very similar, and though it is difficult to identify the one true peak of the ultrasound signal, it is easier to try to match up several peaks (and valleys) of one signal with the peaks of the next one (Lawson et al., 1983).

In recent years there has been great interest in applying the theory of nonlinear dynamics to understanding variations in heart rates in adults and fetuses. Investigators have applied chaos theory to derive a number known as the "fractal dimension" that describes heart-rate variability in a much better way than can be done with classical descriptive statistics (Goldberger and West, 1987; Shono et al., 1991). Work with this technique in adults has shown that there are changes in the fractal dimension immediately prior to certain pathological condi-

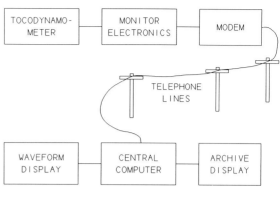

Figure 11.10. Block diagram for a home system to monitor uterine activity.

tions. These approaches are just beginning to be applied to the fetal heart rate.

Another analytical approach that may have some promise for evaluating fetal heart-rate variability is a derived variable known as "approximate entropy" (Pincus, Gladstone, and Ehrenkranz, 1991). Both approximate entropy and the fractal dimension are somewhat complicated to calculate, requiring several minutes of continuous heart-rate information and a dedicated computer to arrive at the results. At the present time, these techniques do not have any clinical utility, but they offer some unique research opportunities aimed at understanding the nonlinear relationships involved in cardiac control and the possibility of providing a clinically useful tool at some time in the future.

Uterine-activity monitoring at home

The indirect uterine-activity channel of a cardiotocography has been used alone to act as a simple uterine-activity monitor that can be used by patients at increased risk for premature birth to monitor their uterine activity at home. The basic system is illustrated in Figure 11.10. The patient is trained in how to place a tocodynamometer on her abdomen and is instructed to rest quietly for about an hour twice a day, with the tocodynamometer in place and connected to a small monitor in her home. The monitor contains a computer memory that stores the signals obtained by the tocodynamometer as the recording is being made. Usually, home uterine-activity monitors do not have any display, because no clinician is present to interpret the results. Instead, the monitor can be connected to the telephone line, and after a day's worth of recording is stored in memory, it can be downloaded over the telephone lines to a central computer, where the data can be plotted out for a clinician to interpret. The monitor itself contains a modem that allows the information stored in memory to be transmitted over the telephone lines. Recordings of the data are prepared at the central station, and a clinician looks at the recordings to determine if the uterine activity is above a level that might indicate the early stages of preterm labor. If that is the case, the clinician reading the chart can contact the patient and her physician and ask her to come to the physician's office, clinic, or hospital for further evaluation and possible tocolysis. Some investigators have reported that if the monitor is routinely used each day, there can be a reduction in cervical changes that may lead to premature delivery (Mou et al., 1991). There is some controversy, however, whether the reduction in preterm deliveries results from use of the home uterine-activity monitor or from the increased clinical attention given to patients who use the monitor (Iams, Johnson, and O'Shaughnessy, 1988). Thus, the true utility of this instrumentation in reducing prematurity is not presently known. The technique has, however, demonstrated the usefulness of simplified home monitoring and use of the telephone system to provide intensive and, possibly, cost-effective surveillance of patients at increased risk.

T-QRS changes in the fetal ECG

Recent work in animals (Greene et al., 1982) and humans (Westgate et al., 1993) has shown that there is information in the actual configuration of the fetal ECG, as well as the heart-rate response to uterine activity. By measuring the amplitude of the QRS complex and that of the T wave of the fetal ECG, taken using the direct method, and calculating the ratio of the T-wave amplitude to that of the QRS complex, it was possible to show a relationship between that ratio and induced ischemia in fetal sheep preparations (Greene et al., 1982). That work has now been expanded to human studies, which have shown a 46% reduction in operative deliveries for fetal distress when the method has been used along with the fetal cardiotocogram to assess patients in labor. An evaluation of 2,434 high-risk patients in labor in England also showed a trend, although not statistically significant, to less metabolic acidosis in patients who were followed using the ST-segment analysis along with the cardiotocogram, as

compared with patients studied with conventional methods (Westgate et al., 1993). It is important to point out, however, that this kind of analysis can be done only with signals obtained using the invasive, direct fetal ECG, and so it is limited to patients in labor.

Clinical utility of the cardiotocogram

Use of the cardiotocogram for management of high-risk pregnancies has become well established. There are many clinicians who feel strongly that failure to use a cardiotocograph to assess patients in labor falls short of the best standard of care and can be grounds for malpractice complaints. Nevertheless, there have been few, if any, studies that have carefully evaluated the clinical utility of this technology. As a matter of fact, there have been indications of some clinical limitations on cardiotocography. It is clear that if one looks only at the fetal heart and its relationship to uterine contractions, one has a very limited view of a complicated physiological system. It is not difficult to imagine that information about additional variables would be helpful in differentiating between abnormalities and normal physiology. Miller has shown that when using fetal cardiotocography alone to identify fetal distress, as indicated by acidosis, one is correct only about 50% of the time (Miller, 1982). On the other hand, by adding fetal blood sampling to determine pH (see Chapter 10), one is able to get an independent measure to help further discriminate the fetus in distress. A paper by Havercamp et al. (1979) questioned the specificity of cardiotocography for identifying fetal distress. Although it has been almost 30 yr since fetal monitoring was introduced, investigators are only beginning to realize the importance of critically evaluating electronic fetal monitoring before it becomes widely applied. Thus, as with any other new technology introduced into medicine, it is important that we carefully assess the clinical utility of the new technique through careful clinical trials before its widespread adoption occurs.

REFERENCES

Aladjem, S., and Vidyasagar, D. (1982). *Atlas of Perinatology*. Philadelphia: W. B. Saunders.
Alvarez, H., and Caldeyro-Barcia, R. (1950). Contractility of the human uterus recorded by a new method. *Surgery, Gynecology and Obstetrics* 91:1.
Bergveld, P., Koülling, A. J., and Peuscher, J. H. J. (1986). Real-time fetal ECG recording. *IEEE Transactions on Biomedical Engineering* 33:505–9.
Bernstine, R. L. (1968). Fetal heart studies with the ultra-

sonic Doppler technique. *American Journal of Obstetrics and Gynecology* 102:961.

Bishop, E. H. (1968). Ultrasonic fetal monitoring. *Clinics in Obstetrics and Gynecology* 11:1154.

Csapo, A. (1970). The diagnostic significance of the intrauterine pressure. *Obstetrical and Gynecological Survey* 25:403, 515.

Devoe, L. D., Gardner, P., Dear, C., and Searle, N. (1989). Monitoring intrauterine pressure during active labor. A prospective comparison of two methods. *Journal of Reproductive Medicine* 34:811–14.

Devoe, L. D., Smith, R. P., and Stoker, R. (1993). Intrauterine pressure catheter performance in an in vitro uterine model: a simulation of problems for intrapartum monitoring. *Obstetrics and Gynecology* 82:285–9.

Fanaroff, A. A., and Martin, R. J. (1992). *Neonatal-Perinatal Medicine*, 5th ed. St. Louis: Mosby.

Freeman, R. K. (1982). Contraction stress testing for primary fetal surveillance in patients at high risk for uteroplacental insufficiency. *Clinics in Perinatology* 9:265–70.

Gagnon, R., Patrick, J., Foreman, J., et al. (1986). Stimulation of human fetuses with sound and vibration. *American Journal of Obstetrics and Gynecology* 155:848.

Ginsburg, S. J. (1964). A fetal phonocardiotachometer for use in labor. *IEEE Transactions on Biomedical Engineering* 11:35.

Goldberger, A. L., and West, B. J. (1987). Fractals in physiology and medicine. *Yale Journal of Biology and Medicine* 60:421–35.

Goodlin, R. C., and Fabricant, S. (1970). A new fetal scalp electrode. *Obstetrics and Gynecology* 35:646.

Greene, K. R., Dawes, G. S., Lilja, H., and Rosèn, K. G. (1982). Changes in the ST waveform of the fetal lamb electrocardiogram with hypoxemia. *American Journal of Obstetrics and Gynecology* 144:950–7.

Hammacher, K. (1962). Neue Methode zur selektiven Registrierung der fetalen Herzschlagfrequenz. *Geburtshilfe und Frauenheilkunde* 22:1542.

Haverkamp, A. D., (1979). Orleans, M., Langendoerfer, S., McFee, J., Murphy, J., and Thompson, H. E. (1979). A controlled trial of differential effects of intrapartum fetal monitoring. *American Journal of Obstetrics and Gynecology* 134:399–412.

Herbert, W. N., Bruninghaus, H. M., Barefoot, A. B., and Bright, T. G. (1987). Clinical aspects of fetal heart auscultation. *Obstetrics and Gynecology* 69:574–7.

Hon, E. H. (1963). Instrumentation of fetal heart rate and fetal electrocardiography. II. A vaginal electrode. *American Journal of Obstetrics and Gynecology* 86:772.

(1968). *An Atlas of Fetal Heart Rate Patterns*. New Haven: Harty Press.

Hon, E. H., Paul, R. H., and Hon, R. W. (1972). Electrode evaluation of the fetal heart rate. XI. Description of a spiral electrode. *Obstetrics and Gynecology* 40:362.

Hutchins, C. J. (1978). Scalp infection after fetal monitoring in labour. *New Zealand Medical Journal* 87:390–2.

Iams, J. D., Johnson, F. F., and O'Shaughnessy, R. W. (1988). A prospective random trial of home uterine activity monitoring in pregnancies at increased risk of preterm labor. Part II. *American Journal of Obstetrics and Gynecology* 159:593–603.

Knoke, J. D., Tsao, L. L., Neuman, M. R., and Roux, J. F. (1976). The accuracy of measurements of intrauterine pressure during labor: a statistical analysis. *Computers and Biomedical Research* 9:177–86.

Lawson, G. W., Belcher, R., Dawes, G. S., and Redman, C. W. (1983). A comparison of ultrasound (with autocorrelation) and direct electrocardiogram fetal heart rate detector systems. *American Journal of Obstetrics and Gynecology* 147:721–2.

Macrae, D. J. (1962). Heart monitoring in the foetus and newborn. *Journal of Obstetrics and Gynaecology of the British Commonwealth* 69:1031.

Mannor, S. M., Serr, D. M., Tamari, I., Meshorer, A., and Frei, E. H. (1972). The safety of ultrasound in fetal monitoring. *American Journal of Obstetrics and Gynecology* 113:653–61.

Manseau, P., Vanquier, J., Chavinic, J., et al. (1972). Le rhythme cardiac foetal sinusoidal. Aspect evocateur de souffrance foetale au cours de la grossesse. *Journal de Gynecologie, Obstetrique et Biologie de la Reproduction* 1:343.

Miller, F. C. (1982). Prediction of acid–base values from intrapartum fetal heart rate data and their correlation with scalp and funic values. *Clinics in Perinatology* 9:353–61.

Mou, S. M., Sunderji, S. J., Gall, S., How, H., Patel, V., Gray, M., Kayne, H. L., and Corwin, M. (1991). Multicenter randomized clinical trial of home uterine activity monitoring for detection of pre-term labor. *American Journal of Obstetrics and Gynecology* 165:858–66.

Neuman, M. R. (1977). Pressure measurements in obstetrics. In *Indwelling and Implantable Pressure Transducers*, ed. D. G. Fleming, W. H. Ko, and M. R. Neuman (pp. 85–95). Boca Raton: CRC Press.

(1983). Electronic monitoring of the fetus. *Clinics in Perinatology* 10:237–52.

(1988). Fetal monitoring. In *Encyclopedia of Medical Devices and Instrumentation*, ed. J. G. Webster. New York: Wiley.

Neuman, M. R., Critchfield, F. H., and Lin, W. C. (1970). An intravaginal fetal ECG telemetry system. *Obstetrics and Gynecology* 35:96.

Neuman, M. R., Jordan, J. A., Roux, J. F., and Knoke, J. D. (1972a). Validity of intrauterine pressure measurements with transcervical intra-amniotic catheters and an intra-amniotic miniature pressure transducer during labor. *Gynecologic Investigation* 3:165.

Neuman, M. R., and O'Connor, E. (1980). A two-channel radiotelemetry system for clinical fetal monitoring. *Biotelemetry and Patient Monitoring* 7:104–21.

Neuman, M. R. Picconnatto, J., and Roux, J. F. (1972b). A wireless radiotelemetry system for monitoring fetal heart rate and intrauterine pressure during labor and delivery. *Gynecologic Investigation* 1:92.

Paul, R. H. (1982). The evaluation of antepartum fetal well being using the non-stress test. *Clinics in Perinatology* 9:253–63.

Paul, R. H., and Hon, E. H. (1970). A clinical fetal monitor. *Obstetrics and Gynecology* 35:161.

Pincus, S. M., Gladstone, I. M., and Ehrenkranz, R. A. (1991). A regularity statistic for medical data analysis. *Journal of Clinical Monitoring* 7:335–45.

Reynolds, S. R. M., Heard, O. O., Bruns, P., and Hellman, L. M. (1948). A multi-channel strain-gauge tokodynamometer: an instrument for studying patterns of uterine contractions in pregnant women. *Bulletin of the Hospital for Joint Diseases* 82:446.

Roux, J. F., Neuman, M. R., and Goodlin, R. C. (1975).
  Monitoring of intrapartum phenomena. *CRC Critical
  Reviews in Bioengineering* 2:119–58.
Shenker, L. (1966). Fetal electrocardiography. *Obstetrical
  and Gynecological Survey* 21:367.
Shono, H., Yamasaki, M., Muro, M., Oga, M., Eto, Y.,
  Shimomura, K., and Sugimori, H. (1991). Chaos and
  fractals with 1/f spectrum below 10^{-2} Hz demon-
  strates full term fetal heart rate changes during active
  phase. *Early Human Development* 27:111–17.
Strong, T. H., Paul, R. H., Park, G. D., Cheng, Y.,
  Lewis, D. E., McCart, D. F., and Mueller, E. A.
  (1991). The intrauterine probe electrode. *American
  Journal of Obstetrics and Gynecology* 164:1233–4.
Tam, H.W., and Webster, J. G. (1977). Minimizing electrode motion artifact by skin abrasion. *IEEE Transactions on Biomedical Engineering* 24:134–9.

Vanderschoot, J., Callaerts, D., Sansen, W., Vandewalle,
  J., Vantrappen, G., and Janssens, J. (1987). Two
  methods for optimal MECG elimination and FECG
  detection from skin electrode signals. *IEEE Transactions on Biomedical Engineering* 34:233–43.
Vintzileos, A. M., Antsaklis, A., Varvarigos, I., Papas,
  C., Sofatzis, I., and Montgomery, J. T. (1993). A randomized trial of intrapartum electronic fetal heart
  rate monitoring versus intermittent auscultation. *Obstetrics and Gynecology* 81:899–907.
Westgate, J., Harris, M., Curnow, J. S. H., and Greene,
  K. R. (1993). Plymouth randomised trial of cardiotocogram only versus ST waveform plus cardiotocogram for intrapartum monitoring in 2400 cases.
  American Journal of Obstetrics and Gynecology 169:1151–
  60.

12

Cardiopulmonary monitoring

MICHAEL R. NEUMAN, Ph.D., M.D.

INTRODUCTION

Cardiopulmonary monitoring involves the use of electronic devices to provide continuous or quasi-continuous assessment of the cardiovascular and pulmonary systems. It provides the clinician quantitative and qualitative information on heart and breathing functions in a patient at times when this information may be important in assessing the patient's clinical course. This technique is most frequently applied in critical-care situations, such as the neonatal intensive-care unit, and for perioperative monitoring. It is also applied in less critical medical circumstances, such as a step-down units, where the use of this equipment can help to minimize personnel requirements in caring for patients while still providing intensive surveillance of cardiopulmonary functions.

Cardiopulmonary monitoring can be used outside of the hospital as well. Premature infants can be discharged from the hospital at an earlier age and sent home with a monitor, after the parents or caregivers are adequately trained in the use of the monitor and what to do when alarms sound, thus reducing the high costs associated with the care of preterm infants.

Cardiopulmonary monitors are used in the home in an attempt to detect and perhaps prevent apparent life-threatening episodes (ALTE) or sudden infant death syndrome (SIDS). Home monitors have been used to detect prolonged apnea and heart rates that may have some association with SIDS. Although specific evidence that home monitoring can prevent such incidents is not yet available, many home cardiorespiratory monitors are currently in use in the United States.

Cardiopulmonary monitors for use with infants should be capable of detecting the physiological conditions listed in Table 12.1. Cardiac monitoring provides continuous data on heart rate and rhythm. Specific conditions that warrant sounding an alarm include tachycardia and bradycardia. Sophisticated cardiac monitors can also identify certain arrhythmias and trigger an alarm when they occur. Pulmonary monitors allow one to continuously observe breathing rate and waveform and ideally should present a signal that is roughly proportional to tidal volume, so that conditions suggesting hypoventilation can be detected, triggering an alarm. Pulmonary monitors should be able to detect central, obstructive, and mixed apneas, sounding an alarm when the duration of such apneas exceeds a predetermined threshold.

Monitors should also be able to perform certain checks on their own functioning. They should indicate when there are functional problems, such as a disconnected sensor or a decrease in battery power. Those monitors that store data in an internal memory should also indicate when that memory is approaching capacity, so that measure can be taken to avoid any data loss.

Blood-pressure monitors should be capable of showing the blood-pressure waveform and sounding an alarm when systolic, diastolic, or mean pressures fall outside of predetermined limits.

A general design for a cardiopulmonary monitor is shown in Figure 12.1. The cardiac data and pulmonary information are obtained from the patient by sensors that convert the physiological signals into electrical signals that can be processed by the rest of the monitor. The processing block of the monitor carries out electronic functions to bring the signals to a form that can be used to detect alarm conditions and display the appropriate information.

Table 12.1. *Conditions detected by cardiopulmonary monitors*

Cardiac
 1. Heart rate (beat-to-beat and/or average)
 2. Tachycardia
 3. Bradycardia
 4. Life-threatening arrhythmias

Pulmonary
 1. Breathing rate
 2. Tidal volume (approximate)
 3. Apnea (central, obstructive, and mixed)

Other
 1. Monitor dysfunction
 2. Memory status

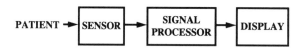

Figure 12.1. Block diagram for general electronic patient monitoring.

The display and recording functions of the monitor provide the necessary information to the clinician, in addition to establishing an archive of that information for later use.

We can further classify monitors as being invasive or noninvasive, depending on how the sensor is interfaced with the patient. Noninvasive sensors are placed on the surface of the patient's skin and do not violate the integrity of the skin, whereas invasive sensors require penetration of the skin or other epithelium to obtain the physiological measurement.

Monitors can continuously report on the variable under consideration, or they can periodically sample the variable. They can be used for diagnostic purposes by providing data on the variable over a relatively long period of time, or they can be set up to provide alarms so that therapeutic measures can be taken as soon as certain conditions occur. Frequently, cardiopulmonary monitors embody all of these functions, so as to provide the most effective patient care.

CARDIAC MONITORING

The primary input signal for cardiac monitoring is the electrocardiogram (ECG). Unlike the practice in diagnostic electrocardiography, limb leads are seldom used for cardiac monitoring. Instead, modified limb leads are used, with the signals being obtained from electrodes placed on the chest rather than on the limbs. These electrode positions are, however, generally described by the Eindhoven triangle, in the same way as the limb leads.

Electrodes

There are several different types of electrodes that can be used with a cardiac monitor (Webster, 1992, ch. 5). Although electrodes frequently were reused when cardiac monitors began to be employed in clinical care, today disposable electrodes are employed almost exclusively. Figure 12.2 illustrates some of the types of disposable electrodes that are used. Usually a silver/silver chloride electrochemical electrode provides the actual contact between the electrical system and the biological system. It is necessary, however, to couple this electrochemical electrode to the skin by means of a solution containing the electrolytes sodium (Na^+) and chloride (Cl^-). In the older, reusable electrodes, those electrolytes were contained in the electrode gel or paste. They are the principal ions found in the body's extracellular fluid and are maintained in the electrolytic solution at concentrations similar to those in the body. In some infants these concentrations (especially of chloride) have been said to cause skin irritation, and special electrolytic solutions with lower ionic concentrations have been developed to avoid this problem. In the disposable wet electrodes, the electrolytic solution is held in a sponge that is placed between the Ag/AgCl electrochemical electrode and the skin. Medical adhesive tape around the periphery of the structure holds the electrode, and hence the fluid-filled sponge, in good contact with the skin. As the water content of the electrolytic solution evaporates, the amount of fluid between the electrode and the skin can diminish to the extent that good contact is not maintained, and reliable signals can no longer be obtained. Most monitors can detect this condition and activate the alarm "Lead Off." In some cases, wet electrodes can dry out in storage and not function properly when placed on a patient. Electrodes are packaged to minimize this problem, but it is always a good idea to verify that the sponge is well saturated with fluid before placing any electrode on an infant.

Another type of disposable electrode shown in Figure 12.2 is the hydrogel electrode. In this case, instead of a sponge saturated with electrolyte, there is a slab of hydrogel in that position. Hydrogel is a solid-appearing polymer of such structure that it looks like a sponge at the microscopic level. Water containing sodium and chloride ions is trapped in

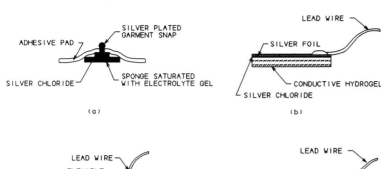

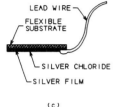

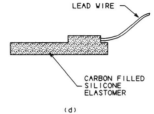

Figure 12.2. Examples of various types of electrodes used with cardiopulmonary monitors shown in cross section: (a) disposable wet electrode, (b) hydrogel electrode, (c) thin-film electrode, (d) carbon-filled silicone rubber dry electrode.

its matrix, turning the hydrogel into a compliant material with a consistency similar to that of soft rubber. Other substances are added to give the hydrogel a sticky surface. Thus, hydrogel serves two purposes on the electrode: (1) It functions as the electrolyte gel, ensuring good contact between the patient's skin and the electrochemical electrode, and (2) it serves as the adhesive tack holding the electrode against the skin. With hydrogel electrodes, no additional adhesive tape or adhesive rings are needed to keep the electrode against the skin. There have been anecdotal reports that motion artifacts are reduced when hydrogel electrodes are used, as compared with wet electrodes. That is understandable, in that when a hydrogel electrode is used, there is no differential movement between the skin surface and the electrode as the patient moves. With a conventional wet electrode, the sponge does not adhere to the skin surface, and there can be differential movement between it and the skin when the patient moves. Such differential movement can result in electrical artifacts being generated.

Other types of electrodes are also used with cardiopulmonary monitors. If the metal electrode on either the wet electrode or the hydrogel electrode is made very thin, it can be transparent or translucent to x rays. These thin-metal-film electrodes are also very flexible and do not need to be removed when it is necessary to x-ray the chest. Their properties are essentially the same as those of the electrodes previously described.

Carbon-filled silicone-rubber electrodes, on the other hand, are quite different. These electrodes, as shown in Figure 12.2, consist of a thin slab of silicone rubber, a soft elastomer material that has been

specially prepared by mixing in finely divided carbon particles while the rubber material is still liquid during manufacture. This carbon makes the silicone rubber electrically conductive. A lead wire is attached to the back of the material, and the carbon-filled rubber acts like the metal part of a conventional electrode. This type of electrode generally has a larger surface area than the electrodes described earlier, and because of its flexibility it is able to closely approximate the skin surface. Because the electrode material is impervious to moisture, as compared with the skin, a thin layer of moisture collects on the skin surface just under the electrode and acts like electrolytic gel to couple the electrode to the skin. These electrodes can be used "dry," without the need for gel, and they will not dry out as can the wet electrodes. Thus, these electrodes may be used for a relatively long period of time, and they are reusable. If the surface of the electrode becomes dirty or contaminated, it need only be washed off to make it ready for reuse. Carbon-filled silicone-rubber electrodes are held in place against the chest by an elastic band, rather than tape. This also helps to make the electrode reusable and to make it convenient for use by nonprofessional caregivers. Although this type of electrode is not widely used in hospitals, it is quite popular for use with home infant apnea monitors.

A discussion of infant electrodes would not be complete without some consideration of the lead wires that connect the electrodes to the patient cable, which in turn is connected to the monitor. There have been reports of incidents in which lead wires have been accidentally connected to the power mains, rather than a patient cable, leading to electrocution of the infants on whom the electrodes were placed (Anonymous, 1993). The possibility of such an occurrence today has been greatly reduced by the use of special connectors on the lead wires, designed so that it is not possible to plug them into anything other than the connector on the patient cable for which they were designed. It is important that all electrode lead wires have these special connectors, rather than the older pin-type connectors, to preclude the risk of electrocution.

One should also consider the connector on the end of the lead wire that is attached to the electrode. Some electrodes come with their lead wires already attached, whereas others have a snap, similar to that used on clothing, to which the lead wire is attached. The lead wires are connected to the snaps either by pressing the connection against the snap until it snaps into place or by means of a connector on the lead wire that is a clip, similar in structure to a spring-loaded clothespin. When the former type of connector is used, it is important to attach the electrode to the lead wire before the electrode is placed on the infant's chest, so that making the connection to the lead wire will not exert excessive force against the infant's chest. On the other hand, the clip-type connectors can be attached when the electrode is in place on the infant, because very little force is transmitted to the infant during this procedure.

Signal processing

The ECG signal sensed by the electrodes is very faint and must be increased in strength before it can be utilized in the monitor. Thus, one of the most important steps in the signal-processing section of a cardiac monitor is amplification of the signal to a usable level. Unfortunately, electrical signals other than just the ECG signal are provided by the electrodes. Extraneous signals or noise, especially during patient movement, will accompany the ECG signal, and these are amplified along with the ECG signal. This noise can interfere with the signal of interest and make it impossible for the monitor to carry out its intended function. Thus, the signal processor must also include a means to minimize this noise. Filtering the signal is a method frequently used to do this. Mathematical analysis of any signal that varies over time, such as the ECG signal, shows that the signal can be decomposed into a series of sinusoidal signals of specific frequencies. Often these frequencies will fall within a band of frequencies characteristic of a specific signal, such as the ECG. Noise, on the other hand, is more

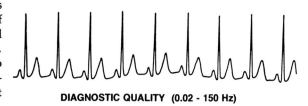

DIAGNOSTIC QUALITY (0.02 - 150 Hz)

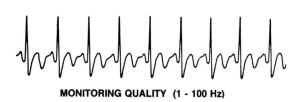

MONITORING QUALITY (1 - 100 Hz)

Figure 12.3. Examples of diagnostic-quality and monitor-quality ECG signals.

broadly distributed over the frequency spectrum, although some types of noise, such as motion artifacts, have dominant components at lower frequencies. Thus, by selectively passing frequencies of a particular band corresponding to a specific signal, it is possible to minimize the effects of noise when the noise includes frequencies outside of that band. Signal processing on cardiopulmonary monitors attempts to do just that. Unfortunately, much of the noise spectrum overlaps the ECG frequencies, and this is especially true at the lower frequencies in the ECG band of frequencies. In some cardiac monitors, a compromise is made wherein some of the lower frequencies of the ECG signal are removed from the signal in an effort to also reduce the effect of noise. This causes some distortion in the ECG, especially around the baseline, but it allows many aspects of the cardiac rhythm to be determined from the filtered signal with much less interference from noise. This type of filtered signal produces what is known as a monitor-quality ECG, whereas the signal covering the full frequency range yields what is sometimes referred to as a diagnostic-quality ECG. The former signal is best used for monitoring a patient who will be engaging in a significant amount of movement during the monitoring period, whereas the diagnostic ECG is best used over a short period of time while a patient is resting quietly. Figure 12.3 shows an ECG as seen with a monitor-quality system and a diagnostic-quality system. Although filtering helps to reduce the effects of motion artifacts on signal quality, the noise problem can never be completely eliminated.

Cardiac monitors determine the heart rate. This is

done by detecting each heartbeat and precisely measuring the time interval between successive beats (Webster, 1992, ch. 6). An important function of the signal-processing section of a cardiac monitor is the detection of the peak of the R wave as a fiduciary mark for each cardiac cycle. Once the time intervals between successive R waves have been determined, the cardiotachometer uses this information to determine the heart rate. An instantaneous heart rate is determined by measuring the interval between successive R waves and applying the following formula to get the heart rate in beats per minute:

$$R_i = \frac{60,000}{T} \qquad (12.1)$$

where R_i is the beat-to-beat heart rate in beats per minute, and T is the R-R interval in milliseconds. This heart rate is the number of beats per minute that would be seen if every successive R-R interval were the same as that currently being measured by the monitor. Of course, the heart usually does not beat with every R-R interval exactly the same, and so the next interval probably will be different from the one just measured. For that reason, the heart rate is recalculated for each R-R interval by the beat-to-beat cardiotachometer, and so the heart-rate value is likely to change by a small amount following each heartbeat, even when the infant being monitored is resting quietly. This beat-to-beat variability is reported only when a beat-to-beat cardiotachometer (sometimes called an instantaneous cardiotachometer) is used.

The averaging cardiotachometer calculates the heart rate in a manner similar to the way a clinician does it. The number of R waves occurring during a predetermined interval (e.g., 15 s) are counted, and this number is entered into the formula

$$R_a = \frac{60N}{I} \qquad (12.2)$$

where R_a is the averaged heart rate, N is the number of beats counted in the measured interval, and I is the duration of the measured interval, in seconds. If the interval is 15 s long, then the monitor can multiply the number of R waves within that interval by 4 to get the heart rate in beats per minute. Of course, a clinician usually will measure the pulse over a full minute to determine the heart rate, but most averaging cardiotachometers use a time interval of less than 15 s. Thus, some variation in heart rate is detected using this system, but certainly not the same heart-rate variability seen with the beat-to-beat cardiotachometer.

The sophisticated monitors used with adults often have computers that can recognize certain cardiac arrhythmias when they occur and alert the clinical staff to the onset of these life-threatening episodes (Jenkins, 1983). That degree of sophistication is not normally used in infant monitors, there being less clinical need. Nevertheless, in clinical situations this aspect of cardiopulmonary monitoring can be an important aid in the clinical care of infants.

Cardiac monitors not only can display the ECG and heart rate of the patient but also can detect when certain clinically significant conditions arise and sound an alarm. For most cardiac monitors, these conditions include bradycardia and tachycardia. When the heart rate exceeds the tachycardia threshold or falls below the bradycardia threshold for a preset time duration (usually on the order of 5 s), an alarm is activated, calling the clinician's attention to this condition. This is a very important function of a cardiac monitor, and it is strongly dependent on how well the monitor is able to detect R waves and how well the cardiotachometer measures heart rate.

Display and recording functions

We often think of the human interface with a cardiopulmonary monitor as being just the interface between the patient and the monitor's sensors. There is, however, another interface that is equally important: the interface between the monitor and the clinical caregivers. This human–machine interface is essential for efficient transmission of critical information, so that the monitored data can be acted on as quickly as possible. The display and recording functions of a clinical monitor are important aspects of this interface. Just as is the case for other features of the monitor, display and recording functions can vary from being very simple to something that is extremely complex.

The simplest display function for a cardiac monitor is a light or a sound source that will produce a flash or a "beep" each time an R wave is detected. This unpretentious display contains a lot of information and can be quite useful in critical clinical situations. A flashing light can be a good way to determine if the monitor is functioning properly. By comparing the flashing light with other measures of pulse rate, such as palpation or auscultation, one can quickly establish that the monitor is functioning properly. The sound device that produces a beep for each heartbeat can be very useful when caregivers are busy carrying out a critical procedure on the infant. Even though the sound of a regular heart rate tends to fade into the background, an acceleration or deceleration of the heart rate will immediately catch the attention of the clinicians without requiring them to watch the monitor. This can be quite valuable in critical situations, when everyone's attention should be directed toward the patient.

Most monitors provide more information than just an indication of when an R wave occurs. A monitor must also indicate the heart rate and rhythm, in addition to indicating when alarm conditions arise. The heart rate is usually presented on a digital display; that is, a set of numbers corresponding to the heart rate in beats per minute is displayed on a screen. This display is usually used to show only averaged values for heart rate. When used to display beat-to-beat heart rate, the numbers on digital displays usually change with each heartbeat, which makes them difficult to read. Heart-rate information can also be presented on an analog display. In that case, the length of a bar or the deflection of a pointer is proportional to the heart rate. The actual rate is determined by comparing this analog signal to a fixed scale. Although averaged heart rates are usually displayed by this type of analog readout, the beat-to-beat heart rate can also be displayed in this way, because the observer can effectively average the display to determine the heart rate, and changes in the display from one beat to the next are not as distracting as they are with the digital display.

Cardiac rhythm is determined from a display of the actual waveform of the ECG on a screen. The display is designed to appear the same as if the ECG were printed out on paper.

Some cardiac monitors also have trending displays. These generally are plots on the monitor screen of data such as the heart rate as a function of time. The time scale for such plots varies from a few minutes to 24 h. Usually the longer time scales are described as trend displays only in that they show long-term changes in the heart rate. Other methods of showing long-term summaries of heart-rate data include plotting histograms of beat-to-beat heart rate or R-R interval or presenting the power spectrum of the heart rate. Both of these techniques help clinicians to see the heart-rate variability and can be useful in evaluating the status of the infant's autonomic nervous system. These techniques, however, are still considered to be experimental and are not generally used with clinical monitors.

BLOOD-PRESSURE MONITORING

Some cardiac monitors include modules for blood-pressure monitoring. These are generally for continuous, direct blood-pressure monitoring, as opposed to the indirect cuff method. Direct blood-pressure monitoring involves a fluid connection between a pressure sensor and the arterial circulation. Indirect monitoring of blood pressure is a sampling procedure and involves measuring the pressure within a cuff placed around a limb. It implies that the pressure within the cuff is the same as the arterial pressure in the infant when special conditions are met.

Details on blood-pressure monitoring can be found in Chapter 14. Basically, the blood-pressure section of a cardiac monitor carries out many of the same functions as the ECG section. For direct blood-pressure monitoring, the technique that is usually used in intensive-care units, a fluid-filled arterial catheter is coupled to an external pressure transducer that converts the pressure signal to an electrical signal. In neonates, the catheter often can be placed within an umbilical artery, and other arteries can also be cannulated for measuring blood pressure. Disposable pressure sensors are the sensors of choice in most recently developed systems for blood-pressure monitoring; they are small and relatively inexpensive and feature accuracy and precision as good as those obtained with reusable sensors. Another advantage of the disposable sensor is that it is not necessary to sterilize it between uses.

Signal processing from direct blood-pressure sensors involves amplification and filtering, as in the case of the ECG. Different frequencies, however, are involved in the blood-pressure signal, and so the actual circuits are different from those used for the ECG. Although a heart rate can be determined from the blood-pressure signal by detecting when the blood-pressure peak occurs and using that as the fiduciary mark of the cardiac cycle, this peak determination is not nearly as accurate as the R-wave determination described in the preceding section. Nevertheless, the blood-pressure monitor still needs to determine the peak in the pressure signal (the systolic pressure) and the minimum value of the pressure signal (the diastolic pressure). Most blood-pressure monitors also calculate the mean arterial pressure by electronically averaging the waveform over one complete cardiac cycle.

The display function of the blood-pressure monitor provides the waveform of the arterial pressure along with digital presentations of systolic, diastolic, and mean arterial pressures. In some monitors, these three quantities are plotted as functions of time in a trend type of display as well. Monitors can be set to alarm when pressures exceed or fall below predetermined levels.

Noninvasive blood-pressure measurement is generally not used for continuous or quasi-continuous monitoring in infants. Instead, the electronic devices for obtaining this signal are used for periodic measurements and are operated by clinical staff. Details on how these devices operate can be found in Chapter 14.

PULMONARY MONITORING

The pulmonary portion of the cardiopulmonary monitor is similar to the cardiac portion in that it can be divided into three major components: the sensor, the processor, and the display. These will be considered next.

Breathing sensors

There are direct and indirect sensors for measuring breathing. In the direct method, the sensor is coupled to the airway and measures the movement or other properties of air transported into and out of the lungs. Indirect sensors, on the other hand, look at variables related to air movement, but do not sense the air movement itself. These methods involve no contact with the airway or the air being moved into or out of the lungs. Although there are invasive and noninvasive sensors in both categories, the direct methods are generally more invasive than the indirect.

There are many different sensors for direct and indirect measurements of breathing (Little et al., 1987). Although any of these can, in principle, be used as the sensor for a patient monitor, most are used only for laboratory studies or under specialized intensive-care situations. In the following paragraphs we shall examine those sensors that are used frequently with cardiopulmonary monitors, as well as those that can be used as standards to calibrate these monitoring systems. Other sensors that are not frequently used for monitoring will be listed in the tables, but will not be described.

Direct sensors of breathing

Direct methods of sensing respiration usually are reserved for special studies, rather than clinical monitoring, because they involve obtrusive connections to the patient. Thus, these methods are more frequently found in the pulmonary-function laboratory or the sleep laboratory, rather than the intensive-care unit. Some of the methods are, however, useful as standards against which other types of monitoring sensors can be tested. Some of the methods listed in Table 12.2 are described in more detail in the following paragraphs.

Table 12.2. *Direct methods for detecting breathing patterns*

1. Pneumotachygraph
2. Spirometry
3. Airway carbon dioxide sensor
4. Airway temperature sensor
5. Anemometry
6. Airflow sound sensor

Pneumotachygraph. Any gas flowing in a tube will encounter some resistance due to that tube. If there is some partial obstruction in the tube, such as a wire screen or a narrowing of a portion of the tube's lumen, the resistance will be increased. It can be shown from basic physical principles that the pressure difference between the two ends of a tube with resistance through which gas is flowing is proportional to the flow through that tube. This is the basic principle of the pneumotachygraph, and it can be applied to monitoring patients when direct connection to the airway is possible (Comroe et al., 1962). A small tube or an added resistance to an existing tube placed in the flowing air, either through the use of a tightly fitting face mask or through an endotracheal tube, represents a known, fixed resistance to the flow of air. The pressure drop across this resistance can then be measured by a differential pressure transducer, and this pressure difference will then be proportional to flow through the sensor. If the added resistance and volume are kept as small as possible, this sensing system will not require any significant increase in breathing effort, nor will it significantly increase dead space. It must be pointed out, however, that when this condition is satisfied, the pressure differences will be very small, and a very sensitive differential-pressure sensor must be used with the system. The flow signal determined by this method can be integrated to give a volume signal. Electronic instruments designed for use with the pneumotachygraph frequently have the capability of providing this integration function.

Carbon dioxide sensor. Air expired from the lungs has a higher percentage of carbon dioxide than does inspired air. Thus, by placing a sensor of carbon dioxide in the airway, it is possible to detect expired air (Rigatto and Brady, 1972). This can be done to determine respiration rate. If the carbon dioxide sensor's response time is fast enough and its connection to the airway is tight, it is possible to determine the carbon dioxide content of alveolar gas. This is known as end-tidal determination of carbon dioxide.

Usually it is not possible to have a carbon dioxide sensor small enough to be located within the airway, nor external devices, such as a face mask, attached to the airway, and so a remotely located sensor must be used. This is coupled to the airway through a fine-bore flexible tube. Gas is sampled from the airway by this tube and transported to the carbon dioxide sensor. There is a delay time associated with the propagation of the air sample down the length of the tube, such that the carbon dioxide from a particular expired breath will be detected 1–2 s (typically) later. Because of the requirement that the sampling tube be placed in or near the airway, this technique is generally used only for in-hospital studies, such as those carried out in the sleep laboratory.

Nasal temperature sensor. A small temperature sensor located within or near the airway can detect breathing by monitoring the temperature differences between inspired air and expired air. This sensor must have a low thermal mass so that it can respond rapidly to temperature changes, possibly resulting from rapid breathing in infants. Temperature sensors can consist of thermistors, very small semiconductor devices that register a large change in electrical resistance as a result of a temperature change, or they can be thin- or thick-film temperature-sensitive elements that are not as sensitive as the thermistor, but have a large surface-area-to-mass ratio, so that they can respond very rapidly. Commercial products are available using either of these technologies, generally consisting of a structure with one sensor located under each nostril and a third over the mouth to detect oral breathing. Relatively inexpensive versions of this device have been produced, and therefore these sensors can be considered disposable items.

Nasal temperature sensors have been used for monitoring breathing in research studies and in the sleep laboratory, but they have not been utilized for clinical monitoring. Their major limitations are the need for a secure method for attachment to the face and the fact that a lead wire connecting the sensor on the face to the monitor must be used. Although sensors incorporating radiotelemetry, to obviate the need for the lead wire, have been developed (Neuman, 1986), it is not recommended that these devices be used for routine clinical monitoring, because they are small and are located near the mouth. It would be easy for an infant to remove the sensor-telemeter, swallow it, and choke on the device.

The advantages of nasal-oral temperature sensors

Table 12.3. *Indirect methods for detecting breathing patterns*

1. Transthoracic electrical impedance
2. Contacting motion sensors
   (a) Compliant strain gauge
   (b) Air-filled capsule
   (c) Displacement magnetometer
   (d) Inductance respirometry
3. Noncontacting motion sensors
   (a) Motion-sensing pad
   (b) Radiation reflection
   (c) Variable capacitance
4. Electromyography
5. Breath sounds
6. Intraesophageal pressure
7. Whole-body plethysmography

are that they are relatively inexpensive and not highly complex from the technical point of view. Such devices are capable of making direct measurements of ventilation and can detect obstruction, but they are not easy to use. At the present time, as far as cardiopulmonary monitoring is concerned, nasal and oral temperature sensors should be considered for use in verifying the functioning of other types of respiration monitors, rather than being used as the primary monitor itself.

Indirect sensors of breathing

Indirect sensors of breathing patterns have the advantage that their attachment to the subject is often simpler than that for the direct sensors described in the preceding section. Indirect sensors are also less likely to interfere with breathing patterns, because they are more remote from the airway and are attached to the patient in areas where there is not likely to be direct interference with the control of breathing. Table 12.3 lists many of the indirect methods for sensing breathing patterns. Of these, transthoracic electrical-impedance monitoring is the most frequently applied, both in the intensive-care unit and outside of the hospital. Other types of indirect sensors, such as the noncontacting motion sensors, are beginning to appear on the market, and these will no doubt grow in popularity as clinicians become familiar with them. The following paragraphs give more detailed descriptions of some of these indirect sensors of breathing patterns.

Transthoracic electrical impedance. The electrical impedance of a circuit is a measure of how difficult it is for an electric current to pass through that circuit. It

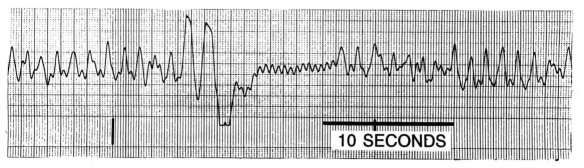

Figure 12.4. Signal from an apneic episode monitored with the transthoracic electrical-impedance method, showing cardiogenic artifact during the apnea.

is more difficult to pass a current through a high-impedance circuit than through a low-impedance circuit. The electrical impedance is a general property that covers all types of signals, whereas electrical resistance is a special case of impedance for signals that do not vary over time (dc signals). The electrical impedance measured between electrodes attached to the chest of an infant will undergo small variations during the infant's breathing cycle and cardiac cycle because of changes in the air and blood volumes in the thoracic structures (Olsson, Daily, and Victorin, 1970). These impedance variations can be measured electrically by special electronic circuits and used to monitor breathing. Investigators have also shown that the cardiac component of these impedance variations can be used to estimate cardiac output. The impedance variations seen with breathing are primarily due to changes in the electrical impedance of the lungs as they fill with air. It would therefore be best to measure these impedance changes by placing electrodes directly on the lungs. That, of course, is not possible, and so electrodes must be placed on the skin surface. Such placement means that the impedance measured between skin electrodes will show much less variation with breathing than they would if they could be placed directly on the lungs. This is because much of the current from the electrodes will be shunted around the lungs through the skin and other subcutaneous tissues. In practice, the breathing component of the impedance measured between electrodes on the skin surface is only about 0.5% of the total impedance measured between these electrodes. Obviously, this small variation is difficult to measure, but there are sophisticated electronic circuits that allow this to be done with reasonable precision.

There is another limitation of transthoracic impedance measurement that is much more serious. Because the component of the impedance due to

breathing is so small, changes in electrical impedance arising from other sources can be of the same size or larger and can interfere with the measurement of breathing. We have already mentioned one such interference: impedance variations over the cardiac cycle. These variations are generally smaller than the variations due to breathing, but in some cases they can still be large enough to produce significant interference. Figure 12.4 is an example of such interference during a brief episode of apnea. Note that the impedance variations due to cardiac activity remain in the signal, even though the respiration variations cease during the apnea.

Relatively large impedance variations will be registered when the subject moves. These variations can be of biologic origin or can result from electrical changes in the interface between the electrodes and the skin. In extreme cases, these movement-induced impedance changes can be so much larger than the breathing-induced changes that they will completely obliterate the signal that we wish to obtain. These impedance variations are known as motion artifacts and represent a major limitation on the transthoracic electrical-impedance technique for infant monitoring. Figure 12.5 illustrates a typical example of how motion artifacts can interfere with a normal breathing signal.

The choice and placement of electrodes for transthoracic electrical-impedance measurement can be important in obtaining the best possible signal quality with minimal artifact. The electrodes used with transthoracic electrical-impedance monitors are the same as those used with the cardiac monitors described earlier in this chapter. Many clinicians have adopted the hydrogel-type electrodes for this use, because they adhere well to the skin, and motion artifacts seem to be reduced when they are used. It is important to note that for a cardiopulmonary monitor, this single set of electrodes can be used to

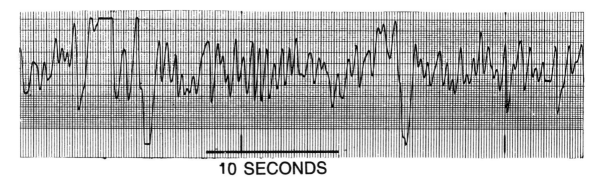

10 SECONDS

Figure 12.5. Example of a transthoracic electrical-impedance recording showing motion artifact along with the respiration signal.

pick up the cardiac signal and the respiration signal. When this is done, however, the optimal placement of the electrodes for one signal may be different from the optimal placement for the other. Baird and co-workers evaluated some of the common electrode placements used in neonatal intensive-care units and found that the best overall position for electrodes for infant cardiopulmonary monitoring was a modified lead II (Baird, Goydos, and Neuman, 1989). In this configuration, the electrodes are placed on the chest in a lead II position, rather than on the limbs. The optimal position, however, varies from one infant to another, and the modified lead II positioning should be considered as a starting point, rather than a fundamental biomedical law.

The frequency of the electrical signal that the monitor uses to measure the transthoracic impedance is also important. At low frequencies, electrode effects can dominate, and this can result in an increase in motion artifact. At frequencies that are too high, the current through the body is primarily in the skin and subcutaneous tissue, and so the effect of impedance changes in the lungs is minimized, thereby reducing the sensitivity of the system. Optimal excitation frequencies for transthoracic electrical-impedance monitors for infant respiration are found in the range from 20 to 100 kHz.

Some clinicians, on first learning that transthoracic electrical-impedance monitors pass a current through the body, have been concerned that such a current might cause electric shock or burning. Two aspects of the monitor design ensure that this cannot happen. First, the current that the monitor passes through the body is kept at a very low level, so that it is below the threshold of sensation. Second, the sensitivity of electrically excitable tissue to electric currents decreases as the frequency of the electric current increases. In the range of frequencies used by infant apnea monitors, there is very

little possibility of any electrical stimulation of tissue (electric shock) because of this. Thus, it can be stated categorically that there is no risk of electric shock or burning from the excitation currents used in transthoracic electrical-impedance monitors.

Contacting motion sensors. As seen from Table 12.3, there are several types of motion sensors that can be used to detect infant breathing. Those that are placed on the body and make contact with it are known as contacting sensors, and those that can sense breathing movements remotely compose the noncontacting category.

Strain-gauge sensors. A strain gauge is a sensor that responds to changes in its length by changing its electrical resistance. Most strain gauges are used to measure very small displacements, and so they are not highly compliant mechanically. Such a strain gauge placed on an infant's chest or abdomen might interfere with breathing and require the infant to exert more effort in breathing, because of having to stretch the strain gauge as well as do the work of breathing. A special type of strain gauge consisting of a compliant thin-walled rubber capillary tube filled with mercury was developed by Whitney (1953) as a limb plethysmograph. In this case, as the tube is stretched, the mercury column lengthens and decreases in cross-sectional area, since the total volume of the mercury cannot change. This results in an increase in the electrical resistance of the mercury column between the ends of the tube. Wires connected to the mercury column at each end of the tube allow the resistance of the sensor to be measured, and if the sensor is placed on the chest or abdomen of an infant, such that breathing movements cause it to stretch and contract, it can be used to detect those breathing movements. Because this type of strain gauge is compliant, it places little mechanical constraint on the breathing efforts of the infant, as compared with conventional strain gauges. This type of strain gauge is used primarily for research, and in some cases for in-hospital monitoring and sleep studies. Its utilization is limited by the fact that it contains a toxic substance that might escape from the sensor if it were used in an unsupervised situation. Also, the long-term stability of these sensors is not good, with sensors often becoming noisy after a few days of use.

McIntyre and co-workers designed a sensor based on the strain-gauge principle that combines the best properties of the conventional strain gauge and the Whitney strain gauge (McIntyre and Neuman, 1989). Their device consists of a corrugated piece of plastic material, such as Mylar or polyimide, with strain gauges deposited on it using microelectronic techniques. The corrugated structure can be easily stretched, and it is springy enough to return to its original position. As it is stretched, the conventional strain gauges on its surface are also stretched, but by a much smaller amount, because of the corrugated nature of the structure.

Inductance plethysmography. Inductance is an electromagnetic property of a loop or coil of wire that is affected by the area of the surface enclosed by the coil or loop. Inductance can be measured using a relatively simple electronic circuit, and so if a coil of wire is placed around the abdomen of an infant, and the wire is made in such a way that it is very compliant, then as the infant inhales, the area within the coil will increase, and the opposite will occur as the infant exhales. If a compliant wire is placed within an elastic belt and one of these belts is placed around the chest and another around the abdomen of an infant, it has been reported that the inductance signals from these two belts can be processed in such a way as to give a measure of tidal volume (Adams et al., 1993). This would make it possible to monitor obstructive apneas as well as central apneas using this technology. This technology is available as a commercial product for monitoring in the intensive-care unit.

Air-filled capsule or vest. The breathing efforts of an infant can be detected from the chest or abdominal movements by a sensor consisting of an air-filled compliant tube, disc, or entire vest attached to the infant (Milner and Allen, 1973). As this structure is stretched or compressed by the infant's breathing movements, the pressure of the air within the structure will increase or decrease. This pressure can be measured by coupling the sensor to a sensitive pressure transducer through a flexible tube, and the pressure variations can be monitored in a way similar to the direct monitoring of blood pressure described in the preceding section. The major advantage of this system is its simplicity. Inexpensive structures for attachment to the infant can be produced economically and made to be interchangeable, with a single pressure-sensor electronic instrument. As long as these structures can be maintained in place on the infant's skin, it should be possible to measure pressure variations resulting from breathing. There is a commercial device based on this principle, used primarily in the United Kingdom.

Motion-sensing pad. Although noncontacting motion sensors of breathing and apnea have great appeal because they do not require that anything be put on the infant, few, if any, have been demonstrated to be viable competitors for sensors requiring contact with the patient. One that has seen some clinical application is the motion-sensing pad that is placed under the infant or under the mattress on which the infant sleeps (Lewin, 1969). The sensitive portion of the pad is usually smaller than the infant and is placed under either the thoracic or lumbar region of the infant. The breathing efforts of the infant result in varying forces being applied to the pad as the center of mass of the infant shifts with respiratory motion. These forces cause the pad to generate a periodic electrical signal related to the breathing effort of the infant.

The major limitation of the motion-sensing pad is that it is sensitive to any movement, whether it derives from the infant's breathing effort or from some extraneous source. This means that such a sensor has great sensitivity to artifacts and is not useful unless the infant is resting quietly. Other body movements can be picked up by the sensor, and the device can even respond to movements that are not associated with the infant at all, such as an adult walking near or bumping the infant's bassinet or crib. In the author's laboratory, a motion-sensing pad is used to detect an infant's movements when studies are being performed with other sensors to detect breathing activity, rather than to detect breathing effort. In this type of application, the sensor is a very reliable method for collecting the information.

Signal processing

The signal-processing section of the pulmonary portion of a cardiopulmonary monitor carries out many of the same functions as the signal-processing section of the cardiac portion of the monitor. These are listed in Table 12.4. The overall purpose of the sig-

Table 12.4. *Functions of the signal processors in a cardiopulmonary monitor*

Cardiac	Pulmonary
1. Amplification	1. Amplification
2. Filtering	2. Filtering
3. R-wave detection	3. Breath detection
4. Heart-rate determination	4. Breathing-rate determination
5. Arrhythmia detection	5. Apnea detection
6. Detect alarm conditions	6. Apnea alarm
7. Calculation of heart-rate variability	

nal-processing section is to determine if a breath has been taken by the infant, just as the purpose of the signal processing in the cardiac portion is to determine if there has been a heartbeat. Because the signal from the breathing-sensor portion of the monitor is generally weak and frequently contains a substantial amount of noise and artifact, amplification and filtering play important roles in the signal processing. Unfortunately, there is more overlap between the frequencies contained in noise and artifact and the frequencies of the breathing signal than there is for the ECG, and so it is often difficult to remove enough of this noise to allow reliable detection of breaths. Thus, motion artifacts can have much more serious effects when determining a respiration rate than when determining a heart rate.

Cardiogenic artifacts in the respiration waveform can also make it difficult to identify breaths. Because it is possible for infants to breath at rates that correspond to their heart rates in some situations, the signal-processing section of a monitor can have difficulty in determining whether a particular signal is due to breathing or to cardiogenic artifacts. Because the rates of the breathing and heart signals can be similar, it is not possible to separate these signals by filtering, and another approach must be taken: anti-coincidence detection. If the monitor indicates that there is a breath every time there is heartbeat, this is usually the result of the monitor detecting cardiogenic artifacts as breathing signals. This can occur during apnea and can cause the monitor to fail to identify that apnea. Monitors are able to avoid this problem by simultaneously looking at the cardiac and breathing signals. If the cardiac section of the monitor detects a heartbeat at or near the same time that the pulmonary section detects a breath, and this occurs for several cardiac cycles, it is most likely that this is the result of detecting cardiogenic artifacts, and the monitor ignores the breath-detection signal. This approach usually prevents the monitor from incorrectly registering cardiogenic artifacts as

breaths, but it also has the potential to overlook infant breathing when the breathing rate is the same as the heart rate and breaths occur at about the same time as the QRS complex.

There are several strategies that can be built into a monitor for actual breath detection (Neuman, 1984). Because the waveforms of individual breaths sensed by the monitor can vary from one breath to the next, in terms of amplitude, duration, and general configuration, it is not as easy to detect breaths as it is to detect heartbeats, where the QRS complexes are almost always very similar from one beat to the next. Several sophisticated breath-detection strategies have evolved for use in the signal-processing section of a pulmonary monitor to get around this problem. Nevertheless, breaths can be overlooked, or "extra" breaths erroneously detected, when there are large variations in configuration from one breath to the next or when noise is present. Thus, monitors that detect and report breathing rates frequently make errors because of these overlooked breaths or extra breaths. Although breath-rate determination can be carried out by an averaging or a breath-to-breath technique (as in the case of the cardiotachometer), because of these errors there can be artifactual variations in the instantaneous breath rate. These errors generally are not as severe when the breath rate is averaged.

The most important aspect of the signal-processing function in the pulmonary portion of a monitor is determination of the duration of apnea. This involves measuring the time between successive breaths. If the time exceeds a preset threshold, the measured interval can be considered an apnea. An alarm function is built into the apnea detector, so that if the apnea exceeds a predetermined duration (e.g., 20 s), an alarm will be sounded. Monitors with the capability to record events often have a shorter-duration trigger for the recording of apnea than for activation of the apnea alarm. This is an effort to aid in the diagnosis of breathing problems in infants

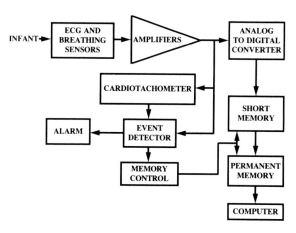

Figure 12.6. Block diagram for a cardiopulmonary monitor. The ECG and breathing signals are detected by sensors on the infant, and these signals are processed by amplifiers and filters. A cardiotachometer determines the heart rate, and an event detector looks at the heart-rate and respiration signals to determine if any significant events are occurring. If it is found that there are significant events, the memory control circuit will store these events in permanent memory and, if appropriate, sound an alarm. The analog-to-digital converter circuit puts the signals in digital format so that they can be stored in the short memory, which is constantly updating itself with the actual data being monitored. When an event occurs, the memory control moves the information from the short memory to the permanent memory, and this information can be read by computer or presented as a permanent paper printout at a later time.

while at the same time avoiding excessive, unnecessary use of the alarm.

Display

Pulmonary monitors have display requirements similar to those previously described for cardiac monitors. In the simplest form, a display should indicate that a breath has been detected. This can be done using a flashing light or another kind of indicator on a computer screen. For monitors that determine the respiratory rate, there should be some type of digital or analog display of that rate. Most monitors that are used in intensive-care units also show the respiratory waveform on a computer screen. This is useful to help identify significant events and their causes, so that appropriate therapeutic measures can be taken Apnea-alarm conditions should also be indicated both visually and audibly when they occur. In cases where a visual display of the waveform is provided, it is useful to have the onset of the alarm indicated on the waveform so that the caretaker can identify the cause of

the alarm and quickly rule out an alarm that was incorrectly triggered while the infant continued to breathe.

CARDIOPULMONARY MONITOR

The cardiac and pulmonary portions of a cardiopulmonary monitor are integrated together in the actual monitor. Figure 12.6 shows a general block diagram for such a monitor. Certain functions of the integrated monitor can be carried out by common components. For example, when a cardiac monitor is used with a transthoracic electrical-impedance breathing monitor, the same electrodes can be used for sensing the ECG and for introducing the current for the transthoracic impedance determination. A circuit connected to these electrodes will separate out the two signals and send them to the appropriate parts of the monitor. Similarly, an integrated display can be used to show cardiac and pulmonary signals together. Waveforms can be plotted alongside one another, and other data can be integrated on the monitor front panel or screen so that information can be presented to the clinician in the most efficient way.

Event-recording monitors include computer memory in their internal circuits, so that data associated with predetermined conditions can be stored for later analysis. This memory makes it possible to have a permanent record of the event that set off a monitor alarm. The record of the event and the data surrounding it are stored in the monitor's memory so that they can be downloaded into a computer at a later time. The computer contains software that allows that event to be displayed on the computer screen and/or printed out on paper for inclusion in the infant's chart. Because most monitors, at some time or other, will indicate that an alarm threshold has been crossed when in fact the infant is breathing normally, it is useful to have this event-recording function. By observing the actual data that triggered the alarm, one can identify a false alarm and discount it. This is especially useful for monitors used in the home, because it provides hard evidence of the events described by the caregiver. With some monitors it is possible to set the threshold for activation of this event-recording capability using a set of conditions different from those used to sound an alarm. These conditions are generally less stringent than the alarm conditions; for example, an apnea monitor might be set to record apneic episodes lasting longer than 15 s, but be set to trigger its alarm only if the apnea exceeds 20 s.

A monitor's memory functions generally are integrated so that when an alarm condition or a recording condition occurs for either the cardiac or the pulmonary portion of the monitor, signals from both will be recorded for the time interval leading up to the event, during the event, and for a short time following the resolution of the event. Often, if other variables, such as the degree of oxygen saturation in the hemoglobin of arterial blood, are being monitored along with the cardiopulmonary variables, these signals will also be stored in memory, so that the clinician reviewing the signals at a later time can get a full picture of what occurred.

In addition to these features, monitors also have certain capabilities for evaluating their own functioning. Monitors that are used with electrodes have internal circuits that determine when an electrode lead wire has come loose or when the contact between the electrode and the skin has deteriorated to the point that it can interfere with the quality of the signals being recorded. This is an alarm condition, with an indicator to point out that a lead is not functioning correctly and needs to be replaced.

Monitors that are used for infants at home have an additional feature: a compliance record. This is a portion of the monitor's memory that indicates when the monitor is being used. When the memory of the monitor is downloaded, this information is provided to the clinician responsible for the patient being monitored. It can help the clinician determine how frequently the monitor is being used, as well as provide medical-legal protection. Such a system may also prompt better compliance by the parents using the monitor at home, in that they will know that a record of how often they have used the monitor will be provided to their physician.

Monitor safety and efficacy

There are two general considerations in determining whether or not a monitor is useful in the clinical setting. The device must be safe, and it must be effective. Manufacturers of monitoring equipment must be able to demonstrate that both of these conditions are met before they are allowed to market their products. The U.S. Food and Drug Administration has undertaken preparation of a set of standards and testing procedures to evaluate infant apnea monitors. These standards will mandate safety features for all monitors and help to clarify the electrical and environmental conditions appropriate for a monitor's use. They should also address the approaches to be taken to demonstrate the clinical effectiveness of infant monitoring technology. Although the final version of these standards has

not yet been published, a draft version covers the clinical and laboratory tests that can be used to demonstrate the effectiveness of these monitors. Such tests will use electronic simulations of signals from patients to represent real or hypothetical data from infant cardiopulmonary monitoring.

There have been few publications concerning the effectiveness of infant cardiopulmonary monitors. Weese-Mayer and colleagues evaluated one type of home monitor for infant apnea (Weese-Mayer et al., 1989; Weese-Mayer and Silvestri, 1992). Their findings indicate that a large proportion of the alarms coming from event-recording transthoracic electrical-impedance cardiopulmonary monitors are in fact false alarms. Many of these alarms result from equipment failures, such as loose leads. The data for those studies were collected in the late 1980s, and since then there have been many improvements in monitor design, especially with regard to signal processing. So it is anticipated that performance ratings will be better for the more recently developed monitors. Nevertheless, the clinician should not expect perfect performance from electronic cardiopulmonary monitors.

CONCLUSIONS

Cardiopulmonary monitoring has played an important role in neonatal intensive care since the mid-1960s. It has made close surveillance of infants possible, so that life-threatening events such as prolonged apnea can be quickly detected and treated. Today, cardiopulmonary monitoring has moved beyond the hospital and is being used at home in caring for recently discharged premature infants and as a possible preventive strategy for dealing with infants at risk for SIDS. Cardiopulmonary monitors detect signals related to the heart and breathing and process those signals to yield rate and rhythm information. These monitors also have the capability of triggering an alarm when a condition of clinical concern arises, such as prolonged apnea. Although these devices have been of great assistance to clinicians and have extended the venues in which care can be given, it is important to remember that they are not perfect. It is possible, because of the presence of noise and the artifacts so often associated with movement of the patient, that there will be sufficient interference with the signals being monitored that reliable operation will not be possible. Thus, clinicians should rely on such monitors to supplement the information gathered with their own senses. One should never consider the monitor a replacement for a well-trained, caring clinical staff.

REFERENCES

Adams, J. A., Zabaleta, I. A., Stroth, D., Johnson, P., and Sackner, M. A. (1993). Tidal volume measurements in newborns using respiratory inductive plethysmography. *American Review of Respiratory Disease* 148:585–8.

Anonymous. (1993). Hazard: risk of electric shock from patient monitoring cables and electrode lead wires. *Health Devices* 22:301–3.

Baird, T. M., Goydos, J., and Neuman, M. R. (1989). Optical lead placement for monitoring the ECG and breathing in infants. *Pediatric Pulmonology* 7:276.

Comroe, J. H., Forster, R. E., Dubois, A. B., Briscoe, W. A., and Carlsen, E. (1962). *The Lung*. Chicago: Year Book.

Jenkins, J. M. (1983). Automated electrocardiography and arrhythmia monitoring. *Progress in Cardiovascular Diseases* 25:367–408.

Lewin, J. E. (1969). An apnoea-alarm mattress. *Lancet* 2:667–8.

Little, G. A., and members of the NIH Consensus Development Panel. (1987). Apnea monitoring: technical aspects. In *Infantile Apnea and Home Monitoring*, U.S. Department of Health and Human Services, NIH publication 87-2905.

McIntyre, T., and Neuman, M. R. (1989). Thin film sensor for infant respiration. In *Proceedings of the 11th IEEE-EMBS Annual International Conference*, ed. Y. Kim and F. A. Spelman (pp. 1115–16). New York: IEEE.

Milner, A. D., and Allen, D. G. (1973). The respiratory jacket: a method for measuring tidal and minute volumes in the newborn. *Guy's Hospital Reports* 122:109–13.

Neuman, M. R. (1984). Optimal detection of respiration and apnea by infant monitors. In: *Medical Technology for the Neonate* (pp. 49–54). Arlington, VA: Association for the Advancement of Medical Instrumentation.

(1986). A microelectronic biotelemetry system for monitoring neonatal respiration using thermistors. Paper presented at the 21st annual meeting of the Association for the Advancement of Medical Instrumentation, Chicago, April 14.

Olsson, T., Daily, W., and Victorin, L. (1970). Transthoracic impedance: theoretical considerations and technical approach. *Acta Paediatrica Scandinavica* [Suppl.] 207:1–27.

Rigatto, H., and Brady, J. P. (1972). A new nose piece for measuring ventilation in preterm infants. *Journal of Applied Physiology* 32:423–4.

Webster, J. G. (ed.). (1992). *Medical Instrumentation: Application and Design*, 2nd ed. Boston: Houghton Mifflin.

Weese-Mayer, D. E., Brouillette, R. T., Morrow, A. S., et al. (1989). Assessing validity of infant monitor alarms with event recording. *Journal of Pediatrics* 115:702.

Weese-Mayer, D. E., and Silvestri, J. N. (1992). Documented monitoring: an alarming turn of events. *Clinics in Perinatology* 19:891–906.

Whitney, R. J. (1953). The measurement of volume changes in human limbs. *Journal of Physiology* (London) 121:127.

Cerebral electrophysiology: Visual, auditory, and somatosensory evoked potentials

MARGOT J. TAYLOR, Ph.D.

INTRODUCTION

Evoked potentials (EPs) are averaged electrical responses that can be recorded from peripheral and central branches of the nervous system, via surface electrodes, to reflect the functional integrity of the sensory pathways. EPs provide nonpainful, noninvasive means to examine various aspects of the nervous system. The latencies and amplitudes of the various EP waveforms can index specific types of damage or dysfunction along these sensory pathways from periphery to cortex. The EPs are obtained in response to repetitive sensory stimulation (auditory, visual, or somatosensory). The individual responses have to be averaged so that the EP, which is constant relative to the stimulus, will emerge from the background noise [electroencephalogram (EEG), electromyogram (EMG)] which is of a higher amplitude than the EP, but random relative to the stimulus.

Recording EPs is a standard part of the investigation in numerous medical applications, but EPs are underutilized in pediatrics, especially in neonatology. This results in part from a general misconception that EPs are more difficult to record in infants, whereas in fact EPs are easier to record in infants, as the potentials generally are much larger, and usually there are fewer artifacts in infants, so that fewer trials per average are needed. A more significant difficulty is that many laboratories are not equipped to do studies in infants (i.e., they do not have

appropriate norms). This is critical, because EP patterns undergo very rapid development in the neonatal period, and without age-matched norms, studies are of little use. Thus, the paucity of studies employing EPs in some neonatal populations has not resulted from technical problems, by and large, but from the fact that relatively few investigators have taken EP monitoring into neonatal wards. EPs provide objective, noninvasive measures of the functioning of the central nervous system (CNS), which in neonates can be difficult to obtain by standard clinical assessments. For sick neonates, the lack of information is even more acute, and the EP findings are more important as an adjunct to the clinical examination. This chapter outlines the methods for recording neonatal EPs and their early developmental changes in the auditory, visual, and somatosensory modalities and then gives an overview of some of the applications of EP recordings in neonatology.

METHODOLOGY AND EARLY DEVELOPMENT

Recording EPs in neonates is generally similar to recording them in children and adults, although some methodological details differ. In neonates, the electrodes should be fixed on the scalp using nonirritating tape and saline jelly, and the electrodes need to be applied gently to avoid unnecessary agitation or irritation. In older infants, the electrodes can be at-

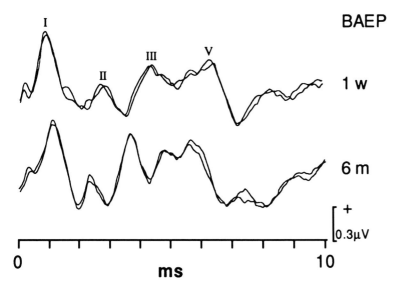

Figure 13.1. BAEP recordings from two infants. That for the 1-wk-old infant (top tracings) shows clear definition of waves I, II, III, and V, but a plateau effect between waves III and V. In the lower tracings, a BAEP from a 6-mo-old shows clearer definition of wave IV and significant shortening of all the latencies, apart from wave I. The BAEP is almost mature by this age, although some latency decreases continue until about 18 mo of age.

tached using an adhesive paste (e.g., EC2 from Grass Instruments) and gauze (or cotton ball). Although electrodes held with paste can fall off of a restless infant, they are easily replaced. If an infant is so restless that the electrodes will not stay on with paste, then that infant probably is not calm enough to have EPs recorded. However, even in infants who are quite restless, cortical EPs usually can still be obtained, because of the large-amplitude responses in this population. Replicating averages is absolutely essential when recording EPs. In other words, at least two averages, using identical recording parameters, must be collected, and the averages superimposed. If the EPs do not replicate (i.e., look very similar, with the peaks occurring at the same latencies), further averages need to be collected. Only when reproducible or replicable peaks are obtained can the EPs be reliably interpreted.

The designations for the component waves of the various EPs differ from one laboratory to another, even within a country, and internationally there is little consensus as to the names or the polarity with which the EPs are recorded. Typically, an "N" followed by a number (e.g., N70) denotes a negative wave occurring at 70 ms after stimulus presentation. Similarly, a "P" (e.g., P200) denotes a positive peak occurring at 200 ms. However, some laboratories code only the order of successive peaks (e.g., N1,

P1, N2, P2), whereas others use the mean latency for the age group with which they are working (e.g., the P35 in an adult is the P28 in children). The exception is the brain-stem auditory evoked potential, as virtually all laboratories use roman numerals to denote the positive components, regardless of their latencies. Unfortunately, for the visual and somatosensory evoked potentials, it is only familiarity with the literature and the EPs themselves that enables one to recognize that an N1 in one study is the same as the N20 or N35 in another. In this chapter, the peaks for the visual and somatosensory evoked potentials are labeled using the nomenclature from established adult norms.

Brain-stem auditory evoked potentials

Brain-stem auditory evoked potentials (BAEPs) typically are elicited in response to the stimulus of a brief broadband "click," and the recorded waveforms reflect conduction along the auditory brainstem pathway. The BAEP has five component waves that are routinely measured (Figure 13.1): Waves I and II arise from the distal and rostral portions of the eighth nerve, respectively; wave III is from the pons, and waves IV and V are from the midbrain. In normal neonates, all of these waves occur within 10 ms after stimulus presentation. The

BAEPs are the smallest of the EPs reviewed in this chapter (about half a microvolt) and require considerably more trials per average (approximately 1,000) than the EPs in the other modalities before a replicable response will emerge from the background noise.

Recording parameters

The BAEP is recorded from electrodes placed on the vertex and the ipsilateral mastoids or earlobes. In young infants, the vertex electrode is best located midline, anterior to the fontanelle. Because an infant's response will be slower than that of a child or an adult, the recording sweep needs to be long (15–20 ms) and the low-frequency cutoff for the filters should also be low (~20–30 Hz), particularly if responses to low-intensity stimuli are being examined. A second recording channel is recommended between the vertex and the contralateral ear, as it can give better IV-V differentiation. If a third channel is available, an ear-to-ear montage is also recommended, as it will provide a clearer wave I. The value of using these three channels for BAEPs is evident particularly in neonates with abnormal BAEPs, in which wave definition may be poor, and the use of three channels facilitates reliable clinical interpretations.

Clicks presented through earphones are the only stimuli for which there are extensive normative data for infants; the standard stimuli in most labs are rarefaction clicks. If alternating clicks are used for neonates, the latency differences between the responses to condensation and rarefaction clicks may distort wave I (Stockard and Westmoreland, 1981). Because an infant's responses will be more sensitive to the rate of stimulation than will an adult's, rate- and age-specific normative data are necessary for comparison. The intensity of the click should be calibrated relative to normal hearing thresholds or levels (nHL) for adults in the laboratory, and one must ensure that the earphones do not slip off the ear or occlude the ear canal, both of which can alter the intensity delivered. In babies, it is best to hold the earphone on the ear by hand; in premature babies it should be held above the ear, as their ear canals can be collapsed by the weight of the earphone.

Frequency-specific thresholds can be determined with techniques utilizing masking (Picton, Stapells, and Campbell, 1981), and they may provide more information about infant hearing than is obtained using the more usual broadband clicks (Hyde, 1985), but the accuracy of frequency-specific BAEPs in terms of threshold determination is lower (Hyde, Matsumoto, and Alberti, 1987). Concerns also remain about the specificity of frequency-specific BAEPs (Hyde, 1988).

Maturation of the BAEP

A recognizable BAEP can be recorded in premature infants by 28–30 wk of gestational age (Schulman-Galambos and Galambos, 1975; Starr et al., 1977), but only with stimuli presented at high intensities and slow rates. The BAEP amplitude is smaller than in full-term neonates, and the latencies of all of the components decrease with increasing conceptional age as the auditory pathway matures (Fawer and Dubowitz, 1982; Mayer, 1990). Wave V shows greater latency decreases with age than does wave I; thus the I-V interpeak latency also decreases with age. A few recent studies have shown slightly different maturational rates in the extrauterine versus intrauterine environment (Collet et al., 1989; Yamamoto et al., 1990), although the explanation does not appear to lie in accelerated maturation of the sensory system itself (Collet et al., 1989).

The BAEP in a term newborn is also generally smaller than a child's; wave I can be double-peaked, and wave II is often replaced by a prominent negativity after wave I. The wave I : V amplitude ratio is also much higher in infants, and waves III, IV, and V are somewhat merged, producing a plateau-like effect (Figure 13.1). As the relative amplitudes of the BAEP waves change rapidly during infancy (Salamy, Mendelson, and Tooley, 1982; Mochizuki et al., 1983), the I : V amplitude ratio requires extensive age-matched normative data. When establishing amplitude norms, it is essential to keep the bandpass constant; a 150-Hz low-frequency cutoff (which is fine for children or adults) results in a very small wave V in neonates (Weber, 1982).

The BAEP matures to the adult pattern in normal children by 18–24 mo (Hecox and Galambos, 1974; Mochizuki et al., 1983), although the various waves mature at different rates, with the peripheral components maturing earlier. Wave I latency reaches adult values by 2–6 mo, whereas waves III and V show a rapid decrease in latency over the first 3 mo and then a slower decrease, to reach normal adult values by the middle to end of the second year.

As with other EPs, the most important measurements are the latencies. There are considerable differences between the norms reported by various laboratories because of factors such as intensity, stimulation rate, and the difficulty of wave I identification in neonates. Thus, it is mandatory that one establish one's own laboratory norms or follow very carefully the methods of the laboratory whose norms one is using. In the neonatal period, the variability of wave latencies is quite large (much greater than in older infants and children), such that one must be cautious about overinterpreting latency abnormalities in this age group (Hyde et al., 1987). There have been conflicting reports whether or not there are sex differences in neonatal BAEPs (Durieux-Smith et al., 1985; Hyde et al., 1987; Chiarenza, D'Ambrosio, and Cazzullo, 1988), although they are certainly present from early childhood (Mochizuki et al., 1983).

Visual evoked potentials

Visual evoked potentials (VEPs) are cortical responses to various visual stimuli measured over the occipital lobes. Subcortical aspects of the visual pathway cannot be measured reliably with EPs, but differentiation between anterior and posterior aspects of the visual pathway can be achieved using electroretinograms (ERGs) and monocular stimulation, recording over both occipital lobes. The primary components measured are the N70 and P100, and both are cortically generated (although these components occur at much longer latencies in babies). The flash and pattern VEPs probably are generated from different but overlapping neuronal populations; for a review, see Regan (1989).

VEPs can be elicited by a flashing light [stroboscopic lamps or goggles with light-emitting diodes (LEDs)] or by pattern stimuli (reversing, or onset/offset, checks, bars, or pinwheels). Pattern stimuli provide far more sensitive measures of visual function and are the only means to accurately estimate visual acuity neurophysiologically. However, in neonates, pattern VEPs often are not feasible. The flash VEPs yield valuable information in this population and are more widely used, because of the difficulty or impossibility of using pattern VEPs in sick neonates.

Recording parameters

Flash VEPs. Flash VEPs are usually recorded in response to the stimulus of red-light-emitting diodes (LEDs) mounted in goggles. Goggles are far easier to use than a stroboscopic flash and are readily employed in neonatal intensive-care units. There are significant differences between the latencies, amplitudes, and distributions of VEPs elicited by LEDs and by stroboscopic flashes (Mushin et al., 1984;

Taylor and Farrell, 1987), and therefore one must have norms specific to each stimulus. The variability for both types of flash VEPs is high, and the range of "normal" is wide, particularly when rapid maturational changes in responses are occurring.

The VEP is usually recorded from occipital electrodes referenced to either F_z or the earlobes. For routine flash VEPs, a single active electrode at O_z is usually sufficient. For neonates, a sweep of 1,000 ms and a stimulus rate of 0.5 Hz are recommended. A bandpass of 1–100 Hz is used, and 40–60 trials per average typically are collected, although replicable responses often can be obtained with fewer trials. In premature infants, the number of trials per average required is even less, because of a much larger signal-to-noise ratio. We have found 20–30 trials quite adequate; Pryds, Greisen, and Trojaborg (1988) reported reliable VEP recording in premature infants using only 3 trials, with very long interstimulus intervals.

Pattern-reversal VEPs. High-contrast reversing checkerboards are the most commonly used pattern stimuli for infants. Several adaptations to the standard testing procedures using pattern VEPs are almost essential to obtain high-quality recordings of pattern VEPs in very young patients: (1) The infant is held seated in front of the stimulus screen in an area away from distracting objects; (2) an observer (screened from view) holds the infant's interest with sounds and/or small objects in front of the stimulus and uses an interrupt switch so that VEPs will be recorded only when the infant is looking at the stimulus; and (3) a large stimulus field is used, so that small changes in gaze will not be important. A check size subtending 60 min of arc should produce clear recordings of VEPs from a cooperative infant; if not, larger check sizes should be employed. Because of the large-amplitude VEPs recorded in young infants, usually only 20–50 trials will be required to obtain a reproducible response (McCulloch and Skarf, 1991); in preterm infants, the number is also low, about 20 trials (Grose et al., 1989). The bandpass should be 1–100 Hz (although 1–30 and 1–50 Hz are also commonly used), the rate $2\,\text{s}^{-1}$, and the sweep 300–500 ms. Because the latencies of the VEP components change significantly with alterations in the filters, norms need to be established with the bandpass used for clinical testing.

Although both binocular testing and monocular testing are possible in young infants, usually only binocular testing is done, because of limited cooperation and attention spans. Monocular testing is par-

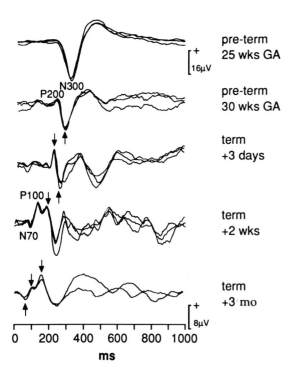

Figure 13.2. VEPs recorded in response to LED-goggle stimulation in neonates. The top tracings show responses from a preterm infant, containing only a late slow negative wave at 300 ms (N300). By 30 wk GA in some infants, particularly those born more prematurely, an earlier positive component emerges at around 200 ms (P200). In the term neonate (3rd trace), the P200 is the most prominent of the components. Shortly after term, an earlier positivity also emerges (P100), and the N70 becomes clearer. In the early postterm period (3 months), the latencies of all three of these components (N70, P100, P200) decrease very rapidly.

ticularly difficult in infants who have unequal vision in the two eyes, as they tend to become upset when the better eye is patched; however, a recent study reported reliable monocular VEP recording from birth onward (McCulloch and Skarf, 1991).

Maturation of the VEP

Flash VEPs. The LED-flash VEPs show remarkable developmental changes during the premature and early postnatal periods. VEPs can be recorded in premature infants starting at about 24 wk of gestational age (GA), but at that age there is only a single late negative peak at 300 ms (N300) (Figure 13.2). At about 26 wk GA, a later positivity emerges (P450), and by 37 wk GA an earlier positivity at 200 ms (P200) is seen (Mushin et al., 1984; Taylor et al.,

1987). These morphological changes are believed to reflect maturational changes in structure and cortical organization in the occipital lobes (Kurtzberg and Vaughan, 1986; Taylor et al., 1987). Among premature neonates, we found evidence suggesting that there is more rapid maturation of the visual pathway in the extrauterine environment than in the intrauterine environment. This requires that VEP norms be established for specific ages of infants in the premature period as a function of GA at birth. After 40 wk of age, rapid maturation is still reflected in the recorded VEPs. The P200 becomes a bifid, with an earlier positivity emerging between birth and 4 wk of age. There is a gradual shortening in the latency of these peaks over the next couple of months (Taylor et al., 1987).

Stroboscopic-flash VEP recordings also show rapid maturation over the premature period, with a similar pattern of emerging components with increasing GA (Kurtzberg and Vaughan, 1986; Stanley, Fleming, and Morgan, 1987). The waveform develops adultlike morphology between birth and 4 mo of age, varying with recording parameters and varying among laboratories. This maturational process does not appear to be affected by prematurity (Ellingson, 1986). There are striking latency decreases over the first 3 mo of life (Ellingson et al., 1972; Laget et al., 1977; Harden, 1982), whereas the reported latency and amplitude changes in the primary components subsequent to that age have been slight. Thus, there are some differences in the maturational patterns of these two types of flash VEPs, emphasizing the need for stimulus-specific norms, but the rapid developmental progressions are similar; the aspect of the visual system assessed by flash stimuli matures very early.

Pattern-reversal VEPs. The maturational changes seen with pattern VEPs differ from those seen with flash VEPs and are dependent on the size of the checks used to elicit the VEPs (Sokol, Moskowitz, and Towle, 1981). VEPs to large check sizes (i.e., 120 min of arc) can be recorded in the late premature period, as well as from birth onward (Sokol, 1982; Fiorentini, Pirchio, and Spinelli, 1983; Harding et al., 1989; Grose et al., 1989; McCulloch and Skarf, 1991). In the first month of life, the VEPs are simple waveforms with only a large, slow positive component, unlike the large negative component first seen with flash VEPs. The maturational changes to large check sizes are quite rapid, with the negative components preceding and following the large positivity appearing at 2 mo of age. An adultlike VEP is recorded by 6 mo to 1 yr of age (Moskowitz and

Sokol, 1983). For small check sizes (i.e., 15 min), the maturational pattern is slower, and VEPs to these small stimuli cannot be recorded in the neonatal period. A simple slow positive component is recorded by 3 mo of age.

A number of other aspects of visual function can be assessed with VEPs in infants, and although they are not widely studied in clinical laboratories, they deserve mention. Contrast sensitivity can be measured by steady-state VEPs to contrast gratings, although such sensitivity is quite immature in the neonatal period (Atkinson, Braddick, and French, 1979). VEPs also provide a reliable means for assessing the development of cortical binocularity (Braddick, Atkinson, and Wattam-Bell, 1986). Measurable VEPs to binocular stimuli appear between 5 and 20 wk of age (Braddick, Wattam-Bell, and Atkinson, 1984; Eizenman, Skarf, and McCulloch, 1988, 1989b), and orientation specificity can be assessed in infants (Braddick et al., 1986) from 5 to 6 wk of age onward. Temporal and spatial properties of the pattern VEP can also be assessed in the neonatal period (Porciatti, 1984). Thus, these several aspects of striate cortical function can be tested, and maturational changes can be monitored if there is concern about their development.

Somatosensory evoked potentials

Somatosensory evoked potentials (SEPs) provide an objective tool with which to assess the neuraxis from peripheral nerve through to the cerebral cortex. In infants, the use of SEPs is particularly relevant, as a clinical examination of the somatosensory system is very difficult. The SEPs are technically the most difficult of the EPs to record, and the techniques have to be changed between testing in very young infants and in older infants. SEP studies are generally very well tolerated by infants. The SEPs (like the VEPs) are larger in infants than in adults; thus, the number of trials required to obtain reproducible results is considerably less than that in adults.

The usual eliciting stimuli are electrical pulses applied over a peripheral nerve, most commonly the median nerve. The recorded potentials from this nerve reflect the afferent volley through the brachial plexus (N9) and entry into the cervical spine (N12), cuneate nucleus (N13), subcortical structures (medial lemniscus and thalamus) (P16, N18), and postcentral somatosensory cortex (N20, P22). Similar localization can be obtained with posterior tibial or peroneal nerve stimulation. The N19 and P22 (N22), recorded over the lumbar spine, reflect the afferent volley in the cauda equina and probably postsynaptic activity in the spinal gray matter, respectively. Spinal SEPs can also be recorded along the entire length of the spinal cord, with increasing latencies as distance from the point of stimulation increases. The N30 can be recorded over the cervical cord or can be seen in the cortical recordings and reflects subcortical activity, possibly in the gracile nucleus, and the P35 (P37) is the primary cortical response. Thus, abnormalities in the recorded SEPs can pinpoint damage or dysfunction anywhere along this pathway, although some of the subcortical components, in particular, are poorly delineated in neonates.

Recording parameters

Median nerve SEPs. A number of investigators have studied SEPs in neonates (Desmedt, Brunko, and Debecker, 1976; Willis, Seales, and Frazier, 1984; Gallai et al., 1986; Laureau et al., 1988), although there is no consensus on the recording parameters to be used in this population. A major concern with some of those reports is that the recordings yielded no identifiable components in a certain percentage of studies in normal infants: 15% in the study by Laureau et al. (1988), 30% for Willis et al. (1984). Hence, some authors have considered that in infants, an absence of responses falls within the range of normal. For SEPs to be clinically useful in neonatal populations, it is essential to use a recording method that is able to obtain reproducible responses in all normal babies. Studies using slow stimulation rates, long sweep times, and lower filters appear to have been the most successful in obtaining infant SEPs (Desmedt et al., 1976; Laget et al., 1976). A recent study investigated combinations of these factors in a neonatal population and recommended a low bandpass (1–100 Hz) and few stimuli (25–50) for recording cortical SEPs (Bongers-Schokking et al., 1989).

George and Taylor (1991) found that two different recording paradigms were useful (5–1,500 Hz, with the usual gain used for SEPs, and a sweep of 200 ms; 30–3,000 or 30–1,500 Hz, with a higher gain, and a sweep of 80–100 ms). If replicable responses are obtained with the second setting, then the 5–1,500-Hz setting need not be used. However, in some infants, particularly ill neonates, the only recordable SEP response is a late positive slow wave (at about 90 ms), seen with the longer sweep and lower bandpass. For both settings, only 50–60 trials per average are needed. Gibson, Brezinova, and Levene (1992) also recorded SEPs in normal neonates with a higher bandpass (10–3,000); it is recommended, however, that a lower bandpass be included for neonates. A slow rate of stimulation (1.1 Hz) is necessary in order to obtain SEPs of acceptable amplitude in babies. The stimulation intensity usually needs to be considerably higher than that used in children and adults, in order to produce a motor response. This is, however, easily tolerated by the babies; most seem quite indifferent to the procedure.

Peripheral SEPs (i.e., those from Erb's point and the cervical spine) are best obtained with the same recording parameters as used in older infants and children: 30–3,000-Hz bandpass, at most a 50-ms sweep, and a stimulation rate of about 4 s^{-1}. However, for peripheral recordings, the infant needs to be asleep and in a fixed position in order to obtain reliable responses (Willis et al., 1984). Difficulties in recording the peripheral potentials in neonates can arise because of their very short latencies and because of interference from stimulus artifacts, which on some EP systems extend beyond the latency range of these potentials in neonates. Also, the N9 is often a bifid component in neonates and young infants, and that needs to be taken into account when establishing normative values.

Posterior tibial nerve SEPs. Relatively little work has been reported on lower-limb SEPs in neonates. Gilmore et al. (1987) first reported SEP recording from premature babies, using bilateral stimulation, a 30–1,500-Hz bandpass, and 1,000–3,000 trials per average. They were able to record the primary cortical component from only 55% of preterm infants, and never from those of less than 31 wk GA. Unilateral nerve stimulation does not yield reliable SEPs in a significant proportion of normal infants. Similarly, Tranier et al. (1990) were able to record posterior tibial nerve SEPs from only 57% of neonates, and that percentage decreased with neonates born prematurely. Cindro, Prevec, and Beric (1985) found that 31% of term infants showed no recordable cortical SEPs to posterior tibial nerve stimulation, and Georgesco et al. (1982) found the same for 23% of infants up to 3 mo of age. Also, with a high bandpass (20–2,000 Hz), Laureau and Marlot (1990) were able to record cortical posterior tibial nerve SEPs from 73% of term infants, and spinal SEPs from 98%. In contrast, White and Cooke (1989) reported that with a 1–100-Hz bandpass and a 100–200-ms sweep, cortical SEPs could be recorded from 93% of infants born between 26 and 41 wk GA and tested within the first weeks of life; spinal SEPs

were recorded from 89%. Likewise, A. Pike and N. Marlow (personal communication, 1993), using a 1–100-Hz bandpass and 25–100 stimuli per average (at a rate of 0.5 Hz), reliably obtained unilateral posterior tibial nerve SEPs from all ($N = 93$) normal preterms from 26 wk GA and on. Their greater success likely was due to their use of a lower bandpass than other researchers, much as has been found useful for median nerve SEPs in preterm infants. Thus, with these recording techniques, posterior tibial nerve SEPs can be reliably recorded in all normal neonates, both term and preterm, and hence their use may now be extended to clinical populations.

Maturation of the SEP

SEPs are recorded from pathways that are known to myelinate and mature at varying rates (Yakovlev and Lecours, 1967). Hence, SEPs recorded from the peripheral and central aspects of the nervous system change differentially with growth and development. The latencies of the responses also vary with the length and conduction velocity of the pathways and the number of synapses traversed. Thus, there are numerous factors that contribute to the maturational changes of the SEP, and it is absolutely essential that one have age-matched normal controls.

Median nerve SEPs. During the early neonatal period, the latencies of the peripheral responses change very little; the SEP from Erb's point does not change at all, and the cervical response shows only minimal decreases in latency (Willis et al., 1984; Gallai et al., 1986; Laureau et al., 1988). Increases in size (which increase latencies) and developmental changes (which decrease latencies) balance each other over the first months of life.

The cortical SEPs in preterm neonates have N20 latencies of more than 70 ms for infants under 30 wk GA (Klimach and Cooke, 1988a) (Figure 13.3). Studies have consistently reported rapid decreases in latencies over the premature and early postnatal periods, such that significant differences were seen over 2-wk periods (e.g., 39–41 wk) (Gallai et al., 1986; Klimach and Cooke, 1988a; Karniski, 1992). Karniski et al. (1992), in an extensive topographic analysis of preterm SEPs, found that the components themselves had changed little during the preterm period. This appears to be a consistent finding even in the early portion (<32 wk) of the preterm period. The components are constant in their appearance in normal preterms from 27 wk on; it is primarily latency changes that are observed between 27 and 40 wk (Karniski, 1992; Taylor, Boor,

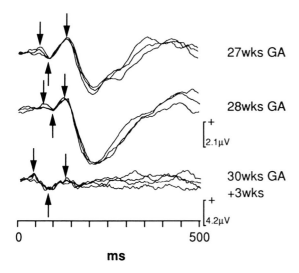

27wks GA

28wks GA

[+
2.1µV

30wks GA
+3wks

[+
4.2µV

0   500

ms

Figure 13.3a. SEPs in three preterm neonates (27 and 28 wk GA, and one born at 30 wk GA, but 3 wk old) showing a late, slow positive-negative-positive complex peaking between 60 and 135 ms. Note that the sweep time for these tracings is 500 ms, and the bandpass is 1–500 Hz.

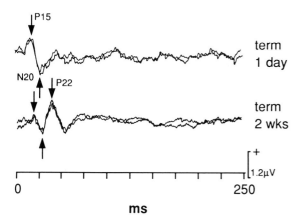

P15

N20   P22

term
1 day

term
2 wks

[+
1.2µV

0   250

ms

Figure 13.3b. SEPs from a term infant (top trace) showing the prominent subcortical component P15 and a subsequent negativity, N20, and SEPs from an infant shortly post-term (bottom trace), showing the clear P22, which emerges in the first month of life; at this age the morphology is similar to that for an adult. Note that the sweep is 200 ms, and these were recorded using a high bandpass of 30–3,000 Hz.

and Ekert, 1994). After the first week of life (Pierrat et al., 1990), differences between term and preterm infants tested at the same conceptional age have not been found (Bongers-Schokking et al., 1990a; Majnemer et al., 1990); thus, this aspect of the somatosensory pathway matures at a constant rate that is independent of an intrauterine or an extrauterine environment. After term, more complex waveforms

are recorded (Gallai et al., 1986; Bongers-Schokking et al., 1990a; Gibson et al., 1992).

Several studies have reported on the postterm maturation of the infant cortical SEP (Cullity et al., 1976; Willis et al., 1984; Tomita, Nishimura, and Tanaka, 1986; Laureau et al., 1988). Across all of the studies, decreasing latencies were reported with increasing age. Laget et al. (1976) found that a mature waveform (i.e., with all the same deflections as seen in the adult waveform) was recorded between 7 and 16 wk of age. We have also found significant changes in the latency, amplitude, and morphology of the cortical SEP over the early neonatal period (George and Taylor, 1991). At birth, the major deflections are the subcortical component, the P15, and the following negative component, the N20, occurring at about 30 ms (Figure 13.3b). Over the first 3 wk of life, the major components become the N20 and a subsequent P22, which emerges during the first 2 wk of life. There is a rapid decrease in the latency of these cortical components over the first 3 mo of life, particularly the first 3 wk. The N20 and P22 continue to decrease during infancy and early childhood, until the myelination of the pathways is complete (Bartel et al., 1987; Zhu, Georgesco, and Cadilhac, 1987; Taylor & Fagan, 1988).

Posterior tibial nerve SEPs. Maturational changes of the SEPs from the lower limb appear to occur at a slower rate than those from median nerve stimulation. It has also been reported that prematurity affects the posterior tibial nerve SEPs (Tranier et al., 1990), unlike the median nerve SEPs. There is no consensus in the literature whether or not the morphology changes over the preterm and early postterm periods. Latencies of the spinal SEP decrease steadily over the preterm and postterm periods (Gilmore et al., 1987; White and Cooke, 1989). Thus, despite the increasing size of the neonates, the latencies decrease, reflecting the marked effect of myelination and maturation of this pathway. The cortical components also decrease in latency over the preterm and early postterm periods, related to the postmenstrual ages of the infants (White and Cook, 1989; A. Pike and N. Marlow, personal communication, 1993; cf. Gilmore et al., 1987); thereafter, they stabilize, as growth and pathway maturation balance each other out.

State of arousal

The state of arousal of the neonate during EP testing can affect the results. The exception is the BAEP, which is unaffected by sleep, general anesthetics, and most drugs. It is far preferable to record BAEPs while an infant is asleep, as the BAEP is the smallest of the EPs and the most difficult to record from restless infants (McCall and Ferraro, 1991). The majority of reports on the flash VEP say that it is unaffected by the sleep state in term infants, although individual exceptions to this general rule can be seen. Careful monitoring of the arousal state has been shown to reduce intraindividual VEP variability (Apkarian, Mirmiran, and Tijssen, 1991). That study was one of the few that found significant effects of sleep on the flash VEP in term infants. In premature infants, the sleep state affects the amplitude of the recorded response: The P200 component can disappear in those premature infants who already have shown this component, and the N300 can also be seriously reduced in amplitude. Thus, in the preterm population, VEPs need to be recorded when the infants are awake or in active sleep (Watanabe, Iwase, and Hara, 1972; Whyte, Pearce, and Taylor, 1987; Grose et al., 1989). As it is difficult to record pattern VEPs without the infant alert and looking at the stimulus, these are routinely done with cooperative, awake babies.

Sleep produces a flattening and lengthening of the cortical median nerve SEPs in neonates (George and Taylor, 1991), such that they need to be recorded from awake infants. Sedation also affects the cortical SEPs, but this should not be an issue in the neonatal population, as sedation should not be necessary. Among preterm infants, the studies in the literature have not reported that sleep adversely affected the recordings. Why this differs between the term and preterm populations is not clear. Sleep does not seem to be a major factor in recording posterior tibial nerve SEPs from term babies. Gilmore et al. (1987) found the lower-limb SEPs easier to obtain from one-third of preterm infants when they were sleeping, although occasionally the cortical response disappeared with sleep. White and Cooke (1989) recorded all of their preterm SEPs from sleeping infants.

Thus, the arousal state needs to be taken into consideration in interpreting EP results. For the SEPs and VEPs, if abnormally small or dispersed responses are recorded from a sleeping infant, it is advisable to wake the baby and repeat the testing. For the BAEPs, the opposite is true: Poor responses from a restless infant can become quite normal if testing is repeated when the infant is sleeping.

CLINICAL APPLICATIONS

Audiology

Hearing impairment early in life can significantly affect the normal development of speech and language. Even a mild hearing loss that is undetected for longer than 6 mo can interfere with normal language development (Davis et al., 1986). It is therefore extremely important to detect any hearing impairment as early as possible. Thus, all newborn infants who are considered at risk for hearing impairment (i.e., a family history of deafness, congenital perinatal infection such as rubella or herpes, prematurity, birth asphyxia, head or neck malformations) should be evaluated during the neonatal period (Picton, Taylor, and Durieux-Smith, 1992). These high-risk factors can be found in 10–12% of all newborn infants, up to 5% of whom will have significant hearing loss. High-risk registers detect about 75% of hearing-impaired infants (Feinmesser and Tell, 1976), but the remaining 25% can be identified only by observant parents and medical staff, who should request audiological evaluation when there is any question about an infant's ability to hear. The reflex responses to loud sounds that are used in early infancy are not at all reliable if the baby is unresponsive because of sickness or if there is a mild or moderate hearing loss. Otoacoustic-emission tests are currently being developed for assessing cochlear impairment in neonates (e.g., Zwicker and Schorn, 1990), and although they are easily performed with appropriate equipment, they have a higher error rate than BAEP recordings and do not pick up sensorineural hearing losses. Thus, they may play a role in neonatal screening, but currently the BAEP recording is the only accurate technique for fully assessing hearing in young infants.

Neonatal screening

For screening neonates, replicate BAEP averages should be obtained for each ear using 70-dB nHL clicks presented in a standard recording paradigm. If clear BAEPs are not obtained, then testing should be repeated at 80 dB or, if necessary, 90 dB. The hearing threshold is then assessed using 30- or 40-dB clicks presented at a rate of 31–61 s^{-1} and averaging at least 4,000 responses. If recognizable BAEPs are not seen, then intensities should be increased until an auditory threshold is obtained. The BAEP can be recorded in normal newborn infants down to at least 30 dB nHL (Hyde et al., 1984; Durieux-Smith et al., 1985; Adelman et al., 1990), provided the testing is technically adequate. Although neonates' thresholds may be somewhat elevated immediately after birth (relative to adults), they will decrease to adult levels by 2 wk of age (Adelman et al., 1990). Thresholds higher than 40 dB nHL are very good predictors of moderate hearing loss and quite good predictors of mild hearing loss. Use of a threshold cutoff of 30 dB nHL will detect more babies who will be found to have mild hearing loss at follow-up, but will also increase the false-positive rate (Hyde, Riko, and Malizia, 1990). Any infant not showing BAEPs at 30 or 40 dB should be retested 3–4 mo later. Although many of these infants will have developed normal thresholds by that time, because a transient perinatal conductive loss will have resolved (Balkany et al., 1978), continued BAEP threshold abnormalities strongly suggest a permanent hearing loss, and therapy should be started (Pollack, 1982). Very few children who pass the BAEP neonatal screening procedure will have auditory impairments at long-term follow-up (Durieux-Smith and Picton, 1988; Hyde et al., 1990).

Several studies have reported the incidence of hearing loss as detected by BAEP screening of all graduates of neonatal intensive-care units (e.g., Alberti et al., 1983; Galambos, Hicks, and Wilson, 1984; Jacobson and Morehouse, 1984) and 1–5% have had sensorineural hearing losses that required hearing aids. That yield is sufficient to justify the screening program. Although screening at 3–6 mo would be more accurate than screening in the neonatal period, it is better to assess infants while they are in the hospital than to risk their not returning for BAEP testing several months later. Of the high-risk infants tested, up to 20% will show audiological abnormalities on BAEP recordings (Guinard et al., 1989).

BAEPs and hearing

It is important to remember that the BAEP recording does not really allow one to assess "hearing." Cortical aspects of the auditory pathway can be assessed with long-latency auditory EPs (AEPs), which when elicited by speech sounds may provide information on the higher-order auditory processing necessary for language development (Kurtzberg et al., 1984). Although technically more difficult to record than the BAEPs, the long-latency AEP can be recorded in infants from term onward, and it is indicated for those infants who have normal BAEPs but evidence of auditory impairment.

There are also infants with good hearing who have abnormal BAEPs. As there are many parallel pathways in the auditory system, there may be some dysfunction that affects the pathways, or synchrony within the pathways, generating the BAEP, while sparing other pathways that are sufficient for hearing. Using the BAEP to evaluate auditory thresholds in infants with neurological disorders must be done cautiously, although about two-thirds of infants with neurologically abnormal BAEPs

show normal BAEP thresholds (Galambos et al., 1984). A history of perinatal anoxia or prematurity should also warn of a possible disorder of the BAEP that can improve with age. In these patients, repeated testing is required before any decision can be made as to their hearing.

Ophthalmology

Assessing visual acuity

Accurate assessment of visual function in infants is critical. Uncorrected visual-system disturbances early in life can result in permanent visual loss, because cortical development in the visual system is strongly influenced by visual experience during critical periods early in life. Even for infants with uncorrectable visual impairment, early assessment is important for diagnosis and prompt referral to appropriate programs to assist with the early development of visually impaired children. The VEP is not usually the first test for assessing ocular causes of decreased visual acuity, but it is useful if other tests indicate abnormality or if they do not explain behavioral visual loss. The pattern VEP can be recorded from birth onward, providing an objective measure of visual function and a quantifiable index of visual impairment (Taylor and McCulloch, 1992).

Visual thresholds can be determined directly from the parameters (e.g., visual angle) of stimuli that elicit just-detectable VEP signals. However, VEPs elicited by near-threshold stimuli are small and difficult to record reliably. Nevertheless, a common clinical technique for estimating visual acuity is to determine the smallest pattern size that will elicit an identifiable VEP. An empirical judgment of visual impairment is based on the stimulus required to elicit the VEP. Several more rigorous methods of estimating visual acuity from VEPs are currently being used: (1) extrapolation of the VEP amplitude-versus-pattern-size function to zero or to the noise level (Campbell and Maffei, 1970; Sokol et al., 1983); (2) sweep techniques presenting a sequence of pattern stimuli with rapidly decreasing pattern sizes (the threshold pattern size is measured where the signal-to-noise ratio of the VEP is unity) (Tyler et al., 1979; Norcia and Tyler, 1985); (3) statistical detection of near-threshold VEP signals in response to small stimuli (Eizenman et al., 1989a).

Disorders of the visual system

The pattern VEP is recorded from the visual cortices, which predominately process information from the central 10° of visual field; hence, its use is in the evaluation of macular pathways and macular vision. In contrast, as the flash ERG is unaffected by localized areas of retinal dysfunction, a normal flash ERG can be recorded even when there is a lesion affecting the entire macular area. Thus, it is useful to record both potentials to differentiate between generalized retinal disorders and disorders affecting only the macula. ERGs should also be recorded from infants who are visually unresponsive, to rule out retinal abnormalities.

Media opacities such as congenital cataracts or persistent hyperplastic primary vitreous (PHPV) prevent examination of the retina and optic nerve. Flash stimuli are transmitted through these opacities, and normal flash VEPs indicate that at least some portions of the visual pathways from the retina to the visual cortex are functioning. In many ocular abnormalities, including optic nerve hypoplasia, macular lesions, congenital glaucoma, and retinal disorders, degrees of visual acuity vary greatly among patients. The use of VEP recordings for assessment of acuity allows a reliable estimate of visual function in infants and can help guide treatment or monitor changes in vision caused by a disorder.

In infants who do not appear to see (i.e., they do not fix and follow), VEP recordings can assist in the differential diagnosis of delayed visual maturation versus visual impairment. Delayed visual maturation is reduced visual responsiveness from birth that subsequently improves. VEPs may reflect delayed maturation (i.e., prolonged latency for age), but are clearly recordable and distinguish these infants from those with serious visual impairments (Fielder et al., 1985). Visual immaturity may be secondary to other neurological disorders (e.g., Gambi et al., 1980; Guthkelch et al., 1984; Placzek, Mushin, and Dubowitz, 1985) or may appear to be only a visual-system disturbance (Fielder et al., 1985; Lambert, Kriss, and Taylor, 1989). VEPs can be used to monitor maturation in such cases and to determine whether or not and when a baby's visual system normalizes.

Clincial neonatology

The neonatal population is a particularly difficult group in which to obtain accurate clinical assessments of sensory and neurological functions, and EPs can provide invaluable information during the postnatal course. This is especially true in sick neonates, in whom the clinical examination may not accurately reflect the likely outcome. Given the appropriate recording techniques, as outlined earlier, the recording of multimodal EPs is relatively straightforward, even in the neonatal intensive-care unit. Recording can be repeated on a daily basis without adversely affecting the infant or the interpretability of the data.

Sensory function

As discussed in the section on audiology, BAEPs provide the only reasonably accurate means for assessing hearing function in neonates. However, in order to have useful predictive power in terms of hearing function, the BAEPs need to be studied in infants at term who are not ill, and the tests should be repeated after several months if the findings are abnormal (Stockard et al., 1983; Picton et al., 1992). Visual acuity can be assessed with pattern VEPs in neonates (as described in ophthalmology), but in order to produce reliable results, this assessment also must be carried out in full-term babies who are not critically ill. If there is concern about the integrity of the somatosensory pathways in infants, because of brachial plexus or cord injury perinatally or postnatally, median nerve SEPs can help to distinguish between complete and incomplete lesions (Wark et al., 1987; Fagan, Taylor, and Logan, 1987). The SEPs can be recorded in the acute stage, and repeat SEP recordings can monitor the recovery of function.

Neonatal asphyxia

Birth asphyxia is the major cause of neonatal mortality and morbidity and is the single largest cause of nonprogressive neurological deficits in childhood. Because of rapid advances in the care and treatment of high-risk newborns, their survival rate has increased considerably, but it has been difficult to establish an accurate prognosis protocol for neurodevelopmental outcomes.

A number of authors have investigated EPs as means for assessing cortical damage and predicting outcomes in asphyxiated newborns. Hrbek et al. (1977) reported that VEPs and SEPs were valuable prognostic indicators in asphyxiated infants; however, the gestational ages of the infants and the duration of follow-up were not discussed. Hakamada et al. (1981) studied VEPs and AEPs in infants with a range of perinatal disorders. They found that abnormal EPs, particularly long-lasting abnormalities, were related to the severity of the outcome for those infants. However, they still had a misclassification rate of 28–30%, probably because of their inclusion of infants with a wide variety of medical and surgical problems. Also, they did not analyze the utility of the AEPs and VEPs separately.

A number of investigators have also studied the BAEP as a prognostic measure in high-risk infants (Salamy et al., 1980; Hecox and Cone, 1981; Stockard et al., 1983). In the ill neonatal population, however, transient abnormalities in the BAEP are quite common and necessitate repeat BAEP testing at least 1 mo after the initial study before any accurate prognostic indication can be determined (Stockard et al., 1983; Picton et al., 1992). Karmel et al. (1988) reported that more detailed analyses of BAEPs in conjunction with cranial ultrasound could predict neurological sequelae, yet they still had a misclassification rate of 23%. Guinard et al. (1989) also reported BAEPs to be of only limited value for assessing neurological abnormalities in high-risk neonates. Thus, the BAEP is not useful early in the neonatal period for predicting neurological outcome.

In contrast, VEPs correlate well with both short- and long-term neurological outcomes in asphyxiated infants (Whyte et al., 1986; Taylor et al., 1989; Muttitt et al., 1991); VEPs also have some prognostic value regarding visual outcome (McCulloch, Taylor, and Whyte, 1991). All the neonates included in those studies were full-term asphyxiated infants who had VEPs recorded within the first 3 d of life. The VEP recordings were repeated several times within the first week of life and then at weekly intervals until discharge. The infants were all enrolled in an intensive follow-up program that included return visits (during which VEP recordings were repeated) until 24 mo of age. VEPs were divided into the normal (which included consistently normal VEPs and those that were transiently abnormal, i.e., they normalized within the first week of life) (Figure 13.4a) and the abnormal (those that were consistently abnormal in the first week or were absent at any time during the first week) (Figure 13.5a). The VEPs had a predictive accuracy of 87% for the group as a whole, and 93% for the group of moderately asphyxiated infants (Sarnat stage II) (misclassifications of 13% and 7%, respectively). An absence of VEPs at any time during the first week or persistently abnormal VEPs throughout the first week of life were always (100%) associated with death or severe neurological sequelae. Thus, despite the simplicity of this measure of CNS function, in that population the VEPs provided an accurate prognostic indicator of neurological sequelae.

SEPs have also been recorded in term asphyxiated neonates. Willis, Duncan, and Bell (1987) and Majnemer et al. (1987) reported that SEPs were reliable predictors of outcome in high-risk neonates, al-

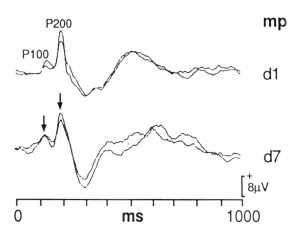

Figure 13.4a. VEPs in a moderately asphyxiated neonate recorded on days 1 and 7 showing normal responses and the presence of the P100 and P200 even on the first day of life. This infant developed normally and had normal neurodevelopmental assessment at 2 yrs of age.

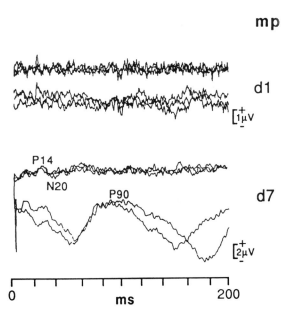

Figure 13.4b. SEPs for the same infant as in Figure 13.4a showing absence of responses on the first day of life and small responses by day 7. Two bandpasses were used to record SEPs in the neonatal period. The top tracing of each pair used a bandpass of 30–3,000 Hz, and the bottom tracing of each pair used a 5–1,500-Hz bandpass.

though Willis et al. (1987) recorded the SEPs at 2 mo after birth, when clinical assessments are also accurate predictors, and Majnemer et al. (1987) included asphyxiated, preterm, and small-for-gestational-age babies in their series and also tested them at some

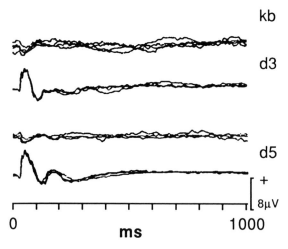

kb

d3

d5

+

8μV

0   ms   1000

Figure 13.5a. VEPs and ERGs from a severely asphyxiated neonate showing the presence of ERGs but absence of VEPs on both days 3 and 5. This baby died at the end of the first week of life.

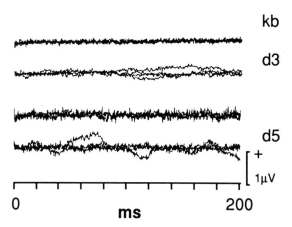

kb

d3

d5

+

1μV

0   ms   200

Figure 13.5b. SEPs from the same infant as in Figure 13.5a showing complete absence of any recordable components on both days 3 and 5.

variable interval after birth. Taylor, Murphy, and Whyte (1992) recorded SEPs within the first 3 d of life and then at regular intervals thereafter. The findings showed the SEPs to be more variable during the critical first week of life (Figure 13.4b) and less accurate as indicators of neurological outcome than were the VEPs. However, normal SEPs within the first week of life were virtually always (97%) positive prognostic signs (Figure 13.4b), whereas consistently abnormal SEPs were usually (85%) indicators of poor outcomes (Figure 13.5). These findings replicate those of de Vries et al. (1991), who also studied term asphyxiated neonates with repeat

SEP testing within the first week of life. They found that normal SEPs were always associated with normal outcomes, and consistently abnormal responses were associated with abnormal outcomes in 90% of cases. Thus, both VEPs and SEPs should be routinely available for assessing the asphyxiated term population, as they provide a very powerful adjunct to the neurological examination. This accuracy requires, however, that the EPs be repeated within the first week of life; a single EP result should always be replicated, preferably 2 d later, as neonates can, on occasion, show remarkable recovery or deterioration in their EPs. In the term asphyxiated neonate, it is recommended that the VEPs be recorded first. If they are abnormal, recording should be repeated by day 3 of life. If still abnormal, the prognostic power is very high, and the prognosis is poor. If the VEPs are normal, then SEPs should be recorded (to try to separate out the 13% who have normal VEPs, but do poorly).

Sequelae of prematurity

A number of authors have utilized EPs to predict outcomes in the high-risk premature population. Placzek et al. (1985) found that VEPs correlated with visual-acuity measures in preterm infants, as well as neurological development, although their follow-up period was very short. Klimach and Cooke (1988b) found a close relation between SEPs recorded close to term and outcomes at 6–16 mo in infants with head ultrasound abnormalities. Infants with asymmetrical SEPs developed hemiplegia, which was not necessarily the case for infants with unilateral lesions. Bilateral SEP abnormalities always predicted neurological sequelae. The head ultrasound and clinical examinations were less reliable prognostically. However, in a larger series, de Vries et al. (1992) found the SEPs at term, in infants born prematurely, to be no more reliable than ultrasonography. Consistently abnormal SEPs did not always predict sequelae, nor did normal SEPs guarantee normal outcomes, although the specificity of the SEPs was 92%. In infants with extensive cystic leukomalacia, absence of VEPs predicted cortical blindness (de Vries et al., 1987), but the median nerve SEPs recorded at term did not predict neurological outcomes (Pierrat et al., 1993). Serial studies in the preterm period may be necessary to increase prognostic power (as is found with term asphyxia). As sequelae of prematurity more often affect the lower limbs than the upper limbs, posterior tibial nerve SEPs may prove to be valuable predictors of outcomes in these infants. There have been no published reports, although A. Pike and N. Marlow (personal communication, 1993) are encouraged by early findings of an apparent association between outcomes and posterior tibial nerve SEPs recorded early in the postnatal period in premature infants, independent of ultrasound findings. A study of VEPs in the preterm population has shown that they are not reliable predictors of neurodevelopmental outcome at 2–3 yr (Ekert, Taylor, and Whyte, 1994). A comparison between these modalities for prognostic utility has yet to be published, but perhaps SEPs will be more useful prognostically than VEPs in infants born prematurely.

Hydrocephalus

Early diagnosis and treatment of hydrocephalus are important to minimize the risk of neurological sequelae. A number of studies have investigated EPs in patients with hydrocephalus in attempts to find a sensitive measure of increased intracranial pressure, associated pathological changes, or an indication of the need for neurosurgical intervention (Ehle and Sklar, 1979; Guthkelch, Sclabassi, and Vries, 1982; Guthkelch et al., 1984; York et al., 1984). Ehle and Sklar (1979) found that all 15 infants they studied had abnormally delayed VEPs, which improved quickly after shunting. Guthkelch et al. (1982) found that increased latencies were observed only when the hydrocephalus was accompanied by increased head size (above the 98th percentile); neonates who were normocephalic had normal VEPs, more often than not. They also reported that the hydrocephalic infants showed slower maturation of the VEP (Guthkelch et al., 1984). On repeat post-shunt testing in infants of less than 4 mo, they found only small decreases in latency. Frequently, BAEPs have also been shown to be abnormal in hydrocephalic infants, many having threshold as well as neurological abnormalities, but the abnormalities have been nonspecific and have not been related to etiology, head size, or brain-stem symptoms (Edwards, Durieux-Smith, and Picton, 1985; Lary et al., 1989).

George and Taylor (1987) studied a series of hydrocephalic infants and recorded VEPs and SEPs when the infants first entered the hospital, and again following shunting if they underwent that procedure. Among infants less than 10 wk of age, most (83%) had abnormal flash VEPs, whereas less than half had abnormal median nerve SEPs. Those abnormalities did not correlate with head circumference or clinical status (Figure 13.6). However, the EP abnormalities improved dramatically within a few days after shunting in all of those infants in

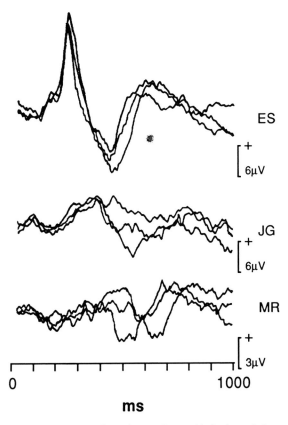

Figure 13.6. VEPs from three infants with hydrocephalus, showing a normal VEP (top trace), a delayed-latency VEP (middle trace), and a complete absence of VEP (bottom trace). The VEPs in the neonatal period are not reliably associated with clinical symptoms, but do show rapid recovery with surgical correction of the hydrocephalus.

whom the shunting procedure was successful. De Vries et al. (1990) found a positive correlation between SEPs and cerebrospinal-fluid pressure in a small series of infants, and they also noted marked improvement following shunting. In another series of neonates with hydrocephalus (>65 infants), we found that the VEPs ranged from normal to absent, and both normal and abnormal VEPs were seen in babies with enlarged head circumferences and in normocephalic infants. Again, the abnormal VEPs improved quickly after shunting, except in those infants who did not improve clinically.

Thus, currently EPs appear to have only limited usefulness acutely in the diagnosis of hydrocephalus or shunt malfunction; their value lies in the monitoring of successful shunting. The variability of the EP findings in hydrocephalic infants probably relates to the range of precipitating factors and to whether the hydrocephalus began prenatally or postnatally, in term or preterm infants. Stretching of the sensory tracks can produce either no sensory-system dysfunction or a mixture of demyelinization and axonal loss, resulting in a combination of latency delays and amplitude reductions, both of which could be confounded in some cases with the mass effects of a tumor. More detailed analyses, with careful documentation of such clinical factors as cerebrospinal-fluid pressure, are needed to increase the utility of EPs in this population.

Arnold-Chiari malformation

Arnold-Chiari malformation is present in infants with myelomeningocele, although only a certain portion will become symptomatic, typically in the first months of life (Park et al., 1983). Because an Arnold-Chiari malformation displaces cerebellar tissue into the upper cervical canal and produces a dislocation of the lower pons, medulla, and fourth ventricle, a number of studies have investigated BAEPs to determine if they have predictive power regarding the emergence of clinical symptoms. Hydrocephalus is commonly associated with Arnold-Chiari malformation and may be secondary to downward compression on the fourth ventricle or an aqueductal anomaly. The application of EP recordings in hydrocephalus was discussed earlier. Holliday et al. (1985) studied 12 patients and found that normal BAEPs always were associated with a failure to develop symptomatic Arnold-Chiari malformation and usually were associated with lumbosacral rather than thoracic myelomeningoceles. Lutschg, Meyer, and Jeanneret-Iseli, (1985) studied 27 children with myelomeningocele and found the longest central conduction times in the patients with hydrocephalus and neurological symptoms. Mori et al. (1988) found BAEPs not predictive, although they tested patients from 1 d to 33 yr of age and found the BAEPs to be more frequently abnormal in younger children. They suggested that the BAEPs may be more valuable if recorded and repeated within the first year of life.

We recorded VEPs and BAEPs in a series of 44 infants presenting with myelomeningocele (2 d to 3 mo of age). The VEPs were normal in 64%, but the BAEPs were normal in only 45%. The BAEPs tended to have a typical morphology, with clear waves I and/or II and then poorly reproducing and/or delayed later waves (Figure 13.7). This was despite technically good testing conditions. The later waves (i.e., III, IV, and V) were often of low amplitude. I-V interpeak latency delays were seen in 29%, and low-amplitude later waves in 52%, with a number of in-

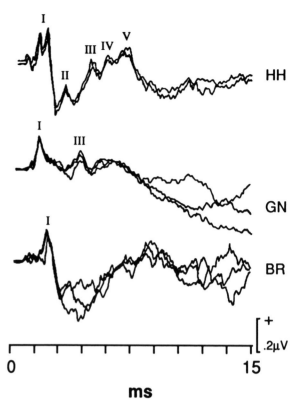

Figure 13.7. BAEPs from three infants with Arnold-Chiari malformations. The top trace shows a normal BAEP, which is seen in about 40% of these patients. The second trace shows normal I and III, in morphology and latency, but very poorly formed and delayed IV and V; this is seen in 25% of these patients. The bottom trace shows a BAEP with a normal wave I and very poorly formed and delayed waves III and V; this type of response is seen in about 45% of these patients, often in conjunction with delayed interpeak latencies.

fants having both abnormalities. The outcomes at 2 yr did not appear to be associated with the early VEPs, whereas abnormal BAEPs were very often associated with neurological sequelae.

Hyperbilirubinemia

Neonatal hyperbilirubinemia can lead to serious neurological sequelae and auditory impairment (Johnston et al., 1967; de Vries, Lary, and Dubowitz, 1985), but the CNS toxicity of bilirubin and the outcome cannot be accurately predicted. Thus, the guidelines for therapeutic intervention in jaundiced newborns have limited value. Investigators have examined EPs, particularly BAEPs, in infants with hyperbilirubinemia in the hope that the EPs might give some indication whether or not an infant would benefit from exchange transfusion and whether or not an infant was likely to suffer neurological or audiological impairment. A concern, particularly in preterm infants, is to determine what bilirubin levels are safe. Prolonged BAEP interpeak latencies while infants are hyperbilirubinemic, with improvement following exchange transfusions, have been widely reported (Perlman et al., 1983; Chin, Taylor, and Perlman, 1985; Nakamura et al., 1985; Streletz et al., 1986). In those studies, however, the BAEP abnormalities did not always covary with bilirubin levels (i.e., only some of the infants with very high bilirubin levels had abnormal BAEPs), and follow-up data were not obtained in those studies to determine if those transient abnormalities were significant (transient BAEP abnormalities are frequently seen in the neonatal population) (e.g., Picton et al., 1992). Soares et al. (1989) found only 8 of 72 hyperbilirubinemic neonates to have BAEP abnormalities. Those authors found no relation between either prematurity or actual bilirubin levels and the BAEPs. They concluded that there was no obvious application for BAEP recordings in this population. A more recent study also showed no relation between BAEP and serum bilirubin concentration, but a significant inverse relation between serum reserve albumin concentration and BAEP (Esbjörner et al., 1991). Those findings may explain the lack of clinical relevance of BAEP abnormalities in earlier studies, and they suggest that the otoneurological toxicity of bilirubin is related to the bilirubin-binding properties of serum albumin. A replication of those data with a larger series would be important to confirm the role of BAEPs in hyperbilirubinemia. Only one study has investigated SEPs in hyperbilirubinemic neonates (Bongers-Schokking et al., 1990b), showing a close association between SEP abnormalities and bilirubin levels in a fairly large series of infants. Those authors suggested that the SEPs could be used as a daily monitor of the effect of bilirubin on the CNS.

Small size for gestational age

Distinguishing between small-for-gestational-age (SGA) infants and preterm neonates (which they resemble in size and weight) is clinically important, as the risk factors are higher for SGA infants than for preterm infants. Reliable criteria for this differentiation can be based on neurological development, an aspect of which can be assessed with EP recordings. Watanabe et al. (1972) found that VEP latencies correlated with postconception age in SGA infants as well as in normal preterm infants, suggesting that neurological development in SGA infants progresses relatively normally and independently of

the unfavorable intrauterine conditions that cause the slower physical growth. In contrast, Hrbek, Iversen, and Olsson (1982) found that although the VEPs of SGA infants generally corresponded to those of age-matched normal neonates, there was a tendency toward longer latencies in the SGA infants, as well as the presence of late slow waves, which those authors believed to be a sign of neurological immaturity. Both of those features, however, were transient. Pryds et al. (1989) examined eight SGA infants and found no abnormalities or unusual patterns of findings. Pettigrew, Edwards, and Henderson-Smart (1985), as well as Soares et al. (1988), found that the BAEP interpeak latencies were in fact shorter in SGA infants that in age-matched controls, although Soares et al. (1988) suggested that that was not due to precocious development of the auditory brain-stem pathway, but to immaturity of the cochlea. Sarda, Dupuy, and Boulot Prieu (1992) further investigated the phenomenon and found that the BAEP latencies were closely associated with the presence or absence of maternal hypertension. That suggests that the cause of the growth retardation affects the EPs, which may also explain the variable findings in the literature to date.

Gallai et al. (1986) found no differences in SEPs between preterm and term populations nor between SGA and normal babies. More recent studies, however, found a significant proportion of SGA infants to have abnormal SEPs (L. S. de Vries, personal communication). Those abnormalities were not associated with neurological sequelae in infants with normal findings on head ultrasound studies, but in a smaller number in whom cerebral palsy was seen, both abnormal ultrasound findings and abnormal SEPs were recorded.

EPs appear to index the maturational stage of the CNS, and SGA infants are distinguishable from preterms in that their EPs reflect their ages, not their sizes. However, growth retardation does not appear to be affecting the CNS uniformly, according to these measures (perhaps because of etiological factors) (Sarda et al., 1992), but because some authors have found abnormalities in the EPs not associated with nervous system disorders, caution must be exercised in interpreting abnormal findings in this population.

Respiratory distress

A few studies have examined the role of EPs in neonates suffering respiratory distress. Graziani, Weitzman, and Pineda (1972) studied 13 premature infants during periods of severe respiratory difficulty and found abnormal VEPs or no VEPs in all cases; the abnormalities were associated with blood gas levels. After repeated or prolonged hypoxemia, only the absence of VEPs was registered, and most of those infants died. Gambi et al. (1980) studied VEPs in infants with respiratory distress, graded from slight to severe. Slight respiratory distress did not affect the VEPs, whereas in infants with moderate to severe respiratory distress the VEPs were abnormal, and in some cases the abnormalities persisted until the 9-mo testing. Pryds et al. (1989) studied 75 infants who required either ventilation or continuous positive airway pressure. They found no differences in VEPs between those infants and their normal controls; the babies requiring ventilation tended to be more premature. Their data would suggest that the infants included in their series did not suffer severe respiratory distress. Our experience has been consistent with that of Gambi et al. (1980), in that among those who have suffered mild or transient respiratory distress, the VEPs have been normal, for both term and preterm neonates. As for those with severe respiratory distress, they usually have suffered significant hypoxic episodes, and the VEPs are more often abnormal. However, the rapid recovery of VEPs following a hypoxic event is a positive prognostic indicator. Continuing VEP abnormalities raise an ominous sign, regardless of cause.

CONCLUSIONS

This chapter has reviewed both the techniques most commonly used for recording EPs in the newborn and the early developmental changes. The very rapid maturational changes in the EPs, including morphological changes in the preterm and early postterm periods and the very rapid latency changes within the first months of life, provide an invaluable means for assessing and monitoring development within the CNS. The maturational changes are such that normative values are absolutely necessary for comparison, and such norms must take into account both the gestational age at birth and the postnatal age, as maturation in the nervous system can be accelerated in preterm infants.

EPs are important in a range of neonatal applications, because of the difficulty of accurate neurological evaluation of infants. EPs also provide a means for reliable assessment of sensory-system functions in neonates. Early identification of infants with hearing loss or visual impairment allows referral to early intervention programs, which can ameliorate the long-term consequences of the disability. VEPs and SEPs provide reliable prognostic information in

asphyxiated term neonates, and EPs can aid in the assessment of various other conditions, such as respiratory distress, myelomeningocele, and delayed intrauterine growth, that can affect the newborn and may lead to neurological sequelae. EP recordings offer a valuable adjunct in the examination of newborn infants, and their place in neonatology units is now well established.

REFERENCES

Adelman, C., Levi, H., Linder, N., and Sohmer, H. (1990). Neonatal auditory brain-stem response threshold and latency: 1 hour to 5 months. *Electroencephalography and Clinical Neurophysiology* 77:77–80.

Alberti, P. W., Hyde, M. L., Riko, K., Corbin, H., and Abramovich, S. (1983). An evaluation of BERA for hearing screening in high-risk neonates. *Laryngoscope* 93:1115–21.

Apkarian, P., Mirmiran, M., and Tijssen, R. (1991). Effects of behavioural state on visual processing in neonates. *Neuropediatrics* 22:85–91.

Atkinson, J., Braddick, O., and French, J. (1979). Contrast sensitivity of the human neonate measured by the VEP. *Investigative Ophthalmology and Visual Science* 18:210–13.

Balkany, T. J., Berman, S. A., Simmons, M. A., and Jafek, B. W. (1978). Middle ear effusions in neonates. *Laryngoscope* 88:398–405.

Bartel, P., Conradie, J., Robinson, E., Prinsloo, J., and Becker, P. (1987) The relationship between median nerve somatosensory evoked potential latencies and age and growth parameters in young children. *Electroencephalography and Clinical Neurophysiology* 68:180–6.

Bongers-Schokking, C. J., Colon, E. J., Hoogland, R. A., Van den Brande, J. L. V., and de Groot, C. J. (1989). The somatosensory evoked potentials of normal infants: influence of filter bandpass, arousal state and number of stimuli. *Brain Development* 11:33–9.

(1990a). Somatosensory evoked potentials in term and preterm infants in relation to postconceptional age and birth weight. *Neuropediatrics* 21:32–6.

(1990b). Somatosensory evoked potentials in neonatal jaundice. *Acta Paediatrica Scandinavica* 79:148–55.

Braddick, O., Atkinson, J., and Wattam-Bell, J. (1986). VER testing of cortical binocularity and pattern detection in infancy. *Documenta Ophthalmologica Proceedings* 45:107–15.

Braddick, O., Wattam-Bell, J., and Atkinson, J. (1984). The onset of binocular function in human infants. *Human Neurobiology* 2:65–9.

Campbell, F., and Maffei, L. (1970). Electrophysiologic evidence for the existence of orientation and size detectors in the human visual system. *Journal of Physiology* 207:635–52.

Chiarenza, G. A., D'Ambrosio, G. M., and Cazzullo, A. G. (1988). Sex and ear differences of brain-stem acoustic evoked potentials in a sample of normal full-term newborns. Normative study. *Electroencephalography and Clinical Neurophysiology* 71:357–66.

Chin, K. C., Taylor, M. J., and Perlman, M. (1985). Improvement in auditory and visual evoked potentials in jaundiced preterm infants after exchange transfusion. *Archives of Disease in Childhood* 60:714–17.

Cindro, L., Prevec, T. S., and Beric, A. (1985). Maturation of cortical potentials evoked by tibial-nerve stimulation in newborns, infants and children aged four and eight years. *Developmental Medicine and Child Neurology* 27:740–5.

Collet, L., Soares, I., Morgon, A., and Salle, B. (1989). Is there a difference between extrauterine and intrauterine maturation on BAEP? *Brain and Development* 11:293–6.

Cullity, P., Franks, C. I., Duckworth, T., and Brown, B. H. (1976). Somatosensory evoked cortical responses: detection in normal infants. *Developmental Medicine and Child Neurology* 18:11–18.

Davis, J. M., Elfenbein, J., Schum, R., and Bentler, R. A. (1986). Effects of mild and moderate hearing impairments on language, educational, and psychosocial behavior of children. *Journal of Speech and Hearing Disorders* 51:53–62.

Desmedt, J. E., Brunko, E., and Debecker, J. (1976). Maturation of the somatosensory evoked potentials in normal infants and children, with special reference to the early N1 component. *Electroencephalography and Clinical Neurophysiology* 40:43–58.

de Vries, L. S., Connell, J., Dubowitz, L. M. S., Oozeer, R. C., Dubowitz, V., and Pennock, J. M. (1987). Neurological electrophysiological and MRI abnormalities in infants with extensive cystic leukomalacia. *Neuropediatrics* 18:61–6.

de Vries, L. S., Eken, P., Pierrat, V., Daniels, H., and Casaer, P. (1992). Prediction of neurodevelopmental outcome in the preterm infant: short latency cortical somatosensory evoked potentials compared with cranial ultrasound. *Archives of Disease in Childhood* 67:1171–81.

de Vries, L. S., Lary, S., and Dubowitz, L. M. S. (1985). Relationship of serum bilirubin levels to ototoxicity and deafness in high-risk low-birth-weight infants. *Pediatrics* 76:351–4.

de Vries, L. S., Pierrat, V., Eken, P., Taketsugu, M., Daniels, H., and Casaer, P. (1991). Prognostic value of early somatosensory evoked potentials for adverse outcome in full-term infants with birth asphyxia. *Brain and Development* 13:320–5.

de Vries, L. S., Pierrat, V., Minami, T., Smet, M., and Casaer, P. (1990). The role of short latency somatosensory evoked responses in infants with rapidly progressive ventricular dilatation. *Neuropediatrics* 21:136–9.

Durieux-Smith, A., Edwards, C. G., Picton, T. W., and MacMurray, B. (1985). Auditory brainstem responses to clicks in neonates. *Journal of Otolaryngology [Suppl.]* 14:12–18.

Durieux-Smith, A., and Picton, T. W. (1988). Predictive value of BERA in the assessment of hearing loss in high-risk infants. *Audiology in Practice* 2:4–6.

Edwards, A. D., McCormick, D. C., Roth, S. C., Elwell, C. E., Peebles, D. M., Cope, M., Wyatt, J. S., Delphy, D. T., and Reynolds, E. O. R. (1992). Cerebral hemodynamic effects of treatment with modified natural surfactant investigated by near infrared spectroscopy. *Pediatric Research* 32:532–6.

Edwards, C. G., Durieux-Smith, A., and Picton, T. W. (1985). Auditory brainstem response audiometry in neonatal hydrocephalus. *Journal of Otolaryngology* 14:40–6.

Ehle, A., and Sklar, F. (1979). Visual evoked potentials in infants with hydrocephalus. *Neurology* 29:1541–4.

Eizenman, M., McCulloch, D., Hui, R., and Skarf, B. (1989a). Detection of threshold visual evoked potentials, non invasive assessment of the visual system. *1989 Technical Digest Series* (Optical Society of America, Washington, DC) 7:88–91.

Eizenman, M., Skarf, B., and McCulloch, D. (1988). Detection of early development of binocular fusion in infants. *Investigative Ophthalmology and Visual Science [Suppl.]* 29:25.

— (1989b). Development of binocular vision in infants. *Investigative Ophthalmology and Visual Science [Suppl]* 30:313.

Ekert, P. G., Taylor, M. J., and Whyte, H. E. Visual evoked potentials (VEPs) for prediction of neurodevelopmental outcome in preterm infants. Presented at the Fifth International Evoked Potential Symposium, Milan, Italy, Sept. 1994.

Ellingson, R. J. (1986). Development of visual evoked potentials and photic driving responses in normal fullterm, low-risk premature, and trisomy-21 infants during the first year of life. *Electroencephalography and Clinical Neurophysiology* 63:309–16.

Ellingson, R. J., Lathrop, G. H., Nelson, B., and Danahy, T. (1972). Visual evoked potentials of infants. *Review of Electroencephalography and Clinical Neurophysiology* 2:395–400.

Esbjörner, E., Larsson, P., Leissner, P., and Wranne, L. (1991). The serum reserve albumin concentration for monoacetyldiaminodiphenyl sulphone and auditory evoked responses during neonatal hyperbilirubinaemia. *Acta Paediatrica Scandinavica* 80:406–12.

Fagan, E. R., Taylor, M. J., and Logan, W. J. (1987). Somatosensory evoked potentials. Part II: A review of clinical applications in paediatric neurology. *Pediatric Neurology* 3:249–55.

Fawer, C., and Dubowitz, L. M. S. (1982). Auditory brain stem response in neurologically normal preterm and fullterm newborn infants. *Neuropaediatrics* 13:200–6.

Feinmesser, M., and Tell, L. (1976). Evaluation of methods for detecting hearing-impairment in infancy and early childhood. In *Early Identification of Hearing Loss*, ed. G. T. Mencher (p. 102). Basel: Karger.

Fielder, A. R., Russell-Eggitt, I. R., Dodd, K. L., and Mellor, D. H. (1985). Delayed visual maturation. *Transactions of the Ophthalmological Society of the United Kingdom* 104:653–61.

Fiorentini, A., Pirchio, M., and Spinelli, D. (1983). Development of retinal and cortical responses to pattern reversal in infants: a selective review. *Behavioural Brain Research* 10:99–106.

Galambos, R., Hicks, G. E., and Wilson, M. J. (1984). The auditory brain stem response reliably predicts hearing loss in graduates of a tertiary intensive care nursery. *Ear and Hearing* 5:254.

Gallai, V., Mazzotta, G., Cagini, L., Del Gatto, F., and Agnelotti, F. (1986). Maturation of SEPs in preterm and full-term neonates. In *Maturation of the CNS and Evoked Potentials*, ed. V. Gallai (pp. 95–106). Amsterdam: Elsevier.

Gambi, D., Rossini, P. M., Albertini, G., Sollazzo, D., Torrioli, M. G., and Polidori, G. C. (1980). Follow-up of visual evoked potential in full-term and pre-term control newborns and in subjects who suffered from perinatal respiratory distress. *Electroencephalography and Clinical Neurophysiology* 48:509–16.

George, S. R., and Taylor, M. J. (1987). VEPs and SEPs in hydrocephalic infants before and after shunting. *Clinical Neurology and Neurosurgery [Suppl. 1]* 89:96 (abstract).

(1991). Somatosensory evoked potentials in neonates and infants: developmental and normative data. *Electroencephalography and Clinical Neurophysiology* 80: 94–102.

Georgesco, M., Rodiere, M., Seror, P., and Cadilhac, J. (1982). Les potentiels cerebraux somesthesiques evoques a partir du membre inferieur chez le nouveau-ne et le nourisson. *Review of Electroencephalography and Clinical Neurophysiology* 12:123–8.

Gibson, N. A., Brezinova, V., and Levene, M. I. (1992). Somatosensory evoked potentials in the term newborn. *Electroencephalography and Clinical Neurophysiology* 84:26–31.

Gilmore, R., Brock, J., Hermansen, M. C., and Baumann, R. (1987). Development of lumbar spinal cord and cortical evoked potentials after tibial nerve stimulation in the preterm newborns: effects of gestational age and other factors. *Electroencephalography and Clinical Neurophysiology* 68:28–39.

Graziani, L. J., Weitzman, E. D., and Pineda, G. (1972). Visual evoked responses during neonatal respiratory disorders in low birth weight infants. *Pediatric Research* 6:203–10.

Grose, J., Harding, G. F. A., Wilton, A. Y., and Bissenden, J. G. (1989). The maturation of the pattern reversal VEP and flash ERG in pre-term infants. *Clinical and Visual Sciences* 4:239–46.

Guinard, C., Fawer, C. L., Despland, P. A., and Calame, A. (1989). Auditory brainstem responses and ultrasound changes in a high-risk infant population. *Helvetica Paediatrica Acta* 43:377–88.

Guthkelch, A. M., Sclabassi, R. J., Hirsch, R. P., and Vries, J. K. (1984). Visual evoked potentials in hydrocephalus: relationship to head size, shunting and mental development. *Neurosurgery* 14:283–6.

Guthkelch, A. M., Sclabassi, R. J., and Vries, J. K. (1982). Changes in the visual evoked potentials of hydrocephalic children. *Neurosurgery* 11:599–602.

Hakamada, S., Watanabe, K., Hara, K., and Miyazaki, S. (1981). The evolution of visual and auditory evoked potentials in infants with perinatal disorder. *Brain Development* 3:339–44.

Harden, A. (1982). Maturation of the visual evoked potentials. In *Clinical Application of Cerebral Evoked Potentials in Pediatric Medicine*, ed. G. A. Chiarenza and D. Papakostopoulos (pp. 41–59). Amsterdam: Excerpta Medica.

Harding, G. F. A., Grose, J., Wilton, A., and Bissenden, J. G. (1989). The pattern reversal VEP in short-gestation infants. *Electroencephalography and Clinical Neurophysiology* 74:76–80.

Hecox, K. E., and Cone, B. (1981). Prognostic importance of brainstem auditory evoked responses after asphyxia. *Neurology* 31:1429–33.

Hecox, K. E., and Galambos, R. (1974). Brainstem auditory evoked responses in human infants and adults. *Archives of Otolaryngology* 99:30–3.

Holliday, P. O., Pillsbury, D., Kelly, D. L., Jr., and Dillard, R. (1985). Brain stem auditory evoked potentials in Arnold-Chiari malformation: possible prognostic value and changes with surgical decompression. *Neurosurgery* 16:48–53.

Hrbek, A., Iversen, N., and Olsson, T. (1982). Evaluation of cerebral function in newborn infants with fetal growth retardation. In *Clinical Applications of Evoked Potentials in Neurology*, ed. J. Courjon, F. Mauguiere, and M. Revol (pp. 89–95). New York: Raven Press.

Hrbek, A., Karlberg, P., Kjellmer, I., Olsson, T., and Riha, M. (1977). Clinical application of evoked electroencephalographic responses in newborn infants. I: Perinatal asphyxia. *Developmental Medicine and Child Neurology* 19:34–44.

Hyde, M. L. (1985). Frequency-specific BERA in infants. *Journal of Otolaryngology* 14:19–27.

(1988). Evoked potential audiometry. In *Scott-Brown's Otolaryngology*, ed. A. G. Kerr and J. Groves (pp. 80–103). London: Butterworth-Heinemann.

Hyde, M. L., Matsumoto, N., and Alberti, P. W. (1987). The normative basis for click and frequency-specific BERA in high-risk infants. *Acta Oto-laryngologica* 103:602–11.

Hyde, M. L., Riko, K., Corbin, H., Moroso, M., and Alberti, P. (1984). A neonatal hearing screening research program using brainstem electric response audiometry. *Journal of Otolaryngology* 13:49–54.

Hyde, M. L., Riko, K., and Malizia, K. (1990). Audiometric accuracy of the click ABR in infants at risk for hearing loss. *Journal of the American Academy of Audiology* 1:59–66.

Jacobson, J. T., and Morehouse, C. R. (1984). Electrophysiologic techniques in audiology and otology: a comparison of auditory brain stem response and behavioural screening in high risk and normal newborn infants. *Ear and Hearing* 5:247–53.

Johnston, W. H., Angara, V., Baumal, R., Hawke, W. A., Johnson, R. H., Keet, S., and Wood, M. (1967). Erythroblastosis fetalis and hyperbilirubinemia, a five-year follow-up with neurological, psychological, and audiological evaluation. *Pediatrics* 39:88–92.

Karmel, B. Z., Gardner, J. M., Zappulla, R. A., Magnano, C. L., and Brown, E. G. (1988). Brain-stem auditory evoked responses as indicators of early brain insult. *Electroencephalography and Clinical Neurophysiology* 71:429–42.

Karniski, W. (1992). The late somatosensory evoked potential in premature and term infants. I. Principal component topography. *Electroencephalography and Clinical Neurophysiology* 84:32–43.

Karniski, W., Wyble, L., Lease, L., and Blair, R. C. (1992). The late somatosensory evoked potential in premature and term infants. II. Topography and latency development. *Electroencephalography and Clinical Neurophysiology* 84:44–54.

Klimach, V. J., and Cooke, R. W. I. (1988a). Maturation of the neonatal somatosensory evoked response in preterm infants. *Developmental Medicine and Child Neurology* 30:208–14.

(1988b). Short-latency cortical somatosensory evoked responses of preterm infants with ultrasound abnormality of the brain. *Developmental Medicine and Child Neurology* 30:215–21.

Kurtzberg, D., Hilpert, P. L., Kreuzer, J. A., and Vaughan, H. G. (1984). Differential maturation of cortical auditory evoked potentials to speech sounds in normal fullterm and very low-birthweight infants. *Developmental Medicine and Child Neurology* 26:466–75.

Kurtzberg, D., and Vaughan, H. G. (1986). Preterm and post-term regional maturation of flash and pattern

ERPs. In *Maturation of the CNS and Evoked Potentials*, ed. V. Gallai (pp. 9–15). Amsterdam: Elsevier.

Laget, P., Flores-Guevara, R., D'Allest, A. M., Ostre, C., Raimbault, J., and Mariani, J. (1977). La maturation des potentiels evoques visuels chez l'enfant normal. *Electroencephalography and Clinical Neurophysiology* 43:732–44.

Laget, P., Raimbault, J., D'Allest, A. M., Flores-Guevara, R., Mariani, J., and Thieriot-Prevost, G. (1976). La maturation des potentiels evoques somesthesiques (pes) chez l'homme. *Electroencephalography and Clinical Neurophysiology* 40:499–515.

Lambert, S. R., Kriss, A., and Taylor, D. (1989). Delayed visual maturation. A longitudinal clinical and electrophysiological assessment. *Ophthalmology* 96:524–9.

Lary, S., De Vries, L. S., Kaiser, A., Dubowitz, L. M., and Dubowitz, V. (1989). Auditory brain stem responses in infants with posthaemorrhagic ventricular dilatation. *Archives of Disease in Childhood* 64:17–23.

Laureau, E., Majnemer, A., Rosenblatt, B., and Riley, P. (1988). A longitudinal study of short latency somatosensory evoked responses in healthy newborns and infants. *Electroencephalography and Clinical Neurophysiology* 71:100–8.

Laureau, E., and Marlot, D. (1990). Somatosensory evoked potentials after median and tibial nerve stimulation in healthy newborns. *Electroencephalography and Clinical Neurophysiology* 76:453–8.

Lutschg, J., Meyer, E., and Jeanneret-Iseli, C. (1985). Brainstem auditory evoked potentials in meningomyelocele. *Neuropediatrics* 16:202–4.

McCall, S., and Ferrar, J. A. (1991). Pediatric ABR screening: pass–fail rates in awake versus asleep neonates. *Journal of the American Academy of Audiology* 2:18–23.

McCulloch, D. L., and Skarf, B. (1991). Development of the human visual system: monocular and binocular pattern VEP latency. *Investigative Ophthalmology and Visual Science* 32:2372–81.

McCulloch, D. L., Taylor, M. J., and Whyte, H. E. (1991). Visual evoked potentials and visual prognosis following perinatal asphyxia. *Archives of Ophthalmology* 109:229–33.

Majnemer, A., Rosenblatt, B., Riley, P., Laureau, E., and O'Gorman, A. M. (1987). Somatosensory evoked response abnormalities in high-risk newborns. *Pediatric Neurology* 3:350–5.

Majnemer, A., Rosenblatt, F., Willis, D., and Lavallee, J. (1990). The effect of gestational age at birth on somatosensory-evoked potentials performed at term. *Journal of Child Neurology* 5:329–35.

Mayer, M. (1990). *Potentiels Evoqués et Electromyographie en Pédiatrie.* Paris: Masson.

Mochizuki, Y., Go, T., Ohkubo, H., and Motomura, T. (1983). Development of human brainstem auditory evoked potentials and gender differences from infants to young adults. *Progress in Neurobiology* 20:273–85.

Mori, K., Uchida, Y., Nishimura, T., and Edhwrudajakpor, P. (1988). Brainstem auditory evoked potentials in Chiari-II malformation. *Child's Nervous System* 4:154–7.

Moskowitz, A., and Sokol, S. (1983). Developmental changes in the human visual system as reflected by the pattern reversal VEP. *Electroencephalography and Clinical Neurophysiology* 56:1–15.

Mushin, J., Hogg, C. R., Dubowitz, L. M. S., Skouteli, H., and Arden, G. B. (1984). Visual evoked responses to light emitting diode (LED) photostimulation in newborn infants. *Electroencephalography and Clinical Neurophysiology* 58:317–20.

Muttitt, S. C., Taylor, M. J., Kobyashi, J., and Whyte, H. E. (1991). Serial evoked visual potentials and outcome in full term birth asphyxia. *Pediatric Neurology* 7:86–90.

Nakamura, H., Takada, S., Shimabuku, R., Matsuo, M., Matsuo T., and Negishi, H. (1985). Auditory nerve and brainstem responses in newborn infants with hyperbilirubinemia. *Pediatrics* 75:703–8.

Norcia, A. M., and Tyler, C. W. (1985). Spatial frequency sweep VEP: visual acuity during the first year of life. *Vision Research* 25:1399–408.

Park, T. S., Hoffman, H. J., Hendrick, E. B., and Humphreys, R. P. (1983). Experience with surgical decompression of the Arnold-Chiari malformation in young infants with myelomeningocele. *Neurosurgery* 13:147–52.

Perlman, M., Fainmesser, P., Sohmer, H., Tamari, H., Wax, Y., and Pevsmer, B. (1983). Auditory nerve–brainstem evoked responses in hyperbilirubinemic neonates. *Pediatrics* 72:658–64.

Pettigrew, A. G., Edwards, D. A., and Henderson-Smart, D. J. (1985). The influence of intra-uterine growth retardation on brainstem development of preterm infants. *Developmental Medicine and Child Neurology* 27:467–72.

Picton, T. W., Stapells, D. R., and Campbell, K. B. (1981). Auditory evoked potentials from the human cochlea and brainstem. *Journal of Otolaryngology [Suppl. 9]* 10:1–41.

Picton, T. W., Taylor, M. J., and Durieux-Smith, A. (1992). Brainstem auditory evoked potentials in pediatrics. In *Electrodiagnosis in Clinical Neurology*, 3rd ed., ed M. J. Aminoff (pp. 537–67). London: Churchill-Livingstone.

Pierrat, V., de Vries, L. S., Minami, T., and Casaer, P. (1990). Somatosensory evoked potentials and adaptation to extrauterine life: a longitudinal study. *Brain and Development* 12:376–9.

Pierrat, V., Eken, P., Duquennoy, C., Rousseau, S., and de Vries, L. S. (1993). Prognostic value of early somatosensory evoked potentials in neonates with cystic leucomalacia. *Developmental Medicine and Child Neurology* 35:683–690.

Placzek, M., Mushin, J., and Dubowitz, L. M. S. (1985). Maturation of the visual evoked response and its correlation with visual acuity in preterm infants. *Developmental Medicine and Child Neurology* 27:448–54.

Pollack, D. (1982). Amplification and auditory/verbal training for the limited hearing infant 0 to 30 months. *Seminars in Speech, Language and Hearing* 3:52–67.

Porciatti, V. (1984). Temporal and spatial properties of the pattern-reversal VEPs in infants below 2 months of age. *Human Neurobiology* 3:97–102.

Pryds, O., Greisen, G., and Trojaborg, W. (1988). Visual evoked potentials in preterm infants during the first hours of life. *Electroencephalography and Clinical Neurophysiology* 71:257–65.

Pryds, O., Trojaborg, W., Carlsen, J., and Jensen, J. (1989). Determinants of visual evoked potentials in preterm infants. *Early Human Development* 19:117–25.

Regan, D. (1989). *Human Brain Electrophysiology: Evoked Potentials and Evoked Magnetic Fields in Science and Medicine.* Amsterdam: Elsevier.

Salamy, A., Mendelson, T., and Tooley, W. (1982). Developmental profiles for the brainstem auditory evoked potential. *Early Human Development* 6:331–9.

Salamy, A., Mendelson, T., Tooley, W., and Chalin, E. (1980). Contrasts in brainstem function between normal and high risk infants in early postnatal life. *Early Human Development* 4:179–85.

Sarda, P., Dupuy, R. P., and Boulot Prieu, D. (1992). Brainstem conduction time abnormalities in small for gestational age infants. *Journal of Perinatal Medicine* 20:57–63.

Schulman-Galambos, C., and Galambos, R. (1975). Brainstem auditory evoked responses in premature infants. *Journal of Speech and Hearing Research* 18:456.

Soares, I., Collet, L., Delorme, C., Salle, B., and Morgon, A. (1989). Are click-evoked BAEPs useful in case of neonate hyperbilirubinemia? *International Journal of Pediatric Otorhinolaryngology* 17:231–7.

Soares, I., Collet, L., Morgon, A., and Salle, B. (1988). Effect of brainstem auditory evoked potential stimulus intensity variations in neonates small for gestational age. *Brain and Development* 10:174–7.

Sokol, S. (1982). Infant visual development: evoked potential estimates. *Annals of the New York Academy of Sciences* 388:514–23.

Sokol, S., Hansen, V., Moskowitz, A., Greenfield, P., and Towle, V. (1983). Evoked potential and preferential looking estimates of visual acuity in paediatric patients. *Ophthalmology* 90:152.

Sokol, S., Moskowitz, A., and Towle, V. L. (1981). Age-related changes in the latency of the visual evoked potential: influence of check size. *Electroencephalography and Clinical Neurophysiology* 51:559–62.

Stanley, O. H., Fleming, P. J., and Morgan, M. H. (1987). Developmental wave form analysis of the neonatal flash evoked potential. *Electroencephalography and Clinical Neurophysiology* 68:149–52.

Starr, A., Amlie, R. N., Martin, W. H., and Sanders, S. (1977). Development of auditory function in newborn infants revealed by auditory brainstem potentials. *Pediatrics* 60:831–9.

Stockard, J. E., Stockard, J. J., Kleinberg, F., and Westmoreland, B. F. (1983). Prognostic value of brainstem auditory evoked potentials in neonates. *Archives of Neurology* 40:360–5.

Stockard, J. E., and Westmoreland, B. F. (1981). Technical considerations in the recording and interpretation of the brainstem auditory evoked potential for neonatal neurologic diagnosis. *American Journal of EEG Technology* 21:31–54.

Streletz, L. J., Graziani, L. J., Branca, P. A., Desai, H. J., Travis, S. F., and Mikaelian, D. O. (1986). Brainstem auditory evoked potentials in fullterm and preterm newborns with hyperbilirubinemia and hypoxemia. *Neuropediatrics* 17:66–71.

Taylor, M. J., Boor, R., and Ekert, P. G. (1994). Preterm maturation of the somatosensory evoked potential. Presented at the Fifth International Evoked Potential Symposium, Milan, Italy, Sept. 1994.

Taylor, M. J., and Fagan, E. (1988). SEPs to median nerve stimulation: normative data for paediatrics. *Electroencephalography and Clinical Neurophysiology* 71:323–30.

Taylor, M. J., and Farrell, E. J. (1987). Latency, morphological and distributional changes in VEPs with various stimuli. *Canadian Journal of Neurological Sciences* 14:244 (abstract).

Taylor, M. J., and McCulloch, D. L. (1992). Visual evoked potentials in infants and children. *Journal of Clinical Neurophysiology* 9:357–72.

Taylor, M. J., Menzies, R., MacMillan, L. J., and Whyte, H. E. (1987). VEPs in normal full-term and premature neonates: longitudinal versus cross-sectional data. *Electroencephalography and Clinical Neurophysiology* 68:20–7.

Taylor, M. J., Murphy, W. J., and Whyte, H. E. (1992). Prognostic reliability of SEPs and VEPs in asphyxiated term infants. *Developmental Medicine and Child Neurology* 34:507–15.

Taylor, M. J., Muttitt, S. C., MacMillan, L. J. and Whyte, H. E. (1989). Longitudinal VEPs and neurological outcome of full-term birth asphyxia. *Canadian Journal of Neurological Sciences* 16:246–7.

Tomita, Y., Nishimura, S., and Tanaka, T. (1986). Short latency SEPs in infants and children: developmental changes and maturational index of SEPs. *Electroencephalography and Clinical Neurophysiology* 65:335–43.

Tranier, S., Chevallier, B., Lemaigre, D., Liot, F., Lagardere, B., and Gallet, J. P. (1990). (Somatosensory evoked potential of the lower extremity in the premature neonate). *Neurophysiologie Clinique* 20:463–79.

Tyler, C., Apkarian, P., Levi, D., and Nakayama, K. (1979). Rapid assessment of visual function: an electronic sweep technique of the pattern visual evoked potential. *Investigative Ophthalmology of Visual Sciences* 18:703–13.

Wark, J. E., George, S. R., Armstrong, D., and Whyte, H. E. (1987). Clinical course and investigations in neonatal high cervical cord injuries resulting from forceps delivery. *Canadian Journal of Neurological Sciences* 14:239 (abstract).

Watanabe, K., Iwase, K., and Hara, K. (1972). Maturation of visual evoked responses in low-birthweight infants. *Developmental Medicine and Child Neurology* 14:425–35.

Weber, B. A. (1982). Comparison of auditory brain stem response latency norms for premature infants. *Ear and Hearing* 3:257.

White, C. P., and Cooke, R. W. I. (1989). Maturation of the cortical evoked response to posterior-nerve stimulation in the preterm neonate. *Developmental Medicine and Child Neurology* 31:657–64.

Whyte, H. E., Pearce, J., and Taylor, M. J. (1987). Changes in the VEP in preterm neonates with arousal states as assessed by EEG monitoring. *Electroencephalography and Clinical Neurophysiology* 68:223–5.

Whyte, H. E., Taylor, M. J., Menzies, R., Chin, K., and MacMillan, L. J. (1986). Prognostic utility of visual evoked potentials in term asphyxiated neonates. *Pediatric Neurology* 2:220–3.

Willis, J., Duncan, C., and Bell, R. (1987). Short-latency somatosensory evoked potentials in perinatal asphyxia. *Pediatric Neurology* 3:203–7.

Willis, J., Seales, D., and Frazier, E. (1984). Short latency somatosensory evoked potentials in infants. *Electroencephalography and Clinical Neurophysiology* 59:366–73.

Yakovlev, P. I., and Lecours, A. R. (1967). The myelogenetic cycles of regional maturation of the brain. In *Regional Development of the Brain in Early Life*, ed. A. Minkowski (pp. 3–70). Oxford: Blackwell.

Yamamoto, N., Watanabe, K., Sugiura, J., Okada, J., Nagae, H., and Fugimoto, Y. (1990). Marked latency change of auditory brainstem response in preterm infants in the early postnatal period. *Brain and Development* 12:766–9.

York, D. H., Legan, M., Benner, S., and Watts, C. (1984). Further studies with a noninvasive method of intracranial pressure estimation. *Neurosurgery* 14:456–61.

Zhu, Y., Georgesco, M., and Cadilhac, J. (1987). Normal latency values of early cortical somatosensory evoked potentials in children. *Electroencephalography and Clinical Neurophysiology* 68:471–4.

Zwicker, E., and Schorn, K. (1990). Delayed evoked otoacoustic emissions – an ideal screening test for excluding hearing impairment in infants. *Audiology* 29:241–51.

14

Blood-pressure monitoring

ROBERT A. DARNALL, M.D.

INTRODUCTION

Arterial blood pressure is determined by many factors, including ventricular function, filling of the arterial system, and flow through peripheral resistance. Accurate, direct measurements of arterial pressure, often considered the "gold standard," must also take into consideration reflections of wave energy, the effects of natural oscillation or resonance, and the many variables introduced by the external tubing, transducer, and monitor system.

Most noninvasive methods that are said to measure pressure really do not measure pressure at all, but *estimate* pressure by analyzing various artifacts that result from changes in flow produced by first compressing an artery in an extremity with a pressure cuff and then monitoring various phenomena that occur as the pressure in the cuff is reduced. These phenomena can be detected by palpation or auscultation, or with some externally placed transducer. The almost forgotten flush technique depends on observing color change (flush) in the skin. The palpation methods depend on feeling a pulse. The auscultation technique involves listening for sounds of turbulence generated by flow in a partially compressed vessel. Doppler techniques look at the motions of vessel walls or the movement of blood cells. Oscillometry analyzes the pressure oscillations transmitted to the cuff by the pulsation of the underlying artery. It is not surprising, therefore, that simultaneous measurements of blood pressure using different techniques often produce different values for systolic, diastolic, and mean pressure, and the values obtained with noninvasive methods do not always closely agree with directly measured pressure.

The importance of serial blood-pressure measurements can also be questioned on the basis of the observation that changes in peripheral vascular resistance, rather than pressure, seem to constitute the dominant mechanism to alter perfusion over wide ranges of both physiological and pathologic conditions. Regional vascular resistance is, for the most part, determined by local metabolic needs, and the changes in that resistance affect venous return and cardiac output. Thus, the regulatory system appears to be designed to maintain a relatively constant pressure despite wide variations in regional resistance. Some extreme examples of this in nature can be seen in diving birds and mammals, in which, during submersion, peripheral perfusion is markedly reduced, with little change in mean arterial pressure. One could argue, therefore, that measurements of blood pressure may not offer the best assessments of the physiological processes we would like to monitor, namely, regional perfusion and metabolic needs.

Nevertheless, qualitative inferences often can be drawn from changes in arterial pressure. In a sick neonate, there are many situations in which low blood pressure correlates with a low-flow state. Conversely, hypertension in newborn infants is increasingly becoming recognized as a significant problem. In these situations we rely faithfully on the numbers provided by our monitors to help us make accurate clinical assessments and therapeutic decisions. All too frequently, however, we tend to expect the equipment to do its work and give us the correct result without further effort on our part. More than 20 yr ago, Lenfant observed that

. . . any researcher spends considerable time learning about and checking the instruments that he is going to use; this is, in fact, the first requirement of research apprenticeship. Each physician, no matter how busy he might be, must assure that he or anyone else responsible to him will learn about his equipment. It is fallacious to believe that a fool-proof instrument . . . can be developed. (Lenfant, 1973)

The purpose of this review is to acquaint physicians, nurse practitioners, nurses, respiratory therapists, and other caretakers with the technology involved in direct and indirect measurements of blood pressure in newborn infants. It is hoped that increased knowledge of how various devices function, as well as increased understanding of the many variables that can affect the accuracy of any measurement, will promote a logical, commonsense approach to their use.

BACKGROUND AND DEFINITIONS

The first recorded measurement of blood pressure was made by Hales in 1731, by inserting tubing into an artery in the neck of a horse and observing the height of the blood column (about 9 ft in that case). The U-shaped mercury manometer was introduced by Poiseuille almost 100 yr later, making it possible to take direct measurements within a reasonable space. The sphygmograph was developed shortly thereafter, and in 1856 Faivre measured the blood pressure in a man for the first time. Oscillometry is actually the oldest noninvasive technique, first described by Marey in 1876. Riva-Rocci introduced the blood-pressure cuff about 20 yr later, and in 1905 Korotkoff described indirect measurement of blood pressure by auscultation. Ultrasound methods to measure blood pressure are based on observations made by Doppler in 1842, but they were not actually used for blood-pressure measurements until the 1950s (Darnall, 1985).

To begin, it may be helpful to provide some definitions of commonly used terms, taken from Bruner (1978). *Pressure* is force per unit area, usually measured in dynes; millimeters of mercury (mm Hg) or centimeters of water (cm H_2O) are the units most frequently used in the clinical setting. These units of measure are valid only if the force exerted by gravity is constant. A more general unit, the torr, named after the Italian physicist Torricelli, was established to compensate for variations in the force exerted by gravity, as might occur in space or on another planet. On earth, 1 torr is the same as 1 mm Hg. Pressure is measured as the differential force per unit area between two specified points, or "across" one or more components of the system. In clinical situations, one of the "points" is almost always atmospheric pressure.

A *wave* is a traveling disturbance that carries energy. The medium through which the wave moves is disturbed, but does not necessarily travel with the wave. The medium, however, can have both velocity and direction different from those of the wave. Thus, the direction of *flow* of the medium is not necessarily related to the direction of the wave traveling through it. Waves are characterized by frequency, intensity or amplitude, direction, and velocity. The *frequency* is the number of wave peaks that occur in a given period of time. The *amplitude* is a measure of the perturbation of the medium from its resting state. For each type of wave disturbance (sound, for example), there is a fixed *velocity* in a given medium (water, air, etc.).

Every physiological and mechanical system that has the properties of inertia and compliance will have a characteristic *resonant frequency* (f_n) at which it will naturally vibrate. Such an oscillating system will vibrate with greater intensity if one adds to it small increments of energy whose frequency matches the resonant frequency. Simple examples include rocking a vehicle to get it out of a snow bank, and the functioning of a child's backyard swing. *Damping* is a measure of the tendency of such an oscillating system to come to rest. An underdamped system tends to "ring" or oscillate at its resonant frequency when excited by an external force. In contrast, an overdamped system will have a lower frequency response.

Impedance is a measure of resistance to change. It is an index of the change in force associated with a change in activity in a system. For the purpose of this discussion, impedance can be defined as the ratio of change in pressure associated with a change in flow. Impedance is important with respect to the efficiency of the transfer of energy between the components of a system. When two systems are in series, energy is transferred most efficiently when the output impedance of the first matches the input impedance of the second. When the impedance of the second system is higher than that of the first, energy that is not transferred, owing to an impedance mismatch, is reflected. Thus, *amplification* of a pressure-wave disturbance occurs as it moves into narrower and narrower channels (a tapered tube). The amplification occurs because of reflections of energy produced by the increasing impedance encountered by the wave.

DIRECT MEASUREMENT OF ARTERIAL BLOOD PRESSURE

The pressure pulse

Arterial blood pressure is measured directly by analyzing the pressure pulse. The pressure pulse is a

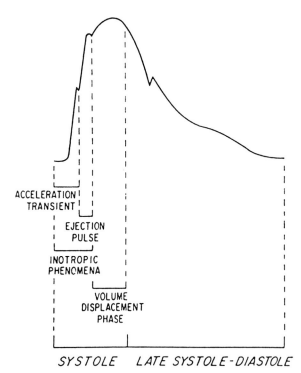

ACCELERATION
TRANSIENT

EJECTION
PULSE

INOTROPIC
PHENOMENA

VOLUME
DISPLACEMENT
PHASE

SYSTOLE   LATE SYSTOLE-DIASTOLE

Figure 14.1. Components of the pressure pulse. The time divisions are arbitrary approximations for descriptive purposes. (From Bruner, 1978, with permission.)

complex "waveform" composed of several components (Figure 14.1), and measurements of its characteristics will vary according to where and how they are measured (Table 14.1). The amplitude and time relationships of these components will change as the pulse travels to the periphery of the vascular tree, to be further modified by interfacing with the measuring system and by the measuring system itself. The waveform of a peripheral pressure pulse obtained from a radial artery and seen on the monitor screen may therefore be very different from the waveform measured at the root of the aorta.

The pressure pulse can be described mathematically as a series of sine waves of different frequencies. The different components of the pulse can be described in terms of a range of frequencies. The fundamental frequencies of the pressure pulse bear little relationship to the repetition rate of the event (i.e., heart rate). The range of frequencies that make up the pressure pulse will be the same regardless of pulse rate. The pressure pulse also travels much faster than the blood flows: 3–14 m $\cdot$ s^{-1}, or 15–100 times the velocity of blood flow (Park, Robotham, and German, 1983).

As the pressure pulse travels from the aortic root to the periphery, the several components become spaced out in time. The amplitudes of some components will increase, other components will be damped or will drop out, and new components may be added. Figure 14.2 illustrates changes in the pressure pulse measured at various distances from the heart in a group of dogs. Note that the pressure pulse measured some distance from the aorta is narrower and has a greater amplitude than the pulse measured in the proximal aorta. This is caused by a gradual increase in impedance toward the periphery, which causes a progressive increase in amplitude as the pressure pulse travels distally. Thus, the amplitude of the pressure wave (measured as systolic pressure) is actually greater in the more peripheral vessels.

In practice, this means that the systolic pressure measured peripherally (particularly in the dorsalis pedis or radial artery) will tend to be greater than that measured centrally (in the aorta). Diastolic and mean pressures are less affected and will be similar in the aorta and the more peripheral arteries (Park et al., 1983). Figure 14.3 shows pulse pressure waveforms measured in the radial and pedal arteries in a young child. Note the differences in the pressure waveforms for the radial and pedal arteries. In addition, mean pressure calculated using the commonly used formula (diastolic pressure plus one-third of the pulse pressure) will give falsely high mean pressures in the periphery, where the pressure pulse is narrower and of greater amplitude. Mean pressure calculated correctly as the time-weighted average of a series of instantaneous measurements will not be greatly affected as the measurement site moves peripherally (Figure 14.3).

Recent comparisons of aortic and radial artery pressures suggest that peripheral amplification may not be as prominent in neonates as in older children and adults. (Butt and Whyte, 1984). Such studies need to be confirmed in a large number of newborns over a wide range of gestational ages, body weights, and arterial pressures, with the measuring systems carefully matched for resonant frequencies and damping characteristics. For example, the smaller catheters used peripherally may damp an otherwise "amplified" amplitude, reducing the difference in the systolic pressures measured centrally and peripherally. Until such studies are done, one should be cautious in assuming that radial or dorsalis pedis pressures (particularly systolic) are equivalent to aortic pressures measured using an umbilical arterial catheter.

Table 14.1. *The pressure pulse*

Phase	Phenomena	Manifestations
Systolic events		
Phase One	Early systolic or inotropic phase	Probably relate to peak acceleration in ascending aortic blood flow
	Acceleration transient	Sound wave, "knocking"
	Ejection pulse	Pressure wave
Phase Two	Volume-displacement phase, volume-displacement component	Fills out and sustains pressure pulse
Late-systolic plus diastolic events		
Phase Three	Reflection and resonance	Duration of pressure systole
	Discharge of capacitance	Downstroke, "dicrotic notch"
	Runoff	Diastolic waves

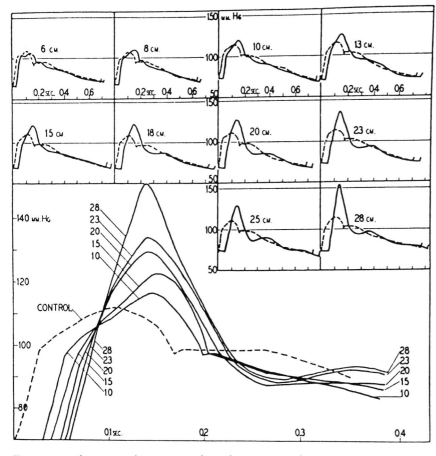

Figure 14.2. Alteration in the pressure pulse with increasing distance from the aortic arch in dogs: aortic arch tracings (dotted lines) compared with simultaneous recordings (solid lines) at various distances from the aortic arch; 5 of the 10 are superimposed in the lower part of the diagram. (From Hamilton and Dow, 1939, with permission.)

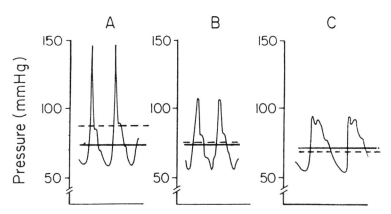

Figure 14.3. Pressure waveform tracings at different locations in children. (A) Greatly amplified pressure pulse from a pedal artery. (B) Slightly amplified pressure pulse from a pedal artery. (C) Nonamplified pressure pulse from a radial artery. Solid lines drawn across the tracings indicate mean pressure calculated by a time-weighted average of the instantaneous signal. Dashed lines indicate mean pressure calculated as diastolic pressure plus one-third of pulse pressure. Note that the actual mean pressure does not change significantly with the change in waveform configuration, whereas it is falsely elevated when the waveform is greatly narrowed and amplified (A). (From Park et al., 1983, with permission.)

Catheters, tubing, and transducers

In early animal experiments, Hales observed that blood-pressure changes measured with a manometer lagged behind the true pulsatile pressure changes. This is because a fluid column cannot respond rapidly enough to accurately reflect the actual pressure pulse. Instead of the long, open-ended tube used in the original measurements of blood pressure, we now use a system of catheters, tubing, flushing devices, stopcocks, and electronic transducers. Pressures must be converted to electrical signals to be displayed on bedside monitors. *Transduction* is the term used to describe the process of changing energy from one form (pressure) to another (electric current or voltage). In addition, each catheter-tubing-transducer system has unique frequency-response characteristics that will determine not only its ability to report the actual pressure changes in the circulation but also how much the signal will be distorted. An ideal pressure-monitoring system should accurately reflect the pressure pulse so that the recorded waveform will be the same as at the tip of the catheter. Transducers and monitors that are marketed for clinical use are generally capable of accurately reporting the pressure changes delivered to them, including the distortion introduced by the tubing and related equipment.

Fluid-filled tubing systems can be described mathematically as underdamped, second-order dynamic systems that are influenced by the compliance of the conductive system, the mass of the fluid moving in the system, and the friction between the tubing and the fluid (Gardner, 1981). These factors determine the natural resonant frequency (f_n) and the degree of damping in the system. Gardner (1981) has compared this phenomenon to a bouncing tennis ball: "When a tennis ball is dropped on a hard, flat floor, it bounces several times and comes to rest on the floor. With each successive bounce it does not rise as high as on the previous bounce. Each bounce has a characteristic frequency, and the time it takes the ball to come to rest is related to the damping coefficient."

The resonant frequency can be measured using a variety of methods. A practical way to calculate f_n is to pull and quickly release the "pigtail" on the Intraflo (Abbott Laboratories) fast-flush valve and record the resulting oscillation in the system. From these recordings, one can easily obtain the resonant frequency using the formula f_n (Hz) = paper speed (mm · s^{-1})/one cycle length (mm). The damping coefficient can be obtained by measuring the amplitudes of two successive peaks of the "ringing" oscillation (in millimeters), calculating the ratio of the smaller to the larger, and determining the coefficient using graphic techniques. Figure 14.4 illustrates the technique. Usually, clinical measurement systems will have an f_n of 15–25 Hz and a damping coefficient of 0.1–0.4.

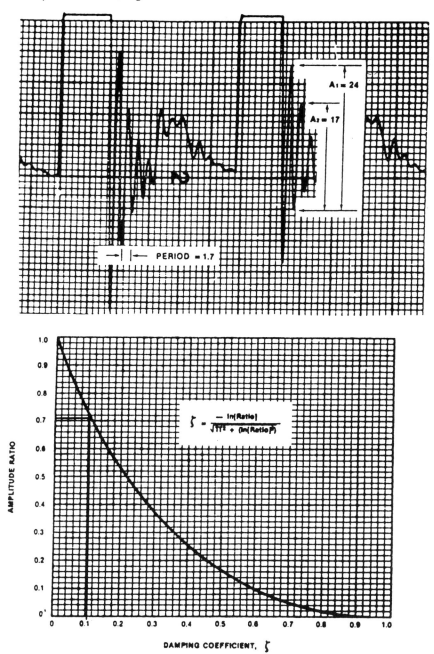

Figure 14.4. Method for determining the natural resonant frequency and damping coefficient by introducing "ringing" in the pressure signal by pulling and releasing the "pigtail" on the intraflow fast-flush valve. *Top:* Resonant frequency (f_n) can be determined by measuring the period of the "ringing" oscillation, in this case 1.7 mm, and dividing this into the paper speed (25 mm · s^{-1}); $f_n = 25/1.7 = 15$ Hz. The damping coefficient can be estimated by taking the ratio of any two successive peaks of the oscillations, in this case $A_2/A_1 = 17/24 = 0.71$. Then, by using the graph (bottom), the damping coefficient can be determined, in this case 0.11. (From Gardner, 1981, with permission.)

When the f_n of the tubing system is higher than the component frequencies of the pressure pulse, there will be less distortion of the transmitted pressure changes. Ideally, the resonant frequency of an underdamped recording system should be considerably greater ($\times 5$) than the highest significant frequency in the signal imposed on the system (Bruner et al., 1981). Unfortunately, the significant frequencies of the pressure pulse have not been adequately defined. Some have suggested that frequencies as high as 20 Hz may be important! Most important, the fluid-filled system coupling the catheter to the electronic transducer (tubing, stopcocks, flushing devices) will resonate at frequencies in the 10–25-Hz range and may therefore be limiting. Tubing length is an important contributor to the potential maximum resonant frequency of a hydraulic system. Figure 14.5 illustrates the effect the length of pressure tubing on the pressure pulse in a critical-care setting. From a practical point of view, a reasonably flushed system incorporating a 4-ft length of tubing can be expected to have a resonant frequency of about 20 Hz and a damping coefficient of about 0.2.

Gardner and associates studied dynamic responses using 3.5 and 5.0 Fr catheters in the usual umbilical artery setup used in most neonatal intensive-care units (NICUs). They found that both sizes of catheters produced natural frequencies and damping coefficients sufficient for adequate recording of pressure (Gardner, Parker, and Feinauer, 1982). There have been no similar studies of the smaller cannulas of various sizes commonly used for peripheral blood-pressure measurements.

Given the limitations described earlier, most of the commercially available systems (monitor, transducer, tubing, intraflow devices) have response characteristics adequate to reproduce the pressure pulse, taking the usual precautions. In general, problems in pressure-monitoring systems occur in the fluid-filled part of the system, rather than in the electronics. There are two major sources of error that one may encounter: (1) A catheter of very small diameter will act as a low-pass filter, causing loss of higher frequencies, resulting in underestimation, particularly of systolic pressure. (2) Introduction of small air bubbles into the system will result in excessive damping (Weindling, 1989).

Other common practical problems are related to errors introduced by the dynamic and static components of the energy of the pressure pulse. For example, the measured systolic pressure will be increased if an end-hole catheter is pointed upstream into the flow. Although a side-hole catheter will eliminate this problem, it may be more prone to thrombotic complications. The static component can

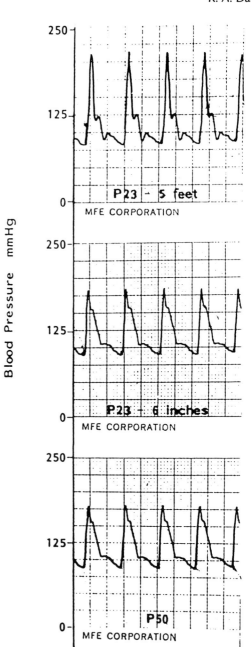

Figure 14.5. Simultaneous recordings of blood-pressure waveforms by three transducer-tubing systems using 5 ft of tubing, 6 in. of tubing, and no tubing. Resonant frequencies were 7 Hz, 34 Hz, and 45 Hz, respectively. (From Boutros and Albert, 1984, with permission.)

be minimized by being careful to place the transducer at the level of the catheter tip.

A discussion of invasive monitoring would not be complete without some consideration of the risks of umbilical and peripheral arterial catheterization. Besides the more common problems of thrombosis, vasospasm, hemorrhage, and infection, there have been recent concerns about occlusion of the radial artery after catheter removal in newborns (Hack et al., 1990) and bacterial and fungal contamination of blood-pressure transducers (Solomon et al., 1986; Weems et al., 1987). Clearly, an indwelling arterial catheter must be cared for with meticulous attention to detail and not left in place any longer than necessary. Frequently, difficult decisions must be made, balancing the risks of catheterization and the need for the information that can be gained from pressure measurements and arterial blood gas determinations.

INDIRECT MEASUREMENT OF BLOOD PRESSURE

Comparisons of indirect and direct measurements

Advances in technology have introduced a number of new, easy techniques for measuring blood pressure. Also, it is generally advantageous to replace invasive methods with noninvasive ones. A sensitive balance must be achieved between the risk to the patient and the accuracy and clinical usefulness of the information obtained. Further, noninvasive measurement of blood pressure involves analyzing different "artifacts" that may be only indirectly related to the physiological processes being investigated. A better understanding of how various blood-pressure devices operate and what they actually measure will facilitate greater appreciation of the differences between methods and will allow decisions whether or not such differences are clinically important.

A very important consideration is that most noninvasive measurement usually are referenced to direct measurement via an arterial catheter. Pressure-pulse analysis, however, as described earlier, is not as straightforward as it first appears. It may make sense to use directly measured blood pressure as a reference, but one should remember not to regard the direct or any particular noninvasive method as an absolute gold standard.

Almost all noninvasive techniques involve occlusion of a vessel with an external cuff. The relationship between the size of the cuff and the size of the extremity has an important effect on the values obtained. In general, if the cuff is too narrow, values will be too high, and if the cuff is too wide, values will be too low. There appear to be greater errors associated with narrow cuffs than with wider cuffs. Most comparative studies seem to agree that within the accuracy obtainable in most clinical situations,

the cuff bladder should completely encircle the extremity, and its width should be about one-half of the circumference or 1.2 times the diameter of the extremity (Park, Kawabori, and Guntheroth, 1976; Lum and Jones, 1977). Even though the effects of cuff size are well recognized, few comparative studies have reported the ratio between cuff width and arm circumference. In some cases, the "cuff size recommended by the manufacturer" has been used, or "the smallest cuff available." Meaningful comparisons are difficult without this information.

When comparing direct and indirect methods, it is important to appreciate that the accuracy of a direct pressure measurement is affected by the resonance and damping characteristics of the conductor-tubing system. Unfortunately, very few comparative studies have discussed the resonance and damping characteristics of direct measurement systems. This is particularly true of studies in newborn infants. In addition, systolic pressure can be highly dependent on the site of measurement and can be particularly vulnerable to significant and unpredictable amplification by the conducting-tubing system. One must therefore be especially cautious when interpreting comparisons of direct and indirect systolic pressure measurements in newborns. Also, most of the early comparative studies of newborns were performed with methods that best estimated systolic pressure, such as palpation or ultrasound. Early studies with oscillometric techniques were also concerned primarily with systolic pressure. In contrast, comparisons of mean pressure should be less influenced by catheter-tubing-transducer dynamics (Gardner, 1981).

Estimates of diastolic pressure using noninvasive methods have been even more arbitrary and controversial than those for systolic pressure. With the use of auscultation methods in children, "true" diastolic pressure is believed to be close to but lower than that seen at the fourth Korotkoff sound and higher than that at the fifth sound (Park and Menard, 1987). Palpation and ultrasound techniques do not provide diastolic values. Diastolic pressures estimated with oscillometry probably are more accurate than those from auscultation, but they do not correlate with directly measured pressures as well as do mean and systolic pressures (Park and Menard, 1987).

In the case of comparison between oscillometric techniques and direct measurements, there has been some confusion about when simultaneous measurements should be taken (Park, 1987). Automated oscillometric devices such as the Dinamap determine pressures over several cardiac cycles. In addition, during a single measurement cycle, systolic, mean, and diastolic pressures are not determined simultaneously, but at different times as the cuff is deflated. The precise times are hidden from the user, and therefore comparisons between the indirect and direct values cannot be made simply by recording a single intraarterial value at the point that the indirect value is displayed. Direct pressure measurements used for comparison must be taken over a relatively long period during the cuff deflation, at intervals corresponding to the systolic, mean, and diastolic pressure determinations. Although there have been many studies comparing the values obtained with these devices to directly measured pressures, only a few have taken this factor into account.

Finally, the statistical methods used to compare direct and indirect pressure measurements have not always been optimal. Most comparative studies have reported mean differences between direct and indirect methods and have used regression analysis to correlate the measurements. Thus, the results often have been based on averages of many measurements. The clinician, however, often bases therapeutic decisions on one, or at most a few, blood-pressure determinations. Few studies have reported on the error associated with a single measurement or have provided enough information to calculate such an error. In most studies in which the data have been graphically displayed, although the correlations may have appeared excellent, there has been considerable scatter, suggesting relatively large errors for single measurements. A practical method for specifying the maximum error for a single measurement ("error bound") is the absolute value of the mean error plus two standard deviations of the mean. If the errors are normally distributed, fewer than 5% of all measurements will have errors that will fall outside this error bound. In addition, if one knows the error associated with a single measurement, confidence can be increased by making multiple measurements and taking the average. The error bound can be reduced by dividing it by the square root of the number of measurements. Only a few comparison studies have reported these or other similar statistics that could be so valuable to the clinician.

Older methods

Palpation and auscultation

The earliest palpation technique consisted of a rough estimate of the digital force required to compress a peripheral artery. Early attempts to quanti-

tate that force using counterpressure directly led to the development of the oscillometric techniques widely used today. In 1986, Riva-Rocci developed the blood-pressure cuff, and in 1905 Korotkoff described the method of auscultation using the sounds produced by blood flow distal to a partially compressed artery. Because Korotkoff sounds are rarely audible in newborns, palpation of the initial pulsatile flow has been used to estimate systolic pressure. Because the generation of turbulence or a pulse is dependent on flow, conditions inhibiting flow (i.e., reduction of cardiac output, volume depletion, or increased peripheral vascular resistance) will make palpation or auscultation of turbulent flow difficult, if not impossible. The classic studies of Woodbury and associates in 1938 revealed good correlation between brachial palpation pressure and directly measured umbilical systolic pressure in 37 infants. They noted that cuff size affected the measurements and that a small (2.5-cm) cuff was required (Woodbury, Robinow, and Hamilton, 1938).

The chief advantage of the palpation method is its simplicity and minimum equipment requirements. The obvious disadvantages include the inability to make continuous measurements and its limitation to assessing only systolic pressure. In addition, in a critically ill neonate with a low perfusion state, decreased cardiac output, or increased peripheral vascular resistance, pulses may be impossible to detect. Nevertheless, in non-intensive-care settings, or in situations where no other methods are available, this method offers a simple means to detect trends in systolic pressure.

Flush technique

Largely because of the difficulties encountered with the auscultation and palpation techniques, a simple, rapid method using the "flush" principle, first described by Gaertner in 1899, was introduced by Goldring and Wohltmann in 1952. Reinhold and Pym gave the method wider publicity in 1955. Forfar and Kibel further established the method in a study of 513 blood-pressure estimations in 143 newborn infants (Darnall, 1985). For many years this technique was the standard method used in newborn infants. The technique depends on the principle of vessel occlusion, described earlier, except that the end point is the pressure at which a flush first appears in a previously blanched extremity.

Although rarely used today, it is interesting that as recently as 1974, Virnig and Reynolds compared direct aortic and flush pressures obtained in a group of "sick" newborns. The frequency response of the recording system for direct measurement was not described, and infants known to have conditions or attributes that would adversely affect recognition of an end point were excluded from the study. In their selected group of patients, regression analysis produced excellent correlation, and they calculated that a single flush measurement would be within 9 mm Hg of the direct mean pressure 95% of the time (Virnig and Reynolds, 1974). In the only study in which the characteristics of the recording system for direct measurements were described, Moss and Adams found that flush reading occupied a wide range between the directly recorded systolic and diastolic pressures. The approximation of the flush readings to either systolic or mean pressure was highly dependent on the speed of cuff deflation, and flush readings were closest to mean pressures when the cuff was deflated at a rate of about 5 mm Hg per second (Moss and Adams, 1964).

That method clearly has serious limitations for use in infants requiring intensive care. The method is highly dependent on peripheral perfusion and the skill of the operator. The end point depends not only on flow in a relatively large vessel but also on the time it takes for blood to perfuse to the smaller vessels and capillaries of the skin. Also, the pressure reading at which the flush occurs is highly dependent on the speed of cuff deflation. In situations of high peripheral vascular resistance, or low flow, blood-pressure estimations will be significantly lower than centrally measured pressure and probably can give little more information than blanched-skin refill time.

Newer methods

Ultrasound

Ultrasound methods to measure blood pressure depend on a phenomenon described in 1842 by Christian Doppler. He observed that as a vehicle approaches and then leaves an observer, there is a change in the pitch of the sound emanating from the vehicle. The application of this principle involves the use of a sensor that is placed distal to an inflatable cuff or between it and the limb over a major artery. The sensor consists of a transmitter that sends ultrasound into the limb and a transducer that picks up reflected sound waves from the various soft-tissue interfaces. Most of these interfaces will not be moving, and therefore the frequency reflected from them will be the same as the frequency transmitted. The frequencies of the sound waves reflected from the soft-tissue interfaces that are mov-

ing will be shifted in proportion to that component of the velocity of the interface that is in the direction of the ultrasound path. Electronic circuits are used to distinguish between moving interfaces and stationary ones. The ultrasound reflected from moving interfaces is converted to an audible sound, from which the listener can determine the maximum cuff pressure that will allow blood flow distal to the cuff. Ultrasound can therefore be used to sense moving blood cells distal to an inflatable cuff on a limb or to sense the arterial wall motion distal to the cuff. Systolic blood pressure can be estimated by noting when blood first starts to flow or when the vessel wall starts to pulsate distal to the cuff.

Satomura first applied the Doppler principle for diagnosing cardiovascular abnormalities in human subjects in 1957. Ware adopted the principle for indirect measurement of human blood pressure in 1965, and Stegall, Kardon, and Kemmerer suggested the use of Doppler sphygmomanometry in infants in 1968. Subsequently, a number of reports appeared in the literature comparing Doppler techniques with other noninvasive and invasive measurements.

Doppler measurements of systolic pressure tend to be more reliable than estimates of diastolic pressure, and they indicate higher values then either the palpation or flush technique (Kirkland and Kirkland, 1972). Like other indirect techniques, Doppler measurements are highly dependent on cuff size (Kirkland and Kirkland, 1972; Hill and Machin, 1976; Lum and Jones, 1977). When proper cuff sizes are used, Doppler measurements of systolic pressure are consistently lower in the lower extremities than in the upper extremities (Kirkland and Kirkland, 1972; de Swiet, Peto, and Shinebourne, 1974).

Of particular importance with respect to measurements of systolic pressure, most comparisons of Doppler and direct methods have not described the characteristics of the direct recording systems used. Nevertheless, comparisons of Doppler and aortic systolic pressures have consistently found good correlation, with a tendency for Doppler measurements to be slightly lower than directly measured aortic pressures (Hernandez, Goldring, and Hartmann, 1971; Black, Kotrapn, and Massie, 1972; Dweck, Reynolds, and Cassady, 1974; Reder et al., 1978). In one study, the best correlation was obtained when Doppler measurements were obtained in the leg rather than in the arm (Dweck et al., 1974). Although diastolic pressure can be measured with most, but not all, Doppler devices (Reder et al., 1978), the correlations are not as good as for systolic pressure. The Doppler devices have been shown to produce good results with inexperienced as well as experienced operators (Dweck et al., 1974).

Although Doppler blood-pressure estimation has become less widely used because of the introduction of reliable automated oscillometric techniques, there is still a range of units available in the marketplace, and all work similarly. It appears that systems that use separate cuffs and transducers give more accurate results than systems that have an integrated cuff-transducer (Reder et al., 1978). Although a reasonable approximation of systolic pressure can be obtained with the Doppler devices, their main disadvantages are that they cannot easily record diastolic pressure and mean pressure and cannot measure pressure either continuously or in an automated fashion. In addition, the transducers are easily broken, and considerable time is consumed for each measurement.

Oscillometry

Other than palpation techniques, oscillometry is the oldest method for noninvasive blood-pressure measurement. In addition, this technique has clearly become the most widely used noninvasive means to measure blood pressure in newborns. In 1876, Marey placed a liquid-filled occluding chamber around an artery and found that the arterial pulsations were transferred to the fluid in the chamber. Subsequent investigators attempted to define the relationship between the amplitude of the externally measured pressure oscillation and the pressure within the vessel. The method employs a cuff similar to that used in other noninvasive methods. As the cuff pressure is reduced and the vessel begins to pulsate, these pulsations are transmitted either to the primary cuff or to a second cuff that has been placed proximal to the primary inflating cuff. The oscillations in the cuff are then sensed and recorded. Prior to Korotkoff's description in 1905, palpation and oscillometry were widely used for clinical determinations of blood pressure, and an oscillometer for use in infants was described by Balard as early as 1913 (Darnall, 1985). During the 1950s and 1960s, several oscillometric devices were introduced to estimate systolic pressures in newborns (Ashworth, Neligan, and Rogers, 1959; Rice and Posener, 1959; Goodman, Cumming, and Raber, 1962; Nelson, 1968).

It was initially thought that the pressure at which pulsations were first detected correlated with systolic pressure and that the pressure at which oscillations were maximal correlated with diastolic pres-

sure. As early as 1916, however, it was suggested that maximum oscillation occurred above diastolic pressure, perhaps above mean pressure (Brooks and Luckhardt, 1916). Subsequently, others, using liquid-filled (Pachon and Fabre, 1921) and air-filled (Gley and Gomez, 1931) chambers, independently reported that the minimum occlusive pressure for maximum oscillation was very close to mean arterial pressure. That conclusion was supported in more sophisticated studies (Posey et al., 1969; Geddes et al., 1970). The oscillometric method, therefore, is the only noninvasive method that primarily estimates mean arterial pressure.

In 1979, Ramsey reported on a new instrument utilizing oscillometry for automated, indirect, noninvasive measurement of mean arterial pressure. The device did not require an external microphone or transducer and could automatically make determinations as often as every few minutes without operator involvement. Figure 14.6 illustrates how the automated oscillometric device (Dinamap) developed by Ramsey functions. Although there may be some variations, depending on the manufacturer, the basic principles remain the same. In the subsequent discussion, I shall refer to the automated oscillometric technique as the "Dinamap" technique. The following description is taken from Ramsey's original report. The major components of the instrument include a microprocessor (central processor or CPU), an air pump to inflate the cuff, a bleed value to deflate the cuff by discrete pressure decrements, a pressure transducer, and an overpressure switch to prevent the pressure in the system from exceeding approximately 300 mm Hg at any time.

The cuff is inflated through one tube from the pump. The pressure is sensed through another tube that leads from the cuff to the pressure transducer within the instrument. The electronic signal from the pressure transducer is processed in two ways: (1) After suitable scaling, it is digitized by an analog-to-digital converter (A/D converter) and used by the CPU to measure the actual pressure in the cuff, and thus to control inflation and deflation. (2) After signal processing, the pulsatile component is digitized and used by the CPU for determining the amplitude of the cuff-pressure oscillations. The mean pressure is chosen as the lowest cuff pressure at which the oscillations are maximum.

The instrument repeatedly measures the mean arterial pressure at user-selected cycle times. Each cycle consists of cuff inflation, pressure determination, and cuff deflation and can range between 1 min and 8.5 min in 0.5-min increments. At the end

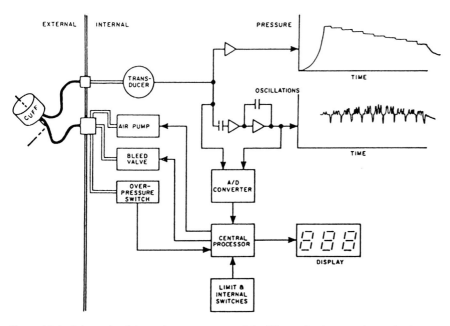

Figure 14.6. Schematic of the major components of the Dinamap. The waveforms that occur during a single determination are shown in the upper right-hand corner. (From Ramsey, 1979, with permission.)

of the delay, the system automatically measures and compensates for any drift in the transducer zero setting before a new pressure determination is made.

Motion artifacts are reduced by requiring two successive oscillations of almost equal amplitudes and by constraining the rise time and maximum slope of an oscillation to be within allowable limits at each level of cuff deflation. When all of these criteria are met, the two oscillation amplitudes are averaged, and the cuff pressure is reduced in increments of 3–6 mm Hg. This process is repeated until an oscillation maximum is found, and then five more cycles of deflating the cuff by decrements in pressure and measuring the oscillation amplitude are executed to be certain that the true maximum has been found, not a premature maximum. A logic diagram for the Dinamap is shown in Figure 14.7. Over the years, the specifications have changed slightly, but the basic principles have not changed. Table 14.2 shows the operating specifications for a recent Dinamap, model 8100.

In Ramsey's report of 1979, he also compared measurements of mean arterial pressure made with the Dinamap to directly measured mean pressure in adult subjects. Excellent correlation was found between mean Dinamap measurements and direct measurements, but the accuracy for a single Dinamap measurement was not discussed.

In the same year. Yelderman and Ream (1979) published a sophisticated study comparing the Dinamap technique to directly measured mean pressure in adult patients undergoing open heart surgery. They used an elaborate computer-assisted technique identical with that used by Ramsey in the Dinamap. The process involved digitizing the outputs from both the arterial and Dinamap transducers and storing the data on magnetic tape for later analysis. During the analysis, the baseline cuff pressure for each interval between cuff decrements was defined as the cuff pressure without superimposed oscillations. For each indirect determination of mean pressure, the average magnitude of the oscillation of cuff pressure at each value of baseline cuff pressure was calculated. Indirect mean arterial pressure was defined as the minimum baseline cuff pressure at which maximum cuff-pressure oscillation occurred (this is the value displayed as mean arterial pressure on the Dinamap). Direct mean intraarterial pressure was obtained by averaging the intraarterial pressures over a period of three sequential baseline intervals. Thus the second interval contained the minimum baseline cuff pressure for maximum oscillation. These periods of arterial averaging ranged from 8 to 12 s and contained a discrete number of complete heart cycles. Figure 14.8 shows the typical intervals for one measurement. The

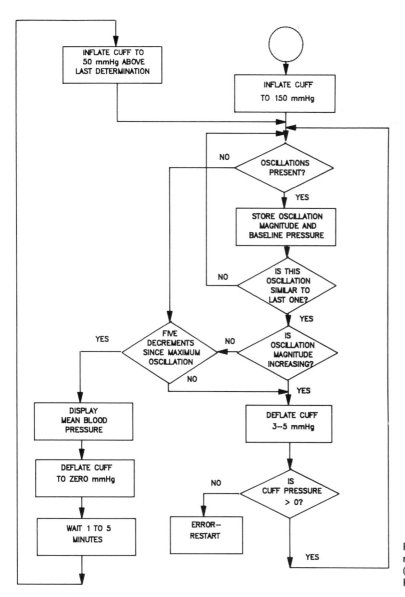

Figure 14.7. Logic diagram for a Dinamap mean pressure determination. (Courtesy of M. Yelderman and A. K. Ream.)

mean difference for the pooled data was 1.4 torr, with a standard deviation of 6.22 torr. The error for an individual oscillometric measurement was calculated using both the pooled data, and regression analysis and was found to be 14 torr.

Working closely with Yelderman and Ream, Kimble and associates compared Dinamap mean arterial pressures with directly measured pressures in a group of 14 newborn infants requiring umbilical artery catheters (Kimble et al., 1981). The same computerized techniques were used that had been used in adults by Yelderman and Ream, and both the accuracy of the method and the effect of cuff size were

evaluated. In each infant, 10 simultaneous measurements of indirect and direct mean arterial pressures were made using each of four different-sized cuffs. A fourth-order regression, of measurement error (intraarterial pressure − Dinamap pressure) on the ratio of cuff width to arm circumference (CW/AC), showed that the smallest error occurred when the CW/AC ratio was between 0.45 and 0.70. Figure 14.9 shows the relationship between CW/AC and measurement error. Subsequent analysis was done on 250 determinations in which CW/AC was between 0.45 and 0.70. The regression analysis for those data is shown in Figure 14.10. The mean error

Table 14.2. *Performance specifications for the model 8100*

Specification	Compliance	
Cuff-pressure range	Adult/pediatric:	0–250 mm Hg
	Neonatal:	0–235 mm Hg
Initial cuff inflation	Adult/pediatric:	178 ± 15 mm Hg
	Neonatal:	125 ± 15 mm Hg
Determination ranges	Systolic:	30–245 mm Hg (adult/pediatric)
		30–190 mm Hg (neonates)
	Diastolic:	10–210 mm Hg (adult/pediatric)
		10–160 mm Hg (neonates)
	Map:	20–225 mm Hg (adult/pediatric)
		20–170 mm Hg (neonates)
	Pulse:	40–200 bpm (adult/pediatric)
		40–220 bpm (neonates)
Blood-pressure accuracy	Blood-pressure accuracy meets and exceeds proposed AAMI standards for noninvasive blood-pressure accuracy (AAMI standard: ± 5 mm Hg mean error; <8 mm Hg standard deviation, as compared with central aortic pressure)	
Static-pressure accuracy	Displayed pressures will not vary by more than the greater of ± 3 mm Hg or ± 2% from that of a mercury manometer in the range of 0–250 mm Hg	
Pulse-rate accuracy	± 3.5%	
Determination time	20–45 typical; 120 maximum	
Overpressure cutoff	310 ± 45 mm Hg (adult/pediatric)	
	235 ± 10 mm Hg (neonates)	
Battery charging	At least 90% capacity in 16 h; unit will operate and charge battery simultaneously when connected to an ac power source	
Battery operating time	6 h minimum operation (5-min cycle time with adult cuff at 25°C)	

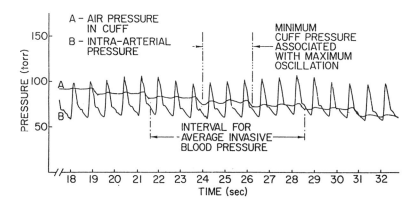

Figure 14.8. Selected example from actual recordings used by Yelderman and Ream (1979) to estimate mean pressure via the Dinamap technique and to calculate simultaneous mean arterial pressure: A, air pressure within the blood-pressure cuff; B, direct arterial pressure. The interval over which arterial pressure was averaged for comparison is marked. The same technique was used by Kimble et al. (1981). (From Yelderman, and Ream, 1979, with permission.)

for the data was −0.2 torr, with a standard deviation of 3.8 torr. The 95% error bound for a single Dinamap measurement in those studies was 7.7 torr. Although the f_n and damping characteristics of the system for direct measurement of arterial pressure were not stated, that would not be expected to greatly affect the measurement of mean arterial pressure (Gardner, 1981).

There have been several subsequent studies comparing Dinamap pressure determinations with direct pressure measurements. Unfortunately, they are difficult to compare, for a number of reasons. One important factor is that the studies of Kimble and associates and those of Yelderman and associates remain the only two that have compared Dinamap pressure with directly measured pressure

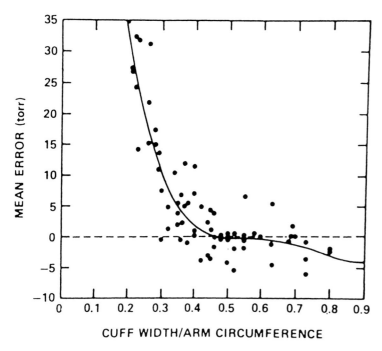

Figure 14.9. Nonlinear-regression analysis comparing error (between Dinamap and intraarterial) with CW/AC ratio. Each point represents the average of 10 determinations with the same cuff in a given patient. (From Kimble et al., 1981, with permission.)

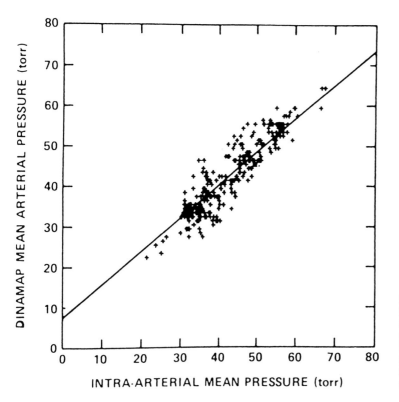

Figure 14.10. Comparison of intraarterial and Dinamap mean blood-pressure determinations in a group of patients in whom CW/AC ratios were between 0.45 and 0.70 (linear-regression analysis). Each point represents a single comparison. (From Kimble et al., 1981, with permission.)

averaged over the period of oscillometric determination. Most studies did not report how "simultaneous" values were obtained. Some simply used the readout directly from the pressure monitor at the time the Dinamap displayed update. Others used a method that involved determining the range of directly measured pressures over the period of the Dinamap determination. Using that method, if the Dinamap value were to fall within the range, the mean pressure would be taken to be equal to the Dinamap reading. If the Dinamap reading were above or below the range, the upper or lower limit of the range, respectively, would be recorded as the direct pressure (Park and Menard, 1987). To complicate matters further, some studies compared mean pressures, others compared only systolic and diastolic pressures, and others compared all three.

Another important issue involves the statistics generally used to evaluate the comparisons. Only three studies in newborns reported the confidence level associated with a single or a few averaged Dinamap determinations, which would seem to be the most important statistic for the clinician. Kimble and co-workers reported that 95% of the time, a simultaneously measured direct mean arterial pressure would be within the range described by the Dinamap reading (± 7.7 mm Hg). Wareham et al. (1987) reported the 95% predictive intervals for a single Dinamap measurement in 15 premature infants (six measurements in each infant) to vary from 17 torr for mean pressure to 20 torr for systolic and diastolic pressures. Stated in another way, there would be a 95% chance that a simultaneously measured direct mean pressure would be within the range described by the Dinamap reading [± 8.5 (17/2) mm Hg]. Those results are very close to the findings of Kimble and co-workers. The slightly greater error bound found by Wareham and co-workers may have resulted from the different methods used to make "simultaneous" comparisons. Wareham and co-workers used a single direct pressure reading occurring at the time of the Dinamap readouts, whereas Kimble and co-workers used the average mean pressure recorded over the Dinamap determination period. In addition, Wareham and co-workers used cuff widths according to the manufacturer's recommendation, whereas Kimble and co-workers first determined the range of CW/AC that would minimize the error in their study population (0.45–0.70) (Table 14.2) and then analyzed only those comparisons in which CW/AC fell within that range.

In one other study, involving a group of 15 low-birth-weight infants weighing 730–1,400 g, Sones-son and Broberger compared directly measured and Dinamap mean pressures and reported the 95% confidence intervals for the average of two Dinamap measurements. Using a CW/AC of 0.44–0.55, they reported a mean error of -1.0 ± 2.3 mm Hg, with the confidence intervals associated with two measurements being -6 mm Hg to $+4$ mm Hg (Sonesson and Broberger, 1987). The error bound for two averaged measurements (calculated from mean error and standard deviation using the same method as Kimble and co-workers) was 5.6 mm Hg. The error was considerably greater using CW/AC ratios of 0.3–0.37 recommended by some cuff manufacturers. Those authors concluded that if one averages two measurements, and uses a CW/AC ratio of 0.44–0.55, the Dinamap is reasonably accurate in the blood-pressure range of 25–50 mm Hg in preterm infants weighing less than 1,500 g. If one multiplies this error bound for two averaged measurements by the square root of 2 (1.4142), the resulting approximate error bound for one measurement is 7.9 mm Hg, which is very close to that reported by Kimble and co-workers.

It has been suggested that a clinical instrument for measuring blood pressure should have a mean error of less than 5 mm Hg and a standard deviation of the mean of less than 7 mm Hg (Ramsey, 1980). Certainly the Dinamap falls well within that range (-0.2 ± 3.8 mm Hg for Kimble and co-workers; -1.6 ± 4.4 mm Hg for Wareham and co-workers). However, there is a relatively large predictive interval for a single determination, and the clinician must take this into consideration before making therapy decisions based on a single measurement or a few measurements. For example, an error bound of 7.7 mm Hg may be reasonable when the mean pressure is 40–60 mm Hg, but could be unacceptable in a very small premature infant, where a normal mean pressure may be 25–30 mm Hg.

This potential for large errors has been pointed out in several studies. In 1986, Briassoulis studied six infants using two cuff sizes and reported that with the cuff recommended by the manufacturer (Omega 1100) (CW/AC ratio = 0.35–0.44) and with a cuff one size larger (CW/AC ratio = 0.50–0.64), 34% and 33% of oscillometric determinations of mean arterial pressure varied more than 5 torr from the direct measurements, and 3.8% and 5.7% varied more than 10 torr (Briassoulis, 1986). As would be expected from the design of the Dinamap, which best determines mean pressure, there was a wider variation when systolic or diastolic pressure was measured. From those data, Briassoulis concluded that especially in the low ranges of blood pressure below 50 torr, the error may be dangerously large to be relied on in an intensive-care situation. Interestingly, however, the accuracy of those measurements is close to the error bounds reported by Kimble and co-workers and Wareham and co-workers.

Diprose et al. (1986) reported that the Dinamap "failed to detect hypotension in very low birthweight infants" during a study of 417 paired measurements made in 12 infants weighing between 700 and 1,470 g. Although they carefully analyzed paired measurements only where the direct blood pressure (recorded on a chart recorder) was undamped, they did not report the point at which the pressures were compared. They used the smallest available cuff size for all infants, but did not report the actual CW/AC ratios. They used contingency tables to show that especially when the pressure was in the low range, the Dinamap overestimated both systolic and diastolic directly measured pressures. Although they did not report the error for an individual measurement, the correlation coefficients for systolic and diastolic pressures were 0.67 and 0.49, respectively. It is interesting that the authors did not report on the mean pressure determinations, which are best suited for the Dinamap.

There is a suggestion, then, that the Dinamap may be less accurate than direct measurement in small premature infants, particularly when the mean pressure is less than 50 mm Hg. One should be cautious in interpreting these studies. Nevertheless, we would benefit from careful studies done in very small premature infants. Future studies should pay careful attention to the cuff size used and should average directly measured pressures over the period of Dinamap determination. Such studies should use statistics designed to show the predictive value of a single measurement or a few Dinamap measurements and ideally should relate these statistics to specific pressure ranges.

CLINICAL STRATEGIES

Continuous invasive monitoring of arterial blood pressure has become standard care for critically ill newborns. Indications for the insertion of an arterial cannula include anticipation of hypotension and/or myocardial dysfunction requiring continuous infusion of vasoactive drugs, hypertensive crises in postoperative cardiac patients, and the need for frequent arterial blood gas measurements to adjust ventilator settings. The ability to sample blood without disturbing the infant is an important reason for placing an indwelling arterial line. Oxygenation can

decrease dramatically when a compromised infant in crying and struggling during repeated arterial or venous punctures.

In the immediate neonatal period, umbilical arteries usually are cannulated using a 3.5 or 5.0 Fr catheter. The umbilical catheter is placed either at the level of the diaphragm or between the L-3 and L-4 vertebrae, below the origin of the renal and mesenteric arteries. When the umbilical arteries are no longer available, more peripheral arteries can be used. The artery of choice is usually a radial artery, because most infants will have sufficient collateral circulation to the hands. The adequacy of the collateral circulation should be verified with an Allen or similar test prior to cannulation. The dorsalis pedis artery is relatively superficial and straight and usually courses between the second and third metatarsals. It can be cannulated after documentation of adequate collateral blood supply to the foot from the posterior tibial artery, using a modified Allen test. The posterior tibial artery is used less frequently because of its proximity to the posterior tibial nerve and its more winding course, making it more difficult to cannulate. Although easy to palpate, the brachial and temporal arteries generally are not used in the NICU for continuous monitoring. The brachial artery does not have adequate collateral circulation, and the temporal artery site has been associated with cerebral infarcts. Generally, the femoral artery should be used only as a last resort during severe hypotension or resuscitation efforts when no other pulses are palpable.

After placement of the catheter, the system must be calibrated to obtain accurate blood-pressure measurements. The most frequent problems arise in the tubing/stopcock/flushing system and usually are manifest as excessive damping. A practical way to determine if there is damping is to note the presence or absence of the dicrotic notch on the recording. Its absence may indicate excessive damping and should initiate a search for bubbles.

General guidelines for reliable tubing/stopcock/flushing systems include the following: (1) Keep tubing lengths as short as possible, less than 3–4 ft if possible. (2) Use large-bore tubing. This must be balanced against the need for the low dead space needed for sampling purposes in newborns. (3) Use stiff, noncompliant tubing. Soft tubing will absorb pressure variations and cause excessive damping. (4) Use continuous-flush devices. (5) Use the simplest system possible for connection to the transducer. Manifolds and extra connectors are places for air bubbles to collect.

When invasive monitoring is no longer practical

because of problems of arterial access, or after the acute period is over and invasive monitoring is no longer indicated, a noninvasive method such as the Dinamap can be used to monitor pressure. Just as with invasive monitoring, certain precautions should be taken to minimize the errors of measurement: (1) The correct cuff size should be selected. This is easily done by measuring the circumference of the arm or leg and choosing a cuff with a width (include only the bladder width) closest to one-half the circumference. If the resulting CW/AC ratio is less than 0.45, the next larger cuff should be chosen. The ideal CW/AC ratio is 0.45–0.70. (2) Measurements should be made when the infant is quiet, or asleep if possible. Pressures measured in awake infants can be as much as 10 mm Hg greater than those measured in asleep infants (de Swiet, Fayers, and Shinebourne, 1980). (3) If measurements are made infrequently, or are being used for diagnostic reasons, such as upper- and lower-extremity pressures to diagnose coarctation, an average of two or three measurements should be taken. (4) Mean pressure should be used, if possible, as it is less subject to variation. Although it is unclear whether or not systolic or diastolic pressure is more valuable than mean pressure in influencing patient management, measurement of mean pressure may be particularly useful in assessing perfusion (Yelderman and Ream, 1979). (5) In very immature infants, in whom mean pressures may be in the range of 25–35 mm Hg, the Dinamap may overestimate actual pressure and may not reliable detect hypotension or low perfusion states.

In clinical practice, trends in blood pressure are monitored within broad ranges of "normal." When blood pressure drifts outside such ranges, often that signals the need for some therapeutic response. For example, when blood pressure drifts below the lower limit of "normal" in an ill infant, that may call for an infusion of colloid and/or a vasoactive drug such as dopamine. The upper limits are used to determine whether or not an infant is hypertensive. Another set of limits is generally used to determine whether or not one should treat the hypertension. In the absence of large population-based studies of neonatal systemic blood pressure, especially in preterm infants, many clinicians rely on Lieberman's arbitrary criteria, which define neonatal hypertension as systolic pressure greater than 90 mm Hg or diastolic pressure greater than 65 mm Hg in term infants, and systolic pressure greater than 80 mm Hg or diastolic pressure greater than 45 mm Hg in preterm infants (Elliott and Hansen, 1990).

The ranges of "normal," particularly for very im-

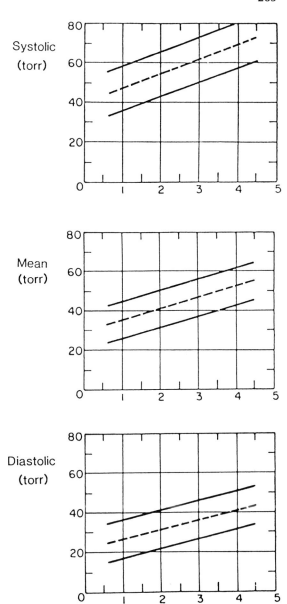

Figure 14.11. Linear regressions (broken lines) and 95% confidence limits (solid lines) for systolic, mean, and diastolic aortic blood pressures on birth weight for 61 healthy newborn infants during the first 12 h after birth. (From Versmold et al., 1981, with permission.)

mature newborns, are large and not well established. Figures 14.11 and 14.12 show normal values for systolic, mean, and diastolic aortic pressures in the first 12 h of life, as reported by Versmold et al. (1981). Less is known about "normal" values in the first few days of life in critically ill neonates. Because

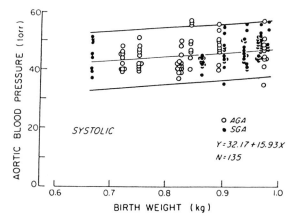

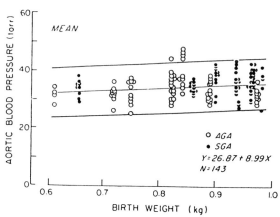

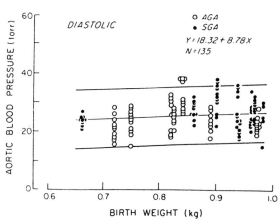

Figure 14.12. Regressions of systolic, mean, and diastolic aortic blood pressures on birth weights during hours 1–12 of age for eight AGA and eight SGA infants whose birth weights were less than 1,000 g. The regression line (thin solid lines) and 95% confidence limits (thick solid lines) are shown. (From Versmold et al., 1981, with permission.)

of the uncertainties of blood-pressure measurement, one must be cautious about interpreting any particular value shown on the LED readout on the monitor. In a given situation, any single blood-pressure measurement probably is no more accurate than ±5 mm Hg, and in most cases is less accurate. After taking the precautions described earlier for invasive or noninvasive monitoring, clinical judgment should be used to interpret trends within the broad range of normal values. Most important, therapeutic decisions should not be made on the basis of changes in blood pressure alone, but should take into consideration other clinical signs and symptoms. For example, taken together, capillary refill time, urine output, and skin color may be as important as blood pressure in determining a low-perfusion state. In the case of diagnosis and management of hypertension, the situation is more difficult, because it is common for neonates with hypertension to exhibit no symptoms (Adelman et al., 1978).

REFERENCES

Adelman, R. D., Merten, D., Vogel, J., Goetzman, B. W., and Wennberg, R. P. (1978). Nonsurgical management of renovascular hypertension in the neonate. *Pediatrics* 62:71–6.

Ashworth, A. L., Neligan, G. A., and Rogers, J. E. (1959). Sphygmomanometer for the newborn. *Lancet* 1:801.

Black, I. F. S., Kotrapn, N., and Massie, H. (1972). Application of Doppler ultrasound to blood pressure measurement in small infants. *Journal of Pediatrics* 81:932–5.

Boutros, A., and Albert, S. (1984). The effect of the dynamic response of transducer-tubing system on accuracy of direct pressure measurement in patients. *Critical Care Medicine* 11:124.

Briassoulis, G. (1986). Arterial pressure measurement in preterm infants. *Critical Care Medicine* 14:735–8.

Brooks, C., and Luckhardt, A. (1916). The chief physical mechanisms concerned in clinical methods of measuring blood pressure. *American Journal of Physiology* 40:49–74.

Bruner, J. M. R. (1978). *Handbook of Blood Pressure Monitoring.* Littleton, MA: PSG Publishing Co.

Bruner, J. M. R., Krenis, L. J., Kunsman, J. M., and Sherman, A. P. (1981). Comparison of direct and indirect methods of measuring arterial blood pressure. Part IV. *Medical Instrumentation* 15:182–8.

Butt, W. W., and Whyte, H. (1984). Blood pressure monitoring in neonates: comparison of umbilical and peripheral artery catheter measurements. *Journal of Pediatrics* 105:630–2.

Darnall, R. A. (1985). Noninvasive blood pressure measurement in the neonatal. *Clinics in Perinatology* 12:31–49.

de Swiet, M., Fayers, P., and Shinebourne, E. A. (1980). Systolic blood pressure in a population of infants in the first year of life: the Brompton study. *Pediatrics* 65:1028–35.

de Swiet, M., Peto, J., and Shinebourne, E. A. (1974). Difference between upper and lower limb blood pressure in normal neonates using Doppler technique. *Archives of Disease in Childhood* 49:734–5.

Diprose, G. K., Evans, D. H., Archer, L. N. J., and Levene, M. I. (1986). Dinamap fails to detect hypotension in very low birthweight infants. *Archives of Disease in Childhood* 61:771–3.

Dweck, H. S., Reynolds, D. W., and Cassady, G. (1974). Indirect blood pressure measurement in newborns. *American Journal of Diseases of Children* 127:492–4.

Elliott, S. J., and Hansen, T. N. (1990). Neonatal hypertension. In *Fetal and Neonatal Cardiology*, ed. W. W. Long (pp. 492–8). Philadelphia: W. B. Saunders.

Gardner, R. M. (1981). Direct blood pressure measurement – dynamic response requirements. *Anesthesiology* 54:227–36.

Gardner, R. M., Parker, J., and Feinauer, L. R. (1982). System for umbilical artery monitoring. *Critical Care Medicine* 10:456–8.

Geddes, L. A., Moore, A. G., Garner, H., et al. (1970). The indirect measurement of mean blood pressure in the horse. *Southwestern Veterinarian* 23:289–94.

Gley, P., and Gomez, D. M. (1931). La determination des pressions moyenne et minima par la methode oscillometrique. *La Presse Medical* 39:294.

Goodman, H. G., Cumming, G. R., and Raber, M. B. (1962). Photocell oscillometer for measuring systolic pressure in newborn. *American Journal of Diseases of Children* 103:152–9.

Hack, W. W. M., Vos, A., van der Lei, J., and Okken, A. (1990). Incidence and duration of total occlusion of the radial artery in newborn infants after catheter removal. *European Journal of Pediatrics* 149:275–7.

Hamilton, W. F., and Dow, P. (1939). An experimental study of the standing waves in the pulse propagated through the aorta. *American Journal of Physiology* 125:48–59.

Hernandez, A., Goldring, D., and Hartmann, A. F., Jr. (1971). Measurement of blood pressure in infants and children by the Doppler ultrasound technique. *Pediatrics* 58:788–94.

Hill, G. E., and Machin, R. H. (1976). Doppler determined blood pressure recordings: the effect of varying cuff sizes in children. *Canadian Anaesthesiology Society Journal* 23:323–6.

Kimble, K. J., Darnall, R. A., Yelderman, M., Ariagno, R. L., and Ream, A. K. (1981). An automated oscillometric technique for estimating mean arterial pressure in critically ill newborns. *Anesthesiology* 54:423–5.

Kirkland, R. T., and Kirkland, J. L. (1972). Systolic blood pressure measurement in the newborn infant with the transcutaneous Doppler method. *Journal of Pediatrics* 80:52–6.

Lenfant, C. (1973). Medical devices control: a panacea? *New England Journal of Medicine* 289:1310.

Lum, L. G., and Jones, D. M., Jr. (1977). The effect of cuff width on systolic blood pressure measurements in neonates. *Journal of Pediatrics* 91:963–6.

Marey, E. J. (1876). Pression et vitesse du sang. In *Physiologique Experimental*, vol. 2, ch. 8. Paris: Masson.

Moss, A. J., and Adams, F. H. (1964). Flush blood pressure and intra-arterial pressure. *American Journal of Diseases of Children* 107:489–91.

Nelson, N. M. (1968). On the indirect determination of

systolic and diastolic blood pressure in the newborn infant. *Pediatrics* 42:934.

Pachon, V., and Fabre, R. (1921). Sur le criterie de la pression minima dans la methode oscillometrique. *Comptes rendus des seances de la Societe de Biologie* 84:871.

Park, M. K. (1987). Are Dinamap blood pressures in premature infants reliable? *American Journal of Diseases of Children* 142:588.

Park, M. K., Kawabori, I., and Guntheroth, W. G. (1976). Need for an improved standard for blood pressure cuff size. *Clinical Pediatrics* 15:784–7.

Park, M. K., and Menard, S. M. (1987). Accuracy of blood pressure measurement by the Dinamap monitor in infants and children. *Pediatrics* 79:907–14.

Park, M. K., Robotham, J. L., and German, V. F. (1983). Systolic pressure amplification in pedal arteries in children. *Critical Care Medicine* 11:286–9.

Posey, J. A., Geddes, L. A., Williams, H., and Moore, A. G. (1969). The meaning of the point of maximum oscillations in cuff pressure in the indirect measurement of blood pressure. Part I. *Cardiovascular Research Centennial Bulletin* 8:15–25.

Ramsey, M., III. (1979). Noninvasive automatic determination of mean arterial pressure. *Medical and Biological Engineering and Computing* 17:11–18.

(1980). Noninvasive blood pressure monitoring methods and validation. In *Essential Noninvasive Monitoring in Anesthesia*, ed J. S. Gravenstein, R. S. Newbower, and A. K. Ream (pp. 37–51). New York: Grune & Stratton.

Reder, R. F., Dimich, I., Cohen, C. L., and Steinfeld, L. (1978). Evaluating indirect blood pressure measurement techniques: a comparison of three systems in infants and children. *Pediatrics* 62:326–30.

Rice, H. V., and Posener, L. J. (1959). A practical method for the measurement of systolic blood pressures of infants. *Pediatrics* 23:854.

Satomura, S. (1957). Ultrasonic Doppler method for the inspection of cardiac functions. *Journal of the Acoustic Society of America* 29:1181.

Solomon, S. L., Alexander, H., Eley, J. W., Anderson, R. L., Goodpasture, H. C., Smart, S., Furman, R. M., and Martone, W. J. (1986). Nosocomial fungemia in neonates associated with intravascular pressure-monitoring devices. *Pediatric Infectious Disease* 5:680–5.

Sonesson, S. E., and Broberger, U. (1987). Arterial blood pressure in the very low birthweight neonate. Evaluation of an automatic oscillometric technique. *Acta Paediatrica Scandinavica* 76:338–41.

Stegall, H. F., Kardon, M. B., and Kemmerer, W. T. (1968). Indirect measurement of arterial blood pressure by Doppler ultrasonic sphygmomanometry. *Journal of Applied Physiology* 25:793.

Versmold, H. T., Kitterman, J. A., Phibbs, R. H., Gregory, G. A., and Tooley, W. H. (1981). Aortic blood pressure during the first 12 hours of life in infants with birth weight 610 to 4220 grams. *Pediatrics* 67:607–13.

Virnig, N. L., and Reynolds, J. W. (1974). Reliability of flush blood pressure measurements in the sick newborn infant. *Journal of Pediatrics* 84:594–8.

Ware, R. W. (1965). New approaches to the indirect measurement of human blood pressure. Presented at the Third National Biochemical Sciences Instrumentation

Symposium, Instrumentation Society of America (BM-65), Galveston, Texas, April 1965.

Wareham, J. A., Haugh, L. D., Yeager, S. B., and Horbar, J. D. (1987). Prediction of arterial blood pressure in the premature neonate using the oscillometric method. *American Journal of Diseases of Children* 141:1108–10.

Weems, J. J., Chamberland, M. E., Ward, J., Willy, M., Padhye, A. A., and Solomon, S. L. (1987). Candida parapsilosis fungemia associated with parenteral nutrition and contaminated blood pressure transducers. *Journal of Clinical Microbiology* 25:1029–32.

Weindling, A. M. (1989). Blood pressure monitoring in the newborn. *Archives of Disease in Childhood* 64:444–7.

Woodbury, R. A., Robinow, M., and Hamilton, W. F. (1938). Blood pressure studies on infants. *American Journal of Physiology* 133:472–9.

Yelderman, M., and Ream, A. K. (1979). Indirect measurement of mean blood pressure in the anesthetized patient. *Anesthesiology* 50:253–6.

15

Intracranial-pressure monitoring: Tonometry, applanometry, fiber optics, Ladd transducer

ELKE H. ROLAND, M.D.
ALAN HILL, M.D., Ph.D.

INTRODUCTION

An elevation in intracranial pressure (ICP) is a well-recognized phenomenon that accompanies many different neuropathological processes (e.g., hypoxic-ischemic brain injury, hemorrhage, meningoencephalitis, metabolic/toxic encephalopathies, trauma). All of these processes can produce brain injury directly. In addition, there is concern that increases in ICP and the consequent inadequate cerebral blood flow can have secondary effects that will potentiate a brain insult and produce additional cerebral ischemia. Thus, much attention has been directed recently toward early diagnosis of elevated ICP. Nevertheless, it should be emphasized that control of ICP alone is rarely sufficient to ensure a favorable outcome. In each instance, the underlying disease must be treated vigorously, and attention must be given to all aspects of intensive supportive care for each patient.

In a newborn, the presence of unfused sutures and an open fontanelle allows some compensation for elevations in ICP. However, the immature brain is at increased risk related to immature cerebrovascular autoregulation. This mechanism normally ensures fairly constant cerebral blood flow and ICP within a range of mean systemic arterial blood pressures in the healthy, mature brain. It is well recognized that prematurity and even moderate hypoxic-ischemic insult to the immature brain (Lou et al., 1979)) can impair cerebrovascular autoregulatory mechanisms, which in turn can produce major fluctuations in cerebral blood flow and ICP.

In this chapter we shall discuss the major techniques for measuring ICP that have clinical application in the newborn. Furthermore, the major medical conditions in newborns that are commonly associated with elevated ICP will be reviewed briefly.

HISTORICAL BACKGROUND

Measurements of ICP may have originated as early as 3000 B.C., when the use of ventricular puncture was documented on Egyptian papyri (Perkins, 1965). Hippocrates (460–377 B.C.) reported the use of ventricular puncture for the treatment of hydrocephalus. The first lumbar puncture was performed in 1764 by the Italian physician Cotugno, who also speculated on the formation, circulation, and reabsorption of cerebrospinal fluid (CSF). However, CSF physiology was not described in detail until 1842, when the French physiologist Magendie published his classic monograph. Shortly thereafter, in the

Table 15.1. *Noninvasive techniques for measuring ICP in newborns*

Technique	Continuous measurement	Intermittent measurement
Clinical assessment	−	+
Modified Schiotz tonometer	−	+
Applanation transducer	−	+
Fiber-optic (Ladd monitor)	+	+

1870s, Quincke defined the role of lumbar puncture as a clinical diagnostic tool, and Leyden reported a method for intermittent, direct measurement of ICP through a trephined opening, with a sensor placed above the dura (Allen, 1986). Continuous recording of ICP was introduced by Guillaume and Janny (1951), and its importance was subsequently stressed by Lundberg (1960), who demonstrated that estimation of ICP based on clinical signs was unreliable. Techniques for monitoring ICP are now used routinely for management and for determination of prognoses for patients who have major neurological and neurosurgical problems.

TECHNIQUES FOR MEASURING ICP

If a technique for monitoring ICP is to have clinical application, it must provide measurements that are reasonably accurate and reliable. Invasive techniques, which can record ICP from intraventricular, subdural, or subarachnoid spaces, have been used extensively in adult patients with neurological diseases. In newborns, the presence of an open anterior fontanelle provides a unique opportunity for noninvasive measurement of ICP with minimum interference to the patient.

Noninvasive methods

Noninvasive techniques, which include clinical methods and tonometry, as well as the applanation transducer and Ladd monitor, are based on the physical principle of applanation. This principle states that a flexible membrane that separates two compartments (e.g., the skin over the anterior fontanelle) will present a flat, planar surface when the pressures are equal in the two compartments. The major noninvasive techniques for measuring ICP are listed in Table 15.1.

Clinical methods

Careful observation of the contour and palpation of the tension/fullness of the anterior fontanelle may raise suspicion of elevated ICP in a newborn. In addition, an increased rate of head growth is consistent with this diagnosis. In contrast, a widening of cranial sutures, which can be recognized either clinically or radiologically, has been reported to be unreliable for the diagnosis of elevated ICP (Philip, 1979). The major drawback of relying on clinical parameters relates to their inability to quantify changes in ICP.

A semiquantitative clinical method for estimation of ICP has been described (Welch, 1970, 1980), based on observations of changes in the contour of the anterior fontanelle in relation to the position of the infant's head: The infant's head is raised or lowered until the anterior fontanelle appears flat. At that point the ICP is considered to be at atmospheric level. The midpoint of the clavicles is considered to indicate the level at which the systemic venous pressure is atmospheric. The ICP is calculated as the vertical distance between the infant's head and the midclavicular level when the fontanelle is flat. This technique permits estimation of ICP with an error of ±1 cm H_2O. Clearly, if the fontanelle remains convex when the infant is held in an upright position, the ICP will exceed that which can be measured by this method. Furthermore, the use of this technique may be precluded by a small anterior fontanelle or by excessive edema and molding of the scalp.

A discussion of clinical techniques for diagnosis of increased ICP in newborns would be incomplete without brief mention of the role of radiological techniques, such as cranial ultrasonography and computed tomography (CT). Although radiological techniques do not provide actual measurements of ICP, certain observations can be consistent with increased ICP in the context of specific clinical situations. Recognition of these radiological features can lead to more accurate measurements of ICP by other methods. For example, in a term newborn infant, cerebral edema may be suspected if the ventricles are of small size, if diminished tissue attenuation is seen using CT (Figure 15.1), or if increased echogenicity is seen using cranial ultrasonography (Volpe, 1987; Lupton et al., 1988). In premature in-

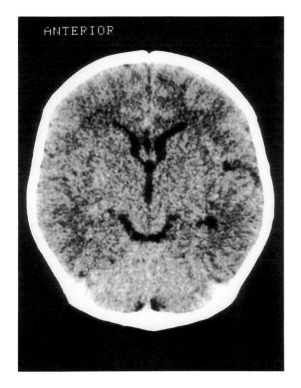

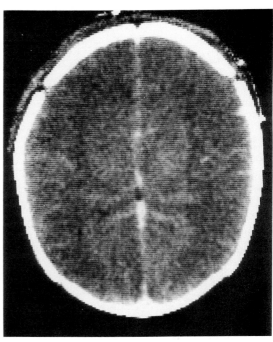

Figure 15.1. *Left:* Normal CT scan of term newborn. Note differentiation between gray and white matter. *Right:* CT scan of severely asphyxiated term newborn. Note diffuse decreased tissue attenuation throughout cerebral hemispheres.

fants, increased ICP may be suspected if there is ventricular enlargement associated with intraventricular hemorrhage or posthemorrhagic hydrocephalus. Focal lesions that are associated with increased ICP can cause lateral shifting of midline structures.

Tonometry

The pneumatic and mechanical tonometers are adaptations of the Schiotz tonometer, an instrument designed originally for estimation of intraocular pressure. The adapted "fontanometer" consists of a flat foot-plate (8 mm wide) that rests on the soft, unsupported scalp tissue of the fontanelle and is surrounded entirely by a rim of fontanelle tissue. A central plunger (4 mm wide) fits through an aperture in the foot-plate and, by virtue of either weight (mechanical force) or gas pressure (pneumatic force), depresses the surface of the fontanelle by a specific amount determined by the ICP and the elasticity of the scalp tissue. The hand-held fontanometer (Figure 15.2) (pneumotonometer, produced by

Digilab Division of Biorad Laboratories, Cambridge, MA) is unaffected by application force over the anterior fontanelle, because it utilizes an air bearing to provide frictionless movement of the piston (Davidoff and Chamlin, 1959; Brett, 1966); Easa, Tron, and Bingham, 1983; Hill, 1985). When the sensor of the pneumatic fontanometer is applied properly, the device produces a continuous whistle, which indicates uniform contact between the sensor and the surface being measured. The restriction of gas flow through the sensor tip causes an increase in pressure in the central chamber that is measured by a pneumatic pressure transducer and is processed by a recording unit to provide continuous permanent chart recordings.

A mechanical tonometer, which depends on weight and gravity, requires that the infant be held in a sitting position, with the surface of the fontanelle in a horizontal plane. In contrast, the pneumotonometer permits measurements while the infant is in a supine position. The hand-held device is easily calibrated and can perform measurements of ICP in approximately 5 s, allowing multiple intemit-

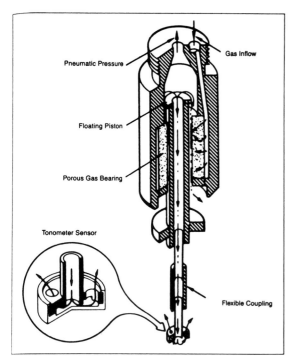

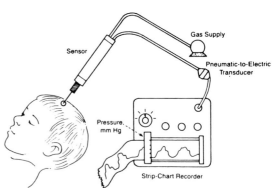

Figure 15.2. *Left:* Pneumotonometer: illustration of technique. *Right:* Schematic diagram of pneumotonometer. (From Easa et al., 1983, with permission.)

tent measurements on several patients within a brief period of time. The major drawbacks of this technique relate to difficulties in obtaining continuous recordings for longer than several minutes and to its dependence on the elasticity of the anterior fontanelle.

The mean ICP measured by pneumotonometer in a series of 35 normal term newborns during the first 3 d of life was 5.3 ± 1.3 mm Hg, with a range of 3–8 mm Hg. In a series of 25 premature infants (26–37 wk gestation), the mean ICP was 5.1 ± 0.9 mm Hg, with a range of 3–7 mm Hg (Easa et al., 1983).

Menke et al. (1982) evaluated the reliability of the pneumatic tonometer in experimental animal studies. Pressure measured with the fontanometer on a surgically created fontanelle in an adult dog correlated well with direct measurements from an epidural balloon catheter (correlation coefficient 0.90).

Applanation transducer

The applanation transducer is constructed of a pressure-sensitive, spring-loaded plunger surrounded by a guard ring. The principle of the applanation technique is that the pressure-sensitive plunger de-

tects the pressure required to prevent a membrane (i.e., the skin over the anterior fontanelle) from bulging into the center of the guard ring that surrounds the plunger. In other words, a force is applied to the plunger until it is in the same plane as the base plate and the membrane (fontanelle) is flat. Under these circumstances, the pressure exerted on the membrane is equal to that beneath the membrane, and there is no effect due to compression of the membrane. Thus, the technique is independent of membrane characteristics, unless the surface area is too small for appropriate placement of the transducer against the fontanelle.

Early clinical studies in newborns using the applanation transducer to measure ICP used the model APT-16 transducer (Hewlett-Packard). Measurements using the technique have been reported to correlate well with direct measurements of ICP obtained by ventricular puncture (Wealthall and Smallwood, 1974; Salmon, Hajjas, and Bada, 1977) and subarachnoid needle insertion (Robinson, Rolfe, and Sutton, 1977). More recently, Whitelaw and Wright (1982) have reported a pneumatic applanation fontanometer that can be used for continuous measurement of ICP (Figure 15.3). This transducer can be applied to the fontanelle using

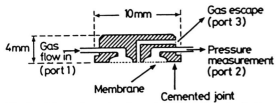

Fig. 1 *Schematic section through the transducer body (for detailed description see text).*

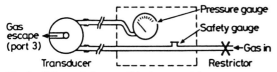

Fig. 2 *Schematic layout of the intracranial pressure monitoring system (for detailed description see text).*

Figure 15.3. Diagrams of applanation transducer technique. (From Rochefort et al., 1987, with permission.)

collodion (Rochefort, Rolfe, and Wilkinson, 1987; Mehta, Wright, and Shore, 1988).

Correct use of the applanation transducer requires that the fontanelle have adequate size for application of the transducer and protude above its bony margins. The positioning of the child is critical, because this particular device measures the pressure of the fontanelle in relation to a chosen reference point (e.g., the right atrium or lowest level of the head). Allowance must be made for the distance between these two points. Furthermore, the attitude of the transducer in relation to the pull of gravity is important. For example, if the infant is supine, with horizontal positioning of the base-plate of the transducer, it must be "zeroed" to that attitude. If these limitations are taken into account, the applanation technique can be useful for continuous, noninvasive measurement of ICP in newborns for prolonged periods of time.

Ladd ICP monitor

The Ladd fiber-optic ICP monitor was originally developed for monitoring ICP in the epidural space. More recently, it has been adapted for noninvasive measurement of ICP in newborn infants (Figure 15.4). This instrument is also based on the applanation principle. It consists of a fiber-optic sensor that uses light to sense the position of a diaphragm that is apposed to the skin of the anterior fontanelle. The sensor is composed of three optical fibers, a pneumatic tube, and a pressure-sensitive diaphragm on which a small mirror is mounted. Air pressure

within the fiber-optic sensor is regulated continuously against the external pressure of the anterior fontanelle acting on the diaphragm. Light is transmitted through one of the optical fibers and reflected back to the other two fibers (output fibers) by a mirror. When the mirror is in a central position, the two output fibers receive equal amounts of light. However, changes in the pressure acting on the diaphragm, related to changes in fontanelle pressure, cause displacement of the mirror and reflection of unequal quantities of light to the two output fibers. These differences in light intensity are monitored by photoelectric detectors, which activate a bellows system, which in turn alters the air pressure within the sensor. The air pressure required to centralize the mirror is equal to the displacing pressure, and therefore provides a measurement of ICP. Using the Ladd ICP monitor, these measurements can be displayed in digital form, or the monitor can be easily interfaced with a strip-chart recorder for continuous recording of ICP (Hill and Volpe, 1981a; Hill, 1985).

The Ladd monitor has the capability to measure absolute pressures between -50 and $+250$ cm H_2O with 1% accuracy, according to the operating manual. The correlations that have been reported for ICP measurements by the Ladd monitor and by direct invasive measurements have varied: Vidyasagar and colleagues (Vidyasagar and Raju, 1977; Vidyasagar, Raju, and Chiang, 1978) reported close correlation between direct measurement of CSF pressure and Ladd ICP measurements ($r = 0.95$; $p < 0.01$). Similarly, close correlations were reported with ICP measurements obtained at lumbar puncture (Purves and James, 1969) or ventriculostomy (Donn and Philip, 1978; Horbar et al., 1980). In contrast, other investigators have disputed the accuracy and reliability of Ladd ICP measurements (Kaiser and Whitelaw, 1987).

The discrepancies between various reports may relate to difficulties in application of the sensor to the fontanelle. Thus, in order to achieve optimal apposition between the diaphragm of the sensor and the fontanelle, it is often necessary to shave the hair overlying the fontanelle. Furthermore, it is of paramount importance that the diaphragm of the sensor be placed on the fontanelle with a *minimum* of external pressure, in order to avoid false elevation of ICP. This problem was investigated by Horbar et al. (1980) with a device that produced serial increases in external application force that were associated with corresponding increases in Ladd ICP measurements and direct ICP measurements obtained by lumbar puncture. Our personal observations confirm that the application force on the sensor can af-

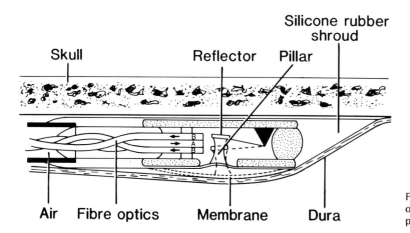

Skull   Reflector   Pillar   Silicone rubber shroud

Air   Fibre optics   Membrane   Dura

Figure 15.4. Diagram of Ladd fiber-optic sensor (From Allen, 1986, with permission.)

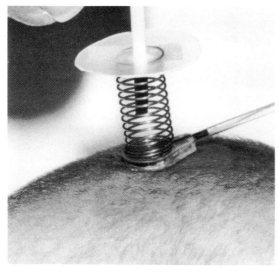

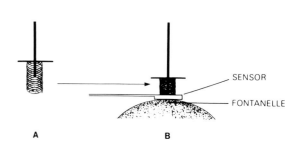

SENSOR

FONTANELLE

A   B

Figure 15.5. *Left:* Spring device for intermittent ICP measurements applied to sensor of Ladd monitor over anterior fontanelle. (From Hill, 1985, with permission.) *Right:* Diagram of application of spring device: A, uncompressed spring attached to rod; B, compression of spring to produce a measured force on sensor. (From Walsh and Logan, 1983, with permission.)

fect ICP values (Hill and Volpe, 1981b; Hill, 1985). In contrast, a study of ICP measurements in monkeys with artificially created fontanelles (Myerberg et al., 1980) demonstrated that measurements by Ladd monitor correlated well with direct ICP measurements, regardless of external application force. The conflicting results may reflect the different methods used in the various studies.

Several techniques have been developed to minimize the effects of external pressure on Ladd ICP measurements. Thus, the sensor can be held gently by hand (Philip, 1979) or apposed to the skin by use of a high-tension spring device attached to a thin rod (Walsh and Logan, 1983; Hill, 1985) (Figure 15.5). For continuous, long-term measurements, various holding devices have been recommended, including adhesive-disc electrocardiography electrodes (Philip, 1979; Finer, 1980) and a plastic frame with a screw device that controls the compression of a calibrated spring that is applied to the surface of the sensor (Figure 15.6, left) (Horbar et al., 1980; Walsh and Logan, 1983). We have used a method for holding the sensor in place with soft, self-adhesive foam material, approximately 4 × 4 cm in size (Reston brand, self-adhering foam roll, no. 1563, 3M Co.); it has high compliance and minimizes external

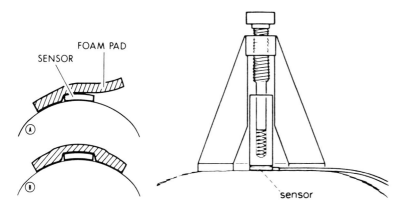

Figure 15.6. *Left:* Diagram of application of sensor of Ladd monitor using a plastic holding device. The force is determined by compression of the spring within the plastic cyclinder by the screw. (From Horbar et al., 1980, with permission.) *Right:* Diagramatic representation of application technique using self-adhesive foam pad. (From Hill and Volpe, 1981a, with permission.)

Table 15.2. *Invasive techniques for measuring ICP in newborns*

Technique	Continuous measurement	Intermittent measurement
Lumber puncture	−	+
Intraventricular catheter	+	+
Epidural screw	+	+
Subdural screw	+	+
Subarachnoid catheter/bolt	+	+

force on the sensor (Hill and Volpe, 1981a) (Figure 15.6, right). To ensure correct application, we recommend the following procedure: Half of the foam material is applied, and the sensor is held gently over the skin to obtain an initial ICP measurement under direct vision. The sensor is then secured in place by application of the remainder of the foam material, and the ICP measurement is repeated. If the second ICP exceeds the initial reading obtained under direct vision, reapplication is necessary (Figure 15.6, right). Adequate contact between the sensor and the skin is confirmed by observation of changes in ICP that correlate with activity of the infant. Thus, spontaneous movements, crying, handling of the infant, or a change in head position can produce twofold or threefold increases in ICP measurements (Perlman and Volpe, 1983a,b; Emery and Peabody, 1983).

It has been demonstrated that the size and shape of the anterior fontanelle, especially in a premature infant, may preclude appropriate application of the sensor of the Ladd monitor for continuous measurement of ICP. Nevertheless, in most of these instances, it is still possible to obtain accurate intermittent measurements of ICP using the hand-held technique (Philip, 1979; Hill and Volpe, 1981a; Hill, 1985).

Invasive methods

Several investigators have reported the use of invasive techniques in newborns, without apparent complications. Sites for invasive measurement of ICP include the lateral ventricles (McWilliam and Stephenson, 1984), subdural space (Goitein and Amit, 1982), and subarachnoid space (Levene and Evans, 1983, 1985; Kaiser and Whitelaw, 1986; Levene et al., 1987; Clancy et al., 1988). Measurements have been obtained by percutaneous insertion of a fine catheter, or placement of a 22-gauge Quick Cath into the subdural space through the fontanelle (Goitein and Amit, 1982). The major clinical applications for invasive techniques are summarized in Table 15.2.

Although invasive techniques have been used in newborns without reports of complications, they do carry the potential for significant risks. The most se-

Table 15.3. *Noninvasive techniques: normal values for ICP in newborns (<1 wk of age)*

Study	Technique	Number of patients	ICP (mm Hg)
Preterm newborns			
Easa et al. (1983)	Digilab pneumotonometer	25	5.1 ± 0.9
Raju et al. (1982)	Ladd monitor	12	7.5 ± 0.9
Vidyasagar & Raju (1977)	Ladd monitor	6	7.14 ± 0.9
Hill & Volpe (1981a)	Ladd monitor	135	6.69 ± 1.65
Term newborns			
Welch (1980)	Clinical assessment	28	3.38 ± 0.9
Robinson et al. (1977)	Applanation transducer	91	8.05 ± 2.3
Salmon et al. (1977)	Applanation transducer	35	7.37 ± 1.45
Menke et al. (1982)	Digilab pneumotonometer	72	7.0 ± 1.9
Easa et al. (1983)	Digilab pneumotonometer	35	5.3 ± 1.3
Vidyasagar & Raju (1977)	Ladd monitor	37	7.67 ± 0.3
Raju et al. (1982)	Ladd monitor	24	8.2 ± 1.0

rious risk relates to intracranial infection (e.g., meningitis or ventriculitis), particularly if continuous monitoring is performed for several days. This risk may be as high as 6% (Allen, 1986). There is a minor risk of intracranial hemorrhage when the dura is opened or the ventricle is punctured. Furthermore, invasive techniques do not yield consistently accurate measurements of ICP. Thus, inaccurate measurements can result from some drainage of CSF at the time of insertion of the catheter. In older patients, it has been reported that ICP measured at extradural sites can be consistently higher than intraventricular ICP. In contrast, subdural measurements can be consistently lower (Allen, 1986). Because invasive techniques are associated with significant risks, without overcoming the problem of inaccurate measurements of ICP, their routine use in newborns cannot be recommended.

SIGNIFICANCE OF ICP IN SPECIFIC NEUROLOGICAL PROBLEMS OF NEWBORNS

Normal values for ICP, which have been reported for both premature and term newborns, are outlined in Table 15.3. In almost all instances, normal ICP is below 10 mm Hg. The major clinical conditions in newborns that can be associated with elevated ICP will be discussed in greater detail.

Premature newborns

Intraventricular hemorrhage

Intraventricular hemorrhage (IVH), which originates from rupture of fragile vessels in the subepen-

dymal germinal matrix, occurs in approximately 30% of premature newborns whose birth weights are less than 1,500 g (Volpe, 1989a,b). Serial cranial ultrasound scans have demonstrated that approximately 90% of IVH occurs prior to 4 d of age, and there is progression in the extent of hemorrhage during the first week of life in 20–40% of cases. Increased ICP is observed in the context of extensive IVH, with dilation of the ventricles and/or extensive hemorrhagic infarction of periventricular cerebral tissue (Figure 15.7). IVH can be recognized clinically on the basis of bulging of the anterior fontanelle and can be associated with a sudden decrease in hematocrit and/or systemic hypotension related to loss of blood volume. Catastrophic deterioration associated with an acute increase in ICP as high as 20–25 cm H_2O has been reported with massive IVH (Kreusser et al., 1984; Volpe, 1987, 1989a). Systemic hypotension combined with elevated ICP can result in decreased cerebral perfusion [cerebral perfusion pressure (CPP) = systemic blood pressure minus ICP], which can produce ischemic injury to cerebral tissue. The precise CPP that is required to prevent ischemic cerebral tissue injury in newborns is not known. However, recent studies with positron-emission tomography suggest that values as low as 5 mm Hg per 100 g per minute may be adequate (Altman et al., 1988). These values are much lower than those reported in older individuals. Several studies (Raju, Doshi, and Vidyasagar, 1982, 1983; Lupton et al., 1988) have reported that CPP values remain normal in newborns despite increased ICP. For example, studies in premature newborns have reported preservation of normal CPP despite the presence of IVH. However, those early studies did not specify the severity of IVH. Nevertheless, re-

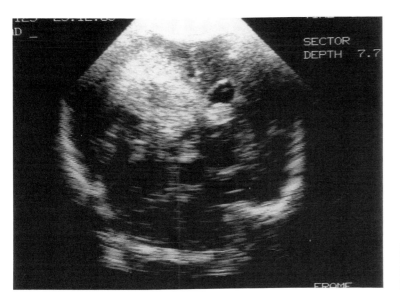

Figure 15.7. Cranial ultrasound scan in coronal plane. Extensive IVH with hemorrhagic infarction of periventricular tissue.

ports of preservation of normal CPP are consistent with current concepts regarding the pathogenesis of another major complication of extensive IVH: periventricular hemorrhagic infarction. This complication is a principal determinant of poor outcome following IVH. It is considered to represent venous infarction related to *localized* obstruction of the medullary and terminal veins at the external angles of the lateral ventricles (Volpe, 1989a), rather than generalized cerebral ischemia.

Posthemorrhagic hydrocephalus

Rapid ventricular dilation and an increase in ICP may take place at the time of occurrence of IVH, as a result of accumulation of excessive quantities of blood within the ventricular system (Kreusser et al., 1984). Subsequently, progressive posthemorrhagic hydrocephalus may develop during the ensuing weeks or months. Potential pathogenetic mechanisms may involve impaired CSF reabsorption, related to an obliterative arachnoiditis in the posterior fossa (communicating hydrocephalus), blockage of arachnoid villi by particulate matter, or obstruction of CSF flow at the level of the aqueduct by blood clot or debris (obstructive hydrocephalus) (Volpe, 1987).

It is important to realize that clinical signs of hydrocephalus (e.g., increased rate of head growth, bulging fontanelle, widening of cranial sutures, distension of scalp veins, and prominence of frontal regions of the skull) may be delayed for weeks following the initial diagnosis of progressive ventriculomegaly by cranial ultrasonography (Volpe, 1987). This delay in the occurrence of the clinical

features of hydrocephalus most probably relates to the relatively large subarachnoid space in a premature infant and the increased compliance of periventricular cerebral tissue in an immature brain, especially if there has been prior hypoxic-ischemic cerebral injury.

Ventriculomegaly may be progressive or may resolve spontaneously (totally or partially) within weeks of the IVH. In approximately 50% of cases there is arrest either with or without resolution of ventriculomegaly (Hill and Volpe, 1982; Volpe, 1987; Dykes et al., 1989). In the remainder there is progressive hydrocephalus that requires drainage of CSF either by serial lumbar punctures (Kreusser et al., 1985) or by surgical intervention (e.g., ventriculoperitoneal shunt, ventriculostomy). The optimal timing for surgical intervention has not been established, because the role of slowly progressive ventricular dilation in the genesis of brain injury has not been clarified. Experimental data suggest that ventricular dilation may be associated with periventricular edema, axonal stretching, and altered molecular composition of the periventricular white matter (Volpe, 1989a). In addition, studies in human newborns demonstrated decreased velocity of cerebral blood flow (using Doppler technique) (Hill and Volpe, 1982) and reversible impaired cerebral perfusion (using positron-emission tomography) in infants with ventriculomegaly (Volpe et al., 1983). Those parameters improved following drainage of CSF (Volpe, 1987). Furthermore, reversible increased latencies of visual-evoked responses have been reported, presumably related to axonal stretching of the optic radiations in the region of the dilated occipital horns of the lateral ventricles (Ehle and Sklar, 1979).

A recent randomized trial involving 157 infants evaluated the potential benefit of early drainage of CSF from the ventricular system by repeated lumbar punctures, as compared with observation without intervention (Ventriculomegaly Trial Group, 1990). Preliminary data regarding neurological outcomes at 12 mo of age demonstrated that the overall incidence of abnormalities was high (85%) and that 62% of infants ultimately required permanent ventricular drainage. There appeared to be no benefit from early intervention for infants who did not have associated parenchymal lesions. Furthermore, among the children who had parenchymal lesions, only motor impairment was reduced by early treatment.

Rarely, newborns may have elevated ICP related to congenital hydrocephalus, which is associated most commonly with aqueductal stenosis. The majority of these infants have associated cerebral dysgenesis, neural tube defects, or genetic syndromes (Volpe, 1987).

Problems in term newborns

Hypoxic-ischemic encephalopathy

Experimental animal studies suggest that an immature brain is relatively resistant to the development of cerebral edema and that tissue necrosis may be a prerequisite for brain swelling (Mujsce, Boyer, and Vannucci, 1987). Increased ICP, related to cerebral edema, is relatively uncommon in asphyxiated human newborns and occurs only in association with severe hypoxic-ischemic encephalopathy at term. It is not usually observed following hypoxic-ischemic insults in premature newborns. In a study in which serial ICP measurements were performed during the first week of life in 32 asphyxiated term newborns (Lupton et al., 1988), increased ICP (>10 mm Hg) was recorded rarely and occurred in only 7 severely asphyxiated newborns. The ICP measurements increased to a maximum between 24 and 72 h of age (Figure 15.8). All infants with increased ICP either died (3 infants) or developed severe neurological sequelae, such as microcephaly or spastic quadriplegia (4 infants). CT scans of the heads of all infants with increased ICP demonstrated diffuse decreases in tissue attenuation (Figure 15.1), which appeared most extensive between 2 and 4 d of age, at a time when the ICP was maximal. Autopsy studies in infants who died confirmed severe brain necrosis. In contrast, infants in whom ICP remained normal had either normal outcomes or only mild

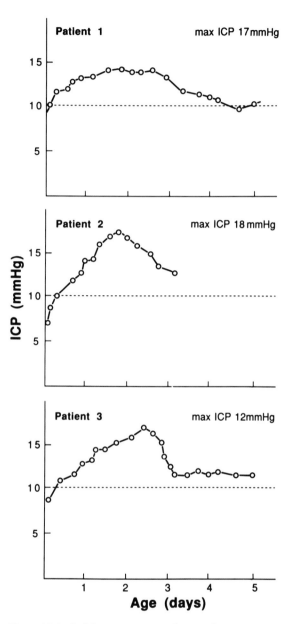

Figure 15.8. Serial measurements of ICP in three term newborns with severe hypoxic-ischemic encephalopathy who died. (From Lupton et al., 1988, with permission.)

neurological abnormalities at 18 mo of age. The autopsy findings, together with the temporal profiles of ICP and CT abnormalities, support the notion that brain swelling is a consequence of extensive cerebral injury (Lupton et al., 1988). Similar observations were made in 10 severely asphyxiated term newborns in whom continuous, direct ICP measurements were obtained using a subarachnoid bolt

(Clancy et al., 1988). Recent studies have demonstrated that increased ICP in asphyxiated term newborns can be reduced by the use of antiedema agents, such as mannitol or dexamethasone (Levene and Evans, 1985; Levene et al., 1987). However, because increased ICP in this context reflects extensive cerebral necrosis, it is unlikely that the reduction of ICP will improve neurological outcomes significantly (Lupton et al., 1988). Nevertheless, clinical recognition of elevated ICP may be regarded as a prognostic factor that indicates poor neurological outcomes following hypoxic-ischemic insults in term newborns.

Miscellaneous conditions

Seizures

Seizures are the most common manifestations of serious neurological disorders in newborns. They can occur in both premature and term newborns in the context of hypoxic-ischemic encephalopathy, IVH, intracranial infection, and metabolic derangements. Transient elevations of ICP above 22 mm Hg during seizures have been documented by Ladd monitor (Philip, 1979; Perlman and Volpe, 1983b). Presumably they reflect increases in cerebral blood flow and elevated systemic blood pressure.

Intracranial infection

Bacterial meningitis and viral encephalitis in both premature and term newborns can be associated with marked increases in ICP (Volpe, 1987). In these instances, the principal mechanisms relate to cerebral edema and hydrocephalus. Complications such as cerebral abscess or subdural effusion occur rarely in neonatal meningitis. Initially, vasculitis may result in cerebral edema secondary to cellular injury, and water retention may be caused by inappropriate secretion of antidiuretic hormone (Reynolds, Dweck, and Cassady, 1972; Kaplan and Feigin, 1978). Increased ICP may persist or worsen during the ensuing days or weeks, because of the development of hydrocephalus related to obstruction of CSF flow by ventriculitis or arachnoiditis. In this context, serial measurements of ICP may detect progressive hydrocephalus and can indicate the optimal timing for external ventricular drainage or serial lumbar punctures.

Viral encephalitis, particularly herpes infection, can be associated with massive cerebral edema related to cerebral necrosis. Recognition of extensive cerebral edema in this context invariably implies a poor prognosis (Volpe, 1987).

CONCLUSIONS

In summary, both invasive and noninvasive techniques are available for continuous and intermittent monitoring of ICP in newborn infants. Early diagnosis of elevated ICP in this age group allows a rational approach to management of newborns with serious neurological conditions and may permit more accurate prognoses.

REFERENCES

Allen, R. (1986). Intracranial pressure: a review of clinical problems, measurement techniques and monitoring methods. *Journal of Medical Engineering and Technology* 10:299–320.

Altman, D. I., Powers, W. J., Perlman, J. M., Herscovitch, P., Volpe, S. L., and Volpe, J. J. (1988). Cerebral blood flow requirement for brain viability in newborn infants is lower than in adults. *Annals of Neurology* 24:218–26.

Brett, E. M. (1966). Measurement of cerebrospinal fluid pressure in infants without puncture. *Developmental Medicine and Child Neurology* 8:207–10.

Clancy, R., Legido, A., Newell, R., Bruce, D., Baumgart, S., and Fox, W. W. (1988). Continuous intracranial pressure monitoring and serial electroencephalographic recordings in severely asphyxiated term neonates. *American Journal of Diseases of Children* 142:740–7.

Davidoff, L. M., and Chamlin, M. (1959). "The Fontanometer." Adaptation of the Schiotz tonometer for the determination of intracranial presssure in the neonatal and early periods of infancy. *Pediatrics* 24:1065–8.

Donn, S. M., and Philip, A. G. S. (1978). Early increase in intracranial pressure in preterm infants. *Pediatrics* 61:904–7.

Dykes, F. D., Dunbar, B., Lazarra, A., and Ahmann, P. A. (1989). Post-hemorrhagic hydrocephalus in high-risk preterm infants: natural history, management and long-term outcome. *Journal of Pediatrics* 114:611–18.

Easa, D., Tron, A., and Bingham, W. (1983). Noninvasive intracranial pressure management in the newborn: an alternate method. *American Journal of Diseases of Children* 137:332–5.

Ehle, A., and Sklar, F. (1979). Visual evoked potentials in infants with hydrocephalus. *Neurology* 29:1541–4.

Emery, J. R., and Peabody, J. L. (1983). Head position affects intracranial pressure in newborn infants. *Journal of Pediatrics* 103:950–3.

Finer, N. N. (1980). Newer trends in continuous monitoring of critically ill infants and children. *Pediatric Clinics of North America* 27:553–66.

Goitein, K. S., and Amit, Y. (1982). Percutaneous placement of subdural catheter for measurement of intracranial pressure in small children. *Critical Care Medicine* 10:46–8.

Guillaume, J., and Janny, P. (1951). Manometric intracranienne continui: interet de la methode et premiers resultats. *Revue Neurologique et Psychiatrie* 84:131–42.

Hill, A. (1985). Intracranial pressure measurements in the newborn. *Clinics in Perinatology* 12:161–77.

Hill, A., and Volpe, J. J. (1981a). Normal pressure hydrocephalus in the newborn. *Pediatrics* 68:623–9.

(1981b). Measurement of intracranial pressure using the Ladd intracranial pressure monitor. *Journal of Pediatrics* 98:974–6.

(1982). Decrease in pulsatile flow in the anterior cerebral arteries in infantile hydrocephalus. *Pediatrics* 67:4–7.

Horbar, J. D., Yeager, S., Philip, A. G. S., and Lacey, J. F. (1980). Effect of application force on noninvasive measurements of intracranial pressure. *Pediatrics* 66:455–7.

Kaiser, A. M., and Whitelaw, A. G. L. (1986). Normal cerebrospinal fluid pressure in the newborn. *Neuropediatrics* 17:100–12.

(1987). Noninvasive monitoring of intracranial pressure – fact or fancy? *Developmental Medicine and Child Neurology* 29:320–6.

Kaplan, S. L., and Feigin, R. D. (1978). The syndrome of inappropriate antidiuretic hormone in children with bacterial meningitis. *Journal of Pediatrics* 92:758–61.

Kreusser, K. L., Tarby, T. J., Kornar, E., Taylor, D. A., Hill, A., and Volpe, J. J. (1985). Serial lumbar punctures for at least temporary amelioration of neonatal post-hemorrhagic hydrocephalus. *Pediatrics* 75:719–24.

Kreusser, K. L., Tarby, T. J., Taylor, D., Kornar, E., Hill, A., Corry, J. A., and Volpe, J. J. (1984). Rapidly progressive post-hemorrhagic hydrocephalus with increased intracranial pressure in the newborn: treatment with internal ventricular drainage. *American Journal of Diseases of Children* 138:633–5.

Levene, M. I., and Evans, D. H. (1983). Continuous measurement of subarachnoid pressure in the severely asphyxiated newborn. *Archives of Disease in Childhood* 58:1013–15.

(1985). Medical management of raised intracranial pressure after severe birth asphyxia. *Archives of Disease in Childhood* 60:12–16.

Levene, M. I., Evans, D. H., Forde, A., and Archer, L. N. J. (1987). The value of intracranial pressure monitoring in asphyxiated newborn infants. *Developmental Medicine and Child Neurology* 29:311–19.

Lou, M. C., Lassen, N. A., and Friis-Hansen, B. (1979). Impaired autoregulation of cerebral blood flow in the distressed newborn infant. *Journal of Pediatrics* 94:118–21.

Lundberg, N. (1960). Continuous recording and control of ventricular fluid pressure in neurosurgical practice. *Acta Psychiatrica et Neurologica Scandinavica* [Suppl. 149] 36:1–193.

Lupton, B. A., Hill, A., Roland, E. H., Whitfield, M. F., and Flodmark, O. (1988). Brain swelling in the asphyxiated term newborn: pathogenesis and outcome. *Pediatrics* 82:130–42.

McWilliam, R. C., and Stephenson, J. B. P. (1984). Rapid bedside technique for intracranial pressure monitoring. *Lancet* 2:73–5.

Mehta, S., Wright, B. M., and Shore, C. (1988). Clinical fontonometry in the newborn. *Lancet* 1:754–6.

Menke, J. A., Miles, R., McIlhaney, M., Bashiru, M., Chua, C., Schuted, E., Menten, T., and Khanna, N.

(1982). The fontanel tonometer – a noninvasive method for measurement of intracranial pressure. *Journal of Pediatrics* 100:960–3.

Mujsce, D. S., Boyer M. A., and Vannucci, R. R. (1987). CBF and brain edema in perinatal cerebral hypoxic-ischemia. *Pediatric Research* 21:494A (abstract).

Myerberg, D. Z., York, C., Chaplin, E. R., and Gregory, G. A. (1980). Comparison of noninvasive and direct measurements of intracranial pressures. *Pediatrics* 65:473–6.

Perkins, J. R., Jr. (1965). The relation of the cerebrospinal fluid to respiration: a brief historical introduction. In *Cerebrospinal Fluid and the Regulation of Ventilation*, ed. C. Brooks, F. F. Kao, and B. B. Lloyd (pp. 7–41). Oxford: Blackwell.

Perlman, J. M., and Volpe, J. J. (1983a). Suctioning in the preterm infant: effects on cerebral blood flow velocity, intracranial pressure and arterial blood pressure. *Pediatrics* 72:329–33.

(1983b). Seizures in the preterm infant. Effects on cerebral blood flow velocity, intracranial pressure and arterial blood pressure. *Journal of Pediatrics* 102:288–93.

Philip, A. G. S. (1979). Noninvasive monitoring of intracranial pressure. A new approach for neonatal clinical pharmacology. *Clinics in Perinatology* 6:123–37.

Purves, M. J., and James, I. M. (1969). Observations on the control of cerebral blood flow in the sheep fetus and newborn lamb. *Circulation Research* 25:651–67.

Raju, T. N. K., Doshi, U., and Vidyasagar, D. (1982). Cerebral perfusion pressure studies in healthy premature and term newborn infants. *Journal of Pediatrics* 100:139–42.

(1983). Low cerebral perfusion pressure: an indicator of poor prognosis in asphyxiated term infants. *Brain Development* 5:478–82.

Reynolds, D. W., Dweck, H. S., and Cassady, G. (1972). Inappropriate antidiuretic hormone secretion in a neonate with meningitis. *American Journal of Diseases of Children* 123:251–3.

Robinson, R. O., Rolfe, P., and Sutton, P. (1977). Noninvasive method for measuring intracranial pressure in normal newborn infants. *Developmental Medicine and Child Neurology* 19:305–8.

Rochefort, M. J., Rolfe, P., and Wilkinson, A. R. (1987). New fontanometer for continuous estimation of intracranial pressure in the newborn. *Archives of Disease in Childhood* 62:152–5.

Salmon, J. H., Hajjas, W., and Bada, H. S. (1977). The fontogram: a noninvasive pressure monitor. *Pediatrics* 60:721–5.

Ventriculomegaly Trial Group (1990). Randomised trial of early tapping in neonatal posthemorrhagic ventricular dilation. *Archives of Disease in Childhood* 65:3–10.

Vidyasagar, D., and Raju, T. N. K. (1977). A simple noninvasive technique for measuring intracranial pressure in the newborn. *Pediatrics* 59:957–61.

Vidyasagar, D., Raju, T. N. K., and Chiang, J. (1978). Clinical significance of monitoring anterior fontanel pressure in sick neonates and infants. *Pediatrics* 62:996–9.

Volpe, J. J. (1987). *Neurology of the Newborn*. Philadelphia: W.B. Saunders.

(1989a). Intraventricular hemorrhage and brain injury in the premature infant: neuropathology and pathogenesis. *Clinics in Perinatology* 16:361–86.

(1989b). Intraventricular hemorrhage in the premature

infant. Current concepts. Part I. *Annals of Neurology* 25:3–11.

(1989c). Intraventricular hemorrhage and brain injury in the premature newborn: neuropathology and pathogenesis. *Clinics in Perinatology* 16:361–86.

Volpe, J. J., Herscovitch, P., Perlman, J. M., and Raichle, M. E. (1983). Positron emission tomography in the newborn. Extensive impairment of regional cerebral blood flow in intraventricular hemorrhage and hemorrhagic intracerebral involvement. *Pediatrics* 72:589–601.

Walsh, P., and Logan, W. J. (1983). Continuous and intermittent measurement of intracranial pressure by Ladd monitor. *Journal of Pediatrics* 102:439–42.

Wealthall, S. R., and Smallwood, R. (1974). Methods of measuring intracranial pressure via the fontanel without puncture. *Journal of Neurology, Neurosurgery and Psychiatry* 37:88–96.

Welch, K. (1970). The emergence of hydrocephalus after ventricular hemorrhage and the estimation of intracranial pressure in infants. *American Journal of Diseases of Children* 131:1203–4.

(1980) The intracranial pressure in infants. *Journal of Neurosurgery* 52:693–9.

Whitelaw, A. G. L., and Wright, B. C. (1982). A pneumatic applanometer for intracranial pressure measurements. *Journal of Physiology* 336:3–4.

PART IV

Machines

Machines have come to dominate perinatal biomedical technology. In this Part IV, two different types of machines are discussed: the ventilator and the heater. Ventilators need to be servocontrolled to regulate blood oxygenation, FIO_2, and blood PCO_2. They also need more "smartness," such as what positive-pressure breathing patterns are best. This is becoming more important as smaller babies and those with more severe lung disease are ventilated with increasingly complex ventilators and ventilatory patterns. These machines are excellent for regulating blood PO_2 and PCO_2, but, especially for very immature infants, we do not know how the machines affect lung development. For example, does the constant distension of high-frequency ventilation promote or inhibit lung growth and neural regulation of breathing? Are some expansion–relaxation cycles necessary for optimal function? How often, and in what patterns, with what pressures?

As for thermoregulation, neonatal medicine had its modern origins near the start of the twentieth century with the public demonstration of surviving premature infants in Pierre Boudin's incubators. Heaters are essential to prevent the adverse metabolic effects of hypothermia in small, preterm infants and increases in metabolic rate in older, more mature infants. Since the development of the first incubators, modern heaters have become far more sophisticated in design and in their ability to control the infant's thermal environment. But they still have not made care as easy and as safe as it should be. Incubators do not allow ready access to the baby, and they take up lots of space. They are poorly designed for filtering out excessive noise and light. Radiant warmers, though they do allow better access, also are inadequate for maintaining proper humidification of the infant's skin. The addition of sensitive scales would be of considerable help as a measure of adequate hydration. If calorimetry could be added, it would be possible also to determine the optimal thermal environment for each infant that would maximize energy balance for maintenance and growth.

16

Neonatal respirators

ROBERT A. deLEMOS, M.D.
GEORGE SIMBRUNER, M.D.
RANGASAMY RAMANATHAN, M.D.

INTRODUCTION

The earliest description of mouth-to-mouth resuscitation of a child is found in the Bible (2 Kings 4:32–5). Since that time, many different approaches to sustaining respiration by artificial means have been attempted. References to early attempts at assisted ventilation appear in the writings of Hippocrates (ca. 400 B.C.) (Daily and Smith, 1971), Paracelsus (1493–1541) (Daily and Smith, 1971), and a number of sixteenth- and seventeenth-century physicians who described tracheostomy, tracheal intubation, and simple forms of continuous artificial ventilation (Thatcher, 1953). The first device specifically designed for resuscitation and short-term ventilation of newborn infants was the *aérophore pulmonaire*, a simple rubber balloon connected to a tracheal tube, described by Gairal in 1879 (Daly and Smith, 1971).

From that beginning, many complex and sophisticated mechanical ventilators have been developed, their designs largely determined by the range of techniques available to gain access to the trachea and by the technology available to produce a ventilator. From the early beginnings to the present time, the major goal has been to provide effective ventilation with minimal side effects.

Prior to the development of safe and effective endotracheal tubes, body-enclosing ventilators similar to the "iron lung" were the primary means of providing prolonged ventilatory support for infants. They produced tidal ventilation by alternately creating positive and negative pressure around the thorax (Doe, 1889). Donald and Lord (1953) developed a negative-pressure ventilator that monitored the breathing movements of an infant with a photocell and used the data obtained to trigger inspiration. That was a major advance, heralding the modern era of mechanical ventilation. Alternative methods attempted during that period included constant thoracic traction (Drinker and Shaw, 1929), body tilting, phrenic nerve stimulation (Cross and Roberts, 1951), and intragastric oxygen inflation (James et al., 1963). None of those approaches proved to be satisfactory for support of infants in respiratory failure. Most made it difficult to gain access to the patient and still maintain adequate ventilation, thus limiting patient examination. In addition, they proved to be ineffective for providing adequate ventilation in infants with anything more than a minimum degree of respiratory failure. There were also serious technical problems with each of the approaches. Even the sophisticated negative-pressure ventilator manufactured by Airshields, Inc., was used infrequently, although in recent years there has been a renewal of interest in this technology (Chernick and Vidyasagar, 1972; Outerbridge and Stern, 1981).

With the development of safe endotracheal tubes and effective mechanical ventilators in the 1950s, positive-pressure ventilation became the method of choice for management of most infants in respiratory failure. These devices achieved their widespread popularity because they allowed the clinician easy access to care for and examine the patient and were simpler in construction (despite offering a wide range of settings and control modes), easier to use, and cheaper to produce than negative-pressure ventilators (Cox, 1974; Hakanson and Stern, 1975;

Delivoria-Papadopoulos and Anday, 1979). Clinicians also began to understand the interaction between ventilatory strategies and their effects on ventilation and oxygenation of patients. Initially, investigators using intermittent positive-pressure ventilation (IPPV) attempted to mimic the intrinsic respiratory patterns of infants with hyaline membrane disease (HMD) by providing high ventilation frequencies, high inspiratory flow rates, and low inspiratory : expiratory ratios. As a result, peak inflation pressures tended to be high (Delivoria-Papadopoulos and Anday, 1979). Subsequently, the beneficial effects of continual distending pressure (Gregory et al., 1971) and inflation-hold were discovered and introduced into clinical practice (McIntyre, Laws, Ramachandran, 1969; Llewellyn and Swyer, 1970). That allowed reductions in the ventilatory rate and peak airway pressure while simultaneously treating or preventing atelectasis.

A major advance in infant ventilation came with the development of intermittent mandatory ventilation (IMV) in the early 1970s (Kirby et al., 1972). That technique provided a continuous flow of fresh gas throughout the respiratory cycle, thereby allowing either spontaneous breathing with continuous positive airway pressure (CPAP) or a slow rate of IPPV with positive end-expiratory pressure (PEEP) within the same system (Kirby et al., 1972; Luce, Pierson, and Hudson, 1981). IMV made it possible to impose a respiratory pattern directed at a particular strategy while allowing the patient's spontaneous breathing to compensate for some of the adverse physiological effects of the ventilator-controlled breaths. The development of IMV was a major advance over controlled ventilation and proved to be particularly useful in weaning infants from assisted ventilation (deLemos and Kirby, 1980).

During the past decade, the interactions among the ventilator, the ventilation strategy, and the patient risks/benefits have become better understood (Rogers, 1972; Simbruner and Götz, 1976; Epstein and Epstein, 1979). Furthermore, the idea that adult ventilators could be adapted for pediatric use (Mushin et al., 1969) was replaced by the understanding that infants required equipment specifically designed to meet their ventilatory requirements. One recent advance has been increased sophistication in the development of ventilators that allow the infant to initiate the ventilator-induced breath. Initially these systems were designed to detect a small negative pressure (<0.5 cm H_2O) generated in the breathing circuit and ventilator at the initiation of spontaneous inspiration. Recently, more responsive technologies have been developed to initiate triggering of the mechanical ventilator. This has made it possible to assist or synchronize ventilation even when high cycling frequencies are required (Epstein, 1971; Greenough and Pool, 1988). Modern infant ventilators have also benefited from technologies involving fluidics (Weitzner and Urban, 1969) and microprocessors (Heller and Heinrichs, 1979). These have allowed the development of sophisticated control modes and created the potential for concurrent monitoring of the patient's respiratory status.

In this decade, recognition of the role of barotrauma in neonatal lung injury has led to developments in ventilator technology directed at the prevention of ventilator-associated lung injury. The category of "high-frequency ventilation" encompasses a group of techniques that have in common their ability to achieve acceptable alveolar ventilation using tidal volumes less than or near to dead-space volumes and supraphysiological respiratory frequencies (Klain and Smith, 1977; Sjöstrand, 1977; Bohn et al., 1980; Butler et al., 1980; Carlon et al., 1981; Marchak et al., 1981; Gerstmann, deLemos, and Clark, 1991). Because high-frequency ventilation (HFV) accomplishes adequate ventilation with minimal volume excursions above and below mean lung volume, it has been particularly efficacious in the treatment and prevention of pulmonary barotrauma in neonates (Froese and Bryan, 1978). Pressure-release ventilation holds the lung at a constant pressure and then intermittently releases the pressure, allowing the lung to collapse to functional residual capacity (FRC). Because the greater portion of the ventilatory cycle is held at peak volume, this technique has been useful in the management of adults with large intrapulmonary shunts, but has not been widely used in neonates. Finally, as mentioned earlier, more sophisticated techniques have been developed to synchronize mechanical-ventilator breaths with the onset of spontaneous ventilation. Preliminary evidence suggests that the use of synchronized IMV may reduce pulmonary barotrauma (Hird and Greenough, 1990).

Newborn infants are prone to respiratory failure and often require mechanical ventilation (Thomas et al., 1965; Norlander, 1968). Therefore, the success or failure of mechanical ventilators in replacing the lost functions of the diseased respiratory system can have an enormous impact on mortality and morbidity among these infants (Delivoria-Papadopoulos, Levison, and Swyer, 1965; Northway, Rosan, and Porter, 1967; Daily, Sunshine, and Smith, 1971; Johnson et al., 1974; Marriage and Davies, 1977; Fitzhardinge, 1978; Heldt et al., 1980; Jacob et al.,

1980; Lindroth et al., 1980; Schreiner et al., 1980; Rothberg et al., 1981).

Numerous ventilators have been built and used to ventilate infants mechanically, often with minimal evaluation before clinical use. As a result, testing procedures have been developed and advocated by the International Standards Organisation (ISO, 1978). Despite this, only a few publications have appeared so far that have critically examined the performances of neonatal ventilators in human infants (Murdock et al., 1970; Llewellyn and Swyer, 1971; Mattila and Suutarinen, 1971; Nordstrom, 1972; Keuskamp, 1974), experimental animals (Amaha et al., 1967; Mattila and Suutarinen, 1971; Nordstrom, 1972; Boros et al., 1977; Downs et al., 1979), and lung models (Epstein, 1971; Mattila, 1974; Abrahams et al., 1975; Simbruner and Gregory, 1981; Boros et al., 1984; Carr et al., 1986; Kirpalani, Santos-Lyn, and Roberts, 1988), or from a theoretical standpoint (Rogers, 1972; Weigl, 1973; Epstein and Epstein, 1979). Unlike other devices, a ventilator cannot be evaluated as a freestanding entity. The ventilator and the patient constitute a system in which each component interacts with and influences the other. How they interact determines how well the lung will be ventilated. The main problems in evaluating neonatal ventilators lie in the complexity of this interaction and in the limitations on our theoretical and practical knowledge of artificial ventilation (Keuskamp, 1974). In this chapter we shall discuss the performance goals for both conventional and high-frequency neonatal ventilators and describe criteria for deciding which ventilator may be best for use in a given clinical setting, realizing that no mechanical ventilator is ideal for all applications.

FUNCTIONS OF A VENTILATOR

The ultimate goal of mechanical ventilation is to provide effective gas exchange (as evidenced by normal oxygenation and normal carbon dioxide elimination), while causing minimal side effects (pulmonary barotrauma, circulatory compromise, and alterations in thermal and energy balances), for as long as necessary for the infant to recover from the primary disease (Reynolds, 1974; Gottschalk, King, and Schuth, 1980). This requires that the ventilator perform a number of functions: move gas into the gas-exchange units, hold it there for the desired amount of time before allowing it to escape, allow unimpeded gas egress to a preset end-expiratory pressure, heat and humidify the inspired gas, provide the desired concentration of inspired oxygen, provide continuous monitoring of ventilator func-

tions that affect the patient–ventilator interaction, and assess the patient's respiratory status (lung mechanics, energy balance, etc.), and all of these must be carried out in a safe and reliable manner. In the following sections we shall examine each of these requirements.

GAS EXCHANGE AND THE RESPIRATORY PATTERN

Gas exchange in the lung takes place by two mechanisms: bulk flow and diffusion. Although traditionally it was thought that gas was transported by bulk flow to the alveoli and by diffusion across the alveolar–capillary membrane, more recent data suggest that other mechanisms (molecular and axial diffusion, *Penduluft*, asymmetrical velocity patterns) also play roles in gas transport and that the relative contributions of these are dependent on both the type of ventilator and the specific strategy employed (Chang, 1984). During HFV, for example, it is believed that the transition between bulk flow and molecular diffusion occurs more proximal in the airway than during normal tidal breathing.

The diffusion of carbon dioxide is about 20 times faster than the diffusion of oxygen from alveoli to capillaries. Thus, elimination of CO_2 is critically dependent on emptying the gas-exchange units and subsequent replacement with fresh gas. To be effective, a ventilator must be able to exchange the volume of gas required for ventilation and expose a large enough lung volume and lung surface area for diffusion by preventing and/or overcoming atelectasis.

The respiratory pattern can be described in terms of the duration of gas flow, the tidal volume, and the pressure required to produce them. All are interrelated: volume/pressure = compliance; pressure/flow = resistance;　volume = flow × time. We begin by describing the respiratory pattern in terms of pressure and time.

Ventilators generate a tidal breath by altering the pressure in the airway relative to atmospheric pressure. The pressure generated can be either positive or negative. The respiratory cycle, generated in either way, consists of five elements: inflation, inflation-hold, exhalation, expiratory pause, and pressure at end-expiration (Figure 16.1). The two functions (pressure differences within the lung and the respiratory-cycle length) required to achieve gas exchange are reflected in these factors. The ventilation volume is the result of pressure differences between the mouth and alveoli (peak inspiratory and end-expiratory pressures and the respiratory-cycle length)

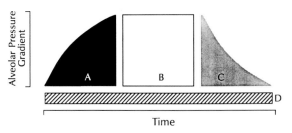

Figure 16.1. Schematic representation of the respiratory cycle: A, inspiration; B, inflation-hold; C, exhalation; D, end-expiratory pressure. The area of each component reflects the contribution of each to the mean airway pressure. The heights of A and B reflect tidal volume; the lengths of A, B, and C indicate cycle durations. Varying the size and shape of any or all of the components will influence the relationships between ventilation and the peak and mean pressures of the ventilator breath.

and the sum of inspiratory time (i.e., the time for inflation plus inflation-hold) and expiratory time (i.e., the time for exhalation plus expiratory pause). Ideally, tidal volume should not be limited by the time necessary for the pressure to develop or decay. The end-expiratory pressure level does not influence tidal volume unless this pressure is increased or decreased without readjusting the peak inspiratory pressure. All four elements of the respiratory cycle are responsible for exposing an adequate lung volume, because they interact to create the alveolar pressures that expand the lung and keep it expanded. The inflation-hold and expiratory pressure level are most important in this regard and are the products of pressure and time. The contribution to mean alveolar pressure due to inspiration and expiration is the integral of pressure over time. The faster that inspiration and expiration are achieved, the less these factors contribute to mean alveolar pressure for a given minute ventilation, and vice versa. If inspiration and expiration become sufficiently short, tidal gas exchange will more or less be the result of a mean alveolar pressure. Positive-pressure ventilators usually are able to achieve the pressures necessary for tidal ventilation, but they may do so by producing high alveolar pressures, which increase the likelihood of barotrauma. Maintaining a low ratio between ventilation and mean alveolar pressure will reduce the number of possible ventilatory patterns and theoretically reduce the resultant degree of barotrauma. Negative-pressure ventilators are limited in their ability to develop large transpulmonary pressure and adequate tidal volumes in patients with severe lung disease (Stern et al., 1970; Outerbridge and Stern, 1981).

During the course of inspiration and expiration, tidal volume and airway pressure increase with inflow and decrease with egress of gas from the lung and ventilator. Before flow changes directionally from inspiration to expiration, or vice versa, there is a brief interval during which gas flow in the system is zero. This is analogous to what occurs during an inflation-hold or an expiratory pause, when volume and pressure in the lung are held constant and there is no gas flow. The points in the respiratory cycle where directional changes in gas flow occur are called turning points. They mark the beginning and the end of an interval and denote its duration. These turning points are associated with a specific volume of gas and/or airway pressure or with zero gas flow.

The concept of turning points in the respiratory cycle is useful in understanding the control mechanisms of specific ventilators. One such mode, the cycling mode, refers to the parameter that causes the direction of gas flow to change. Another, the limiting mode, refers to the parameter that determines where changes cease – for example, the peak airway pressure. Both modes compare one or more measured parameters with a preset value(s). Where the parameter is measured, and whether it is referenced to the airway or to the alveolus, should be specified. Both reference points have been used, but it is more logical to reference to the alveolus, because that is where gas exchange takes place. However, the difficulties in measuring or estimating alveolar pressures have led manufacturers of commercially available ventilators to reference either to proximal-airway pressure or to intratracheal pressure measured through a double-lumen endotracheal tube. Gas flow, tidal volume, and pressure measured in the ventilator circuit and airways can differ from those in the alveoli, depending on the mechanical properties of the lung. Even a volume-cycled ventilator will not necessarily deliver the desired volume of gas to the areas of gas exchange when lung mechanics are abnormal. This is particularly true in immature infants with HMD, where the conducting airways may be the most compliant portions of the respiratory system (Nilsson, Grossmann, and Robertson, 1978). In reality, the only parameter that is the same at all levels of the patient–ventilator system is time.

PHYSICAL CHARACTERISTICS OF VENTILATORS

Ventilators are made up of multiple components that when properly matched and functioning will

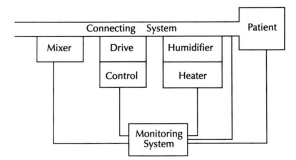

Figure 16.2. Basic components of infant ventilators: drive and control mechanisms, humidifier and heater, gas mixer, connecting system, monitoring system.

work together to provide the desired output. There are basically six such components in modern ventilators: the drive mechanism, the control mechanism, the humidifier and heater, the gas mixer, the connecting system, and the monitoring system (Figure 16.2).

Until recently, most ventilator classifications were based on the physical properties of their drive and/or control mechanisms. That was presumed to be useful in order to understand their behavior and predict performance (Mushin et al., 1969; Grogono, 1972; Baker and Murray-Wilson, 1974; Lough, Doershuk, and Stern, 1974). However, ventilators have now become so complex that all components are of approximately equal importance in understanding the overall performance of the device. Therefore, development of a meaningful hierarchical classification for ventilators is difficult. Instead, it is more reasonable to classify these devices with regard to both a description of physical design and a functional analysis of performance. Because the negative-pressure ventilator currently available for use with infants is used only on a limited basis, we shall confine our discussion to positive-pressure ventilators.

Drive mechanism

The drive mechanism or force generator of a ventilator moves the breathing gas between the ventilator system and the lung. These mechanisms are either electrically or pneumatically powered. Those that are electrically powered use a motor to move a piston (which produces a constant sinusoidal flow pattern), compress a bellows, or activate a compressor. Pneumatically powered ventilators derive the energy for their driving force from a pressure source such as a high-pressure gas reservoir. Drive mecha-

nisms can also be distinguished by whether they use a container or a flow system to generate a tidal volume. A container system is one in which a given volume of gas is contained within a rigid cylinder (piston) or flexible bag (bellows) prior to the initiation of each inflation. The contents of the container are expelled into the ventilator tubing and the lung during inspiration. Container systems produce a volume change under isobaric conditions, either by moving a piston in a rigid container or by compressing a flexible container (bellows). A third type of container system, a rigid container under pressure, moves the gas under isochoric (volume-constant) conditions. The drop in pressure seen with this system corresponds to the volume of gas delivered.

The other type of drive mechanism is the flow system. As in the isochoric container system, a continuous pressure is provided from a high-pressure source to drive the ventilator. These high-pressure, constant-flow generators interpose a resistance between the pressure source and the patient to regulate the amount of flow. This allows gas flow to be routed into the patient or diverted into the environment. If the breathing gas and that used for the driving force come from the same source, the system is described as a primary system; if the gases used for the driving force and breathing are separated, the system is described as a primary-secondary system.

Ventilators can also be classified as to whether or not they produce a constant flow or pressure (Lough et al., 1974). Although both will produce a tidal volume, the mechanism used to produce that volume has an impact on how closely the delivered tidal volume approximates the desired volume and on how expensive it is to produce the tidal volume. In a container system, the size of the container and the speed with which it is refilled limit the tidal volume and the rate at which it can be delivered. The container itself is a compressible gas space that increases the internal compliance of the ventilator. Container systems allow more thorough mixing of the inspired gases, and therefore a more nearly constant concentration of inspired gas, as compared with flow systems. Container systems usually allow the operator more control over the gas flow pattern than is possible with flow systems. They also permit rebreathing of gases purged of carbon dioxide, which allows them to be used for administering anesthesia. This is not possible with flow systems. Flow systems, on the other hand, have the advantage of providing a driving force that is great enough to deliver large tidal volumes at rapid rates. These systems are simpler in design, smaller, and less expensive. Because of this, the latest generation of adult ventilators have been developed using this principle. Motor-powered ventilators are usually larger, noisier, and subject to more technical problems than pneumatically powered ventilators. The drive mechanism in large part determines which power source will be used.

Control mechanism

Control of gas flow in the ventilator–patient system is determined by a controller and a regulator. The controller receives, processes, and stores information for developing the ventilatory pattern. The regulator effects the changes dictated by the controller. Ideally, the controller will permit the operator to influence all elements of the respiratory pattern.

The cycling and limiting modes of the ventilator influence the respiratory pattern of the breathing cycle. The cycling mode determines when the direction of gas flow in the system will change. Volume, pressure, flow, and time can be used to initiate or terminate ventilator cycling. When the chosen parameter reaches its preset value, the ventilator either terminates or initiates inspiration. Multiple factors can be employed simultaneously to control cycling (mixed cycling). For example, a ventilator that uses both volume and time to end inspiration will cycle off when either a predetermined volume of gas has been delivered or a preset time has elapsed.

The limiting mode causes a parameter to remain constant when it reaches its preset value. The same parameters that are used for the cycling modes can be used for the limiting modes. The usual limiting parameters are gas volume and pressure, although theoretically it is also possible to use flow limitation. Although time cannot be used as a limiting factor, it can be used to determine when a turning point will occur.

Cycling and limiting modes can be employed to define turning points from expiration to inspiration and inspiration to expiration. This makes possible many combinations of control modes. First, let us look at inspiratory cycling modes, when the expiratory cycling factor is time. If the inspiratory cycling-mode parameter is volume or time, it is possible to ventilate with a constant tidal volume and respiratory rate, assuming that the gas flow rate during inspiration is constant (gas flow × time = volume). If the ventilator is pressure- or flow-cycled, tidal volume and the maximum frequency of ventilation will depend on lung mechanics, because the compliance and resistance of the lung will determine how rap-

idly a pressure is achieved and when zero flow is reached. The control-mode parameter for terminating expiration is usually time, although the use of other parameters is possible. Flow-cycled expiration is technically feasible and should minimize gas trapping within the lung and its associated inadvertent PEEP (Weigl, 1973). This concept has recently been incorporated into new infant ventilators (Servant et al., 1992).

The control and assist modes refer to the mechanisms used to initiate a breathing cycle. In the control mode, the controller is programmed to initiate a ventilator cycle at set intervals. In the assist mode, some mechanism is used to detect the initiation (or cessation) of spontaneous breaths. This can be accomplished by sensing the development of negative pressure or changes in gas flow within the breathing circuit, or be detection of chest or abdominal-wall motion with pressure sensors or impedance pneumography (Mitchell, Greenough, and Hird, 1989). The ventilator then receives and processes this signal and in response initiates a tidal breath. In the assist-control mode (also called the demand mode), the ventilator initiates inspiration at the start of patient inspiration, or after a preset interval if the patient fails to breathe spontaneously. It is also possible to terminate the assisted breath concurrent with termination of the spontaneous breath.

Most currently available neonatal ventilators provide a continuous source of gas flow, allowing spontaneous breathing and mechanical ventilation in either the control or the assist mode. This allows the use of either synchronized or independent IMV.

In addition to the control modes, there are parameters that are uncontrolled. These uncontrolled parameters represent the degrees of freedom of the patient–ventilator system (Bendixen, 1976). The degrees of freedom determine how many ways the patient–ventilator system can react in response to those parameters that are controlled and determine how many aspects of the respiratory pattern will be altered. For example, when using a volume-cycled ventilator, the tidal volume is preset. The airway pressure needed to deliver the tidal volume is a function of the compliance and resistance of the lung and represents one degree of freedom. When using a pressure-cycled ventilator, the ventilator pressure is controlled, and the delivered tidal volume and length of inspiration are uncontrolled. Thus, there are two degrees of freedom. A flow-generated, time-cycled ventilator delivers a given tidal volume as a function of the inspiratory flow and the inspiratory time. However, the introduction of a limiting parameter, such as pressure, will alter the tidal volume. In this setting, pressure is the controlled variable, and volume is uncontrolled. When ventilators are used in the assist mode, the frequency is uncontrolled. The ideal number of degrees of freedom is still debatable. In general, ventilators that reduce the degrees of freedom as close to unity as possible are desirable because they allow tighter control over, and more knowledge of, the parameters involved in the patient–ventilator system.

Connecting system

The system that links the drive mechanism, the humidifier, and the measuring devices of the ventilator to the patient is critically important to the performance of neonatal ventilators. The connecting system consists of rigid and elastic components that have a finite volume. During inspiration, gas is compressed within this volume (compressible gas volume), causing the volume of gas delivered to the patient with each breath to be reduced. The connecting tubing, the piston or bellows, and the gas-humidification system determine the internal compliance of a ventilator. These components may also offer resistance to gas flow. When they do, they may interfere with either inspiration or expiration or both. For example, if the resistance to exhalation is increased, it will take longer for the expired gas to leave the lung. The length of the connecting system will determine the distance a pressure wave has to travel and thus can delay the appearance of a pressure signal in the machine or in the patient. The dead space of the connecting system depends on the distance between the expiratory opening and the endotracheal tube and on the presence of a continuous flow to wash out exhaled carbon dioxide. Because of changes in internal volume, a highly compliant connecting system can negate many of the advantages of a well-designed ventilator, particularly when lung compliance is low or airway resistance high.

PERFORMANCE OF VENTILATORS

Ultimately it is the interaction between the ventilator and the respiratory system of the infant that must determine the overall performance of a ventilator. The result of that interaction cannot be predicted on the basis of assessing the functioning of single components of the ventilator, such as the drive or control mechanism, but can be determined only by testing the ventilator under conditions similar to those found in the clinical setting. The discrepancy between the expected performance and the actual performance of a ventilator can be assessed by examining (1) its ability to deliver a constant tidal volume, (2) the airway pressure required to generate a tidal volume, (3) the inflation-hold, (4) the gas outflow characteristics of the system, and (5) the effectiveness of the assist mode in synchronizing mechanical- and patient-initiated breaths.

Delivery of a constant tidal volume

It would be relatively easy to deliver a constant tidal volume if the ventilator were as close to the infant's lungs as is the natural respiratory pump (respiratory muscles, rib cage). However, the necessity of using connecting tubes and humidifiers makes that impossible, because these components constitute a buffer in which gases will be compressed when lung mechanics worsen. The compliance of the respiratory system in an infant with HMD can range between 0.3 and 1 ml · (cm H_2O)$^{-1}$ (Cook et al., 1957; Chu et al., 1964; Ahlstrom, 1975; Auld, 1975; Simbruner et al., 1982; Carlo and Maktin, 1983; Cunningham and Desai, 1986), and the internal compliances of ventilators range between 0.3 and 3 ml · (cm H_2O)$^{-1}$ (Rogers, 1972). The tidal volume lost in the connecting system of the ventilator as a result of its internal compliance can be calculated (Okmian, 1963): tidal volume delivered/tidal volume set on the machine = 1/[1 + compliance (internal)/compliance (patient)]. For example, if the machine's internal compliance and the patient's compliance are both 0.5 ml · (cm H_2O)$^{-1}$, only half of the gas volume ejected from the ventilator will actually be delivered to the patient. A 10% change in the respiratory compliance of the patient will cause a 5% change in the original tidal volume. This loss in tidal volume is correctly calculated only when the inspiratory duration is sufficient to allow full inspiration. If not, the delivered tidal volume will be even smaller. Epstein and Epstein (1979) have shown that the flow of gas delivered to the patient is less than that generated by the ventilator at the start of inspiration.

When a constant-flow generator is used, 38–197 ms are required to reach 90% of the final gas flow when the compliance of the connecting system is 0.5 ml · (cm H_2O)$^{-1}$, the lung compliance is between 1 and 3 ml · (cm H_2O)$^{-1}$, and the resistance to flow is between 50 and 200 cm H_2O · l^{-1} · s^{-1} (Kirby et al., 1972). When infants are ventilated with higher respiratory rates, the inspiratory time may be even shorter. A point will be reached at which very little gas flow will occur during a large portion of the inspiratory cycle. The delivery of a constant tidal volume will also be impaired if there is a gas leak in the system.

These theoretical considerations were confirmed by earlier studies in which neonatal ventilators showed considerable variation in their ability to deliver a given tidal volume when the lung mechanics of the test system were systematically altered (Mattila and Suutarinen, 1971; Keuskamp, 1974; Abrahams et al., 1975; Simbruner and Gregory, 1981). Even the more sophisticated ventilators tested delivered only half of the predicted tidal volume when lung mechanics were grossly abnormal. Abrahams et al. (1975) showed that in extreme cases, such as those that might occur in an infant with HMD and a partially occluded endotracheal tube [lung compliance 1 ml · (cm H$_2$O)$^{-1}$, resistance 1,000 cm H$_2$O · l^{-1}·s^{-1}, PEEP 13 cm H$_2$O, and a leak of gas from the system], only 10% of the predicted gas volume would reach the lungs. Though Okmian (1963), Hedenstierna and Oquist (1974), and Forbat and Her (1980) described methods to compensate for this loss of gas volume, those corrections are not reliable when applied to the neonatal lung.

A volume-preset ventilator is better able to deliver a constant tidal volume than is a pressure-preset ventilator. In the latter, decreases in tidal volume are proportional to any decrease in lung compliance and/or increase in resistance. In spite of their theoretical advantages, volume-cycled ventilators have not been widely used in newborns. In part, this is related to problems with delivery-circuit compliance and leaks around the endotracheal tube, both of which lessen the efficiency of the devices. Recently, a new infant volume-cycled ventilator was introduced combining microprocessor technology, integration of pneumatic solenoids and both pressure and flow transducers to allow either time-cycled, pressure-limited ventilation or volume-controlled ventilation with a single device. Although preliminary reports suggest that it may have advantages in selected infants, volume-controlled ventilation has not yet been broadly used in neonatal patients (Bandy, Nicks, and Donn 1992).

Tidal volume, mean and peak alveolar pressures

Ventilators differ considerably in regard to the time required to deliver a tidal volume and to allow gas egress. They also differ in terms of the mean alveolar pressures generated when delivering that tidal volume. The limitations of some ventilators include a diminished capacity to deliver gas flow rapidly and an inability to generate an adequate tidal volume within a short time interval. In most of the available neonatal ventilators, exhalation is prolonged because of high outflow resistance. This has an additive effect on the time limitations imposed by the time constant of the lung (compliance × resistance). Thus, it is necessary to ensure that the expiratory time is equal to or longer than that required for complete exhalation, in order to prevent gas trapping (Weigl, 1973; Simbruner and Gregory, 1981). The more rapidly the tidal volume is delivered, and the less time required for complete exhalation, the shorter the potential breathing cycle, and therefore the higher the ventilator rate can be without causing gas trapping and development of inadvertent PEEP. Differences between ventilators are most pronounced at the extremes of lung compliance and resistance. Ventilators that allow the rapid generation and egress of a tidal volume do so with relatively low mean alveolar pressures. It then follows that these ventilators have advantages over others because they permit the use of a wider range of ventilator settings. Furthermore, they can provide adequate minute ventilation and high mean alveolar pressures while producing relatively low peak airway pressures. Because the time for inspiration is short, there is also adequate time to provide an inflation-hold, if desired. This is one effective way to increase the mean alveolar pressure without increasing the peak airway pressure, although some studies have shown an increased risk of air leak with this approach. Increases in PEEP also increase the mean airway pressure. However, often one must concurrently increase the peak airway pressure to maintain an adequate tidal volume. Finally, it must be remembered that many PEEP devices are flow resistors that increase the resistance to outflow of gas (Simbruner and Gregory, 1981).

Inflation-hold (or pressure plateau)

Ventilators can create a pressure plateau by several different mechanisms. Those that use a container system as the drive mechanism produce an inflation-hold by maintaining a tidal volume within the lung for the duration of the inflation-hold. Ventilators with a flow system as the force generator achieve a pressure plateau by use of the limiting mode and time cycling. Both systems will create an alveolar pressure plateau. When the lung is healthy, both approaches will produce an inflation-hold at about the same time. However, when the lung is diseased and an inflation-hold would be of value, there is some delay in developing an alveolar pressure plateau with flow generators.

Assist mode

In older systems, patient-assist modes required the patient to develop an intraluminal negative pressure as the signal for initiation of inspiratory cycling. For this type of assist mode to be of use in newborns, the ratio of patient effort (the volume of gas that the infant needs to withdraw from the circuit to produce reliable triggering) to tidal volume should be less than 0.01, and the ratio of response time to inspiratory time less than unity (Rogers, 1972). This means that a volume of 0.1 ml and a response time of 50 ms are required for a tidal volume of 10 ml and an inspiratory time of 0.5 s. With this approach to synchronized mechanical ventilation, the triggering mechanism of the ventilator is activated when the patient withdraws a small volume of gas from the breathing circuit, thus producing a negative pressure in the system. The minimal volume of gas that must be withdrawn will depend on the internal compliance of the ventilator, with greater compliance requiring a larger volume of gas to be withdrawn. Thus, the triggering volume, not pressure, is important.

This method of generating the patient's signal has not proved effective in sick newborns. Recently, several alternative approaches have been developed to circumvent these problems. One has been to use a pressure transducer on the abdominal wall to detect its upward displacement following diaphragmatic contraction (Hird and Greenough, 1990). Coupling this signal to a rapid-responding microprocessor-controlled ventilator has in part offset the time lag inherent with this technology. A second technique uses impedance pneumography to detect the onset of spontaneous inspiration. This eliminates the requirement that one be lying on one's back or side to obtain an appropriate signal, but it requires a complex algorithm to eliminate cardiac artifact. Finally, some investigators have used hot-wire anemometers or smaller pressure transducers to increase the sensitivity of the flow/volume-triggered systems. All of these techniques are currently in clinical testing and theoretically are capable of providing an adequate signal for an assisted or synchronized IMV mode, even in small premature infants. Although the preliminary reports suggest that their use reduces air leak and other manifestations of barotrauma, further clinical evaluation is necessary.

The total time required to initiate inspiration (ventilator response time) has several elements: (1) the time it takes for the inspiratory signal from the patient to reach the ventilator, (2) the time needed for the ventilator to react to the signal and begin delivering a tidal volume, (3) the time required for the tidal volume to reach the lungs. In earlier studies, Epstein (1971) showed that the response times of ventilators varied markedly. Of the older ventilators tested in his studies, only the Bourns LS 104-150 was capable of assisting respiration in small infants (Epstein, 1971). That ventilator had been considered state-of-the-art technology until development of the new sensor-triggering systems described earlier. No comparable studies have been performed on the newer generation of ventilators.

Mixing of breathing gases

Basically, there are two kinds of gas-mixing devices in common use: blenders and flow mixers. Blenders provide the breathing gas at high pressure; flow mixers provide it at low pressures. All ventilators that use inspired gases for both breathing and powering the ventilator (systems without a secondary flow system) require blenders for gas mixing. A blender has two throttles that have variable cross-sectional openings. The blender is connected to a high-pressure gas source on the inflow side and to the ventilator on the outflow side. Provided the inflow pressure is constant, the two gases will be mixed in proportion to how wide the throttles are opened. If the inflow pressure to either throttle is unstable or there is no buffer system between the blender and the ventilator to modulate variations in gas demand, the delivered oxygen concentration can be highly variable.

Humidifying and heating the breathing gas

Tracheal intubation prevents the nasopharynx from humidifying and warming the inspired gases. Those functions must therefore be carried out by a device that humidifies and heats the inspired gases to approximately body temperature. Though there is still some debate about the amount of water that should be added to the inspired gases, there is general agreement that the water content of the inspired air should approach 44 mg per liter of gas. To accomplish this, water can be added as steam, microdroplets, or aerosol. Humidifiers often are categorized on this basis, that is, whether they add steam or droplets of water to the inspired gases. Humidifiers of the first type are divided into (1) those in which the breathing gas is either bubbled through water or convected over water and (2) those that add steam to the inspired gases. Although heated humidifiers can produce more than 40 mg of water per liter of gas egress, the water content of the gas inspired by the patient is usually lower, because the gas temperature decreases as the gas passes through the inspiratory side of the breathing circuit. The decrease in temperature causes water to condense in the tubing. To compensate for that, the temperature of the gases leaving the humidifier must be high (usually above 40°C), or the surface area of the heated water must be large, or the gas temperature must be maintained by use of a heated wire in the delivery circuit if the gas inspired by the patient is to contain the appropriate amount of water. Each of these techniques has potential problems. The first must be servocontrolled to the proximal-airway temperature to minimize the danger of overheating the inspired gases. The second results in a large internal compliance (compression volume). Bubble-through humidifiers increase the resistance of the inspiratory circuit. Steam does not increase inspiratory resistance; however, it is difficult to judge the volume of water produced and to control fluctuations in the temperature of the inspired gases.

Humidifiers of the second type add droplets of water to the inspired gas by using an ultrasonic device or high-velocity gas jet. Ultrasonic nebulizers are exceedingly effective at adding water to the inspired gases – so effective, in fact, that they can add as much as 100 mg of water per liter of gas. These devices usually produce a mist of droplets of uniform size. The droplet size depends on the frequency of excitation of the water (e.g., 3.5 Hz will produce droplets 1 μm in diameter). Small droplets are relatively unstable and short-lived, because they evaporate. However, the high density of water in the mist makes it possible to fully saturate the inspired gases at low gas temperatures. The advantages of ultrasonic humidification lie in its ability to saturate the inspired gases with water and the relatively small effect of these devices on compression volume. Their disadvantages lie in the uniform droplet size, the cost of the device, and the potential for overhydrating small infants.

Gas-driven nebulizers force pressurized gas through a fine jet nozzle to produce a spray of droplets 5–20 μm in diameter. These droplets are relatively stable. The number of small droplets present in the fog is dependent on the pressure driving the jet. Therefore, for maximum efficiency, these nebulizers require a high driving pressure. Gas-driven nebulizers often do not perform optimally and therefore fail to fully humidify the inspired gases.

Reliability, safety, and monitoring

It is imperative that ventilators be as reliable and safe as possible. By "reliable" we mean that the apparatus should be constructed in such a way that there is very low probability of the machine malfunctioning or failing altogether. By "safe" we mean that there must be mechanisms to avoid deleterious effects during various failure modes. Although it is necessary to monitor all essential functions of the ventilator in order to warn of system failures, one should realize that each time another safety device is added, the reliability of the machine may decrease owing to an increased potential for system failures. A warning system should provide audible and visible alarms to indicate that a system failure has occurred. Although it is necessary under certain circumstances to disable a particular alarm, provision should be made to limit the time interval over which the inactivation can occur. The alarms that most experts consider obligatory on every ventilator include those that indicate loss of power (electrical and/or gas pressure) and those that indicate high or low airway pressures. It is also desirable to monitor delivered tidal volume or minute ventilation, humidification, oxygen concentration, and gas temperature. Finally, efforts are being directed to develop systems to monitor the ventilator–patient interaction. These will provide data on the uncontrolled parameters (parameters with a degree of freedom), as well as information on additional functions such as lung mechanics, oxygen uptake, and/or carbon dioxide production. We believe that continuing efforts should be directed toward improving the monitoring of these additional parameters.

NEW VENTILATION TECHNOLOGIES

Although the pathogenesis of chronic lung disease in newborn infants is not completely understood, increasingly the data are implicating ventilator-induced pulmonary injury as a major contributing factor. Ramanathan, Mason, and Raj (1990) have demonstrated that barotrauma alters lung permeability. Dreyfus et al. (1988) have shown that even short periods of acinar overdistension can lead to prolonged perturbations of alveolar–capillary permeability. Recent data from studies in premature nonhuman primate, using homologues of HMD and bronchopulmonary dysplasia (BPD), suggest that nonuniform patterns of lung inflation play an important role in the pathogenesis of both long-term and short-term pulmonary injury in premature infants (Meredith et al., 1984; Clark et al., 1992). These observations, coupled with the relative failure of surfactant replacement therapy to markedly diminish the incidence of chronic lung disease in premature infants, have led investigators to develop new techniques of assisted ventilation in which the

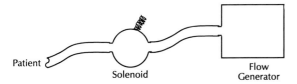

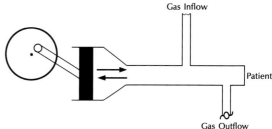

Figure 16.3. Solenoid system, the basic drive/control mechanism for the currently available high-frequency jet and flow interrupters. A source of pressurized gas is delivered from the flow generator and is intermittently interrupted by the solenoid. The delivered volume is dependent on the flow rate and the time during which the valve is open to the patient. In HFJV, the gas is injected into the trachea near the carina. In HFFI, the gas is delivered proximal to the endotracheal tube.

Figure 16.4. Schematic representation of a piston-driven HFOV. A bias-flow system allows a continuous flow of gas distal to the piston and provides all of the fresh gas to the patient. Flow and the resistance at the outflow port determine the mean airway pressure. There is no net delivery of gas from the piston itself.

primary goal is to minimize or prevent pulmonary barotrauma.

High-frequency ventilation

The term "high-frequency ventilation" (HFV) includes a number of ventilatory techniques that have in common the use of low tidal volumes and supraphysiological respiratory frequencies. With the use of tidal volumes that are near to or less than deadspace volumes, pressure excursions around mean pressure are kept minimal, and acinar overdistension can be avoided. HFV allows maintenance of mean lung volume in the desired range, while avoiding cyclical collapse and reexpansion.

Three basic HFV methods are currently available: high-frequency jet ventilation (HFJV), high-frequency flow interruption (HFFI), and high-frequency oscillatory ventilation (HFOV) (Figures 16.3 and 16.4). With both HFJV and HFFI, inhalation is active, and exhalation is a passive process dependent on the recoil of the lung and chest wall. In contrast, during the exhalation phase of HFOV, a negative pressure is created at the airway, producing a pressure gradient that enhances gas egress. Because the time available for exhalation is limited during HFV, gas trapping is a potential problem (Gerstmann et al., 1990). The presence of an active exhalation phase with HFOV enhances air egress from the lung, thus allowing the safe use of higher frequencies with this technique than with HFJV or HFFI.

Principles underlying design of HFV systems

In general, the physical components of an HFV system (drive mechanisms, control mechanisms, and connecting systems) are not different from those of conventional ventilators. However, because effective use of HFV is predicated on delivery of very

small tidal volumes, some aspects of design are more critical than with conventional ventilators.

Both internal compliance and connecting-system compliance must be low, because even minimal expansion of the volume within the delivery system will severely limit the gas volume actually delivered to the patient. The combination of a compliant delivery system and a high-inertance endotracheal tube will decrease HFV efficiency to unacceptable levels. It is therefore necessary to use fairly rigid plastics in the delivery circuit, and every effort must be made to minimize compliance and tubing length. In all HFV systems, the pressures developed within the delivery circuit are relatively high; thus, the less expansile the delivery tubing, the closer the relationships between ejected and delivered tidal volumes.

Likewise, limitation of the compressible gas volume is critical to obtaining adequate volume delivery. In HFJV and HFFI, where humidification systems often are in series with the delivery circuit, volume loss may be substantial, particularly as the fluid level in the humidifier falls. To offset this potential problem, some HFJV manufacturers have developed an in-line nebulization system, taking advantage of the high flow velocity in the jet stream.

HFJV and HFFI work on the same basic principles. A pressurized source of gas is interrupted by one or more solenoid valves, allowing a finite volume of gas to be delivered, the volume determined by flow and inspiratory duration. In HFJV, the gas is delivered through a low-compliance cannula placed in the patient's airway just above the carina. Often this is accomplished by use of a multilumen endotracheal tube that allows simultaneous monitoring of distal-airway pressure. Because this endotracheal tube is relatively thick-walled, its outer diameter may be too large for intubation of very small premature infants. Intratracheal pressure is servo-controlled to the ventilator valving mechanisms, providing precise control of delivered pressures. The high-velocity jet stream entrains additional gas either from the environment or from the delivery system. In the most commonly used neonatal jet ventilator system (Life Pulse, Bunnell, Inc.), HFJV is used in conjunction with a conventional ventilator that provides the background flow and expiratory resistance necessary to maintain a continuous positive distending pressure.

With HFFI, the ventilator volume is delivered proximal to the endotracheal tube, which, in the case of small tubes, acts as a low-pass filter. Because the volume is injected into the delivery circuit proximal to the high-inertance endotracheal tube, substantial volume loss may occur because of distension of the circuit and/or gas compression. The only commercially available high-frequency flow interrupter for use in infants (Infant Star, Infrasonics, Inc.) is, in its present configuration, incapable of providing sufficient volume output to ventilate near-term/term infants using HFFI without adding a background IMV rate. That limits the use of the device for prevention/treatment of barotrauma in relatively large newborn infants. Design modifications have been made to offset this limitation, and the upgraded ventilator is now being evaluated in clinical testing.

Because both HFJV and HFFI theoretically could deliver infinite pressures/volumes should the solenoid-controlled valves fail in the open position, well-conceived algorithms and microprocessor-based systems are essential components of the safety design. Because HFVs are considered "new" technology under current FDA regulations, this safety feature is carefully assessed prior to receiving approval.

The drive mechanism used in HFOVs can be either a piston or a diaphragm or a hybrid combination of the two. The driver displaces a gas volume into the patient and then creates a negative airway pressure during the exhalation phase, enhancing gas egress (Froese and Bryan, 1978). Because this feature minimizes gas trapping at any frequency/tidal-volume combination, HFOV can be safely used at higher frequencies (and lower tidal volumes) than HFJV or HFFI (Froese and Bryan, 1978). The oscillator itself provides no net flow of gas to the patient. Fresh gas is provided via a bias-flow circuit, which, by adding a restrictive valve or low-pass filter on the exhalation side, also allows precise and independent control of mean airway pressure (Figure 16.4). Gas can be humidified prior to entering the bias-

flow circuit, making it easier to isolate the humidification system from the gas volume than is possible with HFJV or HFFI. One unique feature of HFOV is that mean airway pressure is an independently controlled variable rather than a dependent variable. In situations where lung compliance is changing dynamically, the operator must actively decrease mean airway pressure to avoid lung overinflation. Failure to do this will result in increased lung volume and pleural pressure and will increase the risk for periventricular hemorrhage and cardiovascular compromise, particularly in premature infants (Carter et al., 1990; Gerstmann et al., 1991; Clark et al., 1992).

Under clinical conditions, the airway pressure during HFFI and HFOV is highest proximal to the endotracheal tube; it then falls markedly across the endotracheal tube and further attenuates distally in the tracheobronchial tree. Alveolar pressures are extremely low, particularly at frequencies above 10 Hz. Commercially available HFOV (Sensormedics 3100, Sensormedics Inc.) and HFFI ventilators measure pressure at the proximal airway, which provides only qualitative information about distal pressures. Proximal-airway pressures are not measured with the currently available jet ventilators. Although the display representing intratracheal pressure during HFJV reads lower than the proximal pressure displayed with HFFI and HFOV, these numbers are not comparable; under equivalent conditions, alveolar pressures are higher with HFJV than with HFOV or HFFI because of the need to use a lower frequency (and larger tidal volume) during jet ventilation.

Mean airway pressure in the alveoli should be the same as or lower than those in the proximal airway (Gerstmann et al., 1990). However, if insufficient time is available for gas egress, air trapping will occur, resulting in either focal or global increases in alveolar mean pressure (Froese and Bryan, 1978; Gerstmann et al., 1990). In general, the presence of an active exhalation phase with HFOV allows safe use of a higher operating frequency than with the other HFV techniques (Froese and Bryan, 1978). An additional margin of safety can be provided by using a low inspiratory : expiratory (I : E) ratio (Gerstmann et al., 1990). Although this increases the maximum inspiratory flow velocity and theoretically can increase the risk for shear injury in the airway, there is no evidence that this has been of clinical significance (Gerstmann et al., 1988). At a 1 : 2 I : E ratio and frequencies of 20 Hz or less, mean tracheal and alveolar pressures during HFOV are less than those measured at the proximal airway, whereas at a 1 : 1 ratio they are the same or higher (Gerstmann et al., 1990). This is likely related to asymmetrical flow velocities and explains in part why somewhat higher mean proximal-airway pressures are required to obtain equivalent oxygenation with HFOV than with conventional ventilation.

Strategies for use of HFV

Clinical success with HFV is dependent on the development and use of a strategy appropriate for the underlying pathophysiology. When the various HFV systems are used with the same approach in comparable experimental and clinical settings, similar results are obtained.

HFV allows the use of a high mean airway pressure with minimal excursions above and below the mean pressure. Therefore, in contrast to conventional mechanical ventilation, it is possible to use HFV at a high mean airway pressure with minimal risk of barotrauma. This approach is particularly efficacious in the treatment of subjects with diffuse alveolar disease and high closing forces. Both experimental and clinical data support this view. When mean airway pressure is maintained at a level above closing pressure, oxygenation is improved, and lung injury minimized (Froese and Bryan, 1978; Meredith et al., 1984). This "high mean airway pressure" strategy has been shown to be efficacious in management of newborns with HMD, adult respiratory distress syndrome, and pneumonia. In recent studies, more than 50% of near-term/term infants meeting the accepted clinical criteria for extracorporeal membrane oxygenation (ECMO) were rescued with HFOV (Carter et al., 1990). In a controlled trial in premature infants with HMD, HFOV resulted in a decreased incidence of chronic lung disease (Clark et al., 1992; Ogawa et al., 1993).

HFV has also been shown to be efficacious in the management of infants with air-leak syndromes. In this case, the strategy is to use the lowest mean and peak airway pressures possible, to allow the anatomic defects in airways/saccules to heal and any interstitial air to resorb (Clark et al., 1986). The earlier the intervention with HFV is accomplished, the more likely it is that the air leak will resolve.

HFV has not been effective in the management of respiratory failure in infants whose pathophysiology has included substantial lower-airway obstruction. Recent data from our laboratory suggest that superimposition of low-volume oscillations on a tidal waveform leads to significant decreases in both peak pressure and ventilator frequency, as compared with conventional ventilation, in experimental animals following smoke inhalation. The combined use of HFV and conventional ventilation is possible with the commercially available jet and flow interrupters. The role of this combined mode of ventilation in the management of infants with heterogeneous lung disease and respiratory failure needs to be critically evaluated.

Clinical applications of HFV

HFV has been shown to be efficacious in "rescue" management of infants with air leaks and in the management of newborns with diffuse alveolar disease who fail to respond to exogenous surfactant therapy and require high ventilator pressures or who are unmanageable with conventional ventilation. Clinical studies suggest that with an appropriate strategy, HFV can prevent ventilator-induced lung injury in premature infants with or without surfactant deficiency. The combination of HFV and surfactant replacement therapy has been reported to reduce the need for surfactant and to decrease the time on mechanical ventilation, thus improving the outcomes and decreasing the costs in small preterm infants. However, additional studies are needed to determine if HFV should be the ventilatory modality of choice in the management of infants at risk for the development of chronic lung disease.

Liquid ventilation

Studies have been reporting success in the use of oxygenated perfluorocarbons (PFCs) for liquid ventilation of experimental animals since the initial report by Clark and Gollan in 1966 (Calderwood et al., 1975; Curtis, Fuhrman, and Howland, 1990). Immature lambs ventilated with PFCs have shown improved gas exchange and lung mechanics compared with conventionally ventilated controls (Schaffer, 1987). Recently, several successful short-term applications in premature human newborns have been reported (Greenspan et al., 1990). It has been suggested that the elimination of high surface forces in the liquid-filled lung could account for the improved gas exchange, mechanical stability, and decreased lung injury seen with this technique.

Two approaches to liquid ventilation have been used. Until recently, studies using total liquid ventilation incorporated an oxygenator in series with a specially designed computer-controlled liquid ventilator. Total liquid ventilation was maintained for a period of time, following which the subject was returned to air breathing. In limited human studies, liquid ventilation was applied in two 3–5 min cycles separated by 15-min intervals of gas ventilation. Oxygenated PFCs at 15 ml · kg^{-1} were given at a rate of two or three breaths per minute from a reservoir suspended above the infant. Most infants showed improvement in lung mechanics and/or oxygenation.

Fuhrman has proposed an alternative approach, perfluorocarbon-associated gas exchange (PAGE), in which the lung is filled to FRC with PFCs, with the subject being maintained on a conventional ventilator and air breathing (Fuhrman, Paczan, and de Francisis, 1991). In preliminary studies, this technique appears to result in changes in gas exchange and lung mechanics similar to those seen with total liquid ventilation, and it has the added advantage of simplicity of use. It has been shown to be effective for maintaining gas exchange and preventing progression of lung injury in short-term applications using animal models of adult respiratory distress syndrome (Tutuncu, Faithful, and Lachmann, 1993), meconium aspiration syndrome (Thompson, Fuhrman, and Alan, 1993), aspiration pneumonia (Nesti et al., 1993), and HMD (Leach et al., 1993).

Liquid ventilation is still a research tool. Limited data suggest that it is safe when used for periods up to 96 h in preterm baboons. It shows promise as a technique to reduce barotrauma in a variety of experimental settings, and once its safety is established, it likely will be evaluated in clinical trials in infants refractory to surfactant therapy.

CONCLUSIONS

The type of ventilator available to the clinician determines, in part, the range of therapeutic options available. There is general agreement that certain alterations in the settings of ventilators used for infants result in specific changes in gas exchange (McIntyre et al., 1969; Smith et al., 1969; Reynolds, 1971; Boros et al., 1977; Ciszek et al., 1981; Heicher, Kasting, and Harrod, 1981). Ventilation is determined by frequency and delivered tidal volume, and changes in either of these parameters will predictably affect Paco$_2$, provided pulmonary blood flow is adequate and the expiratory interval is sufficient to prevent gas trapping. In infants with diffuse alveolar disease and intrapulmonary shunting, there is general agreement that oxygenation is dependent on mean airway pressure. However, in spite of the acceptance of these principles, there is little agreement regarding the optimal method of mechanically ventilating newborns in respiratory failure. Even in the management of HMD, approaches vary widely: high frequency with small tidal volumes (Bland et al., 1977), low frequency with

large tidal volumes (Boros and Campbell, 1980) and prolonged inspiratory times (Mannino et al., 1976), including inflation-hold, IMV, and synchronous intermittent mandatory ventilation (SIMV) (Smith et al., 1969; Llewellyn and Swyer, 1971; Kirby et al., 1972; Reynolds, 1975; Mannino et al., 1976; Bland et al., 1977; Sjöstrand, 1977). All of these ventilation strategies attempt to minimize barotrauma (Reynolds and Taghizadeh, 1974; Ogata et al., 1976; Stocks and Godfrey, 1976; Nilsson et al., 1978), either by reducing peak inspiratory pressures (Herman and Reynolds, 1973; Reynolds, 1975) or by avoiding asynchronous breathing. Lacking a consensus on what is optimal ventilator management for such patients, and given that lung disease is both heterogeneous and dynamic, it is best to select a ventilator that allows a wide range of settings, which in turn allows the greatest flexibility in the patterns of individual breaths or breathing sequences. Emphasis should be placed on those parameters that can be regulated reliably and precisely, such as time and pressure. In other words, the ability to regulate inspiratory time, expiratory time, inflation-hold, and peak and end-expiratory pressures is essential when using the time-cycling and pressure-limiting modes in conventional ventilators.

Although it might be beneficial to have a ventilator that would truly deliver a constant tidal volume to an infant despite changes in lung mechanics, such an approach has not been adequately evaluated in newborn ventilation. Most volume-cycled ventilators terminate inspiration when a certain tidal volume of gas has been delivered to the connecting tubing of the ventilator, rather than to the infant. Because of this, the tidal volume that must be provided during mechanical ventilation of newborn infants exceeds that during spontaneous breathing, because of compression volume, tubing expansion, losses of gas from the system, and wasted ventilation (Hedley-White, Laver, and Bendixen, 1964; Epstein and Hyman, 1980; Hakanson, 1981). In general, a tidal volume between 7.5 and 10 ml · kg^{-1} is needed to provide adequate ventilation for children weighing 7 kg or less, thus negating some of the theoretical advantages of using a volume-cycled ventilator. Several new-generation volume-cycled ventilators for infants use microprocessor technology interacting with on-line monitoring of lung volumes and mechanics to try to offset these limitations. Insufficient data are available at this time to validate their efficacy, particularly in extremely immature newborns in respiratory failure.

The rapidity with which a tidal volume enters and leaves the lung is of utmost importance. The more quickly the gas can be delivered, the more possibilities there are for varying the patterns of ventilation. When minute ventilation is achieved with high ventilator rates and low tidal volumes, the peak and mean alveolar pressures may be lower, reducing the adverse effects of pressure on the lung (Northway et al., 1967; Ogata et al., 1976; Bland et al., 1977; Sjöstrand, 1977; Marchak et al., 1981) and circulation (Cournand et al., 1948; Lenfant and Howell, 1960; Suter, Fairley, and Schlobohm, 1975; Cassidy et al., 1979; Cassidy and Mitchell, 1981; Simbruner and Gregory, 1981). A minute ventilation that is achieved with high mean airway and alveolar pressures and low peak airway pressures will facilitate oxygenation and minimize barotrauma (Boros et al., 1977; Boros, 1979; Boros and Campbell, 1980). One method of accomplishing this is to keep inspiration short and add an inflation-hold (Ciszek et al., 1981). Alternatively, this goal can be accomplished using HFV with a high-pressure strategy (Froese and Bryan, 1978).

Ventilator designs for use with infants must allow the use of continuous ventilation, IMV, SIMV, and continuous distending airway pressure. The ideal infant ventilator should also have the potential for HFV, both as an independent entity and in a combined mode with conventional ventilation. It should be possible to superimpose HFV on the conventional waveform during inspiration and exhalation and throughout the ventilatory cycle. In addition, the ability to vary the I : E ratio below 1 : 1 during HFV would be desirable.

It is important that the expiratory portion of the delivery circuit not significantly increase resistance to exhalation or prolong the expiratory time constant of a healthy lung by more than 50%. Otherwise, the work of breathing may be excessive during weaning from IMV (Goldman, Brady, and Dumpit, 1979; Simbruner and Gregory, 1981). This may be a major factor in recent observations that premature infants can be more rapidly extubated from a low IMV rate than they can after weaning to CPAP (Greenspan et al., 1990).

Though it is one of the least expensive components of the ventilator, the tubing that connects the patient to the ventilator can have a profound influence on performance. Use of compliant tubing will influence internal compliance, compression volume, and, ultimately, the tidal volume and the pressure waveform. This becomes particularly critical when using extremely low tidal volumes and/or a small endotracheal tube and is of paramount importance during HFV. Under these conditions, even a relatively rigid delivery circuit may be sufficiently distensible to limit tidal-volume delivery by the ventilator. As a general guide, it is desirable that the internal compliance of the ventilator–patient circuit be less than $0.5 \ ml \cdot (cm \ H_2O)^{-1}$.

The control panel of the ventilator should be designed to be as simple and functional as possible. It would be better if the essential elements of the respiratory cycle, such as frequency, inspiratory time, expiratory time, inflation-hold, peak inspiratory pressure, and continuous distending pressure, were displayed directly, with less attention given to certain derived parameters such as I : E ratios. Finally, a number of relatively inexpensive respiratory-function monitors have been developed and are available as integral parts of the ventilator monitoring package or can be purchased as freestanding units. They offer the advantage of direct on-line measurement of tidal volume and lung mechanics and thus introduce another level of sophistication into respiratory management of newborns. However, as of this time there are no data validating the software and hardware for any of these monitors, nor have there been studies suggesting that their use improves respiratory outcome.

Ideally, the physician should know as much about ventilators as possible. This knowledge, coupled with an appropriate ventilation strategy, should yield the best possible results in ventilator management of infants in respiratory failure.

REFERENCES

Abrahams, N., Fisk, G. C., Vonwiller, J. B., and Grant, G. C. (1975). Evaluation of infant ventilators. *Anesthesia and Intensive Care* 3:6–11.

Ahlstrom, H. (1975). Pulmonary mechanics in infants surviving severe neonatal respiratory insufficiency. *Acta Paediatrica Scandinavica* 64:69–80.

Amaha, K., Liu, P., Weitzner, S. W., and Harmel, M. H. (1967). Effects of constant chest compression on the mechanical and physiologic performance of different ventilators. *Anesthesiology* 28:498–509.

Auld, P. A. M. (1975). Concepts of pulmonary physiology. Pulmonary physiology of the newborn infant. In *Pulmonary Physiology of the Fetus and Newborn and Child*, ed. E. M. Scarpelli (pp. 1–36, 140–65). Philadelphia: Lea & Febiger.

Baker, A. B., and Murray-Wilson, A. (1974). Towards a better classification of lung ventilators. *Anesthesia and Intensive Care* 2:151–7.

Bandy, K. P., Nicks, J. J., and Donn, S. M. (1992). Volume controlled ventilation for severe neonatal respiratory failure. *Neonatal Intensive Care* 4:70–3.

Bendixen, H. H. (1976). Rational ventilator modes for respiratory failure. In *The Lung in the Critically Ill Patient*, ed. W. C. Shoemaker. Baltimore: Williams & Wilkins.

Bland, R. D., Kim, M. H., Light, M.J., and Woodson, J. L. (1977). High frequency mechanical ventilation of low birth-weight infants with respiratory failure from hyaline membrane disease. *Pediatric Research* 11:531.

Bohn, D. J., Miyasaka, K., Marchak, B. E., Thompson, W. K., Froese, A. B., and Bryan, A. C. (1980). Ventilation by high frequency oscillation. *Journal of Applied Physiology: Respiratory, Environmental, and Exercise Physiology* 48:710–16.

Boros, S. J. (1979). Variations in inspiratory–expiratory ratio and airway pressure wave form during mechanical ventilation. The significance of mean airway pressure. *Journal of Pediatrics* 94:114–17.

Boros, S., Bing, D., Mammel, M., Hagen, E., and Gordon, M. (1984). Using conventional infant ventilators at unconventional rates. *Pediatrics* 74:487–92.

Boros, S. J., and Campbell, K. (1980). A comparison of the effects of high frequency–low tidal volume and low frequency–high tidal volume mechanical ventilation. *Journal of Pediatrics* 97:108–12.

Boros, S. J., Matalon, S. V., Ewald, R., Leonard, A. S., and Hunt, C. E. (1977). The effect of independent variations in inspiratory–expiratory ratio and end expiratory pressure during mechanical ventilation in hyaline membrane disease. The significance of mean airway pressure. *Journal of Pediatrics* 91:794–8.

Butler, W. J., Bohn, D. J., Bryan, A. C., and Froese, A. B. (1980). Ventilation by high-frequency oscillation in humans. *Anesthesia and Analgesia* 59:577–84.

Calderwood, H. W., Ruiz, B. C., Tham, M. K., Modell, J. H., Saga, S. A., and Hood, C. I. (1975). Residual levels and biochemical changes after ventilation with perfluorinated liquid. *Journal of Applied Physiology* 39:603–7.

Carlo, W., and Maktin, R. (1983). Principles of neontal assisted ventilation. *Pediatric Clinics of North America* 10:205–21.

Carlon, G. C., Kahn, R. C., Howland, W. S., Ray, C., Jr., and Turnbull, A. D. (1981). Clinical experience with high frequency jet ventilation. *Critical Care Medicine* 9:1–6.

Carr, D., Rich, M., Murkowski, K., and Neu, J. (1986). A comparative evaluation of three neonatal ventilators. *Critical Care Medicine* 14:234–6.

Carter, J. M., Gerstmann, D. R., Clark, R. H., Snyder, G., Cornish, J. D., Null, D. M., Jr., and deLemos, R. A. (1990). High-frequency oscillatory ventilation and extracorporeal membrane oxygenation for the treatment of acute neonatal respiratory failure. *Pediatrics* 85:159–64.

Cassidy, S. S., Eschenbacher, W. L., Robertson, C. H., Jr., Nixon, J. V., Blomqvist, G., and Johnson, R L., Jr. (1979). Cardiovascular effects of positive pressure ventilation in normal subjects. *Journal of Applied Physiology: Respiratory, Environmental, and Exercise Physiology* 47:453–61.

Cassidy, S. S., and Mitchell, J. H. (1981). Effect of positive pressure breathing on right and left ventricular preload and afterload. *Federation Proceedings* 40:2178–81.

Chang, H. K. (1984). Mechanisms of gas transport during ventilation by high-frequency oscillation. *Journal of Applied Physiology: Respiratory, Environmental and Exercise Physiology* 56:553–63.

Chernick, V., and Vidyasagar, D. (1972). Continuous negative chest wall pressure in hyaline membrane disease: one year experience. *Pediatrics* 49:753–62.

Chu, J. S., Dawson, P., Klaus, M., and Sweet, A. Y. (1964). Lung compliance and lung volume measured concurrently in normal full-term and premature infants. *Pediatrics* 34:525–32.

Ciszek, T. A., Modanlou, H. D., Owings, D., and Nelson, P. (1981). Mean airway pressure – significance during mechanical ventilation in neonates. *Journal of Pediatrics* 99:121–6.

Clark, L. G., Jr., and Gollan, F. (1966). Survival of mammals breathing organic liquids equilibrated with oxygen at atmospheric pressure. *Science* 1952:1755–6.

Clark, R. H., Gerstmann, D. R., Null, D. M., Jr., and deLemos, R. A. (1992). Prospective randomized comparison of high frequency oscillatory ventilation and conventional ventilation in respiratory distress syndrome. *Pediatrics* 89:5–11.

Clark, R. H., Gerstmann, D. R., Null, D. M., Jr., Yoder, B. A., Cornish, J. D., et al. (1986). Pulmonary interstitial emphysema treated by high-frequency oscillatory ventilation. *Critical Care Medicine* 14:926–30.

Cook, C. D., Sutherland, J., Segal, S., Cherry, R., Mead, J., McIlroy, M., and Smith, C. (1957). Studies of respiratory physiology in the newborn infant. III. Measurements of the mechanics of respiration. *Journal of Clinical Investigation* 36:440–8.

Cournand, A., Motley, H. L., Werko, L., and Richards, D. W., Jr. (1948). Physiological studies of the effects of intermittent positive pressure breathing on cardiac output in man. *American Journal of Physiology* 152:162–74.

Cox, J. M. (1974). Techniques in neonatal ventilation. *International Anesthesiology Clinics* 12:111–40.

Cross, K. W., and Roberts, P. W. (1951). Asphyxia neonatorum treated by electrical stimulation of the phrenic nerve. *British Medical Journal* 1:1043–8.

Cunningham, D., and Desai, N. (1986). Methods of assessment and findings regarding pulmonary function in infants less than 1000 gr. *Clinics in Perinatology* 13:299–313.

Curtis, S. E., Fuhrman, B. F., and Howland, D. F. (1990). Airway and alveolar pressures during perfluorocarbon breathing in infants elambs. *Journal of Applied Physiology* 68:2322–8.

Daily, W. J. R., and Smith, P. C. (1971). Mechanical ventilation of the newborn infant. *Current Problems in Pediatrics* 1:1–37.

Daily, W. J. R., Sunshine, P., and Smith, P. C. (1971). Mechanical ventilation of newborn infants. V. Five years' experience. *Anesthesiology* 34:132–8.

deLemos, R. A., and Kirby, R. R. (1980). Early development. Intermittent mandatory ventilation in neonatal respiratory support. *International Anesthesiology Clinics* 18:39–51.

Delivoria-Papadopoulos, M. D., and Anday, E. K. (1979). Twenty years of mechanical ventilation in the newborn infant. *Respiratory Therapy* 9:73.

Delivoria-Papadopoulos, M., Levison, H., and Swyer, P. R. (1965). Intermittent positive pressure respiration as a treatment in severe distress syndrome. *Archives of Disease in Childhood* 40:474–9.

Doe, O. W. (1889). Apparatus for resuscitating asphyxiated children. *Boston Medical and Surgical Journal* 120:9.

Donald, I., and Lord, J. (1953). Augmented respiration. Studies in atelectasis neonatorum. *Lancet* 1:9–14.

Downs, J. B., Douglas, M. E., Ruiz, B. C., and Miller, N. L. (1979). Comparison of assisted and controlled mechanical ventilation in anesthetized swine. *Critical Care Medicine* 7:5–8.

Dreyfus, D., Soler, P., Basset, G., and Saumon, G.

(1988). High inflation pressure pulmonary edema. *American Review of Respiratory Disease* 137:1159–64.

Drinker, P., and Shaw, L. A. (1929). An apparatus for the prolonged administration of artificial respiration. I. A design for adults and children. *Journal of Clinical Investigation* 7:229–47.

Epstein, M. A., and Epstein, R. A. (1979). Airway flow patterns during mechanical ventilation of infants: a mathematical model. *IEEE Transactions on Biomedical Engineering* 26:299–306.

Epstein, R. A. (1971). The sensitivities and response times of ventilatory assistors. *Anesthesiology* 34:321–45.

Epstein, R. A., and Hyman, A. I. (1980). Ventilatory requirements of critically ill neonates. *Anesthesiology* 53:379–84.

Fitzhardinge, P. M. (1978). Follow-up studies in infants treated by mechanical ventilation. *Clinics in Perinatology* 5:451–61.

Forbat, A. F., and Her, C. (1980). Correction for gas compression in mechanical ventilators. *Anesthesia and Analgesia* 59:488–93.

Froese, A. B., and Bryan A. C. (1978). High frequency ventilation. *American Review of Respiratory Disease* 135:1363–74.

Fuhrman, B. P., Paczan, P. R, and de Francisis, M. (1991). Perfluorocarbon-associated gas exchange. *Critical Care Medicine* 19:712–22.

Gerstmann, D. R., deLemos, R. A., and Clark, R. H. (1991). High-frequency ventilation: issues of strategy. *Clinics in Perinatology* 18:563–82.

Gerstmann, D. R., deLemos, R. A., Coalson, J. J., Clark, R. H., et al. (1988). Influence of ventilatory technique on pulmonary baroinjury in baboons with hyaline membrane disease. *Pediatric Pulmonology* 5:82–91.

Gerstmann, D. R., Fouke, J. M., Winter, D. C., Taylor, A. F., and deLemos, R. A. (1990). Proximal, tracheal and alveolar pressure during high-frequency oscillatory ventilation in a normal rabbit model. *Pediatric Research* 28:367–73.

Goldman, S. L., Brady, J. P., and Dumpit, F. M. (1979). Increased work of breathing associated with nasal prongs. *Pediatrics* 64:160–4.

Gottschalk, S. K., King, B., and Schuth, C. R. (1980). Basic concepts in positive-pressure ventilation of the newborn. *Perinatology/Neonatology* 4:15–19.

Greenough, A., and Pool, J. (1988). Neonatal patient triggered ventilation. *Archives of Disease in Childhood* 63:394–7.

Greenspan, J. S., Wolfsan, M. R., Rubenstein, S. D., and Shaeffer, T. G. H. (1990). Liquid ventilation of human preterm neonates. *Journal of Pediatrics* 117:106–11.

Gregory, G. A., Kitterman, J. A., Phibbs, R. H., Tooley, W. H., and Hamilton, W. K. (1971). Treatment of the idiopathic respiratory-distress syndrome with continuous positive airway pressure. *New England Journal of Medicine* 284:1333–40.

Grogono, A. W. (1972). The classification of intermittent positive pressure ventilators. *British Journal of Anaesthesia* 44:405–7.

Hakanson, D. O. (1981). Positive pressure ventilation: volume-cycled ventilators. In *Assisted Ventilation of the Neonate*, ed. J. P. Goldsmith, and E. H. Karotkin (pp. 128–51). Philadelphia: W. B. Saunders.

Hakanson, D. O., and Stern, L. (1975). Respiratory distress syndrome of the newborn: current status of ventilatory assistance. *Postgraduate Medicine* 58:200–6.

Hedenstierna, G., and Oquist, L. (1974). Insufflation pressure and compressed gas ventilation with the Engstrom respirator. *Acta Anaesthesiologica Scandinavica* 18:41–7.

Hedley-Whyte, J., Laver, M. B., and Bendixen, H. H. (1964). Effect of changes in tidal ventilation on physiologic shunting. *American Journal of Physiology* 206:891–3.

Heicher, D. A., Kasting, D. S., and Harrod, J. R. (1981). Prospective clinical comparison of two methods for mechanical ventilation of neonates: rapid rate and short inspiratory time versus low rate and long inspiratory time. *Journal of Pediatrics* 98:957–61.

Heldt, G. P., McIlroy, M. B., Hansen, T. N., and Tooley, W. H. (1980). Exercise performance of the survivors of hyaline membrane disease. *Journal of Pediatrics* 96:995–9.

Heller, K., and Heinrichs, W. (1979). Ein neues Beatmungsgerät mit Mikroprozessorsteuerung. *Anaesthetist* 28:409–13.

Herman, S., and Reynolds, E. O. R. (1973). Methods for improving oxygenation in infants mechanically ventilated for severe hyaline membrane disease. *Archives of Disease in Childhood* 48:612–17.

Hird, M. F., and Greenough, A. (1990). Causes of failure of neontal patient triggered ventilation. *Early Human Development* 23:101–8.

ISO (1978). International Standards Organisation TC 121–110: Proposed draft for international standards for breathing machines for medical use.

Jacob, J., Gluck, L., DiSessa, T. G., Edwards, D. K., Kulovich, M., Kurlinski, J., Merritt, T. A., and Friedman, W. F. (1980). The contribution of PDA in the neonate with server RDS. *Journal of Pediatrics* 96:79–87.

James, L. S., Apgar, V., Burnard, E. D., and Moya, F. (1963). Intragastric oxygen and resuscitation of the newborn. *Acta Paediatrica Scandinavica* 52:245–51.

Johnson, J. D., Malachowski, N. C., Grobstein, R., Welsh, D., Daily, W. J. R., and Sunshine, P. (1974). Prognosis of children surviving with the aid of mechanical ventilation in the newborn period. *Journal of Pediatrics* 84:272–6.

Keuskamp, D. H. G. (1974). Ventilation of premature and newborn infants. *International Anesthesiology Clinics* 12:281–307.

Kirby, R., Robison, E., Schulz, J., and deLemos, R. (1972). Continuous flow ventilation as an alternative to assisted or controlled ventilation in infants. *Anesthesia and Analgesia* 51:871–5.

Kirpalani, H., Santos-Lyn, R., and Roberts, R. (1988). Some infant ventilators do not limit peak inspiratory pressure reliably during active expiration. *Critical Care Medicine* 16:880–3.

Klain, M., and Smith, R. B. (1977). High frequency percutaneous transtracheal jet ventilation. *Critical Care Medicine* 5:280–7.

Leach, C. L., Fuhrman, B. P., Marin, F. C., III, Rath, M., Herman, L., Holm, B., Papo, M., and Steinhorn, D. (1993). Perfluorocarbon-associated gas exchange (PAGE) with perflubron (Liquivent™) in respiratory distress syndrome. *Pediatric Research* 33:1309.

Lenfant, C., and Howell, B. J. (1960). Cardiovascular adjustments in dogs during continuous pressure breathing. *Journal of Applied Physiology* 15:425–8.

Lindroth, M., Svenningsen, N. W., Ahlstrom, H., and Jonson, B. (1980). Evaluation of mechanical ventilation in newborn infants. I. Techniques and survival rates. *Acta Paediatrica Scandinavica* 69:143–9.

Llewellyn, M. A., and Swyer, P. R. (1970). Positive expiratory pressure during mechanical ventilation in the newborn. Presented to the Society for Pediatric Research, Atlantic City.

(1971). Assisted and controlled ventilation in the newborn period: effect on oxygenation. *British Journal of Anaesthesia* 43:926–31.

Lough, M. D., Doershuk, C. F., and Stern, R. C. (1974). *Pediatric Respiratory Therapy*. Chicago: Year Book.

Luce, J. M., Pierson, D. J., and Hudson, L. D. (1981). Intermittent mandatory ventilation. *Chest* 79:678–84.

McIntyre, R. W., Laws, A. K., and Ramachandran, P. R. (1969). Positive expiratory pressure plateau: improved gas exchange during mechanical ventilation. *Canadian Anaesthetists Society Journal* 16:477–86.

Mannino, F. L., Feldman, B. H., Heldt, G. P., DeLue, N. A., Wimmer, J. E., Fletcher, M. A., and Gluck, L. (1976). Early mechanical ventilation in RDS with a prolonged inspiration. *Pediatric Research* 10:464.

Marchak, B. E., Thompson, W. K., Duffy, P., Miyaki, T., Bryan, M. H., Bryan, A. C., and Froese, A. B. (1981). Treatment of RDS by high-frequency oscillatory ventilation: a preliminary report. *Journal of Pediatrics* 99:287–92.

Marriage, K. J., and Davies, P. A. (1977). Neurological sequelae in children surviving mechanical ventilation in the neonatal period. *Archives of Disease in Childhood* 52:176–82.

Mattila, M. A. K. (1974). The role of the physical characteristics of the respirator in artificial ventilation of the newborn. *Acta Anaesthesiologica Scandinavica [Suppl. 56]* 19:1.

Mattila, M. A. K., and Suutarinen, T. (1971). Clinical and experimental evaluation of the Loosco baby respirator. *Acta Anesthesiologica Scandinavica* 15:229–92.

Meredith, K. S., deLemos, R. A., Coalson, J. J., and King, R. J. (1984). Role of lung injury in the pathogenesis of hyaline membrane disease in premature baboons. *Journal of Applied Physiology* 66:2150–8.

Mitchell, A. Greenough, A., and Hird, M. (1989). Limitations of patient triggered ventilation in neonates. *Archives of Disease in Childhood* 64:924–9.

Murdock, A. I., Linsao, L., Reid, M. M., Sutton, M. D., Tilak, K. S., Ulan, O. A., and Swyer, P. R. (1970). Mechanical ventilation in the respiratory distress syndrome: a controlled trial. *Archives of Disease in Childhood* 45:624–33.

Mushin, W. W., Rendell-Baker, L., Thompson, P. W., and Mapelson, W. W. (1969). *Automatic Ventilation of the Lungs*, 2nd ed. Oxford: Blackwell.

Nesti, F. D., Fuhrman, B. P., Papo, M. C., Steinhorn, D. M., Hernan, L. J., Duffy, L., Leach, C. L., Holm, B., Paczan, P., and Burak, B. (1993). Perfluorocarbon associated gas exchange (PAGE) in gastric aspiration. *Pediatric Research* 33:215.

Nilsson, R., Grossmann, G., and Robertson, B. (1978). Lung surfactant and the pathogenesis of neonatal bronchiolar lesions induced by artificial ventilation. *Pediatric Research* 12:249–55.

Nordstrom, L. (1972). On automatic ventilation. *Acta Anaesthesiologica Scandinavica [Suppl.]* 47:29–56.

Norlander, O. P. (1968). The use of respirators in anesthesia and surgery. *Acta Anaesthesiologica Scandinavica [Suppl.]* 30:5–74.

Northway, W. H., Rosan, R. C., and Porter, D. Y. (1967). Pulmonary disease following respirator therapy of hyaline membrane disease. *New England Journal of Medicine* 276:357–68.

Ogata, E. S., Gregory, G. A., Kitterman, J. A. Phibbs, R. H., and Tooley, W. H. (1976). Pneumothorax in the respiratory distress syndrome: incidence and effect on vital signs, blood gases, and pH. *Pediatrics* 58:177–83.

Ogawa, Y., Miyasaka, K., Kawano, T., Imura, S., Inukai, K., Okuyama, K., Oguchi, K., Togari, J., Nishida, H., and Mishina, J. (1993). A multicenter randomized trial of high frequency oscillatory ventilation as compared with conventional mechanical ventilation in preterm infants with respiratory failure. *Early Human Development* 32:1–10.

Okmian, L. G. (1963). Direct measurement of pulmonary ventilation in newborns and infants during artificial ventilation with the Engstrom respirator. *Acta Anaesthesiologica Scandinavica* 7:155–68.

Outerbridge, E. W., and Stern, L. (1981). Negative pressure ventilators. In *Assisted Ventilation of the Neonate*, ed. J. P. Goldsmith and E. H. Karotkin (pp. 152–62). Philadelphia: W. B. Saunders.

Ramanathan, R., Mason, G. R., and Raj, J. U. (1990). Effect of mechanical ventilation and bartotrauma on pulmonary clearance of 99m technetium diethylenetriamine pentaacetate in lambs. *Pediatric Research* 27:70–4.

Reynolds, E. O. R. (1971). Effect of alterations in mechanical ventilator settings on pulmonary gas exchange in hyaline membrane disease. *Archives of Disease in Childhood* 46:152–9.

(1974). Pressure waveform and ventilatory settings for mechanical ventilation in severe hyaline membrane disease. *International Anesthesiology Clinics* 12:259–80.

(1975). Management of hyaline membrane disease. *British Medical Bulletin* 31:184–90.

Reynolds, E. O. R., and Taghizadeh, A. (1974). Improved prognosis of infants mechanically ventilated for hyaline membrane disease. *Archives of Disease in Childhood* 49:505–15.

Rogers, E. J. (1972). Physics vs. physiology in infant ventilation. A nondimensional analysis approach for determining ventilator–patient suitability. *Respiratory Therapy* 2:45–9.

Rothberg, A. D., Maisels, M. J., Bagnato, S. Murphy, J., Gifford, K., McKinley, K., Palmer, E. A,. and Vanucci, R. C. (1981). Outcome for survivors of mechanical ventilation weighing less than 1,250 gm at birth. *Journal of Pediatrics* 98:106–11.

Schaffer, T. H. (1987). A brief review: liquid ventilation. *Undersea Biomedical Research* 14:169–79.

Schreiner, R. L., Kisling, J. A., Evans, G. M., Phillips, S., Lemons, J. A., and Gresham, E. L. (1980). Improved survival of ventilated neonates with modern intensive care. *Pediatrics* 66:985–7.

Servant, G. M., Nicks, J. J., Donn, S. M., Bandy, K. P., Lathrop, C., and Dechert, R. E. (1992). Feasibility of applying flow-synchronized ventilation to very low birth weight infants. *Respiratory Care* 37:249–53.

Simbruner, G., and Götz, M. (1976). Neonatal respirator

allowing simultaneous ventilation and suction. *Klinische Pädiatrie* 188:532–8.

Simbruner, G., and Gregory, G. A. (1981). Performance of neonatal ventilators: the effects of changes in resistance and compliance. *Critical Care Medicine* 9:509–14.

Simbruner, G., Popow, C., Salzer, H., and Lischka, A. (1982). Fetal respiratory function and perinatal survival. *Lancet* 1:1187.

Sjöstrand, U. (1977). Review of the physiologic rationale for and development of high frequency positive pressure ventilation (HFPPV). *Acta Anesthesiologica Scandinavica* [*Suppl.*] 64:7–27.

Smith, P. C., Daily, W. J. R., Fletcher, G., Meyer, H. B. P., and Taylor, G. (1969). Mechanical ventilation of newborn infants. I. The effect of rate and pressure on arterial oxygenation of infants with respiratory distress syndrome. *Pediatric Research* 3:244–54.

Stern, L., Ramos, A. D., Outerbridge, E. W., and Beaudry, P. H. (1970). Negative pressure artificial respiration: use in treatment of respiratory failure of the newborn. *Canadian Medical Association Journal* 102:595–601.

Stocks, J., and Godfrey, S. (1976). The role of artificial ventilation, oxygen and CPAP in the pathogenesis of lung damage in neonates: assessment by serial measurements of lung function. *Pediatrics* 57:352–62.

Suter, P. M., Fairley, H. B., and Schlobohm, R. M. (1975). Shunt, lung volume and perfusion during short periods of ventilation with oxygen. *Anesthesiology* 43:617–27.

Thatcher, V. S. (1953). *History of Anesthesia*. Philadelphia: Lippincott.

Thomas, D. V., Fletcher, G., Sunshine, P., Schafer, I. A., and Klaus, M. H. (1965). Prolonged respirator use in pulmonary insufficiency of newborn. *Journal of the American Medical Association* 193:183–90.

Thompson, A. E., Furhman, B. P., and Alan, J. (1993). Perfluorocarbon associated gas exchange (PAGE) in experimental meconium aspiration (MAS). *Pediatric Research* 33:1418.

Tutuncu, A. S., Faithful, N. S., and Lachmann, B. (1993). Intratracheal perfluorocarbon administration combined with mechanical ventilation in experimental respiratory distress syndrome. Dose-dependent improvement of gas exchange. *Critical Care Medicine* 21:962–9.

Weigl, J. (1973). A case against high respiratory rates in controlled neonatal ventilation. *Respiratory Therapy* 3:57.

Weitzner, S. W., and Urban, B. J. (1969). A new ventilator using fluid logic. *Journal of the American Medical Association* 207:1126–30.

17

Thermoregulation: The design of incubators and radiant warmers

MICHAEL H. LeBLANC, M.D.
MICHAEL M. DONNELLY, B.E.

INTRODUCTION

It has long been recognized that keeping small infants warm is critical to their survival. Both incubators and radiant warmers are now routinely used for this purpose. In the simplest of terms, an incubator or a radiant warmer provides a controlled amount of additional heat that raises the effective temperature of an infant's environment, keeping the infant from becoming too cold in an otherwise frigid world. The objective of thermal support with either an incubator or radiant warmer is to maintain normal body temperature and to reduce the metabolic energy that must be expended for thermoregulation. The thermoneutral environment encompasses the range of temperatures in which an infant expends minimal energy for thermoregulation.

An incubator is a box, heated by a heater, in which an infant is placed. The heat from the heater is carried into the box by either natural or forced convective flows, and the air in the box and the walls of the box become warm relative to the air in the room in which the incubator is kept.

Current incubators are composed of a heater, a fan to blow air over the heater and through the incubator, and a box made of Plexiglas or Lucite. Much effort has been devoted to the control circuitry to turn the heater's electric current on and off and thus maintain the box at a safe and appropriate temperature for the infant – whenever possible, even under

single-fault conditions (i.e., when one part of the incubator is broken).

Radiant warmers, on the other hand, do not enclose the babies, except to a limited degree, but allow them to be positioned in the relatively cooler environment of an indoor room, subjected to the cold air of the room, but providing enough additional energy in the form of infrared radiation (usually provided by a hot filament) to balance their heat losses to the room around them. Again, great care must be taken to control the heater, providing just the right amount of heat to the babies under normal circumstances, but activating an alarm under single-fault conditions.

A baby produces heat, as does any living thing; however, the heat losses of small infants at normal ambient temperatures can exceed even their maximal heat production. By what means can heat losses be reduced, or extra heat be transferred to a baby to make up for heat losses? The basic forms of heat losses are defined physically. Conduction is discussed first because it is the simplest mathematically.

CONDUCTION

Conduction is the process by which heat flows through a solid body. For example, if one holds one end of a solid steel rod and places the other end in an open fire, initially the rod will be cool, but over time the rod will become too hot to hold. In this case, heat is conducted from the hot end of the rod to the cooler end. The rate of heat flow depends on the temperature gradient across the body and on the thermal conductance, or thermal insulation, of the solid object. That is, $H = KA/t(T_1 - T_2)$, where H is the heat loss by conduction, K is the thermal conductance of the solid through which heat is flowing, A is the cross-sectional area through which the heat is flowing, t is the thickness of the solid, T_1 is the temperature on one side of the solid, and T_2 is the temperature on the other side of the solid. In practice, in the existing incubators and radiant warmers, we attempt to eliminate heat loss by conduction. This is a relatively simple procedure, because the thermal conductivities of solids can vary by a factor of 10,000 from one material to another. Thus, if one chooses a material with a very low thermal conductivity, it is possible to reduce conductive heat loss to near zero. For this purpose, foam-rubber mattresses are used in infant incubators and radiant warmers, because the thermal conductivity of foam rubber is 0.02 W $\cdot$ m^{-1} $\cdot$ °C^{-1}. The surface area in contact with the mattress is about 10% of the baby's total surface area: surface area (m^2) = $W^{0.75}/10.8$, where W is weight (kg). The thickness of the mattress is usually 1 in. (2.5 cm). Thus, if the temperature gradient across the mattress is maintained at less than 10°C, the heat flow across the mattress will be less than 0.08 W, which is only 5% of the minimal heat production of a baby at birth (1.7 W $\cdot$ kg^{-1}).

CONVECTION

Convection is the mode of heat flow that involves the transfer of heat through a moving fluid, such as air. In convective heat transfer, adjacent molecules transfer heat by conduction, but in addition to that conduction process, large numbers of molecules circulate because of buoyancy differences and transfer heat between regions of the fluid. The additional transfer of energy by the movement of large numbers of molecules together is what distinguishes convection from conduction. Convection can be classified as either natural or forced. In natural convection, motion is induced by forces of gravity acting on density differences due to fluid expansion. Heat convection is forced if the motion of the fluid is driven by forces other than natural convection.

Convection is the mechanism of heat transfer when cool air comes into contact with a baby's skin. The air is heated by contact with the baby's skin. The heated air expands and thus becomes lighter or less dense than the colder air around it. The lighter air is then displaced upward by the force of gravity on the surrounding cold air and travels along the edge of the baby where the skin surface is relatively vertical, but leaves the skin as a plume when the surface of the skin begins to curve toward a horizontal position (Lewis et al., 1969). The thickness of the layer of air flowing along the baby's skin because of natural convection will be determined by the wind velocity in the room. If the wind velocity is very low, there will be a relatively thick layer of air flowing in a laminar pattern along the baby's vertical skin surfaces. If the wind velocity in the room is higher, this layer will be thinner, as the air will be swept away from the baby's skin much more quickly. The thicker the layer of relatively still air at the baby's skin surface, the lower the convective heat losses from the baby, and thus convective heat loss is a function of the velocity of the wind traveling at the baby's surface. The approximate equation for convection heat loss is $H = A(T_1 - T_2)(a + bV^{2/3})$, where H is the heat loss by convection, A is the area of contact between the skin and the air, T_1 is the temperature of the surface of the skin, T_2 is the air temperature, V is the velocity of the wind near the baby, and a and b are constants, where a relates to natural convection, and b to forced convection (LeBlanc, 1987).

If heat flow is measured in watts, area in square meters, temperature in degrees Celsius, and wind velocity in meters per second, then for a term infant weighing approximately 3 kg, a will be about 3.5, and b about 14.7. If D is the diameter of the infant, a should vary approximately as $1/D^{0.25}$, and b as $1/D^{0.5}$. Thus, the smaller the infant, the greater the heat loss by convection, even if described per square meter per degree Celsius. Thus, care must be taken not only in controlling the air temperature but also in controlling the wind velocity near the infant to maintain appropriate convective heat losses.

EVAPORATION

The physical process of evaporation is largely analogous to convection. The moisture within an infant diffuses through the waxy layer of the skin and into the dryer surrounding air. The propulsive force for this water flow is the difference between the partial pressure of water vapor at equilibrium at the surface of the skin (100% humidity at skin temperature) and that at the outer edge of the still layer of air next to the baby's body. Because the width of the still layer of air is a function of the velocity of the wind and the pattern of natural convection for a baby, these will influence the evaporation from the baby's skin. The most marked and variable feature of a baby's skin, however, is the thickness of the natural insulation against evaporation: the stratum corneum. The stratum corneum is markedly thinner in very immature infants relative to that in mature infants. Indeed, the evaporation across the skin decreases exponentially with increasing gestational age from approximately 26 wk to approximately 40 wk (Hammarlund, Sedin, and Strömberg, 1982). In very small infants, the rates of evaporative water and heat losses decrease exponentially with the postnatal age as the stratum corneum begins to thicken following exposure to the air (LeBlanc, 1987). This is an important route for heat loss in very small infants and has necessitated the use of methods to increase the humidity of air in incubators in order to keep very immature infants warm. Although the radiant heat from a radiant warmer usually is sufficient to keep babies warm, it causes excessive insensible water losses that may be difficult to manage clinically. Thus, although the currently marketed radiant warmers have no such provision, most clinical uses of radiant warmers for tiny babies involve methods for raising the local humidity around a baby's skin. This can be done either directly, by pouring humid air into an enclosure around the baby, or indirectly, by enclosing the baby and allowing the evaporative water lost from the skin to raise the local humidity. Heat loss due to evaporation is directly proportional to each of three factors: the area of air–skin contact, the hydraulic conductivity of the skin's surface layers, and the gradient of the partial pressure of water vapor across the still layer of air near the skin. Because the amount of water vapor that air can hold varies with its temperature, even in air that is at 100% relative humidity there can be evaporative heat losses, because the partial pressure of water vapor in saturated air (100% humidity) is higher at the higher temperatures at the skin's surface than it is at the lower temperatures of the ambient conditions around the baby. Heat loss by evaporation is approximately 511 calories per gram. The humidity in an incubator is generally controlled by forcing the air flow from the incubator to go over a pool of water, thus absorbing water vapor as it passes. These systems are generally designed so that the path that the air follows over the water will be long enough that the air coming from the chamber containing the water will be saturated with water vapor at the temperature of the water. By heating the water or by placing it in a warmer area within the incubator, one can obtain a greater partial pressure of water vapor in the exit flow. Be-

cause of the demand for very high humidity in many neonatal centers in Europe, many companies are now designing nebulizers that will directly add water to the air, even in excess of that required to saturate the air with water vapor. This results in rainout, or condensation of water on the walls of the incubator, reducing visibility through the walls of the incubator.

RADIATION

Radiation is the form of heat loss most difficult to understand conceptually. All bodies at temperatures greater than zero degrees Kelvin ($-273.15°C$) emit photons of electromagnetic radiation, the principal wavelength of which is determined by the average temperature of the surface. The heat one feels on a sunny day when moving from a shadowed area to a sunny area is heat that is transmitted from the sun by radiation. The sun, whose surface temperature is 10,000°C, emits a large proportion of its energy as visible radiation, which our eyes can detect. On the other hand, objects at temperatures in the 0–100°C range emit electromagnetic radiation, largely in the infrared range, which the human eye cannot detect. All objects we are likely to encounter are both emitting and receiving large amounts of infrared radiation, but what determines the heat flow and net heat flux by these processes? Because both the quantity and wavelength of electromagnetic radiation released are functions of the surface temperature of the source, objects that are hotter are giving off more energy than they are receiving from the world around them, whereas objects that are colder than the world around them experience a net influx of energy by radiation. For a quantitative treatment of these issues, see Kreith and Black (1980), and for application to an infant, see LeBlanc (1983). Radiant exchange goes on across infrared-transparent materials. Air is infrared-transparent over the distances we encounter in incubators, radiant warmers, and even normal rooms. Thus, radiant exchange occurs between an infant and the nearest infrared-opaque solid surface: in the case of an incubator, the Plexiglas walls of the incubator and the mattress on which the infant lies. In the case of the radiant warmer, such surfaces are the walls and ceiling of the room, as well as the mattress on which the infant lies. In addition, the warmer has a hot filament that transmits a large amount of infrared radiant energy, offsetting the infant's large losses of energy radiated to the walls of the room and convected to the cold air of the room. Because radiant exchange occurs with the first surface encountered that is radiopaque to infrared radiation, it is worth considering the relative transparencies of commonly used materials. Plexiglas, which is used for the walls of the incubator, is opaque to infrared radiation but transparent to visible radiation, allowing us to observe infants in their incubators while at the same time not subjecting them to excessive radiant heat losses. Few other plastics are as infrared-opaque as Plexiglas, and thus substitution of other materials for the walls of an incubator often will result in increased radiant losses through those walls. The walls of a single-wall incubator are cooler than the air in the incubator, because at a steady state there will be heat flowing by conduction from the air in the incubator to the air in the room. Generally, single-wall incubators have wall temperatures roughly midway between the air temperature in the room and the air temperature in the incubator. Providing a second insulating wall or directly heating the wall can result in warmer wall temperatures and decreased heat flow due to radiation. In using a radiant warmer, if we attempt to insulate babies from evaporative heat losses by placing some sort of containers over them, we have the opposite task of ensuring infrared flows from the heating element of the warmer directly to the babies. That is, any object placed between a baby and the infrared heater should be infrared-transparent or at least partially so. The way to determine the infrared transparency of a material is to overlay the infrared spectrum of the material (which is available from commonly used tables of infrared spectra for plastics) (Hummel, 1966) onto the emission spectrum for the baby, which can be calculated from Planck's formula for spectral emittance (Sears and Zemansky, 1964), resulting in diagrams such as those shown for polyethylene and saran in Figure 17.1 (LeBlanc, 1982). Polyethylene, commercially available as Glad Wrap, is the most infrared-transparent practical material, but materials that are partially infrared-transparent, such as Saran Wrap, will produce satisfactory results.

Thus, in summary, conductive heat losses can be controlled in incubators and radiant warmers by using an insulating material for the mattress. Radiant and convective losses in an incubator can be reduced by placing a Plexiglas box over the infant, both to contain air warmed by the incubator heater and reduce radiant losses to the walls of the room by interposing a radiopaque wall that is warmer than the walls of the room. A radiant warmer does not attempt to reduce convective and radiant losses to the air and walls of the room, but rather provides a powerful supplemental source of infrared radia-

tion that compensates the baby for heat losses by those routes. In an incubator, evaporative heat losses can be reduced by increasing the humidity within the incubator. As for radiant warmers, the commercial devices provide no method for controlling evaporative heat losses and water losses, and thus users must design their own devices (Baumgart, 1984). In such a design, it is essential that any enclosure over a baby have a radiotransparent upper surface that will allow the radiant heat from the warmer to reach the baby. Although theoretically it is possible to have the radiant warmer heat a radiopaque wall that will secondarily warm the infant, in practice that usually leads to unpredictable results. The control logic for the warmers is not designed to manage this type of configuration.

CONTROL LOGIC

A control system in an incubator or radiant warmer is designed to turn the heater on and off, either totally or partially, in such a way as to maintain the appropriate environmental temperature for an infant. This can be done in incubators by controlling the air temperature or controlling the temperature of the walls of the incubator. Charts are available showing the appropriate temperature for infants, and that can be adjusted according to the individual reactions of infants to the initial temperature setting. From a design standpoint, the temperature probe used to measure the air temperature should be as small and light as possible, with as little thermal inertia as possible, so that it can rapidly sense changes in air temperature. It should be in the center of the incubator compartment, close to the infant, so that it will monitor the air temperature most relevant to the infant. On the other hand, the probe must be strong enough that it cannot be easily broken and must be placed in a position where its temperature will not likely be altered artifactually during the care of the infant. Neither the infant nor any of the accoutrements should be situated so as to be able to touch or blow cold air on the air probe. To a certain extent, these two requirements are mutually exclusive, and some sort of engineering compromise is necessary. It should be remembered by the operator that any probe can report only its own temperature. If that temperature is in some way altered so that it does not reflect the air temperature in the incubator around the infant, then there is no hope that the incubator will operate in an appropriate manner.

Because the skin temperatures of infants are proportional to their environmental temperatures

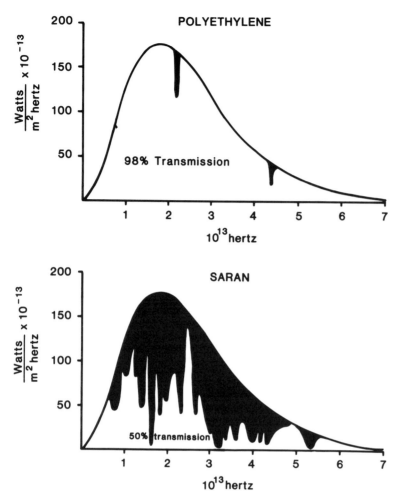

Figure 17.1. Thermal emission from a 37°C blackbody overlaid with the absorption spectra of polyethylene (top) and saran (bottom). Polyethylene absorbed only 2% of the transmissions, whereas saran absorbed 50% of the transmissions. (From LeBlanc, 1982, with permission.)

across a range of temperatures, including the thermal neutral zone, it is possible to control infants' temperatures within their neutral thermal environments by controlling their skin temperatures (LeBlanc, 1984, 1985). Because rectal temperatures are maintained well beyond the neutral thermal environment, to the point of decompensation of an infant's normal thermostatic systems (i.e., heat stroke, or freezing to death), control of rectal temperature will not result in optimal control of an infant's temperature (LeBlanc, 1984, 1985). Skin servocontrol (closed-loop feedback control of the skin temperature) is commonly used in incubators and is the only currently available means for control in radiant warmers. Currently it is not possible, on a

practical basis, to determine the operative temperature in the thermally complex environment of a radiant warmer. In an incubator, the control system should produce a temperature as close as possible to the desired temperature dialed up by the operator, and as stable as possible over time. Temperature instability will result in excursions of an infant's environmental temperature beyond the thermal neutral zone. Thermal instability is generally measured in terms of the stability of the air temperature or the operative or environmental temperature of the incubator or radiant warmer.

The simplest form of control system is an on/off system. As an example, let us consider an on/off system set to control skin temperature at 36.5°C. If

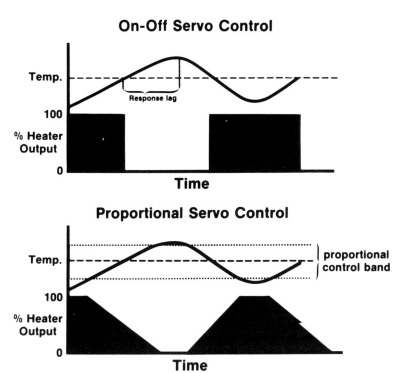

Figure 17.2. Patterns of thermal control for an on/off servocontrol system and a proportional servocontrol system. The set-point temperature is denoted by the dashed line. The controlled temperature is the solid line. The percentage heater output is shown at the bottom of the graph as the darkened area. (From LeBlanc, 1991, with permission.)

the skin temperature is below 36.5°C, then this simple control logic will turn on the current to the heater, and if the skin temperature exceeds 36.5°C, the control logic will turn off the current to the heater (Figure 17.2, upper panel). This kind of system always results in some degree of cyclical variation in the controlled temperature, because of the time delay between turning on the current to the heater and actually seeing an increase in the temperature at the skin probe. In practical terms, the heater coils take time to warm up, then the warm heater must heat the air, which takes additional time, and finally the warm air must heat the skin, which takes additional time. The longer the lag time between turning on the heater and seeing an increase in temperature at the probe, in this case the skin probe, the more unstable the temperatures will be. Because air temperature can be raised more quickly than skin temperature, controlling the air temperature results in a more stable thermal environment than controlling the skin temperature (Figure 17.3, third panel). In a skin-servocontrolled

incubator, the air temperature will be more unstable than the skin temperature. If one were to try to achieve control by monitoring rectal temperature, there would be an even greater lag time, because heat would have to be transferred from the skin surface to the body core. That would add an additional delay between turning on the heater and seeing a response at the control probe and generally would result in unacceptably unstable operation for all of the currently available radiant warmers and incubators. In the case of a radiant warmer, the discussion is analogous, except that the radiant warmer will directly heat the skin probe itself and the skin, rather than relying on transfer of heat to the air and then to the skin. Thus, radiant warmers tend to cycle in heat output at somewhat higher frequencies than incubators. In addition, as can be seen in Figure 17.3, when some intervention necessitates opening the incubator, cooling it below its steady-state operating level, much large excursions in air and skin temperatures will be seen, with gradual oscillations back to the previous steady-state values.

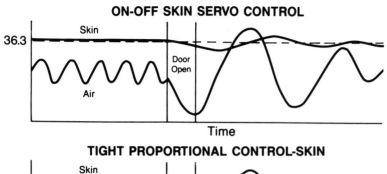

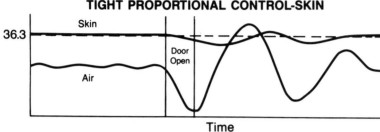

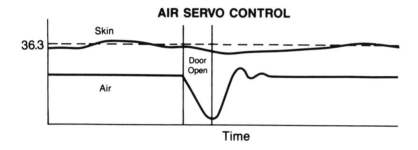

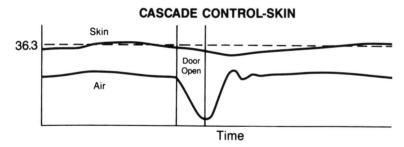

Figure 17.3. Skin temperatures and air temperatures in an incubator under four different types of control. The temperatures of the skin and the air are shown in labeled solid lines. The dashed line shows the set point for the skin temperature. The two vertical lines enclosing "Door Open" show the effect of a thermal disruption, such as opening the front door of the incubator.

Variations in air temperature are bothersome for several reasons:

1. There is an increased incidence of apnea among infants kept in warming devices that have unstable temperatures (Perlstein, Edwards, and Sutherland, 1970).

2. There is an increase in mortality among infants nursed in warming devices that have unstable temperatures (Perlstein et al., 1976).

3. Because most devices have systems to sound an alarm if excursions in temperature become excessive, unstable systems will result in a large number of nuisance alarms (LeBlanc, 1985).

In an incubator, typically there is a control system that sounds an alarm and disconnects the heater whenever the air temperature exceeds some preset value. If a very small, immature infant is nursed in an incubator, then one may need an air temperature that closely approximates that upper limit. How closely one can approximate the upper limit depends on how stable one can maintain the air temperature. That is, during the normal nursing of the infant, if the air temperature, because of temperature variation, frequently exceeds the high-temperature alarm point, one will be forced to lower the temperature setting to maintain stable incubator operation and to avoid excessive nuisance alarms.

In attempts to improve the stability of thermal control in incubators, more sophisticated control logics have been introduced. The most commonly used new development in control logic is called proportional control. With this system, the current to the heater is not turned totally on or off if the monitored temperature falls below the set point or exceeds the set point, but rather is turned up or down gradually as the monitored temperature deviates from the set point (Figure 17.2, bottom panel). Over a range or band of temperatures, the heater can go from being fully on to fully off. This system typically produces more stable temperatures. There is, however, an engineering compromise involved. To produce the most stable temperatures, one needs a rather broad proportioning band over which the heater output can be varied. However, let us hypothesize the situation in which an infant would require only 20% of the heater's output to stay warm. At a steady state, with all temperatures stable, the monitored skin temperature for this infant, with a broad proportioning band, might be substantially below the set point chosen by the clinician caring for the baby. That would require the clinician to adjust the set point upward. The educational requirements involved in marketing such a system (i.e., explaining to clinicians what proportional control means) were thought to be impractical and excessive, and such a system has never been marketed. What, in fact, is done is that the proportioning band is narrowed to the extent that any deviation of the measured skin temperature from the set point at steady state will be so small as to be unnoticed by clinicians. That, however, forces contraction of the proportioning band to such a degree as to compromise the stability of this kind of system. If the controlled temperature is outside of the proportioning band, the proportional incubator acts like an on/off incubator or warmer. Thus, simple proportional-controlled incubators, when operated under skin servocontrol, produce relatively unstable air temperatures in actual nursery conditions when they are subjected to frequent intrusions during the care of an infant (Figure 17.3, second panel). Standard additions to proportional control in other controlling systems include integral and cascade control.

In integral control, a broadband proportional controller is supplemented by a system that increases the output of the heater in proportion to the time integral of the difference between the set point and the monitored temperature (the time integral is the area on a graph of temperature versus time between the actual temperature line and the set point). That is, if a broadband proportional controller settles in on a temperature that is below the set point, an integral controller will gradually increase the set point, without intervention of the clinician, to approach the set point chosen by the clinician. This system has the fault that if a cold infant is placed in such a system and allowed to warm, the system will have a large error function (large value for the time integral) because of the long period of time when the skin was too cold. The system will then overheat the infant for several hours before it will settle down to a normal temperature.

When we branch out from simple control systems into a cascade control system, that is, using one control system to control the set point of another control system, we can achieve very sophisticated control that will adjust for a variety of conditions if the system is well designed. The first such control system was designed at the University of Cincinnati and patented by Perlstein, Edwards, and Atherton (1976; Atherton et al., 1975), following the work of Dr. L. S. James: The controlled temperature was actually the average of the skin and air temperatures in the incubator. The set point was initially chosen to produce a neutral thermal environment, even for a warming infant, and was then adjusted by 0.01°C every minute if the skin temperature was not within an acceptable range. It was found necessary to produce a dead band or a range of acceptable temperatures, rather than a single acceptable temperature, to produce stability in that system. A similar kind of system is currently marketed by Ohmeda Engineering: The air temperature in the incubator is controlled, but the set point for the air temperature is adjusted 0.1°C every 10 min if the infant's temperature is outside of an acceptable range. This kind of system results in much more stable air temperatures during operation of the incubator under skin servo-control in a real nursery environment (Figure 17.3, fourth panel). Obviously, as we enter the era of inexpensive digital controllers, we can expect much experimentation with cascade controllers of various types. As a general word of advice, it is important to understand the logic by which a given controller operates, because they all have quirks that are difficult to deal with unless one understands the logic on which the incubator or warmer system is operating. However, the clinician should not be discouraged by this complexity, because it is generally much easier to deal with the quirks of even a complicated control logic than to assemble a large, well-trained nursing staff with sufficient knowledge of thermal requirements to operate simple incubators well.

The heater current in incubators and warmers typically is controlled by a triac, a form of silicon-controlled rectifier, which has the advantage of being able to reduce the power input to a device without wasting energy though resistive loading. A triac will instantaneously cut the current at any part of an alternating-current (ac) cycle and typically is used to cut off part of the cycle and thus reduce heat output. By a little more complicated engineering, it is possible to cut the current only when there is no current flowing and thus cut out halves or whole ac cycles. This is important, because the collapse of a large current to zero nearly instantaneously will produce a powerful pulse of electromagnetic radiation that can interfere with the performance of electrical instrumentation. Thus, the zero-crossing triac is the current standard for controlling a heater output.

Temperature currently is almost always monitored by a thermistor, which is a semiconductor device whose resistance decreases as the temperature goes up and increases as the temperature goes down. From a clinical perspective, this means if a wire in a thermistor is broken, the temperature reported will be low, typically the lowest temperature the device can record. A short circuit, a somewhat less common condition, will result in a recorded temperature being too high. An unstable temperature recorded by a thermistor typically means that a wire is loose and is making intermittent connections.

When an incubator or warmer or any other electrical device is turned on, engineering standards require that a light come on somewhere on the surface of the instrument. If no light appears, one must verify that the power cord is appropriately plugged into the wall and that all connections are secure. A device such as an incubator or warmer that requires a large amount of power is totally dependent on a continuing source of electric power. If one is forced to operate such devices away from a readily available source of electric power, that is, on batteries, it is important that the time of operation be very short or that the power consumption of the device be very low. One way to reduce power consumption is to use a heavily insulated device, that is, an incubator rather than a warmer, and typically an incubator with thick, well-insulated walls and as little Plexiglas surface as is consistent with adequate visibility of the infant. All Plexiglas surfaces should be double-paned. If one uses radiant warmers with battery power, the battery power typically will not last long, and thus the transit time between one's origin and final destination must be short and carefully calculated. An infant under a radiant warmer will cool very rapidly if the heat output is interrupted. An additional caveat is that extraordinary care should be taken not to interfere with the heat output from the radiant warmer by placing any radiopaque material between the radiant heater and the baby. Radiopaque materials that commonly can be inadvertently placed between the heater and the baby include x-ray machines, the back of a physician's head, and the bag of a bag-and-mask ventilator. In incubators, which are highly dependent on insulation, it is important not to eliminate that insulation. Thus, one should carry out medical procedures though the portholes of an incubator, rather than opening the front wall, or by similarly careful means that will not affect the internal temperature of the incubator. For example, the Ohmeda IC incubator, which does not have portholes, will maintain its temperature when the front is opened to the first detent, but not beyond that point. Should medical procedures require greater access, the infant should be moved to a radiant warmer, rather than attempting them in the incubator with the front wall open for more than a brief time (seconds, not minutes).

SAFETY CIRCUITS

Incubators and radiant warmers serve a vital function in warming babies, but inadequate heating or overheating of these very sensitive patients can have the potential to compromise the quality of their lives throughout their remaining years. Thus, it is important that even if these devices are not operating as they should, nothing should be allowed to occur that could harm an infant.

The first safety circuits were designed to prevent

heating systems from overheating infants – fail-safe systems to control incubator heating if the primary systems for control of heating failed. In an incubator, this is accomplished by having an override system that will activate an alarm and turn the heater off if the incubator air temperature exceeds what is considered safe. For example, suppose that an infant is being cared for in an incubator on skin servo-control, and the sensor comes loose from the skin and falls out of the incubator onto the floor. If there is no safety override, the incubator will heat continuously until the error is discovered. If the incubator temperature and the infant's temperature rise above 108°F or 42°C, the infant may die or be permanently damaged. The system that is set up to prevent such a situation is a combination of a temperature sensor that will sound an alarm when the air temperature exceeds some preset number and a sensor that will cut the power to the heater when the upper limit for air temperature is exceeded. Historically, 38°C was the upper limit allowed for air temperature. As smaller and smaller infants began to be nursed in incubators, especially dry incubators, it became clear that higher numbers would be needed. Some commercial incubators now allow air temperatures up to 39°C, although they usually require one to activate a manual override of the lower-temperature alarm, because 39°C is too hot for a term infant. Radiant warmers, on the other hand, do not have an enclosed environment in which temperature can be controlled, and thus they are generally set to alarm and turn off the heater when there is evidence that the skin-temperature probe, which is used to control the heater, is no longer attached to the infant.

The criterion most commonly used to determine skin-temperature-probe dislodgment is a skin-temperature excursion by more than a certain amount from the set point. That is, if the skin temperature is more than 0.5°C or 1°C from the set point, the alarm will sound, and the heat from the warmer will be cut off. Although this functions primarily as a probe-dislodgment alarm, it also detects rarer malfunctions such as control-system failure and heater-element failure. This probe-dislodgment alarm works well if the skin probe suddenly becomes dislodged and falls into a cooler place. If the skin probe becomes gradually dislodged, then the machine will not always sense the dislodgement, and the potential for overheating will still exist. It is useful to have an alarm cutoff that will allow inactivation of the alarm system during the initial warming of a cold infant using a radiant warmer, when the infant's skin temperature may be below the set point for some period of time. An important feature of these

alarms is that if they are inactivated, for any reason, they will reactivate automatically after a given period of time. This is important, because alarms on radiant warmers are relatively frequent. If a baby has been overheated because a probe fell off, then the skin temperature will continue to be too high for some period, until it cools down again. It would be impractical in an active nursery setting to allow the alarm to sound for that period, which might be 15 min. Thus, there must be a way of silencing the alarm while the baby's skin temperature reequilibrates. However, if the alarm could be permanently silenced, occasionally personnel might forget to reactivate the alarm manually. If that should happen, and a second fault condition should occur, that is, the skin probe might fall off again, then there would be no alarm, and the baby's temperature would increase uncontrolled until death from heat stroke. That would be an unacceptable safety hazard. Therefore, alarm systems that become inactivated, for whatever reason, will reactivate themselves after a fixed period, usually about 15 min. The alarm limits, of course, involve an engineering compromise. The closer the alarm limits are to the skin-temperature set point, the sooner the nursing personnel will be notified of a fault condition, and the less the baby will be overheated or underheated when something causes the radiant warmer to malfunction. However, radiant warmers function in an unstable manner, as they generally are narrowband, proportionally controlled devices. One cannot use a machine that generates too many false alarms. Thus, the alarm limits must be broad enough so as not to generate too many false alarms. This type of alarm system for skin-probe dislodgement has now been added to most incubators. In addition, most incubators now contain an airflow alarm. This is a heated thermistor that is placed in the airflow. If the airflow becomes too low to cool the thermistor, it will overheat and trigger an alarm.

Most incubators also have a battery-powered alarm for loss of electric power. Thus, if an incubator switch is turned on, but no power is reaching the incubator, an alarm will sound briefly to alert the user that the power cord has not been properly attached or that there is some other source of power failure (Perlstein, Edwards, and Atherton, 1976).

Radiant warmers and incubators may also allow a manual mode, wherein the electric current to the heater is controlled by the user. Typically, radiant warmers in the manual mode will alarm at a given interval to make sure that the user checks the baby's temperature frequently enough to prevent death from hyperthermia.

CONCLUSIONS

Accessibility is one of the primary reasons for increasing use of radiant warmers, and it is this feature that today's incubators cannot match. Concern over the increased insensible water losses experienced with radiant warmers will continue to prompt attempts to modify the radiant-warmer environment to reduce this problem. In addition, the thermal environment provided by a radiant warmer is less well controlled and, because of its complexity, has been less well studied than that of an incubator. The enclosed compartment of the incubator offers a level of protection from the nursery environment that can never be achieved with an open-bed radiant warmer. With a radiant warmer, an infant is directly exposed to ambient nursery contaminants (dust, noise). However, it has never been documented that infants cared for using radiant warmers have had a higher incidence of infection than infants cared for in the filtered air of incubators. The radiant-warmer infant is directly exposed to ambient nursery noise, which periodically can be as high as 90 dBA. The incubator, in contrast, dampens and modulates the frequency content of nursery noise. However, infants in incubators can be at risk from high noise levels if maintenance of the fan motor and its associated components is inadequate. The ideal device would combine the access and visibility offered by the radiant warmer with the thermal and environmental control of the closed incubator.

From a mechanical point of view, incubators and warmers are relatively simple devices. Control systems are currently being developed in an attempt to produce greater temperature stability and safety during operation. Understanding the principles behind their operation will aid the clinician in using them more effectively.

REFERENCES

Atherton, H. D., Edwards, N. K., Perlstein, P. H., Sutherland, J. M., and Wee, W. G. (1975). A computerized incubator temperature control system for newborn infants. In *Computer Technology to Reach the People* (pp. 229–32). New York: IEEE.

Baumgart, S. (1984). Reduction of oxygen consumption, insensible water loss and radiant heat demand with use of a plastic blanket for low-birth-weight infants under radiant warmers. *Pediatrics* 74:1022–8.

Hammarlund, K., Sedin, G., and Strömberg, B. (1982). Transepidermal water loss in newborn infants. *Acta Paediatrica Scandinavica* 71:369–74.

Hummel, D. O. (1966). *Polymer Reviews: Infrared Spectra of Polymers* (p. 105). New York: Interscience.

Kreith, F., and Black, W. Z. (1980). *Basic Heat Transfer* (pp. 19–21, 282–380). New York: Harper & Row.

LeBlanc, M. H. (1982). Relative efficacy of an incubator and an open warmer in producing thermoneutrality for the small premature infant. *Pediatrics* 69:439–45.

(1983). Oxygen consumption in premature infants an incubator of proven clinical efficacy. Appendix. *Biology of the Neonate* 44:76–84.

(1984). Skin, rectal or air temperature measurement – Which is the preferred method? In *Medical Technology for the Neonate*, AAMI technology assessment report TAR no. 9 (pp. 15–19). Arlington, VA: Association for the Advancement of Medical Instrumentation.

(1985). Skin, rectal, or air temperature control in the neonate: Which is the preferred method? *Journal of Perinatology* 5:2–7.

(1987). The physics of thermal exchange between infants and their environment. *Medical Instrumentation* 21:11–15.

(1991). Thermoregulation, incubators, radiant warmers, artificial skins and body hoods. In *Clinics in Perinatology: New Technologies in the Neonate*, vol. 18, ed. Y. Brans (pp. 403–22). Philadelphia: W. B. Saunders.

Lewis, H. E., Foster, A. E., Mullan, B. J., Cox, R. N., and Clark, R. P. (1969). Aerodynamics of the human microenvironment. *Lancet* 1:1273–7.

Perlstein, P. H., Edwards, N. K., and Atherton, H. D. (1976). Incubator control with computer assistance. *Perinatology/Neonatology* 1:16–19.

Perlstein, P. H., Edwards, N. K., Atherton, H. D., and Sutherland, J. M. (1976). Computer-assisted newborn intensive care. *Pediatrics* 57:494–501.

Perlstein, P. H., Edwards, N. K., and Sutherland, J. M. (1970). Apnea in premature infants and incubator-air-temperature changes. *New England Journal of Medicine* 282:461–6.

Sears, F. W., and Zemansky, N. W. (1964). *University Physics*, 3rd ed. (p. 381). Reading, MA: Addison-Wesley.

PART V

Blood flow

In this Part V, Doppler ultrasound measurements of cerebral blood flow and fetal circulation represent applications of unique technology that allows determination of "regional blood flow." Regional blood flow has great appeal for technical diagnostic advancement. Cardiac output is variably distributed to organs based on blood oxygenation, locally acting systemic circulating factors, and locally produced factors that mediate changes in vascular tone, organ-specific metabolism, and organ-specific responses to injury or disease. It also would be useful to be able to measure regional blood flow in response to therapeutic efforts to regulate flow (principally, increasing flow to correct hypotension, hypoxia, and ischemia, although there is some interest in decreasing flow to ameliorate reperfusion injury and hemorrhage). It is surprising, in fact, that more has not been tried or accomplished in this area. Physicians have perhaps been too complacent, measuring the results (blood acid–base balance, primarily) of ischemia and its correction, and assuming that changes in blood flow must be directly related to changes in blood biochemistry. But mixed venous or arterial blood hardly represents what is going on in individual tissues and organs. Clearly, there

are many examples of normal systemic acid–base values when specific organs are not well perfused: decreased gut blood flow with a patent ductus arteriosus in preterm infants, and reperfusion injury mixed with edema and local underperfusion following recovery from "asphyxia" and hypoxic-ischemic encephalopathy. And there continues to be evidence, although mixed in interpretation, that altered patterns of fetal blood flow to various organs reflect a balance of acute versus chronic pathophysiological conditions.

The difficulty in further application of this technology appears to concern primarily its relative inaccuracy, its lack of spatial (hence, tissue-specific) localization, and the lack of experimental evidence that correlates measured changes in regional blood flow with altered regional functions. The chapters in this section offer insight into this method, as well as solutions to the problems of applicability. For the future, combining measurements of regional blood flow with measurements of organ functions (niroscopy and positron-emission tomography) should provide a better measure of what a given blood flow to an organ means.

18

Doppler measurement of the velocity of cerebral blood flow

HENRIETTA S. BADA, M.D.

INTRODUCTION

The Doppler principle was first described in 1842 by Christian Johann Doppler in his presentation "Ueber das farbige Licht der Doppelsterne und einiger anderer Gestirne des Himmels" ("On colored light of double stars and certain other stars of the heaven"), which was published the following year (Doppler, 1843). A Dutch mathematician later confirmed the Doppler principle as it applied to sound waves (Buys Ballot, 1845). It was only several years later that the Doppler principle was applied to the field of medicine (Satomura, 1956, 1959; Franklin, Schlegel, and Rushmer, 1961), primarily for flow estimation in the peripheral circulation. Subsequently, the Doppler effect became the underlying principle for external sensing devices, the continuous-wave ultrasound systems, either in the nondirectional mode (Rushmer et al., 1967) or in the directional mode (McLeod, 1967), separating forward flow from reverse flow. That was followed by the introduction of the pulsed ultrasound velocity detector (Peronneau and Leger, 1969; Wells, 1969; Baker, 1970), a technique that determines both the Doppler frequency shift and the distance between the probe and the moving interface. Further developments in technology resulted in ultrasound imaging of the internal dimensions of the peripheral arteries (Hokanson et al., 1972), the duplex Doppler systems (Barber et al., 1974; Phillips et al., 1980), and color-coded vessel images based on differential velocity (White and Curry, 1976). Significant advances in the 1980s were directed toward development of real-time color Doppler imaging (Eyer et al., 1981; Namekawa et al., 1982).

In addition to applications of the Doppler principle in peripheral and extracranial vascular diseases, it has become an accepted method for indirect blood-pressure measurement (Ware, 1965), and its use has been extended into pediatrics (Kirkland and Kirkland, 1972). Other areas of application have included cardiology (Benchimol, Desser, and Gartlan, 1972; Holen et al., 1976; Baker, Rubenstein, and Lorch, 1977; Hatle et al., 1978) and obstetrics, to study the waveforms of umbilical blood flow (Fitzgerald and Drumm, 1977; McCallum et al., 1977; Gill, 1978). Current obstetrical applications have been extended to determinations of fetal cardiac function, placental perfusion, uterine flow, and flow velocity in fetal cerebral arteries.

Some three decades ago, one-dimensional ultrasound scans (A scans) could detect only pulsations of the intracranial vessels (Freund, 1965). Those pulsations were also described with B-mode scanning or imaging of the neonatal head (Pape et al., 1979). The significance of those pulsations could not be assessed, because estimation of flow or velocity was not possible with real-time imaging alone. However, by using the continuous-wave Doppler flowmeter through a transfontanelle approach, it became possible to obtain flow-velocity waveforms from the anterior cerebral arteries (Bada et al., 1979). In 1982, Aaslid, Markwalder, and Nornes measured flow velocities in the circle of Willis through intact skull (i.e., the transcranial Doppler approach). Following introduction of the transfontanelle Doppler technique and transcranial Doppler sonography, many articles have been published in the past decade on applications of the Doppler principle to studies of the neonatal cerebral circulation. The noninvasiveness of the technique has made it an attractive clinical tool.

DOPPLER PRINCIPLE

When a high-frequency sound is directed into tissues, the sound reflected from the moving red cells is shifted in frequency (the observed or echo frequency) by an amount proportional to their velocity. This principle is expressed mathematically as

$$\Delta f = \frac{2f_t V(\cos\ \theta)}{C} \qquad (18.1)$$

where Δf *is the frequency shift*, f_t is the transmitted frequency, V is the velocity of the red cells, θ is the angle of incidence between the sound beam and the object path, and C is the velocity of sound in the tissue. When the equation is rearranged, mean velocity $\overline{V}$ can be calculated:

$$\overline{V} = \frac{C\Delta f}{2f_t \cos\ \theta} \qquad (18.2)$$

The mean velocity is said to be proportional to the mean frequency shift, with the following conditions: The angle of incidence is constant from one study to another, the same transmitting frequency is used, and the velocity of sound in the tissue is assumed to be constant (1.56×10^5 cm · s^{-1}). The accuracy of determining the angle of incidence significantly affects velocity calculations. The maximum frequency shift occurs when the angle is zero; the frequency shift decreases with increasing angles of incidence (Johnston et al., 1981). A change in the angle of incidence from zero to 30° will give a 15% error in the velocity calculation, and a further increase in the angle to 60° will underestimate velocity by one-half.

DOPPLER INSTRUMENTATION

Continuous-wave Doppler instruments

Early Doppler studies were performed using continuous-wave velocity detectors. In that system, the transducer uses two piezoelectric crystals: a transmitter crystal and a receiver crystal. The receiver crystal detects the backscattered sound reflected by the moving red cells. The difference between the transmitted and reflected (or received) frequencies is amplified and recorded as analog waveforms using a zero-crossing detector (frequency–voltage converter) or is processed by a sound-spectrum analyzer. The zero-crossing circuit gives an approxi-

mate estimation of the root-mean-square frequency rather than the mean Doppler-shift frequency or true mean velocity. Thus, the recorded mean velocities from the analog tracings tend to exceed predictions by a maximum of 16% (Woodcock et al., 1972). Also, high velocities tend to be underestimated, and low velocities may be somewhat overestimated (Reneman et al., 1973; Sumner, 1982). Continuous-wave analog recordings, however, are acceptable for clinical purposes. Spectral analysis is carried out either off line or by real-time techniques. Real-time spectrum analyzers display varying frequencies and amplitudes of the Doppler spectrum over time. When using continuous-wave Doppler instruments, the sample volume encompasses the whole cross-sectional area of the vessel being insonated, resulting in a frequency spectrum that is broader than that obtained by the pulsed Doppler system.

The continuous-wave Doppler velocity detectors have the advantage of being less expensive than the pulsed Doppler devices. The large sample volume facilitates localization of blood flow. However, a large sample volume has the disadvantage of detecting blood flow from an artery and a vein at the same time, particularly when these two vessels are close together. Furthermore, vessel-wall artifacts are difficult to eliminate without filtering out low-blood-flow velocities.

Pulsed-wave Doppler velocity detectors

The pulsed-wave Doppler system utilizes a transducer that has a single crystal that acts as both transmitter and receiver. Thus the circuitry differs from that of a continuous-wave Doppler instrument. Included in the circuit are the following: a radio-frequency oscillator (1–20 MHz), a gate or switch to determine the transmission time and pulse length, a timing circuit that opens the receiver for the desired ultrasound echo, an amplifier, a mixer-detector that compares the phase and amplitude of the echo to those of the transmitted Doppler pulse, and an audioamplifier. A short burst of ultrasound is transmitted by the transducer at regular intervals, and after an adjustable delay, the echoed signal is received; the length of the delay in receiving the echo determines the range from which the signals are gathered. The maximum Doppler shift frequency (the Nyquist limit) is equal to one-half the pulse repetition frequency (PRF) and is limited by the depth of the vessel. With a deeper vessel, PRF is decreased to allow adequate time for the crystal to receive the ultrasound echo. Use of the pulsed-wave Doppler instrument allows detection of flow-velocity waveforms from a very small sample volume, described

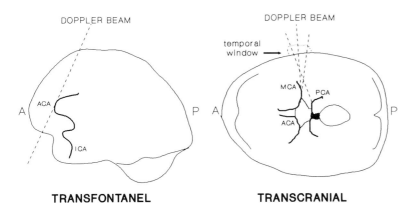

Figure 18.1. Schematic representation of the transfontanelle and transcranial approaches: A, anterior; B, posterior; ICA, internal carotid artery; ACA, anterior cerebral artery; MCA, middle cerebral artery; PCA, posterior cerebral artery.

as "teardrop" in shape. The length of the sample volume is determined by the length of the gate and the sample width is determined by the beam width of the transducer. Thus, velocity profiles can be obtained from different sites within the cross-sectional area of a large vessel (Peronneau et al., 1972). Because the neonatal cerebral arteries are quite small in diameter, the narrowest sample width may actually represent velocity changes from the whole cross section of the artery. The preferred processing of the pulsed Doppler signals is by spectral analysis.

Duplex system

Duplex devices combine a Doppler system and the pulse–echo B-scan system (Barber et al., 1974; Phillips et al., 1980). Thus, Doppler-shift signals are obtained from a determined anatomic location. Whereas earlier systems did not permit simultaneous determination of the Doppler-shift frequency and imaging, recent advances in ultrasound technology allow simultaneous operations of both real-time ultrasound imaging and real-time Doppler studies. An additional improvement in this system is real-time, two-dimensional, color-flow mapping (Mitchell et al., 1988b), wherein the pulse–echo signals are used to produce gray-scale images, and the Doppler-shift information is color-coded to represent different velocities away from or toward the transducer. Forward flow usually appears in red color, and reverse flow in blue.

TECHNIQUE OF VESSEL INSONATION

Transfontanelle approach

With the transfontanelle approach, the Doppler transducer is placed on the anterior fontanelle using a coupling gel and is directed slightly anteriorly so that signals from the anterior cerebral arteries can be obtained (Bada et al., 1979). An angle of almost zero results between the Doppler beam and the anterior cerebral artery segment (distal from its internal carotid artery origin) as it courses upward just before it curves posteriorly along the longitudinal fissure (Figure 18.1). In the absence of imaging, maximal audio signals can be heard by experienced personnel when the angle between the Doppler beam and the anterior cerebral artery is zero or almost zero. When using the currently available instrumentation with combined imaging and Doppler capabilities, the cursor for the Doppler beam is mobilized so that the beam is directed at the location of the pulsating anterior cerebral artery; imaging is best accomplished in the sagittal plane (Figure 18.2; color plate, following page 345). In this plane, insonation of the intracranial segment of the internal carotid artery can also be carried out.

Insonation of the cerebral arteries through the anterior fontanelle can also be accomplished with simultaneous imaging in the coronal plane. The anterior cerebral arteries, the middle cerebral arteries, and the circle of Willis may be localized as one makes a slow sweep from the anterior plane to the posterior plane.

Transcranial approach

Imaging with transcranial Doppler sonography is accomplished in the axial view (Aaslid et al., 1982). The transducer is placed over the temporal area just anterior to the ear and above the zygomatic arch (temporal window). This is represented schematically in Figure 18.1. The probe is directed medially when insonating the middle cerebral artery, and slightly anteriorly when studying the anterior cerebral artery, and the beam is directed posteriorly to insonate the posterior cerebral artery. The velocity

Table 18.1. *Commonly used Doppler variables*

Abbreviations/synonyms	Calculations	References
S: systolic amplitude SV: systolic velocity PSV: peak systolic velocity PSF: peak systolic frequency	Height from zero baseline to highest point (peak) of the waveform	
D: end-diastolic amplitude DV: diastolic velocity EDV: end-diastolic velocity EDF: end-diastolic frequency	Height from zero baseline to the trough of waveform	
Mean, $\bar{V}$ or f MFV: mean flow velocity MF: mean frequency VM: mean velocity	Integrated area underneath the waveform over time, or mean of the frequency shifts underneath the waveform	
Peak-to-peak distance	Distance between peak and trough	Gosling and King (1974)
AUTC per minute: area underneath the curve per minute	Calculated AUTC/time (min)	Rosenkrantz and Oh (1982), Hansen et al. (1983), Batton et al. (1983)

Indices:
  Pourcelot's resistance index
  Gosling's pulsatility index
Other resistance indices:
  A/B or S/D ratio
	RI = (S − D)/S
	PI = peak-to-peak/mean
	
	S/D
		Pourcelot (1975)
		Gosling and King (1974)
		
		Stuart et al. (1980), Trudinger et al. (1985b)

D/S ratio A/B ratio	D/S A, first systolic peak amplitude; B, second systolic peak amplitude	Trudinger et al. (1985a) Baskett et al. (1977), Gosling (1976)
Coefficient of variation (CV)	(standard deviation/mean) × 100	

from the middle cerebral artery usually is higher than velocities from other cerebral arteries. The anterior cerebral artery is more difficult to insonate through the transcranial approach. Forward flow is obtained from the proximal segment of the posterior cerebral artery, whereas the distal segment demonstrates reverse flow. Figures 18.3 and 18.4 (color plates, following page 345) show spectral displays of the velocity changes from the middle cerebral and posterior cerebral arteries, respectively.

DOPPLER WAVEFORM ANALYSIS

Doppler measurements and indices

Most instruments currently available display Doppler waveforms as velocity changes over time. These waveforms, whether displayed as frequency shifts or velocity changes, are analyzed in different ways. Also, the abbreviations used to denote the different Doppler measurements vary from one report to another. Table 18.1 shows Doppler measurements, abbreviations, calculations, and references. Figure 18.5 illustrates how the common measure-

ments are derived from different schematic examples of waveforms obtained from a cerebral artery. The commonly used Doppler measurements are the peak systolic (S or PSV), end-diastolic (D or EDV), and mean ($\bar{V}$ or MFV) velocities. Mean flow velocity is calculated by integrating the area underneath the curve (AUTC) over time (i.e., the mean of the velocities under the waveform). The peak-to-peak measurement represents the distance between the peak and the trough.

In a typical cerebral arterial Doppler waveform (Figure 18.5a), that is, under normal conditions, forward or advancing flow is observed during diastole. This is attributable to the uniquely low cerebrovascular resistance. Such a waveform characteristic differs from the peripheral arterial Doppler waveform, wherein reverse diastolic flow usually is observed. With cerebral vasodilation, the diastolic velocity (D) is increased, so that mean flow velocity is also increased (Figure 18.5b). When cerebrovascular resistance is high, as in conditions associated with increased intracranial pressure, the diastolic component of a cerebral arterial Doppler waveform will decrease to zero or almost zero; at times, the

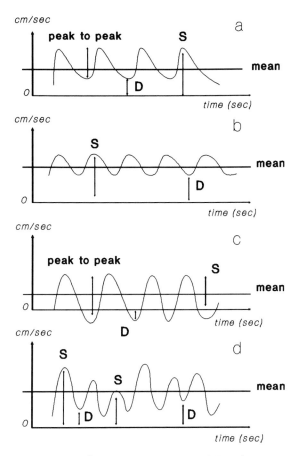

Figure 18.5. Schematic representation of Doppler waveforms obtained from a cerebral artery (a) under normal conditions, (b) when diastolic velocity is increased (vasodilation), (c) when there is retrograde diastolic flow, and (d) when there is significant waveform-to-waveform variability.

flow direction at diastole is reversed (Figure 18.5c), and a negative value for D is calculated. The cerebral arterial velocity pattern can also be affected by changes in cardiac stroke volume or by increases in intrathoracic pressure, because these affect systemic blood pressure. Thus, wide variations in systolic and diastolic components of the cerebral arterial Doppler waveform can be seen in cardiac arrhythmias or in severe respiratory distress (Figure 18.5d). Because of variability from one waveform to another, it is advisable to calculate the means of the Doppler variables from several waveforms.

Aside from the basic Doppler measurements, waveforms can also be analyzed using various indices (Table 18.1). These indices are not dependent on the angle of the probe and therefore offer an attractive means of expressing changes in Doppler

signals. Several of these indices that are said to reflect changes in vascular resistance include Pourcelot's resistance index (Pourcelot, 1975), Gosling's pulsatility index (Gosling and King, 1974), the S/D ratio (Stuart et al., 1980; Trudinger et al., 1985b), and the D/S ratio (Trudinger, Giles, and Cook, 1985a). The A/B ratio (Gosling, 1976) is usually applied in adult carotid diseases. A disadvantage of these indices is that they do not take time into consideration. Indices that include time are the systolic decay-time index (Thompson, Trudinger, and Cook, 1985), the height/width index (Johnston et al., 1984), the path-length index (Johnston et al., 1984), and the relative-flow-rate index (Thompson et al., 1985); these indices are often applied in adults for the study of vascular occlusive diseases. Principal-component analysis of neonatal cerebral Doppler waveforms has been proposed (Evans, Archer, and Levene, 1985) to detect minor changes in waveform shape; this method is, however, quite complex for routine clinical application.

Validation of Doppler measurements

In vitro studies as well as animal studies have been carried out in an attempt to validate the various Doppler measurements and indices that are commonly applied to neonatal cerebral hemodynamic evaluation. At a given angle, S, D, and AUTC will each directly correlate with volume flow (Lundell, Lindstrom, and Arnold, 1984; Miles, 1984; Miles et al., 1987; Spencer et al., 1991). Both Pourcelot's resistance index and Gosling's pulsatility index are correlated inversely with volume flow (Miles et al., 1987; Spencer et al., 1991). If resistance is calculated [i.e., pressure/flow (P/Q)], these indices, including the S/D ratio, correlate directly with resistance, but not necessarily in a linear fashion (Miles, 1984; Spencer et al., 1991). Thus, a poor correlation may be observed between these indices and resistance when the resistance values are all in the low range. This may explain the findings in animal studies (Batton et al., 1983; Hansen et al., 1983) that the Doppler variables S, D, and AUTC per minute correlated well with the volume of cerebral blood flow measured with microspheres, whereas Pourcelot's resistance index did not. Further, in those acute animal studies, the Doppler waveforms showed a high diastolic component, a likely effect of anesthesia or the surgical creation of a large fontanelle. Thus, the values for resistance index (RI) reported were between 0.40 and 0.60, values much lower than the normal values reported in human neonates. In another animal study, using the canine model, RI values from as low as 0.35 to as high as 1.10 varied inversely with cerebral perfusion pressure, which ranged from 20 to 100 mm Hg; an excellent direct correlation was observed between RI and intracranial pressure (Seibert et al., 1989). Also in vivo Doppler measurements of EDV, MFV, and Pourcelot's RI in human neonates, whether obtained by continuous-wave Doppler or by pulsed Doppler instruments, have correlated well with cerebral blood flow measured by the xenon technique (Greisen et al., 1984).

With the current availability of the duplex systems, both velocity and vessel size can be measured (Drayton and Skidmore, 1987). However, volumetric flow determination is best applied to medium-size arteries. With smaller vessels like the neonatal cerebral arteries, measurements of vessel diameters may not be accurate. Furthermore, a cross-sectional area assumes a perfectly circular vessel, which the cerebral arteries are not. The diameter of a cerebral artery does not remain constant, but changes with the cardiac cycle.

The Doppler variables are best regarded as indicators of instantaneous velocity changes, rather than as measurements of flow volume or of the regional or global distribution of blood flow. Because velocity factors into the calculation of the volume of blood flow, correlation between Doppler variables and cerebral blood flow is expected, to a certain degree. However, blood flow can change without velocity change, and velocity can change without resulting in a change in blood flow.

Errors in interpretation of Doppler measurements

The intraobserver and interobserver variabilities seen when obtaining cranial Doppler waveform measurements, even with limited personnel experience, are quite acceptable clinically. In determining Pourcelot's RI from the anterior cerebral artery using the transfontanelle approach, interobserver variability did not exceed intraobserver variability (Moorthy et al., 1990). Intraobserver variability averaged 8.4% (range 6.3–12.6%), whereas interobserver variability was less than 8% (Moorthy, Rees, and Hope, 1989). When insonating the intracranial segment of the internal carotid artery, the reproducibility of the Doppler measurements (S, D, mean, and RI) was quite good; the coefficient of variation was 8–10% (Winberg, Dahlstrom, and Lundell, 1986).

Errors in the analysis of the Doppler waveform and interpretation of the calculations can result from technical difficulties, the inherent characteristics of the vessels, and failure to take into account the infant's physiological and behavioral states. The availability of combined imaging and Doppler capabilities can minimize difficulties in locating the different cerebral arteries. During the procedure, the analog or spectral display of Doppler signals should correspond to the audible audio signals. Discrepancies between the audio signals and the analog or spectral display often can be corrected by appropriate technical adjustments (e.g., the Doppler probe can be redirected to the vessel, the angle of insonation can be changed, or an adequate amount of coupling gel can be used). Errors in the angle of insonation can either overestimate or underestimate velocity measurements. High-pass filters that filter high-energy and low-frequency signals (e.g., vessel-wall motion or "thump") will also eliminate low diastolic Doppler frequencies. A waveform may then be judged to lack a diastolic component, when actually there is a low-velocity flow. On the other hand, with analog waveform tracings from a zero-crossing Doppler flowmeter, an inappropriate signal-to-noise ratio may result in a display of forward diastolic flow velocity when the diastolic component is actually absent (Bada, 1983). Movements, breathing, and awake and sleep states can also affect velocity measurements. Variability in waveforms can be seen with high peak inspiratory pressure or when an infant is breathing out of phase with the ventilator (Cowan & Thoresen, 1987; Rennie, South, and Morley, 1987). Higher velocities can be seen in the awake state compared with the quiet state (Shuto et al., 1987; Jorch, Huster, and Rabe, 1990a).

CLINICAL APPLICATION OF CEREBRAL DOPPLER STUDIES

Normal neonatal measurements

Normal values for the different Doppler measurements will vary with (1) the intracranial artery or segment of the artery that is insonated, (2) the probe/vessel angle, (3) whether a continuous-wave or pulsed Doppler instrument is used, (4) the maturity or gestational age of the infant at the time of the procedure, (5) the postnatal age, (6) the behavioral state of the infant, and (7) changes in $Paco_2$. Velocities obtained from the intracranial segment of the internal carotid artery will be higher than those from the middle, anterior, and posterior cerebral arteries (Raju and Zikos, 1987). The velocities from middle cerebral arteries will be higher than those from either anterior cerebral or posterior cerebral arteries (Raju and Zikos, 1987; Horgan et al., 1989). Peak systolic, end-diastolic, and mean velocities, regardless of the arterial segment insonated, will all increase with gestational age (Horgan et al., 1989) and with postnatal age (Drayton and Skidmore, 1987; Evans et al., 1988; Deeg and Rupprecht, 1989). Term infants, therefore, will have higher velocities from the cerebral arteries than will preterm infants; cerebral arterial velocities will be lower in the first hour of life than in subsequent measurements at 12, 24, and 48 h of age. Changes consistent with velocity changes are also observed with the different indices. Pourcelot's RI, Gosling's pulsatility index, and the A/B ratios will decrease over time (Gray et al., 1983; Drayton and Skidmore, 1987) and will be lower in term infants than in preterm infants (Bada, 1983; Shuto et al., 1987). Cerebral arterial Doppler waveform patterns will be normal in the sleep state; velocities will increase or RI will decrease with active, rapid-eye-movement (REM) sleep (Shuto et al., 1987; Jorch et al., 1990a). In healthy, normal neonates, RI values will fall with increasing end-tidal CO_2 because of an increase in diastolic velocity (Archer et al., 1986a).

Doppler flow patterns in fetal life

Even in fetal life it is feasible to evaluate the cerebral circulation. Fetal values for velocities in the middle cerebral arteries are lower than those in neonates: median of 4.5 cm $\cdot$ s^{-1} in the fetus versus 8.0 cm $\cdot$ s^{-1} in the neonate (Lang et al., 1988). In the normal fetus, the values for Gosling's pulsatility index (PI) from the middle cerebral artery are higher than the values from either the internal carotid or anterior cerebral artery (Mari et al., 1989). Lower-than-normal PI values from the middle cerebral or internal carotid artery suggest intrauterine growth retardation (Mari et al., 1989) or compromised fetal oxygenation (Arduini et al., 1989). The sensitivity, specificity, and negative predictive value of the PI in regard to neonatal postasphyxial encephalopathy in growth-retarded fetuses are 71%, 94%, and 94%, respectively; its positive predictive value is 75% (Rizzo et al., 1989). Lower S/D ratios are also obtained from the intracranial segment of the internal carotid artery in postdate fetuses with abnormal antepartum test findings (Brar et al., 1989).

During labor, with uterine contractions the diastolic flow velocity from the anterior cerebral artery is decreased or can even be zero (Mirro and Gonzalez, 1987). Mean RI during labor is reported to be 0.72 (range 0.52–1.0), with subsequent decreases to

a mean of 0.53 $\pm$ 0.10 (range 0.34–0.68) in the immediate postdelivery period. These low RIs probably reflect abrupt hemodynamic alterations as the cord is clamped and the systemic arterial pressure increases with a consequent increase in cerebral perfusion pressure. As the pulmonary circulation becomes established, with a consequent decrease in pulmonary resistance, left-to-right shunting through the ductus arteriosus may occur, so that a decrease in cerebral arterial flow velocity results, and thus high RI values are calculated in the first hour of postnatal life (Shuto et al., 1987).

Perinatal asphyxia

Animal studies have shown that EDV and PSV, as well as AUTC per minute, correlate inversely with arterial O_2 content (Rosenberg, Narayanan, and Jones, 1985). These Doppler variables also increase with hypercapnia (Batton et al., 1983; Hansen et al., 1983). Human neonates who have suffered perinatal asphyxia have low calculated values for Pourcelot's RI and Gosling's PI; end-diastolic velocities are increased (Bada et al., 1979; Archer, Levene, & Evans, 1986b; Miles et al., 1987). Associated hypoxemia, hypercapnia, and acidosis may explain in part the increase in diastolic velocity suggestive of vasodilation and vasoparalysis. In experimental animals, pial arteriolar vessel diameter increases with asphyxia, and further increases in diameter are observed even after reventilation (Pourcyrous, Leffler, and Busija, 1990); this dilation indicates that resistance proximal to these vessels (i.e., in the cerebral arteries) is also decreased. Low RI values ($\leq$0.55) in neonates with hypoxic-ischemic encephalopathy have been associated with poor outcomes (Archer et al., 1986b; Levene et al., 1989). Some babies with hypoxic-ischemic encephalopathy may actually have low velocities of cerebral blood flow, or they may have high RI or PI values (Anderson and Mawk, 1988; Levene et al., 1989). Whether or not these findings can be attributed to high intracranial pressure, vasospasm, or hypotension needs to be investigated.

Respiratory distress and associated complications

Infants with respiratory distress may have significant waveform-to-waveform variation. This variability can be observed among those at high risk for developing intraventricular hemorrhage, those who require ventilator support with high peak inspiratory pressure, or those whose respiratory effort is not synchronized with the respirator (Perlman et al., 1985; Cowan and Thoresen, 1987; Rennie et al., 1987). Related to hypoxia and hypercapnia, infants with pneumothoraces also demonstrate low RIs or increasing diastolic velocity (Hill, Perlman, and Volpe, 1982). Endotracheal suctioning of infants during mechanical ventilation is associated with increases in AUTC and decreases in RI (Perlman and Volpe, 1983a). These changes in Doppler measurements may be due to increases in mean arterial blood pressure, and thus changes in the velocity of cerebral blood flow tend to be pressure-passive. Measurements of velocities from the intracranial segment of the internal carotid artery have shown direct correlation between MFV and mean arterial blood pressure in ill neonates, especially in preterm infants less than 31 wk of gestational age (Ahmann et al., 1983; Jorch and Jorch, 1987). Significant correlation also exists between the velocity of cerebral blood flow and heart rate. During apnea and bradycardia, diastolic velocity decreases; systolic velocity will also decrease with more severe bradycardic episodes (Perlman and Volpe, 1985).

Seizures

During seizures, RI values from the cerebral arteries will be decreased (Perlman and Volpe, 1983b; Greisen, 1986); mean cerebral arterial velocity will increase with an increase in mean arterial blood pressure. These changes are interpreted to reflect a decrease in cerebral vascular resistance with increases in metabolic rate and cerebral blood flow.

Intraventricular hemorrhage and hydrocephalus

In infants suffering intraventricular hemorrhage, high RI and PI values can be observed; mean flow velocity from the anterior cerebral artery will also be decreased (Bada et al., 1979; Miles et al., 1987; Deeg and Rupprecht, 1989; Seibert et al., 1989). High RI values have also been associated with increased mortality (Bada et al., 1982). Among survivors of intraventricular hemorrhage who develop posthemorrhagic hydrocephalus, particularly when there is an associated increase in intracranial pressure, RI or PI values may be increased, or the diastolic velocity may be decreased. Higher RI values are seen with higher intracranial pressure (Hill and Volpe, 1982; Fischer and Livingstone, 1989). Drainage of cerebrospinal fluid or relief of obstruction will result in normalization of the velocity pattern for cerebral blood flow (Hill and Volpe, 1982; Van Bel et al.,

1988; Chadduck et al., 1989; Fischer and Livingstone, 1989). Changes in RI and in cerebral arterial time-averaged velocity may also indicate autoregulatory responses to the development of posthemorrhagic ventricular dilation (Quinn, Ando, and Levene, 1992).

Brain death

Related to increases in intracranial pressure, as in diffuse cerebral necrosis and edema, cerebral Doppler ultrasound has been found to be a useful tool for determination of brain death. In brain death, the striking finding is the decrease in cerebral arterial diastolic velocity, with subsequent progression to retrograde flow (McMenamin and Volpe, 1983; Kirkham et al., 1987; Bode, Sauer, and Pringsheim, 1988). In neonatal reports of brain death, associated findings were birth asphyxia, increased intracranial pressure, and/or intraventricular hemorrhage (McMenamin and Volpe, 1983; Glasier et al., 1989).

Patent ductus arteriosus and other congenital heart diseases

Reverse diastolic flow is also seen when a large left-to-right shunt occurs through a patent ductus arteriosus (Perlman, Hill, and Volpe, 1981; Lipman, Serwer, and Brazy, 1982; Martin et al., 1982; Snider, 1985; Wu and Hung, 1989). Thus, RI values in the presence of a large left-to-right shunt approach or exceed 1.0. The retrograde diastolic flow in a large left-to-right ductal shunt is likely due to a large diastolic runoff from the carotid and cerebral arteries. Similar changes occur in the peripheral circulation; Doppler velocity patterns with significant retrograde diastolic components are seen in the distal aorta and brachial arteries (Feldtman et al., 1976; Snider, 1985). After ductal closure, the cerebral Doppler flow pattern will return to normal (Lipman et al., 1982; Martin et al., 1982).

Other congenital heart diseases are also associated with cerebral arterial velocity changes (Snider, 1985). In coarctation of the aorta, cerebral arterial RI values are decreased; this is due to the increase in diastolic flow velocity, an increase far greater than the increase in peak systolic velocity. On the other hand, in critical aortic stenosis and in hypoplastic left-heart syndrome, peak systolic velocity is decreased, with normal diastolic component; RI values are low, with a mean of 0.5 ± 0.05. In pulmonary atresia and other cardiac defects with a patent ductus arteriosus, retrograde diastolic flow is seen in the cerebral arterial Doppler waveforms; this reflects changes in the systemic circulation.

Polycythemia/hyperviscosity syndrome and anemia of prematurity

An inverse relationship exists between hematocrit or viscosity and cerebral blood flow. In neonates with polycythemia/hyperviscosity syndrome, altered cerebral arterial Doppler patterns are seen; RI, MFV, and AUTC values indicate a decrease in the velocity of cerebral blood flow (Bada, Korones, and Fitch, 1981; Rosenkrantz and Oh, 1982; Bada et al., 1986). Abnormal cerebral Doppler measurements are usually associated with symptoms (Bada et al., 1986). The MFV and AUTC per minute will increase, while RI values will decrease, and symptoms will decrease following hemodilution. This improvement in the cerebral Doppler measurements with hemodilution probably results from decreases in hematocrit and viscosity and from cerebral autoregulation because of a decrease in O_2 content (Hudak et al., 1986).

Among premature infants with anemia (hemoglobin range 9.4–11.9 $g \cdot dl^{-1}$), blood transfusion will result in a decrease in MFV and a rise in RI (Ramaekers et al., 1988). These changes in Doppler measurements correlate highly with the increases in hematocrit and viscosity.

Cranial arteriovenous malformation

Combined imaging and Doppler modalities have proved useful in the diagnosis of arteriovenous malformation (Soto, Daneman, and Hellman, 1985; Tessler et al., 1989). Vein-of-Galen aneurysms are easily visualized, and rapid swirling or turbulent venous flow is revealed by Doppler ultrasound. Cerebral arteries to which blood is being directed (feeder arteries) have high EDV, greater than 50% of the peak systolic velocity, whereas arteries that do not supply the malformation have low EDV and high RI. Color Doppler imaging has been shown to be useful in assessing flow after embolic or surgical therapy (Tessler et al., 1989)

Treatment modalities

Blood velocities in the arteries of the circle of Willis have been measured before and during extracorporeal membrane oxygenation (ECMO) procedures. With ligation of the right carotid artery, retrograde flow is seen in the right distal internal carotid and right anterior cerebral arteries; RI therefore is increased (Mitchell et al., 1988a; Raju et al., 1989). However, bilateral flow through the middle cerebral arteries is maintained (Mitchell et al., 1988a). During ECMO, the diastolic velocities in the cerebral arteries are increased during high ECMO flow rates (Taylor et al., 1987); nonpulsatile waveforms may be observed.

Changes in cerebral arterial Doppler waveforms may be seen during drug administration. Indomethacin administration results in a decrease in cerebral arterial velocity, with reversal to normal by 12 h after indomethacin administration (Cowan, 1986; Edwards et al., 1990; Van Bel, Van Zwieten, and Ouden, 1990; Mardoum et al., 1991). Indomethacin also attenuates cerebrovascular responses to CO_2 (Levene et al., 1988). The median increase in cerebral blood-flow velocity for a 1-kPa rise in $Paco_2$ is 50% at 10 min after indomethacin, compared with 144% before indomethacin. Caffeine and aminophylline have no effect on cerebral arterial velocity (Ghai et al., 1989; Saliba et al., 1989). Exogenous surfactant instillation results in an increase in MFV (Van de Bor, Ma, and Walther, 1991). No protracted hemodynamic effects have been observed up to 120 h after treatment with surfactant (Jorch et al., 1989). Recent studies, however, have mentioned an associated decrease in cerebral arterial MFV (Cowan et al., 1991); this is likely a result of a decrease in pulmonary resistance, with consequent left-to-right shunting through a patent ductus arteriosus. Administration of surfactant over 30 min appears to attenuate associated hemodynamic changes (Saliba et al., 1992). Intravenous diazepam, when given as a sedative, has no effect on the flow velocities in internal carotid arteries, but is associated with marked increases in flow velocities in anterior cerebral arteries; both PSV and EDV increase, and RI remains unchanged (Jorch et al., 1990b). Phenobarbital does not have an effect on cerebral blood-flow velocity (Jorch, Rickers, and Rabe, 1988). The use of calcium-channel blockers in perinatal asphyxia results in precipitous decreases in both blood pressure and MFV (Levene et al., 1990). Prenatal cocaine exposure is associated with increases in cerebral blood-flow velocities; both diastolic and peak systolic velocities are increased, but RI values do not differ significantly from those in infants with no cocaine exposure (Van de Bor, Walther, and Sims, 1990).

BIOEFFECTS OF ULTRASOUND

The in vitro biological effects of diagnostic ultrasound include thermal effects and acoustic cavitation. An in situ temperature increase to 41°C or higher is considered hazardous in the fetus; the likelihood of damage is greater with longer durations of temperature elevation. Acoustic cavitation can result from short pulses of ultrasound. Pulses with peak pressures greater than 10 MPa (3,300 W · cm^{-2}) can cause cavitation in mammals. The Bioeffects Committee (1988) of the American Institute of Ultrasound in Medicine periodically reviews data on the bioeffects of ultrasound. As of this date, no independently confirmed significant biological effects have been reported in mammalian tissues exposed in vivo to ultrasound, as utilized clinically for diagnostic purposes. There still remains the possibility that adverse biological effects may be recognized in the future. Thus, this calls for prudent use of ultrasound for both imaging and Doppler studies, even though benefits to patients from its use have been reported in the medical literature over the past several decades.

REFERENCES

Aaslid, R., Markwalder, T. M., and Nornes, H. (1982). Noninvasive transcranial Doppler ultrasound recordings of flow velocity in basal cerebral arteries. *Journal of Neurosurgery* 57:769–74.

Ahmann, P. A., Dykes, F. D., Lazzara, A., Holt, P. J., Giddens, D. P., and Carrigan, T. A. (1983). Relationship between pressure passivity and subependymal/intraventricular hemorrhage as assessed by pulsed Doppler ultrasound. *Pediatrics* 72:665–9.

Anderson, J. C., and Mawk, J. R. (1988). Intracranial arterial duplex Doppler waveform analysis in infants. *Child's Nervous System* 4:144–8.

Archer, L. N. J., Evans, D. H., and Levene, M. I. (1985). Doppler ultrasound examination of the anterior cerebral arteries of normal newborn infants: the effect of postnatal age. *Early Human Development* 10:255–60.

Archer, L. N. J., Evans, D. H., Paton, J. Y., and Levene, M. I. (1986a). Controlled hypercapnia and neonatal cerebral artery Doppler ultrasound waveforms. *Pediatric Research* 20:218–21.

Archer, L. N. J., Levene, M. I., and Evans, D. H. (1986b). Cerebral artery Doppler ultrasonography for prediction of outcome after perinatal asphyxia. *Lancet* 2:1116–17.

Arduini, D., Rizzo, G., Romanini, C., and Mancuso, S. (1989). Hemodynamic changes in growth retarded fetuses during maternal oxygen administration as predictors of fetal outcome. *Journal of Ultrasound in Medicine* 8:193–6.

Bada, H. S. (1983). Intracranial monitoring: its role and application in neonatal intensive care. *Clinics in Perinatology* 10:223–36.

Bada, H. S., Hajjar, W., Chua, C., and Sumner, D. S. (1979). Non-invasive diagnosis of neonatal asphyxia and intraventricular hemorrhage by Doppler ultrasound. *Journal of Pediatrics* 95:775–9.

Bada, H. S., Korones, S. B., and Fitch, C. W. (1981). Reversal of altered cerebral hemodynamics by plasma exchange transfusion in polycythemia. *Clinical Research* 29:894A.

Bada, H. S., Korones, S. B., Kolni, H. W., Fitch, C. W., Ford, D. L., Magill, H. L., Anderson, G. D., and Wong, S. P. (1986). Partial plasma exchange transfusion improves cerebral hemodynamics in symptomatic neonatal polycythemia. *American Journal of the Medical Sciences* 29:157–63.

Bada, H. S., Miller, J. E., Menke, J. A., Menten, T. G., Bashiru, M., Binstadt, D., Sumner, D. S., and Khanna, N. N. (1982). Intracranial pressure and cerebral arterial pulsatile flow measurements in neonatal intraventricular hemorrhage. *Journal of Pediatrics* 100:291–6.

Bada, H. S., and Sumner, D. S. (1984). Transcutaneous Doppler ultrasound: pulsatility index, mean flow velocity, end diastolic flow velocity and cerebral blood flow. *Journal of Pediatrics* 104:395–7.

Baker, D. W. (1970). Pulsed ultrasonic Doppler blood-flow sensing. *IEEE Transactions on Sonics and Ultrasonics* SU-17:170–85.

Baker, D. W., Rubenstein, G. A., and Lorch, G. S. (1977). Pulsed Doppler echocardiography: principles and applications. *American Journal of Medicine* 63:69–80.

Barber, F. E., Baker, D. W., Nation, A. W. C., Strandness, D. E., and Reid, J. M. (1974). Ultrasonic duplex echo-Doppler scanner. *IEEE Transactions on Biomedical Engineering* BME-21:109–13.

Baskett, J. J., Beasley, M. G., Murphy, G. J., Hyams, D. E., and Gosling, R. G. (1977). Screening for carotid junction disease by spectral analysis of Doppler signals. *Cardiovascular Research* 11:147–55.

Batton, D. G., Hellmann, J., Hernandez, M. J., and Maisels, M. J. (1983). Regional cerebral blood flow, cerebral blood flow velocity and pulsatility index in newborn dogs. *Pediatric Research* 17:908–12.

Benchimol, A., Desser, K. B., and Gartlan, J. L. (1972). Bidirectional blood flow velocity in the cardiac chambers and great vessels studied with the Doppler ultrasonic flowmeter. *American Journal of Medicine* 52:467–73.

Bioeffects Committee, American Institute of Ultrasound in Medicine (1988). Bioeffects considerations for the safety of diagnostic ultrasound. *Journal of Ultrasound in Medicine* [Suppl. 9] 7:S1–S38.

Bode, H., Sauer, M., and Pringsheim, W. (1988). Diagnosis of brain death by transcranial Doppler sonography. *Archives of Disease in Childhood* 63:1474–8.

Brar, H. S., Horenstein, J., Medearis, A. L., Platt, L. D., Phelan, J. P., and Paul, R. H. (1989). Cerebral, umbilical, and uterine resistance using Doppler velocimetry in postterm pregnancy. *Journal of Ultrasound in Medicine* 8:187–91.

Buys Ballot, C. H. D. (1845). Akustiche Versuche auf der niederlandischen Eisenbahn nebst gelegentlichen Bemerkungen zur Theorie des Hrn. Prof. Doppler. *Pogg Annals* 66:321–51.

Chadduck, W. M., Seibert, J. J., Adametz, J., Glasier, C. M., Crabtree, M., and Stansell, C. A. (1989). Cranial Doppler ultrasonography correlates with criteria for ventriculoperitoneal shunting. *Surgical Neurology* 31:122–8.

Cowan, F. (1986). Indomethacin, patent ductus arteriosus, and cerebral blood flow. *Journal of Pediatrics* 109:341–4.

Cowan, F., and Thoresen, M. (1987). The effects of intermittent positive pressure ventilation on cerebral arterial and venous blood velocities in the newborn infant. *Acta Paediatrica Scandinavica* 76:239–47.

Cowan, F., Whitelaw, A., Wertheim, D., and Silverman, M. (1991). Cerebral blood flow velocity changes after rapid administration of surfactant. *Archives of Disease in Childhood* 66:1105–9.

Deeg, K. H., and Rupprecht, T. (1989). Pulsed Doppler sonographic measurement of normal values for the flow velocities in the intracranial arteries of healthy newborns. *Pediatric Radiology* 19:71–8.

Doppler, C. (1843). Ueber das farbige Licht der Dopplersterne und einiger anderer Gestirne des Himmels. *Abhandlungen der Königlich Bohmischen Gesellschaft der Wissenschaften in Prag* 2:465–82.

Drayton, M. R., and Skidmore, R. (1987). Vasoactivity of the major intracranial arteries in newborn infants. *Archives of Disease in Childhood* 62:236–40.

Edwards, A. D., Wyatt, J. S., Richardson, C., Potter, A., Cope, M., Delpy, D. T., and Reynolds, E. O. R. (1990). Effects of indomethacin on cerebral hemodynamics in very preterm infants. *Lancet* 1:1491–5.

Evans, D. H., Archer, L. N. J., and Levene, M. I. (1985). The detection of abnormal neonatal cerebral haemodynamics using principal component analysis of the Doppler ultrasound waveform. *Ultrasound in Medicine and Biology* 11:441–9.

Evans, D. H., Levene, M. I., Shortland, D. B., and Archer, L. N. J. (1988). Resistance index, blood flow velocity, and resistance-area product in the cerebral arteries of very low birth weight infants during the first week of life. *Ultrasound in Medicine and Biology* 14:103–10.

Eyer, M. K., Brandestini, M. A., Phillips, D. J., and Baker, D. W. (1981). Color digital echo/Doppler image presentation. *Ultrasound in Medicine and Biology* 7:21–31.

Feldtman, R. W., Andrassy, R. J., Alexander, J. A., and Stanford, W. (1976). Doppler ultrasonic flow detection as an adjunct in the diagnosis of patent ductus arteriosus in premature infants. *Journal of Thoracic and Cardiovascular Surgery* 72:288–90.

Fischer, A. Q., and Livingstone, J. N., II (1989). Transcranial Doppler and real-time cranial sonography in neonatal hydrocephalus. *Journal of Child Neurology* 4:64–9.

Fitzgerald, D. E., and Drumm, J. E. (1977). Non-invasive measurement of human fetal circulation using ultrasound: a new method. *British Medical Journal* 2:1450–1.

Franklin, D. L., Schlegel, W., and Rushmer, R. F. (1961). Blood flow measured by Doppler frequency shift of back-scattered ultrasound. *Science* 134:564–5.

Freund, H. J. (1965). Ultraschallregistrierung der Pulsationen einzelner intrakranieller Arterien zur Diagnostik von Gefssverschlussen. *Archiv für Psychiatrie und Nervenkrankheiten Verainigt mit Zeitschrift für die Gesamte Neurologie und Psychiatrie* 207:247–53.

Ghai, V., Raju, T. N. K., Kim, S. Y., and McCulloch, K. M. (1989). Regional cerebral blood flow velocity after aminophylline therapy in premature newborn infants. *Journal of Pediatrics* 114:870–3.

Gill, R. W. (1978). Quantitative blood flow measurement in deep-lying vessels using pulsed Doppler with the Octoson. *Ultrasound in Medicine* 4:341–8.

Gillard, J. H., Kirkham, F. J., Levin, S. D., Neville,

B. G. R., and Gosling, R. G. (1986). Anatomical validation of middle cerebral artery position as identified by transcranial pulsed Doppler ultrasound. *Journal of Neurology, Neurosurgery, and Psychiatry* 49:1025–9.

Glasier, C. M., Seibert, J. J., Chadduck, W. M., Williamson, S. L., and Leithiser, R. E., Jr. (1989). Brain death in infants: evaluation with Doppler US. *Radiology* 172:377–80.

Gosling, R. G. (1976). Extraction of physiological information from spectrum-analyzed Doppler-shifted continuous-wave ultrasound signals obtained noninvasively from the arterial system. In *IEE Medical Electronics Monographs 18–22*, ed. D. W. Hill and B. W. Watson (pp. 73–125). Stevenage, Hertfordshire: Peter Peregrinus.

Gosling, R. G., and King, D. H. (1974). Continuous wave ultrasound as an alternative and complement to x-rays in vascular examination. In *Cardiovascular Applications of Ultrasound*, ed. R. S. Reneman (pp. 266–82). Amsterdam: North Holland.

Gray, P. H., Griffin, E. A., Drumm, J. E., Fitzgerald, D. E., and Duignan, N. M. (1983). Continuous wave Doppler ultrasound in evaluation of cerebral blood flow in neonates. *Archives of Disease in Childhood* 58:677–81.

Greisen, G. (1986). Analysis of cerebroarterial Doppler flow velocity waveforms in newborn infants: towards an index of cerebrovascular resistance. *Journal of Perinatal Medicine* 14:181–7.

Greisen, G., Johansen, K., Ellison, P. H., Fredricksen, P. S., Mali, J., and Friis-Hansen, B. (1984). Comparison of Doppler ultrasound and 133-xenon clearance. *Journal of Pediatrics* 104:411–18.

Hansen, N. B., Stonestreet, B. S., Rosenkrantz, T. S., and Oh, W. (1983). Validity of Doppler measurements of anterior cerebral artery blood flow velocity: correlation with brain blood flow in piglets. *Pediatrics* 72:526–31.

Hatle, L., Brubakk, A., Tromsdal, A., and Angelsen, B. (1978). Non-invasive assessment of pressure drop in mitral stenosis by Doppler ultrasound. *British Heart Journal* 40:131–40.

Hill, A., Perlman, J. M., and Volpe, J. J. (1982). Relationship of pneumothorax to occurrence of intraventricular hemorrhage in the premature newborn. *Pediatrics* 69:144–9.

Hill, A., and Volpe, J. J. (1982). Decrease in pulsatile flow in the anterior cerebral arteries in infantile hydrocephalus. *Pediatrics* 69:4–7.

Hokanson, D. E., Mozersky, D. J., Sumner, D. S., and Strandness, D. E., Jr. (1972). A phase-locked echo tracking system for recording arterial diameter changes in vivo. *Journal of Applied Physiology* 32:728–33.

Holen, J., Aaslid, R., Landmark, K., and Simonsen, S. (1976). Determination of pressure gradient in mitral stenosis with a non-invasive ultrasound Doppler technique. *Acta Medica Scandinavica* 199:455–60.

Horgan, J. G., Rumack, C. M., Hay, T., Manco-Johnson, M. L., Merenstein, G. B., and Esola, C. (1989). Absolute intracranial blood-flow velocities evaluated by duplex Doppler sonography in asymptomatic preterm and term neonates. *American Journal of Roentgenology* 152:1059–64.

Hudak, M. L., Koehler, R. C., Rosenberg, A. A., Traystman, R. J., and Jones, M. D., Jr. (1986). Effect of hematocrit on cerebral blood flow. *American Journal of Physiology* 251:H63–H70.

Johnston, K. W., Cobbold, R. S. C., Kassam, M. S., and Arato, P. G. (1981). Real-time frequency analysis of peripheral arterial Doppler signals. In *Noninvasive Cardiovascular Diagnosis*, 2nd ed., ed. E. B. Diethrich (pp. 233–48). Littleton, MA: PSG Publishing.

Johnston, K. W., Kassam, M., Koers, J., Cobbold, R. S. C., and MacHattie, D. (1984). Comparative study of four methods for quantifying Doppler ultrasound waveforms from the femoral artery. *Ultrasound in Medicine and Biology* 10:1–12.

Jorch, G., Huster, T., and Rabe, H. (1990a). Dependency of Doppler parameters in the anterior cerebral artery on behavioural states in preterm and term neonates. *Biology of the Neonate* 58:79–86.

Jorch, G., and Jorch, N. (1987). Failure of autoregulation of cerebral blood flow in neonates studied by pulsed Doppler ultrasound of the internal carotid artery. *European Journal of Pediatrics* 146:468–72.

Jorch, G., Rabe, H., Garbe, M., Michel, E., and Gortner, L. (1989). Acute and protracted effects of intratracheal surfactant application on internal carotid blood flow velocity, blood pressure and carbon dioxide tension in very low birth weight infants. *European Journal of Pediatrics* 148:770–3.

Jorch, G., Rabe, H., Rickers, E., Bomelburg, T., and Hentschel, R. (1990b). Cerebral blood flow velocity assessed by Doppler technique after intravenous application of diazepam in very low birth weight infants. *Developmental Pharmacology and Therapeutics* 14:102–7.

Jorch, G., Rickers, E., and Rabe, H. (1988). Doppler flow velocities under intravenous phenobarbitone in cerebral arteries in preterm infants weighing 500–1,500 g. *Monatsschrift für Kinderheilkunde* 136:815–18.

Kirkham, F. J., Levin, S. D., Padayachee, T. S., Kyme, M. C., Neville, B. G. R., and Gosling, R. G. (1987). Transcranial pulsed Doppler ultrasound findings in brain stem death. *Journal of Neurology, Neurosurgery, and Psychiatry* 50:1504–13.

Kirkland, R. T., and Kirkland, J. L. (1972). Systolic blood pressure measurement in the newborn infant with the transcutaneous Doppler method. *Journal of Pediatrics* 80:52–6.

Lang, G. D., Levene, M. I., Dougall, A., Shortland, D., and Evans, D. H. (1988). Direct measurements of fetal cerebral blood-flow velocity with duplex Doppler ultrasound. *European Journal of Obstetrics and Gynecology and Reproductive Biology* 29:15–19.

Levene, M. I., Fenton, A. C., Evans, D. H., Archer, L. N. J., Shortland, D. B., and Gibson, N. A. (1989). Severe birth asphyxia and abnormal cerebral blood-flow velocity. *Developmental Medicine and Child Neurology* 31:427–34.

Levene, M. I., Gibson, N. A., Fenton, A. C., Papathoma, E., and Barnett, D. (1990). The use of a calcium-channel blocker, nicardipine, for severely asphyxiated newborn infants. *Developmental Medicine and Child Neurology* 32:567–74.

Levene, M. I., Shortland, D., Gibson, N., and Evans, D. H. (1988). Carbon dioxide reactivity of the cerebral circulation in extremely premature infants: effects of postnatal age and indomethacin. *Pediatric Research* 24:175–9.

Lipman, B., Serwer, G. A., and Brazy, J. E. (1982). Abnormal cerebral hemodynamics in preterm infants with patent ductus arteriosus. *Pediatrics* 69:778–81.

Lundell, B. P. W., Lindstrom, D. P., and Arnold, T. G. (1984). Neonatal cerebral blood flow velocity. I. An in vitro validation of the pulsed Doppler technique. *Acta Paediatrica Scandinavica* 73:810–15.

McCallum, W. D., Olson, R. F., Daigle, R. E., and Baker, D. W. (1977). Real-time analysis of Doppler signals obtained from the feto-placental circulation. *Ultrasound in Medicine* 3B:1361–3.

McCallum, W. D., Williams, C. S., Napel, S., and Daigle, R. E. (1978). Fetal blood velocity waveforms. *American Journal of Obstetrics and Gynecology* 132:425–9.

McLeod, F. D., Jr. (1967). A directional Doppler flowmeter. In *Digest of the 7th International Conference on Medical and Biological Engineering* (p. 213).

McMenamin, J. B., and Volpe, J. J. (1983). Doppler ultrasonography determination of neonatal brain death. *Annals of Neurology* 14:302–7.

Mardoum, R., Bejar, R., Merritt, T. A., and Berry, C. (1991). Controlled study of the effects of indomethacin on cerebral blood flow velocities in newborn infants. *Journal of Pediatrics* 118:112–15.

Mari, G., Moise, K. J., Jr., Deter, R. L., Kirshon, B., Carpenter, R. J., Jr., and Huhta, J. C. (1989). Doppler assessment of the pulsatility index in the cerebral circulation of the human fetus. *American Journal of Obstetrics and Gynecology* 160:698–703.

Martin, G. G., Snider, A. R., Katz, S. M., Peabody, J. L., and Brady, J. P. (1982). Abnormal cerebral blood flow patterns in preterm infants with a large patent ductus arteriosus. *Journal of Pediatrics* 101:587–93.

Matsumoto, J. S., Babcock, D. S., Brody, A. S., Weiss, R. G., Ryckman, F. G., and Hiyama, D. (1990). Right common carotid artery ligation for extracorporeal membrane oxygenation: cerebral blood flow velocity measurement with Doppler duplex US. *Radiology* 175:757–60.

Miles, R. D. (1984). The Doppler pulsatility index and its relation of pressure, flow resistance and angle. *Bruit* 8:274–8.

Miles, R. D., Menke, J. A., Bashiru, M., and Colliver, J. A. (1987). Relationships of five Doppler measures with flow in an in vitro model and clinical findings in newborn infants. *Journal of Ultrasound in Medicine* 6:597–9.

Mirro, R., and Gonzalez, A. (1987). Perinatal anterior cerebral artery Doppler flow indexes: methods and preliminary results. *American Journal of Obstetrics and Gynecology* 156:1227–31.

Mitchell, D. G., Merton, D., Desai, H., Needleman, L., Kurtz, A. B., Goldberg, B. B., Graziani, L., and Wolfson, P. (1988a). Neonatal brain: color Doppler imaging. Part II. Altered flow pattens from extracorporeal membrane oxygenation. *Radiology* 167:307–10.

Mitchell, D. G., Merton, D. A., Mirsky, P. J., and Needleman, L. (1989). Circle of Willis in newborns: color Doppler imaging of 53 healthy full-term infants. *Radiology* 172:201–5.

Mitchell, D. G., Merton, D., Needleman, L., Kurtz, A. B., Goldberg, B. B., Levy, D., Rifkin, M. D., Pennell, R. G., Vilaro, M., Baltarowich, O., Dahnert, W., Graziani, L., and Desai, H. (1988b). Neonatal brain: color Doppler imaging. Part I. Technique and vascular anatomy. *Radiology* 167:303–6.

Moorthy, B., Colditz, P. R., Ives, K. N., Rees, D. G., van't Hoff, W. G., and Hope, P. L. (1990). Reproducibility of cerebral artery Doppler measurements. *Archives of Disease in Childhood* 65:700–1.

Moorthy, M. B., Rees, D. G., and Hope, P. L. (1989). Reproducibility of measurement of pulsatility index by Doppler ultrasound of the anterior cerebral artery of preterm infants. *Journal of the Royal Army Medical Corps* 135:131–4.

Mozersky, D. J., Hokanson, D. E., Baker, D. W., Sumner, D. S., and Strandness, D. E. (1971). Ultrasonic arteriography. *Archives of Surgery* 103:663–7.

Mullaart, R. A., Hopman, J. C. W., Daniels, O., Rotteveel, J. J., De Haan, A. F. J., and Vreuls H. J. M. (1989). Repeatability of Doppler ultrasound measurement of blood flow velocity and its variability in the supraclinoid segment of the internal carotid artery in preterm newborns. *Ultrasound in Medicine and Biology* 15:545–53.

Namekawa, K., Kasai, C., Tsukamoto, M., and Koyano, A. (1982). Realtime bloodflow imaging system utilizing autocorrelation techniques. In *Ultrasound '82*, ed. R. A. Lerski and P. Morley (pp. 203–8). New York: Pergamon Press.

Pape, K. E., Cusick, G., Honang, M. T. W., Blackwell, R. J., Sherwood, A., Thorburn, R. J., and Reynolds, E. O. R. (1979). Ultrasound detection of brain damage in preterm infants. *Lancet* 1: 1261–4.

Perlman, J. M., Goodman, S., Kreusser, K. L., and Volpe, J. J. (1985). Reduction in intraventricular hemorrhage by elimination of fluctuating cerebral blood-flow velocity in preterm infants with respiratory distress syndrome. *New England Journal of Medicine* 312:1353–7.

Perlman, J. M., Hill, A., and Volpe, J. J. (1981). The effect of patent ductus arteriosus on flow velocity in the anterior cerebral arteries: ductal steal in the premature newborn infant. *Journal of Pediatrics* 99:767–71.

Perlman, J. M., and Volpe, J. J. (1983a). Suctioning in the preterm infant: effects on cerebral blood flow velocity, intracranial pressure, and arterial blood pressure. *Pediatrics* 72:329–34.

(1983b). Seizures in the preterm infant: effects on cerebral blood flow velocity, intracranial pressure, and arterial blood pressure. *Journal of Pediatrics* 102:288–93.

(1985). Episodes of apnea and bradycardia in the preterm newborn: impact on cerebral circulation. *Pediatrics* 76:333–8.

Peronneau, P. A., and Leger, F. (1969). Doppler ultrasonic pulsed blood flowmeter. In *Proceedings of the 8th International Conference on Medical and Biological Engineering* (pp. 10–11).

Peronneau, P. A., Xhaard, J., Norwicki, A., Pellet, M., Delouche, P., and Hinglais, J. (1972). Pulsed Doppler ultrasonic flowmeter and flow pattern analysis. In *Blood Flow Measurement*, ed. C. Roberts (pp. 24–8). London: Sector Publishing.

Phillips, D. J., Powers, J. E., Eyer, M. K., Blackshear, W. M., Bodily, K. C., Strandness, D. E., and Baker, D. W. (1980). Detection of peripheral vascular disease using the duplex scanner III. *Ultrasound in Medicine and Biology* 6:205–18.

Pourcelot, L. (1975). Applications cliniques de l'examen Doppler transcutané. In *Velocimetre Ultrasonore Doppler*, ed. P. Peronneau. Paris: INSERM.

Pourcyrous, M., Leffler, C., and Busija, D. (1990). Role of prostanoids in cerebrovascular responses to asphyxia and reventilation in newborn pigs. *American Journal of Physiology* 259:H662–7.

Quinn, M. W., Ando, Y., and Levene, M. I. (1992). Cerebral arterial and venous flow-velocity measurements in post-haemorrhagic ventricular dilatation and hydrocephalus. *Developmental Medicine and Child Neurology* 34:863–9.

Raju, T. N. K. (1991). Cerebral Doppler studies in the fetus and newborn infant. *Journal of Pediatrics* 119:165–74.

Raju, T. N. K., Kim, S. Y., Meller, J. L., Srinivasan, G., Ghai, V., and Reyes, H. (1989). Circle of Willis blood velocity and flow direction after common carotid artery ligation for neonatal extracorporeal membrane oxygenation. *Pediatrics* 83:343–7.

Raju, T. N. K., and Zikos, E. (1987). Regional cerebral blood velocity in infants: a real-time transcranial and fontanellar pulsed Doppler study. *Journal of Ultrasound in Medicine* 6:497–507.

Ramaekers, V. T., Casaer, P., Marchal, G., Smet, M., and Goossens, W. (1988). The effect of blood transfusion on cerebral blood flow in preterm infants: a Doppler study. *Developmental Medicine and Child Neurology* 30:334–41.

Reneman, R. S., Clarke, H. F., Simmons, N., and Spencer, M. P. (1973). In vivo comparison of electromagnetic and Doppler flowmeters: with special attention to the processing of analog Doppler flow signal. *Cardiovascular Research* 7:557–66.

Rennie, J. M., South, M., and Morley, C. J. (1987). Cerebral blood flow velocity variability in infants receiving assisted ventilation. *Archives of Disease in Childhood* 62:1247–51.

Rizzo, G., Arduini, D., Luciano, R., Rizzo, C., Tortorolo, G., Romanini, C., and Mancuso, S. (1989). Prenatal cerebral Doppler ultrasonography and neonatal neurologic outcome. *Journal of Ultrasound in Medicine* 8:237–40.

Rosenberg, A. A., Narayanan, V., and Jones, M. D., Jr. (1985). Comparison of anterior cerebral artery blood flow velocity and cerebral blood flow during hypoxia. *Pediatric Research* 19:67–70.

Rosenkrantz, T. S., and Oh, W. (1982). Cerebral blood flow velocity in infants with polycythemia and hyperviscosity: effects of partial exchange transfusion with Plasmanate. *Journal of Pediatrics* 101:94–8.

Rushmer, R. F., Baker, D. W., Johnson, W. L., and Strandness, D. E. (1967). Clinical applications of a transcutaneous ultrasonic flow detector. *Journal of the American Medical Association* 199:326–8.

Saliba, E., Autret, E., Gold, F., Pourcelot, L., and Laugier, J. (1989). Caffeine and cerebral blood flow velocity in preterm infants. *Developmental Pharmacology and Therapeutics* 13:134–8.

Saliba, E., Autret, E., Nasr, C., Suc, A. L., and Laugier, J. (1992). Perinatal pharmacology and cerebral blood flow. *Biology of the Neonate* 62:252–7.

Satomura, S. (1956). The study of heart function by ultrasound Doppler method. I. Principle. II. Instrumentation. III. Method. IV. Results. *Japanese Circulation Journal* 26:227–8.

(1959). Study of the flow patterns in peripheral arteries by ultrasonics. *Journal of the Acoustical Society of Japan* 15:151–8.

Seibert, J. J., McCowan, T. C., Chadduck, W. M., Adametz, J. R., Glasier, C. J., Williamson, S. L., Taylor, B. J., Leithiser, R. E., Jr., McConnell, J. R., Stansell, C. A., Rodgers, A. B., and Corbitt, S. L. (1989). Duplex pulsed Doppler US versus intracranial pressure in the neonate: clinical and experimental studies. *Radiology* 171:155–9.

Shuto, H., Yasuhara, A., Sugimoto, T., Iwase, S., Kobayashi, Y., and Nakamura, M. (1987). Longitudinal determination of cerebral blood flow velocity in neonates with the Doppler technique. *Neuropediatrics* 18:218–21.

Snider, A. R. (1985). The use of Doppler ultrasonography for the evaluation of cerebral artery flow patterns in infants with congenital heart disease. *Ultrasound in Medicine and Biology* 11:503–14.

Soto, G., Daneman, A., and Hellman, J. (1985). Doppler evaluation of cerebral arteries in a Galenic vein malformation. *Journal of Ultrasound in Medicine* 4:673–5.

Spencer, J. A. D., Giussani, D. A., Moore, P. J., and Hanson, M. A. (1991). In vitro validation of Doppler indices using blood and water. *Journal of Ultrasound in Medicine* 10:305–8.

Stuart, B., Drumm, J., Fitzgerald, D. E., and Duignan, N. M. (1980). Fetal blood velocity waveforms in normal pregnancy. *British Journal of Obstetrics and Gynaecology* 87:780–5.

Sumner, D. S. (1982). Ultrasound. In *Practical Noninvasive Vascular Diagnosis*, ed. R. F. Kempczinski and J. S. T. Yao (pp. 21–47). Chicago: Year Book.

Taylor, G. A., Catena, L. M., Garin, D. B., Miller, M. K., and Short, B. L. (1987). Intracranial flow patterns in infants undergoing extracorporeal membrane oxygenation: preliminary observations with Doppler US. *Radiology* 165:671–4.

Tessler, F. N., Dion, J., Vinuela, F., Perrella, R. R., Duckwiler, G., Hall, T., Boechat, M. I., and Grant, E. G. (1989). Cranial arteriovenous malformations in neonates: color Doppler imaging with angiographic correlation. *American Journal of Roentgenology* 153:1027–30.

Thompson, R. S., Trudinger, B. J., and Cook, C. M. (1985). Doppler ultrasound waveforms in the fetal umbilical artery: quantitative analysis technique. *Ultrasound in Medicine and Biology* 11:707–18.

Trudinger, B. J., Giles, W. B., and Cook, C. M. (1985a). Uteroplacental blood flow velocity–time waveforms in normal and complicated pregnancy. *British Journal of Obstetrics and Gynaecology* 92:39–45.

Trudinger, B. J., Giles, W. B., Cook, C. M., Bombardieri, J., and Collins, L. (1985b). Fetal umbilical artery flow velocity waveforms and placental resistance: clinical significance. *British Journal of Obstetrics and Gynaecology* 92:23–30.

Van Bel, F., Van de Bor, M., Baan, J., Stijnen, T., and Ruys, J. H. (1988). Blood flow velocity pattern of the anterior cerebral arteries. *Journal of Ultrasound in Medicine* 7:553–9.

Van Bel, F., Van Zwieten, P. H. T., and Ouden, L. L. D. (1990). Contribution of color Doppler flow imaging to the evaluation of the effect of indomethacin on neonatal cerebral hemodynamics. *Journal of Ultrasound in Medicine* 9:107–9.

Van de Bor, M., Ma, E. J., and Walther, F. J. (1991). Cerebral blood flow velocity after surfactant instillation in preterm infants. *Journal of Pediatrics* 118:285–7.

Van de Bor, M., Walther, F. J., and Sims, M. E. (1990). Increased cerebral blood flow velocity in infants of mothers who abuse cocaine. *Pediatrics* 85:733–6.

Ware, R. W. (1965). New approaches to the indirect measure of human blood pressure. Presented at the Third National Biomedical Science Instrumentation Symposium, Dallas. Instrumentation Society of America, BM-65.

Wells, P. N. T. (1969). A range-gated ultrasonic Doppler system. *Medical and Biological Engineering* 7:641–52.

White, D. N., and Curry, G. R. (1976). Color-coded differential velocity carotid bifurcation scanner. In *IEEE Ultrasonics Symposium* (pp. 85–7). New York: IEEE.

Winberg, R., Dahlstrom, A., and Lundell, B. (1986). Reproducibility of intracranial Doppler flow velocimetry. *Acta Paediatrica Scandinavica* 329:134–9.

Wladimiroff, J. W., and Van Bel, F. (1987). Fetal and neonatal cerebral blood flow. *Seminars in Perinatology* 11:335–46.

Woodcock, J., Gosling, R., King, D., and Newman, D. (1972). Physical aspects of blood velocity measurement by Doppler-shifted ultrasound. In *Blood Flow Measurement*, ed. V. C. Roberts (pp. 19–23). London: Sector.

Wu, C.-M., and Hung, K.-L. (1989). Pulsatile flow changes in the anterior cerebral arteries in infants with patent ductus arteriosus: measured with Doppler technique. *Acta Paediatrica Sinica* 30:7–14.

19

Ultrasound investigations of fetal circulation

KAREL MARŠÁL, M.D., Ph.D.
HÅKAN STALE, M.D., Ph.D.

INTRODUCTION

The circulatory system of the human fetus in its natural environment, in utero, is relatively inaccessible for direct evaluation. Thus, most of our knowledge of the physiology of fetal circulation has been derived from studies of animal models, in which the use of direct invasive methods is possible (Dawes, 1968). Some additional information has been gained from studies of human umbilical circulation immediately after birth (Stembera et al., 1972).

For a long time, the only way of examining fetal heart action in utero was auscultation of fetal heart sounds. Such examination was improved by the use of phonocardiography, enabling, in addition to estimation of fetal heart rate, analysis of the signal contents of sounds. Later, it became possible to record the fetal electrocardiogram (ECG) either transabdominally or directly from the fetal scalp after rupture of the membranes during labor. However, it was not until the advent of ultrasound techniques that direct evaluation of various features of the fetal circulation became possible.

First, ultrasound studies of the fetal circulation were performed using A-mode techniques, allowing the recording of fetal heart movements through gestation. The M-mode was a substantial improvement in examination of the fetal heart. It allowed exact measurements of the external and internal dimensions of the fetal heart and evaluation of the changes in those dimensions with time. Such information could be related to the various phases of the heart cycle, and secondary variables could be computed, reflecting other heart functions (e.g., myocardial contractility). Development of B-mode real-time imaging allowed evaluation of the structural characteristics of the fetal heart, and its combination with the M-mode facilitated and improved the accuracy of the M-mode recordings (Wladimiroff, Vosters, and McGhie, 1982).

In the late 1970s it was shown that ultrasound Doppler techniques could provide signals from umbilical blood flow (Fitzgerald and Drumm, 1977; McCallum et al., 1978). That immediately aroused interest among both perinatal physiologists and clinicians and initiated an era of intense research in the areas of the fetal and uteroplacental circulations. Combination of the Doppler technique and real-time B-mode imaging made it possible to record the blood velocity in a vessel of interest and to estimate the volume blood flow from the time-averaged mean velocity and the vessel diameter (Gill, 1978; Eik-Nes, Brubakk, and Ulstein, 1980).

Further technical developments brought a number of so-called duplex systems, combining a Doppler velocimeter with a real-time sector scanner, either mechanical or electronic. That made it possible to examine intrafetal and uteroplacental vessels. The addition of color Doppler imaging increased the possibilities, allowing localization and identification of even tiny fetal vessels (e.g., the intracerebral arteries). The improved sensitivity of color Doppler ultrasound instruments of the second and third generations enabled detection of relatively low blood velocities, and that development directed the interest of researchers toward the venous part of the fetal circulation.

In the following sections, the principles of Doppler velocimetry, as applied in antenatal examination of the fetal circulation, will be described. In addition, a new technique based on real-time B-mode ultrasound and time–distance recording (Maršál, Gennser, and Lindström, 1976) will be presented. With this method, pulsatile changes in the diameters of arteries can be recorded and quantified. When it is used on the fetal descending aorta, interesting information is gained regarding vessel-wall properties and changes in fetal blood pressure.

DOPPLER ULTRASOUND VELOCIMETRY

Physical principles and techniques

The Doppler ultrasound technique makes it possible to estimate blood velocity in maternal and fetal vessels in a noninvasive way. According to the Doppler principle, the energy of a sound wave is reflected by a moving reflector, and the wavelength of the reflected wave is different from the emitted wavelength. The change in the wavelength/frequency (i.e., the Doppler shift) is proportional to the velocity of the reflector. In the situation of blood flow measurement, ultrasound at a frequency of 1–10 MHz is transmitted to a tissue and reflected by the moving red cells within a vessel. The frequency of the reflected ultrasound received by a transducer is higher than the emitted frequency when the blood is moving toward the transducer, and lower when the blood is moving away from the transducer. The Doppler shift (f_D) is given by the formula

$$f_D = 2f_0 V \cos \theta / c$$

where f_0 is the emitted ultrasound frequency, V is the blood velocity, θ is the angle between the ultrasound beam and the bloodstream direction, and c the velocity of ultrasound in the tissue. The detected Doppler shift comprises a spectrum of frequencies, rather than a single frequency, as it originates from red cells moving at various velocities within the lumen of the vessel. The Doppler-shift frequencies are within the range of audible sound. They can be analyzed (e.g., by a fast Fourier transform) and displayed as a Doppler-shift spectrum (Figure 19.1). From that spectrum, the mean and maximum velocities can be estimated and further evaluated.

The appearance of the Doppler spectrum is related to the blood velocity profile over the cross section of the vessel. A plug or flat velocity profile (e.g., signals recorded from the fetal aorta during systole) gives a narrow spectrum with no low frequencies; a flow with a parabolic profile (e.g., fetal aortic flow during diastole or flow in the umbilical vein) causes a broadening of the spectrum.

As passage of the ultrasound wave through the tissue causes a partial loss of ultrasound energy, the penetration of ultrasound is limited. The depth of penetration is inversely related to the ultrasound frequency. Accordingly, for measurements of blood flow in deep-lying vessels, low-frequency ultrasound must be used. For use on fetal and uteroplacental vessels, an ultrasound frequency of 2–4 MHz is usually suitable.

Doppler ultrasound can be used in three modes: continuous-wave (CW) Doppler ultrasound, pulsed-wave (PW) Doppler ultrasound, and color-flow imaging. In the first mode, CW Doppler ultrasound is continuously transmitted by one piezoelectric crystal, and the reflected ultrasound is received by another crystal. Signals of blood flow are obtained from all vessels traversed by the ultrasound beam. Application of CW Doppler ultrasound is limited because of lack of range resolution, and the signal-to-noise ratio is usually better with the PW than with the CW Doppler mode. An advantage of the CW Doppler technique is that there is no limitation to the highest blood velocity that can be measured.

In the PW mode, a single piezoelectric crystal is used in turn for both transmission and reception of the ultrasound bursts. By changing the time delay between the transmission of signals and the reception of reflected signals, it is possible to determine the range within the tissue from which the Doppler-shifted signals are received. In other words, it is possible to choose a specific vessel and record signals for its blood velocity. Only the signals returning from a defined region within the tissue, the so-called sample volume, are accepted. The size of the sample volume is determined by the size of the emitting crystal, the shape of the ultrasound beam, and the duration of the pulse. The sample volume is positioned by setting the interval between the transmission and reception of ultrasound signals (i.e., between the opening and closing of the transducer gate). PW ultrasound is often combined with imaging ultrasound (linear array or sector real-time scanner) in order to locate and identify a vessel of interest.

The PW Doppler technique is limited with regard to the maximum detectable velocity. At high Doppler frequencies, the aliasing phenomenon arises (i.e., misinterpretation of high velocities as being of opposite polarity). However, aliasing is seldom a

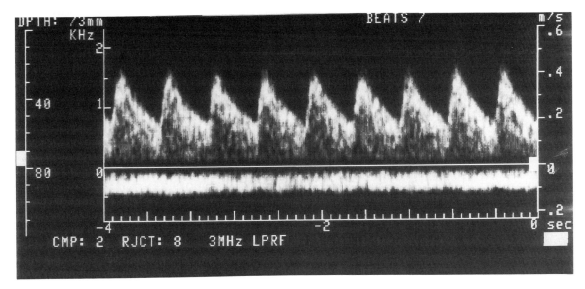

Figure 19.1. Doppler-shift spectrum recorded from the umbilical artery and vein of a 32-wk-old healthy fetus: upper part, pulsatile arterial velocity signals (note the presence of positive flow throughout the heart cycle); lower part, continuous venous velocity signals (the steady pattern indicates that the fetus is in a state of apnea).

problem in obstetrics, as the peak velocities in the fetoplacental and uteroplacental vessels usually do not exceed 1.5–2.0 m $\cdot$ s^{-1}. It is important that the instruments allow optimization of the depth-velocity product, by adjustment of the pulse repetition frequency. Aliasing, when it occurs, can be avoided by changing the insonation angle or the instrument settings (scale, baseline position).

Color-flow imaging enables color coding of the received Doppler signals, usually red for blood flow toward the transducer and blue for flow in the opposite direction. The color signals are then superimposed on the two-dimensional real-time image (Figure 19.2; color plate, following page 345). Color-flow imaging facilitates detection of flow even in very small vessels. For quantification of flow velocity, the color Doppler mode is combined with spectral PW Doppler ultrasound.

Regardless of the Doppler mode used, it is crucial that the primary Doppler signals recorded from the vessel under examination be of good quality if one is to obtain accurate data. The choice of the proper insonation angle, and in the PW mode the size and positioning of the sample volume, must be carefully controlled.

Safety aspects

Because ultrasound at high intensities has known biological effects (e.g., thermal effects and cavita-

tion) (Miller, Church, and Barnett, 1987), it is necessary that the users be constantly alert to the possibility of adverse effects from diagnostic ultrasound. Thus far, no harmful effects of ultrasound on mammalian tissues have been found at the intensities used for diagnostic purposes, and epidemiological follow-up studies have found no evidence of adverse effects from exposure to diagnostic ultrasound in utero (British Institute of Radiology, 1987). Nevertheless, it is recommended that intensities exceeding 94 mW $\cdot$ cm^{-2} of the spatial-peak temporal average in situ be avoided (AIUM, 1988) and that patients be exposed to ultrasound only for appropriate clinical reasons.

It is important that users of Doppler ultrasound be aware of the ultrasound energy put out by the Doppler equipment they are using for examining pregnancies. Some of the PW Doppler devices can put out considerable energy, and therefore it is mandatory that one uses the mode with the lowest energy when examining a fetus. Owing to the specific physical conditions during ultrasound examination of a fetus in utero, Doppler signals of high quality usually can be obtained even when using low-intensity energy.

Volume-flow estimation

Information on the time-averaged mean velocity (V) obtained from a specific vessel, corrected for cos θ,

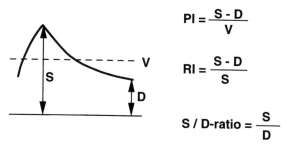

$$PI = \frac{S - D}{V}$$

$$RI = \frac{S - D}{S}$$

$$S / D\text{-ratio} = \frac{S}{D}$$

Figure 19.3. Waveform analysis of maximum blood velocity: S, peak systolic velocity; D, least diastolic velocity; V, mean velocity over the heart cycle; PI, pulsatility index according to Gosling and King (1975); RI, resistance index according to Pourcelot (1974); S/D ratio according to Stuart et al. (1980).

can be used for calculation of the volume flow (*Q*) in milliliters per minute according to the formula

$$Q = Vd^2\pi/(\cos \theta)(4)$$

This assumes that the diameter of the vessel (*d*) is known for the calculation of the cross-sectional area of the vessel.

Measurements of vessel diameters in a two-dimensional ultrasound image are relatively inaccurate and therefore can be used with confidence only for vessels of large caliber – in the fetus, only for the intraabdominal part of the umbilical vein or for the descending aorta (Eik-Nes, Maršál, and Kristoffersen, 1984). Estimation of the volume blood flow also requires knowledge of the insonation angle and uniform insonation of the vessel for reliable estimation of the mean velocity. Because of all these possible sources of error, the method has not found wide application. Nevertheless, it can be expected that further technical developments will enable reliable estimation of flow and that we can expect a revival of this method in perinatology.

Velocity-waveform analysis

The maximum blood velocity (i.e., the envelope of the Doppler spectrum recorded from an artery) can be analyzed for its waveform and characterized by various indices, which are angle-independent. The indices most often used are the pulsatility index (PI) (Gosling and King, 1975), resistance index (RI) (Pourcelot, 1974), and systolic-to-diastolic ratio (S/D ratio or A/B ratio) (Stuart et al., 1980) (Figure 19.3). For waveform analysis, there is no need to know the diameter of the vessel, and the maximum velocity is easier to record than is the mean velocity. Thus, many potential errors in the estimation of blood flow are eliminated. However, this method does not

directly reflect the flow, and the interpretation of the findings is not always obvious.

The diastolic part of the flow-velocity waveform is influenced mainly by the peripheral vascular resistance; an increase in the resistance will lower the diastolic velocity and consequently will increase the values of the waveform indices. However, the waveform and its indices are also influenced by cardiac performance, blood pressure, vessel-wall properties, and the viscosity of blood.

In healthy fetuses during the second half of gestation, diastolic flow is always present in the descending aorta (Lingman and Maršál, 1986) (Figure 19.4) and umbilical artery (Gudmundsson and Maršál, 1988a) (Figure 19.1) during fetal apnea. An absence of diastolic flow is often associated with adverse outcomes of pregnancy, such as intrauterine growth retardation (IUGR) and fetal hypoxia (Laurin et al., 1987; Rochelson et al., 1987; Gudmundsson and Maršál, 1988b). In extreme cases, diastolic flow can even be reversed (Lingman, Laurin, and Maršál, 1986), with the extremely altered velocity waveform sometimes being referred to as ARED flow (absent or reverse end-diastolic flow) (Mandruzzato et al., 1991) (Figure 19.5). A simple semiquantitative evaluation of the waveform recorded from the umbilical artery or fetal descending aorta to determine the presence or absence of end-diastolic flow (yielding blood-flow classes) has been suggested by the Malmö group and has proved to be useful in clinical application (Laurin et al., 1987) (Figure 19.6).

The received Doppler signals usually are passed through a high-pass filter to eliminate signals from slow-moving structures. When a high-pass filter with a high cutoff level is used, a considerable part of the low-velocity-flow signal will be eliminated. This sometimes can result in an erroneous diagnosis of absence of end-diastolic flow. Therefore, it has been recommended that the use of high-pass filters with cutoff levels exceeding 100 Hz be avoided (European Association of Perinatal Medicine, 1989).

Methodological studies

As mentioned earlier, the shape of the arterial-velocity waveform is influenced mainly by the vascular resistance peripheral to the site of measurement. With in vitro and computer models, allowing one to change the resistance to flow while keeping other factors (e.g., pressure and pulse rate) constant, it has been demonstrated that an increase in resistance leads to increases in the values of PI, RI, and S/D ratio (Legarth and Thorup, 1989; Adamson et al., 1989; Thompson and Stevens, 1989). Similar

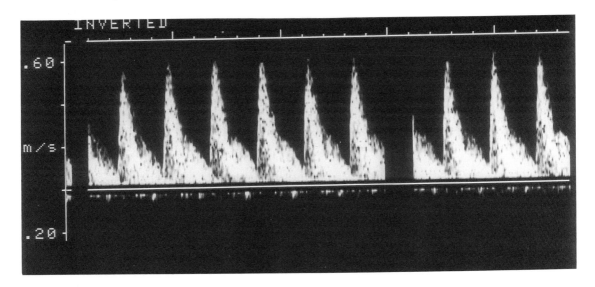

Figure 19.4. Doppler-shift spectrum recorded from the thoracic descending aortat of a 34-wk-old healthy fetus.

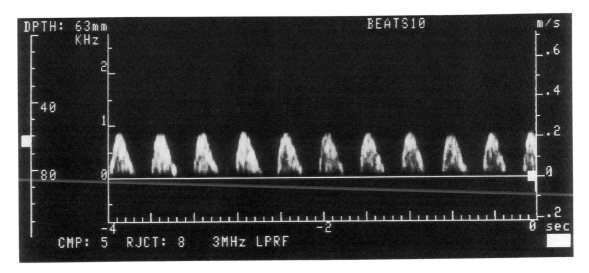

Figure 19.5. Doppler spectrum, with absence of end-diastolic flow in the umbilical artery of a fetus with severe IUGR.

changes in the waveform indices have been obtained when resistance to umbilical flow has been increased in animal experimental models, either by embolizing the fetal side of the placenta using microspheres (Trudinger et al., 1987; Morrow et al., 1989) or by constricting the umbilical vein (Maulik et al., 1989a; Fouron et al., 1991).

The problem of the minimum number of consecutive heart cycles necessary to obtain a representative and reproducible average value for a waveform index has been approached by several authors. On the basis of comparative studies, it has been concluded that five cycles are sufficient, provided that the recording is stable and the waveforms are uniform in shape (Spencer and Price, 1989).

No differences have been found between the values of indices obtained from waveforms recorded using CW and PW Doppler ultrasound (Mehalek et al., 1988; Gudmundsson et al., 1990). The reproducibility of the method has been tested for various waveform indices and various vessels. For the umbilical artery, very good intraobserver and interobserver reproducibility has been reported (Pearce et al., 1988; Maulik et al., 1989b; Gudmundsson

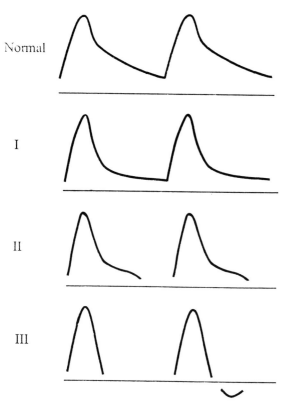

Figure 19.6. Blood-flow classes (BFC): BFC normal, positive flow throughout the heart cycle, and normal PI; BFC I, positive flow throughout the cycle, and PI equal to or greater than the mean + 2 SD for the normal population; BFC II, nondetectable end-diastolic velocity; BFC III, absence of positive flow throughout the major part of diastole and/or reversed flow in diastole.

fetus. For these reasons, fetal Doppler recordings taken during periods of breathing movements or other movements should not be used for waveform analysis.

In fetal vessels, an inverse correlation has been described between the heart rate and the values for PI and RI (Lingman and Maršál, 1986; Mulders et al., 1986; Thompson, Trudinger, and Cook, 1986; Mires et al., 1987). However, for the umbilical artery PI, it has been shown that this correlation is weak as long as the fetal heart rate is within the normal limits, that is, within 120–160 beats per minute (Gudmundsson and Maršál, 1988a). In such a situation, there is no need for PI values to be corrected.

Doppler examination of umbilical and fetal vessels

Umbilical artery

For a healthy fetus, the vascular resistance in the placenta is low, which is reflected in the umbilical artery by the presence of positive flow throughout the heart cycle (Figure 19.1). When recording the umbilical artery Doppler signals, it is important to avoid the parts of the cord close to the fetal abdomen and placenta, as too high and too low PI values, respectively, would be obtained (Sonesson et al., 1993). The placental resistance decreases gradually from midpregnancy toward term, which leads to continuous decreases in umbilical artery PI and RI with increasing gestational age (Gudmundsson and Maršál, 1988a) (Figure 19.7). There seems to be good agreement between the reference curves for umbilical artery waveform indices published by different research groups (Pearce et al., 1988).

In complications of pregnancy associated with increased resistance in the placental vascular bed, such as IUGR, the waveform of umbilical artery velocity is changed in a typical way: The diastolic velocity decreases, which causes an increase in PI. Eventually, the diastolic flow can be missing or even reversed (Figure 19.5). Such a finding is usually associated with fetal hypoxia and other signs of fetal distress (e.g., abnormal cardiotocographic traces).

Fetal descending aorta

The velocity waveforms recorded from the fetal thoracic descending aorta do not change significantly during the last trimester of pregnancy (Lingman and Maršál, 1986). Much as in the case of the umbilical artery, the aortic waveform is influenced mainly

et al., 1990). For the uteroplacental vessels, the reproducibility was less satisfactory (Gudmundsson et al., 1990). However, according to our experience, the use of the color Doppler option has substantially improved the reproducibility of Doppler recordings from the uterine artery.

Several fetal physiological factors can profoundly influence the shape of the velocity waveform and consequently the velocimetry results. Fetal breathing movements can change the intrathoracic pressure and the cardiac output of the fetus (Dawes et al., 1972). In the human fetus, both the venous and arterial circulations are influenced, and blood velocity is modulated by breathing movements (Maršál et al., 1984). Similarly, fetal movements also change the appearance of Doppler velocity signals. Van Eyck et al. (1985, 1987) showed that the values for PI in the descending aorta and internal carotid artery changed with changes in the behavioral state of the

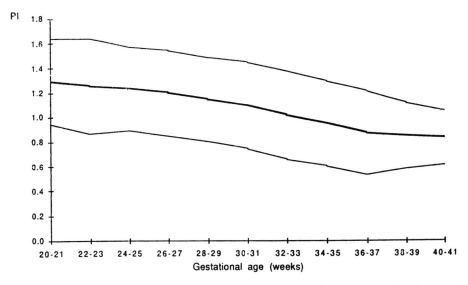

PI

Figure 19.7. Reference values for the PI for umbilical artery velocity waveforms (mean ± 2 SD), based on a cross-sectional study performed at the Malmö laboratory for studies of fetal circulation.

by the placental circulation and normally shows positive diastolic velocity (Figure 19.4). The aorta supplies some other vascular areas in addition to the placenta (e.g., kidneys, splanchnic area, and fetal carcass), with vascular resistance higher than that of the placenta. Therefore, the aortic PI usually is higher than the umbilical artery PI, typically within the range 1.83–2.49 (Maršál, Gudmundsson, and Stale, 1994).

In complicated pregnancies, the changes in the aortic waveform parallel those of the umbilical artery. For clinical purposes, no significant difference has been found between the two vessels (Gudmundsson and Maršál, 1991). However, being much easier to examine in clinical contexts, the umbilical artery is usually preferred.

Fetal middle cerebral artery

Several of the fetal cerebral arteries can be identified using color Doppler systems and the Doppler signals detected using PW Doppler. Among cerebral arteries, the middle cerebral artery is the one most often examined, as its anatomy makes the examination easy (Figure 19.8; color plate, following page 345). The insonation angle can be easily kept to zero, thus providing an optimal signal. In normal pregnancies, the waveform of middle cerebral artery velocities has a positive but relatively low diastolic component (Figure 19.9; color plate, following page 345). PI increases from 20 wk until 28–30

wk of gestation; this increase is then followed by a continuous decrease toward term (Mari and Deter, 1992).

From experimental studies of fetal lambs it is known that hypoxic fetuses redistribute their blood flow and give preferential supply to the brain (Cohn et al., 1974; Kjellmer et al., 1974; Peeters et al., 1979). This is called the brain-sparing phenomenon. It has been shown that the increase in cerebral flow in fetal lambs can be detected using Doppler ultrasound (Malcus et al., 1991): During experimental hypoxia, there was increase in the mean velocity and dilation of the examined vessel (common carotid artery). In a study of the middle cerebral artery in chronically instrumented lamb fetuses in utero, a profound increase in diastolic flow and a decrease in PI were reported (G. Gunnarsson, unpublished data).

In human fetuses, a number of reports have demonstrated decreases in middle cerebral artery PI and RI values in pregnancies with IUGR (Satoh et al., 1989; Mari and Deter, 1992; Arduini, Rizzo, and Romanini, 1992; Gramellini et al., 1992). A significant correlation between fetal hypoxemia and the degree of reduction in the PI was shown in a study analyzing fetal blood gases in samples taken via cordocentesis (Vyas et al., 1990). The abnormally low PI was transiently normalized by distributing oxygen to the mother (Nicolaides et al., 1987; Arduini et al., 1989). In fetuses with severe IUGR, increases in PI values were observed before intrauterine death, possibly because of preterminal cerebral edema (Chandran et al., 1991; Mari and Wasserstrum, 1991).

For practical use, a ratio between the waveform indices in the middle cerebral artery and umbilical artery – the so-called cerebral-placental ratio – has been proposed (Arbeille et al., 1988). This approach has improved the diagnostic accuracy of Doppler velocimetry for predicting adverse perinatal outcomes (Gramellini et al., 1992).

Fetal renal artery

Normally there is positive diastolic flow in the fetal renal artery, and the PI declines toward the end of pregnancy (Mari, Kirshon, and Abuhamad, 1993) (Figures 19.10 and 19.11; color plates, following page 345). Abnormal velocity waveforms have been reported for the renal artery in fetuses with IUGR; however, the predictive value of measurement from this vessel seems low (Vyas, Nicolaides, and Campbell, 1989).

Fetal femoral artery

The Doppler velocity waveforms recorded from femoral arteries in term human fetuses have an appearance resembling that of the waveforms recorded from peripheral arteries in adults, that is, highly pulsatile waveforms with negative velocities in early diastole and high PI values (Mari, 1991). During the third trimester of gestation there is a continuous increase in the PI. In growth-retarded fetuses, no further increase in the PI is observed (G. Gunnarsson, unpublished data), despite the opinion that, hypothetically, the femoral artery might reflect vasoconstriction in the fetal carcass, occurring as a part of flow redistribution in hypoxia.

Fetal venous system

In recent years, Doppler examination of fetal venous velocities has gained the attention of researchers because of the possibility of early detection of changes in heart function. Blood velocities in fetal systemic venous circulation have a characteristic pulsating pattern reflecting changes in central venous pressure (Figure 19.12; color plate, following page 345). At end-diastole, a reversed flow velocity frequently is observed, an expression of atrial contraction. In the umbilical vein and portal circulation, the blood velocity is normally steady, without fluctuations, during fetal apnea (Figure 19.1).

In hypoxic fetuses with increased central venous

pressure and fetuses with incipient or established heart failure, the venous pressure waves are transmitted into the umbilical vein. It has been shown that in fetuses with ARED flow in the umbilical artery, a finding of pulsations in the umbilical vein has been associated with increased perinatal mortality (Lingman et al., 1986; Arduini et al., 1993). In the inferior vena cava in fetuses with heart failure, increased reverse velocities during atrial systole can be observed (Gudmundsson et al., 1991).

Clinical value of fetal Doppler velocimetry

Doppler velocimetry offers the opportunity to evaluate the hemodynamics on both sides of the placenta and in fetal vessels. The method has been successfully applied in patients with various complications of pregnancy, the majority of reports dealing with pregnancies with IUGR. Clinical Doppler velocimetry studies in pregnancies with small-for-gestational-age (SGA) fetuses have improved our understanding of the pathophysiological processes leading to IUGR.

The finding of ARED flow in the umbilical artery and/or in the fetal descending aorta has been shown by many authors to be associated with severe IUGR and high risk for intrauterine death (Mandruzzato et al., 1991). Perinatal mortality among pregnancies with ARED flow is increased almost 10-fold over that observed in the general population. A review of 20 papers reporting 683 fetuses with ARED flow showed an average perinatal mortality among those fetuses of 35% and the incidence of severe IUGR 82% (Maršál et al., 1994). It is now generally accepted that the finding of ARED flow in the umbilical artery and/or fetal descending aorta is a reliable sign of imminent fetal asphyxia and that such a finding should indicate intervention, even in cases where the cardiotocogram findings are still normal.

Changes in the velocity waveform usually occur earlier than the pathological changes seen in conventional cardiotocographic nonstress tests. Therefore, hopes have been raised that Doppler velocimetry might offer a new sensitive clinical method for monitoring fetal health in the presence of IUGR and in high-risk pregnancies in general. As examples of such applications, two studies will be mentioned: In a study of aortic blood flow in 159 SGA fetuses, the sensitivity for predicting IUGR was 41% for PI and 57% for aortic blood-flow classes (BFC); for predicting fetal distress, the corresponding values were 76% and 87% (Laurin et al., 1987). In a study of velocity waveforms from umbilical arteries in 129 fetuses, the sensitivity for predicting IUGR was 56%, and for predicting fetal distress 83% (Gudmundsson and Maršál, 1988b).

The experience from a number of prospective studies suggests that Doppler velocimetry of umbilical and fetal arteries might be a useful diagnostic test for fetal jeopardy. The finding of abnormal velocity waveforms in the umbilical artery and fetal vessels is associated with adverse outcomes of pregnancy: IUGR, increased perinatal mortality, operative delivery for fetal distress (ODFD), acidosis, and low Apgar score. As mentioned earlier, when applied to a preselected population of high-risk pregnancies, Doppler umbilical artery velocimetry proved to be a sensitive diagnostic test, with sensitivity for predicting IUGR of 45–91%, specificity of 30–91%, positive predictive value of 43–82%, and negative predictive value of 58–99% (Maršál et al., 1994), the corresponding values for prediction of fetal distress being sensitivity 62–95%, specificity 79–93%, positive predictive value 54–83%, and negative predictive value 79–99%. The foregoing figures are valid for the use of Doppler velocimetry as a secondary diagnostic test. When applied to a general pregnant population, the method did not prove useful (Beattie, Hannah, and Dornan, 1992).

In recent years, there have been several randomized studies of Doppler velocimetry incorporated into the clinical management of IUGR fetuses. The studies showed that the use of Doppler velocimetry had a positive impact on the outcomes of pregnancies. In a Swedish multicenter study, antenatal surveillance of SGA fetuses by Doppler velocimetry was compared with conventional monitoring using cardiotocography (Almström et al., 1992). In the Doppler group, there were significantly fewer inductions of labor, fewer emergency cesarean sections for fetal distress, and fewer admissions to neonatal intensive-care units than in the cardiotocography group.

A metaanalysis of the first six published randomized trials indicated that the use of Doppler velocimetry led to lower perinatal mortality among high-risk pregnancies (Giles and Bisits, 1992). The typical odds ratio with regard to the effect of Doppler velocimetry of the umbilical artery on perinatal deaths, after exclusion of lethal malformations, was 0.53 (95% confidence interval 0.35–0.82). Thus, the collected clinical experience seems to vindicate the original optimism about the usefulness of the Doppler method in clinical situations.

Incorporation of Doppler velocimetry of fetal cerebral arteries into the clinical management of high-risk pregnancies still awaits evaluation in randomized clinical trials.

Thus far, few studies have evaluated long-term outcomes for fetuses with abnormal intrauterine blood flow. Increased frequencies of neurological sequelae at 6 mo (Weiss, Ulrich, and Berle, 1992) and 2 yr (Valcamonico et al., 1992) were reported in infants who had ARED flow in the umbilical artery in utero. In a follow-up study of 149 children at 7 yr of age, those who had been SGA infants with abnormal patterns of intrauterine aortic flow had a significantly higher frequency of minor neurological abnormalities (Maršál and Ley, 1992). This suggests that Doppler examination of fetal blood flow not only can predict perinatal outcome but also can predict future neurodevelopmental impairment.

PULSE-WAVE ANALYSIS OF VESSEL DIAMETER

Arterial diameter is closely linked to arterial pressure, and the diameter pulse wave has much the same shape as the pressure pulse wave (Busse et al., 1979; Dobrin, 1983). Changes in cardiovascular hemodynamics are reflected in the pressure pulse wave, the contour of which is highly dependent on stroke volume, the viscoelastic properties of the vessel wall, and peripheral resistance (Wiggers, 1952).

As distension of a vessel also implies thinning of its wall, it is essential to know whether the inner or the outer diameter has been recorded, if the findings are to be accurately interpreted (Dobrin, 1978). Early data from in vivo measurements of oscillations in arterial diameter in experimental animals and human adults were obtained primarily with optical methods (Hallock, 1934) or the use of large electromechanical gauges applied directly to surgically exposed vessels (Dobrin, 1978). Exposure of arteries, with removal of surrounding tissue, has been considered to permit abnormal distension of the vessel wall, probably resulting in an accidental shift to the stiffer portion of the characteristic biphasic pressure–diameter curve. In addition, large devices for diameter measurements applied to the outer wall might impede vessel-wall movement (Dobrin, 1978). Angiography does not interfere directly with vessel-wall motion, but has the disadvantages of being invasive and having poor resolution (Kawasaki et al., 1987). In 1968, Arndt introduced ultrasound techniques for noninvasive measurement of the diameter of the intact carotid artery in humans (Arndt, Klauske, and Mersch, 1968).

The introduction of the time–distance (TD) recorder, primarily developed for detection of fetal breathing movements (Lindström et al., 1977), offered the possibility for registering the wall motion of the fetal aorta in situ, with an axial resolution of 0.2 mm (Eik-Nes et al., 1982). Inclusion of the phase-locked echo-tracking principle, as originally described by Hokanson et al. (1972), combined with ultrasound linear-array B-mode equipment, considerably improved the axial-resolution capacity of the TD recorder (Sindberg Eriksen et al., 1985). The phase-locked echo-tracking system has since been used both for animal experiments (Gustafsson et al., 1989) and for human studies of fetal circulation (Sindberg Eriksen, Gennser, and Lindström, 1984; Sindberg Eriksen and Gennser, 1984; Stale, Maršál, and Gennser, 1990; Stale and Gennser, 1991a; Stale et al., 1991) and adult circulation (Imura et al., 1986; Kawasaki et al., 1987; Länne et al., 1992; Sonesson et al., 1993).

Techniques

Development

The phase-locked echo-tracking principle involves locking on the zero-crossing of a selected echo complex, which makes the system independent of the echo amplitude, but also implies the disadvantage of a limited maximum tracking velocity. Thus, the target cannot move more than a certain fraction of a wavelength between each emitted ultrasound pulse if one is to ensure continuous echo tracking. With the analog equipment developed by Hokanson et al. (1972), the tracking velocity was limited to less than a quarter of a wavelength. A modification, introducing a new digital measurement principle that allowed the maximum tracking velocity to be doubled, was developed by Gennser et al. (1981) to study the fetal circulation and later tested in vitro against an independent optical measuring method (Sindberg Eriksen et al., 1985). A further improvement was effected by the introduction of a dual echo tracker that allowed recordings to be made at two levels in the vessel simultaneously, thereby including direct measurements of the pulse propagation velocity (Lindström et al., 1987). The analog output signals from the echo trackers were stored on magnetic tape for subsequent playback on a chart recorder. A digitizer feeding a microcomputer was used for off-line analog-to-digital conversion of the pulse curves. The latest version, now available for commercial use (DIAMOVE, Teltec, Lund, Sweden) (Figure 19.13; color plate, following page 345), includes the capacity to store the recorded diameter curves on a hard disc for later analyses and on-line calculations (Benthin et al., 1991).

Description

The phase-locked echo-tracking system is interfaced with a two-dimensional real-time ultrasound scanner fitted with linear-array transducer probes for three different ultrasound frequencies (3.5, 5, and 7.5 MHz). The number of transducers in each probe is 320. The dynamic focusing system of the scanner improves the ultrasound-image resolution by repeatedly adding new echo information from four different focal distances along each ultrasound-beam line. The scanner is further equipped with a zoom mode, making it possible to enlarge the ultrasound image in three steps: ×1.0, ×1.5, and ×2.0. For the ×1.0 zoom mode, a pulse repetition frequency (PRF) of 3.12 kHz is used, and a PRF of 2.6 kHz for the other zoom modes.

In the standby mode, the scanner can be used for routine diagnostics without any limitations. For recording a diameter pulse wave, the system must be set in the measuring mode. To maintain a sufficient tracking velocity for detection of pulsatile diameter changes at two different sites on the vessel, two measuring lines must be transmitted in between each of the lines giving rise to the ultrasound image. Thereby the original frame frequency will be reduced by two-thirds, and each measuring line will be excited 1,040 or 867 times per second, depending on the zoom mode and thereby the PRF used. By excitation in two sequences (the first frame containing excitation of the ultrasound crystals with odd numbers, and the second frame those with even numbers), a high frame frequency can be preserved, and an ultrasound image with good resolution can be obtained in spite of the reduced number of lines building up each real-time image. This scanning scheme is directed by an interfaced microcomputer function, the programmable read-only memory (PROM), allowing the selection of crystals in two frames or more before the same sequence reappears. To obtain a sufficiently high PRF during the pulse-wave measurement, only one focus should be utilized.

As the target may not move more than a certain fraction of a wavelength between each emitted ultrasound pulse (in the latest version, one-fourth of a wavelength), this implies that the use of a higher ultrasound frequency will reduce the maximum tracking velocity. With an ultrasound transmission speed in human tissue of $1.540 \text{ m} \cdot \text{s}^{-1}$ and a 3.5-MHz transducer, commonly used for fetal examinations, a wavelength of 0.440 mm is obtained. The corresponding maximum tracking velocity (V_{max}) will be

$$V_{max} = 1/(3 \cdot 384 \cdot 10 - 6) \cdot \tfrac{1}{4} \cdot 0.440 = 95 \text{ mm} \cdot \text{s}^{-1}$$

for the $\times 1.5$ and $\times 2.0$ zoom modes (pulse repetition time 384 μs) and will increase to 114 mm · s^{-1} for the $\times 1.0$ zoom mode, where the pulse repetition time is 320 μs. Consequently, the use of 5- or 7.5-MHz transducers will lower the maximum tracking velocity, for the 7.5-MHz transducer to a minimum value of 44 mm · s^{-1} which, however, is more than enough for accurate recording of the proportionately slow diameter oscillations of the fetal and adult arteries.

The microcomputer also controls the 100-MHz sampling system, the analog-to-digital (A/D) and digital-to-analog (D/A) converters, the communication to the personal computer (PC, type 386, Express, Tokyo, Japan), and the remote control. With a 100-MHz sampling frequency using standard electronic logic circuits, diameter changes of 7.8 μm can be detected.

When the measuring procedure starts, the fetus is generally insonated at an oblique anteroposterior angle. The descending aorta is visualized in a longitudinal section with as good an ultrasound image as possible, minimizing disturbing echoes in the lumen of the vessel. With the trackball on the remote control, dual electronic markers are placed inside the vessel and centered between the two sites on the lumen where the image is most distinct and are then aligned with the vessel wall. The automatic search function is then activated, whereupon the markers move laterally in the directions of the anterior and posterior vessel walls. If the vessel is curved or the image at one level is not distinct enough, a separation function makes possible the necessary change in the vertical or horizontal position between the pair of markers. Using only one diameter-pulse-wave curve consequently results in an increase in the PRF, as only one measuring line has to be transmitted.

A peak detector in the microcomputer unit helps to identify the vessel wall by comparing the detected echoes. The output from the peak detector is recorded in the fast 100-MHz random-access memory (RAM). Without disturbing echoes in the lumen, the first peak emanates from the border between the circulating blood and the vessel wall (i.e., the inner vessel wall) and will subsequently be used for the phase-locked tracking. A correct echo-locking procedure is ensured by observing the scanner display to check that the electronic markers attach to the vessel wall (Figure 19.14; color plate, following

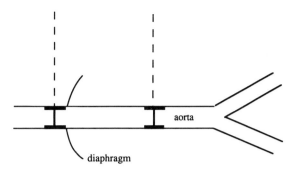

Figure 19.15. Horizontal electronic markers locked to the luminal interfaces of the echo image of the proximal and distal vessel walls at two different levels on the fetal descending aorta. (From Stale and Gennser, 1991b, with permission.)

page 345). The sampled undetected ultrasound signal for the measured line is stored in the RAM. The new positions of the anterior and posterior vessel-wall zero-crossings are calculated in the microcomputer. The differential signals between the simultaneously tracked echoes from opposite vessel walls thereby represent the instantaneous change in vessel diameter on two different levels in a plane perpendicular to the longitudinal axis of the vessel. The new diameter values are continuously transmitted to the PC and the diameter-pulse-wave curves are presented on the monitor with a maximum display time of 11 s (Figure 19.15). The two pulse-wave curves are also available from two analog outputs for recording of longer sequences on a y–t recorder. The calibration function of the remote control gives a calibrated step signal 1 mm in amplitude in 0.1-mm steps to the analog output.

In addition to the two diameter-pulse-wave curves, an external ECG curve can be stored and presented on the monitor screen. The ECG curve is A/D-converted in the DIAMOVE before being transferred to the computer. This conversion is necessary for knowledge of the exact time delay between the ECG signal and the pulse curves if the ECG is to be used as a time reference. Information concerning the three different types of probes is preprogrammed into the PC. During the recording, information about the type of probe used, together with the elapsed time delay between the two transmitted ultrasound beams (depending on the zoom mode and thereby the PRF used), is automatically transmitted to the computer. Information about the probe is vital for a correct calculation of the pulse-wave velocity (PWV), which is based on the exact distance between the two measured lines. Hard-

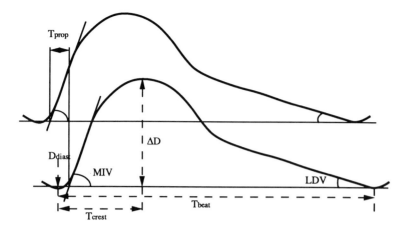

Figure 19.16. Fetal aortic diameter pulse wave: D_{diast}, end-diastolic diameter; ΔD, pulse amplitude; MIV, maximum incremental velocity; LDV, late decremental velocity; T_{beat}, pulse duration, T_{crest}, crest time; T_{prop}, propagation time (for the calculation of pulse-wave velocity, PWV). (From Stale and Gennser, 1991b.)

disc storage of the RAM data makes later viewing and calculations from the pulse curves possible.

The system allows accurate recordings of pulsatile diameter changes in vessels with diameters greater than 2 mm, which approximately corresponds to the diameter of the fetal aorta at 20 wk gestation. Analysis of the diameter pulse waveform is based on evaluation of end-diastolic diameter (D_{diast}), pulse amplitude (ΔD), maximum incremental velocity (MIV), late decremental velocity (LDV), pulse duration (T_{beat}), crest time (T_{crest}), and PWV (Figure 19.16). The calculation of PWV is based on a cross-correlation technique, utilizing only the foot of the pulse wave in every beat, and thereby reducing the interference of reflecting waves from the distal arterial tree.

Methodological studies

In vitro model

The modified system of Gennser et al. (1981), which allows the maximum tracking velocity to be doubled, as developed for the study of the fetal circulation, was tested in vitro against an independent optical method imitating the situation for measurement of the true vessel diameter (Sindberg Eriksen et al., 1985). The instantaneous diameter of a pulsating rubber tube filled with dyed fluid and immersed in water was measured by the echo trackers and simultaneously by a perpendicularly aligned optical system that included a light source

and a silicon photovoltaic cell used as a photodetector. A very high degree of linear correlation was found between the two independent measuring systems ($r = 0.99$).

Animal studies

To determine which information on central hemodynamics could be gained from noninvasively recorded diameter and its pulsatile changes, an animal study was carried out (Gustafsson et al., 1989). Cats were chosen as experimental animals because of their ability to tolerate hemodynamic stress and their suitability for transabdominal recordings of aortic-diameter pulsations without surgical exposure of the vessel. The diameter-pulse-wave characteristics were correlated to hemodynamic parameters measured with intravasal catheters and transducers during a wide variety of cardiovascular states in nonpregnant adult cats.

As a strong correlation between diameter and pressure was obtained both in diastole and in systole in the cat abdominal aorta, noninvasive recording of diameter changes in pulsatile vessels was suggested to give reliable information on the directions and relative magnitudes of blood-pressure changes. Moreover, it was found that some information on ventricular performance, in terms of the direction of change in cardiac output, stroke volume, and aortic-flow acceleration (a measure of inotropy), could be extracted from the variables of the aortic diameter-pulse-wave curve.

Methodological considerations

A high-quality ultrasound real-time image is important for obtaining acceptable pulse-wave recordings. This means distinctly appearing vessel walls and a minimum of disturbing echoes in the vessel lumen. Moreover, the recordings should be carried out during periods of fetal quiescence without breathing movements or other gross movements.

The phase-locked principle, with its extremely high resolution for spatial movements, guarantees high accuracy in estimating the pulsatile changes in diameter. The methodological problems primarily concern the end-diastolic diameter. When the measuring procedure has started, it is necessary to keep the transducer probe steady. If the transducer is not parallel to the longitudinal axis of the vessel, the measured diameter and its changes will falsely increase. In practice, this error will be minimized, because the continuity of vessel visualization will allow the transducer to be kept parallel to the course of the vessel throughout the recording.

If the scanning plane is displaced in relation to the projection of the vessel diameter, which is difficult to detect on the screen, this can result in underestimation of the diameter. However, the width of the beam in relation to the diameter of the fetal aorta presumably makes this error negligible. For a vessel with a larger diameter, locking probably is inhibited by the fact that the intersection between the measuring line and the vessel wall is not perpendicular, thereby impairing the echo quality.

A new locking operation at the same site on the vessel implies the possibility that the locking will not occur at the same zero-crossing in the echo complex and thereby not at the same structure of the vessel wall, which could result in slight differences in end-diastolic diameters. The branching of the fetal aorta, with decreasing diameter in the distal direction, necessitates careful orientation before each measurement to obtain comparable values for end-diastolic diameters.

The manual A/D conversion of the pulse curves by the use of a digitizer that was necessary in earlier versions of the system required a high degree of precision. Owing to the shortness of the segments usually visible on the ultrasound screen (<4 cm) between the two sites of measurement along the fetal aorta, estimation of the propagation time was particularly susceptible to this source of error. That fact probably contributed to the inconclusive results obtained from the calculations of PWV in most of the studies performed earlier. This source of error likely has been eliminated in the latest version, where the manual A/D conversion of the pulse curves has been replaced by the previously described computerized calculation of PWV (Benthin et al., 1991).

The methodological errors in intraobserver and interobserver variations have also been tested, but no significant differences have been found (Sindberg Eriksen et al., 1985).

Clinical experience

Several clinical studies of the fetal circulation based on diameter-pulse-wave recordings using the phase-locked echo-tracking principle have been published. Thus, Sindberg Eriksen et al. (1984) described not only the physiological characteristics of diameter pulses in the fetal descending aorta but also the acute responses of the pulsatile movements in that vessel to maternal smoking (Sindberg, Eriksen and Gennser, 1984). Changes similar to those found in adults after smoking were seen, probably reflecting both increased myocardial contractility and increased afterload. The longitudinal development of the diameter pulse waveform in the abdominal aorta of the human fetus during the second half of gestation suggests a reduction in vessel-wall compliance, probably due to an increase in fetal blood pressure during the third trimester (Stale and Gennser, 1991a). The changes in the aortic diameter-pulse-wave variables in SGA human fetuses indicate diastolic blood pressure to be increased in connection with IUGR (Stale et al., 1991). The system has also been used to study the time relationship between blood-flow velocity and pulsatile vessel diameter (Stale et al., 1990) and to examine the effects of changes in maternal position on the fetal circulation with intact fetal membranes (Luterkort and Gennser, 1986) and after membrane rupture (Stale and Gennser, 1991b).

Interpretation of the diameter pulse waveform is a delicate problem. The typical appearances of the arterial pressure and diameter pulse waves reflect multifactorial relationships, in which cardiac performance, the viscoelastic properties of the vessel wall, peripheral resistance, and reflected waves are the major constituents. Changes in the hemodynamic variables interfere with and influence the contour of the pulse wave more or less in its entirety. Inversely, a change in one of the pulse-wave characteristics is generally a manifestation of complicated changes in cardiovascular hemodynamics, in which individual variables act more or less strongly. However, it seems that the gathered information from noninvasive recordings of aortic pulsatile diameter changes reveals a pattern of responses reflecting cardiovascular adjustments likely to have occurred. Interpreted with caution, this information contributes to an understanding of the complex fetal hemodynamics, but the technique is also suitable for evaluation of great-vessel compliance in adults.

CONCLUSIONS

The noninvasive ultrasound techniques made the fetal circulation accessible for examination in utero. Doppler ultrasound makes it possible to record signals that reveal blood velocities from selected vessels and to estimate from the Doppler-shift spectrum the mean and maximum velocities. Estimation of the volume of blood flow from the data on mean velocity and vessel diameter suffers from inaccuracy and is therefore, at least at present, not suitable for clinical application. The waveform of the maximum blood velocity recorded from the fetal and umbilical arteries contains valuable information on various factors determining fetal blood flow. Waveform indices, especially the PI and RI, are significantly related to the vascular resistance peripheral to the site of measurement. Increased resistance in the placental vascular bed, as indicated by increases in PI and RI values, is associated with adverse outcomes of pregnancy and fetal hypoxia. The finding of ARED flow in the umbilical artery or descending aorta in fetuses is associated with significantly increased perinatal mortality. In hypoxic fetuses, the redistribution of flow, with preferential supply to the brain, is reflected in increased diastolic flow and the consequently decreased values of middle cerebral artery PI and RI values. On the basis of the experience cited, Doppler velocimetry has been successfully applied as a clinical diagnostic test in high-risk pregnancies. Metaanalysis of the published randomized controlled trials has demonstrated that such use of Doppler velocimetry leads to lower perinatal mortality. Continuing technical improvements in Doppler equipment should open new fields of investigation (e.g., evaluation of the fetal venous system) that might, in the future, further increase the sensitivity of the method.

The other method presented – analysis of the fetal aortic diameter pulse waves – gives information on other characteristics of fetal hemodynamics. The shape of the pulse wave is determined by several factors, including the fetal blood pressure. So far, the method should be considered a research tool with great potential for studies of fetal circulatory physiology and pathophysiology. In contrast, Doppler velocimetry can already be considered a useful clinical instrument if properly applied in high-risk pregnancies.

REFERENCES

Adamson, S. L., Morrow, R. J., Bascom, P. A., Mo. L. Y., and Ritchie, J. W. (1989). Effect of placental resistance, arterial diameter, and blood pressure on the uterine arterial velocity waveform: a computer modeling approach. *Ultrasound in Medicine and Biology* 15:437–42.

AIUM (1988). American Institute of Ultrasound in Medicine, Bioeffects Committee: Bioeffects considerations for the safety of diagnostic ultrasound. *Journal of Ultrasound in Medicine* [Suppl. 9] 7:1.

Almström, H., Axelsson, O., Cnattingius, S., Ekman, G., Maesel, A., Ulmsten, U., Årström, K., and Maršál, K. (1992). Comparison of umbilical-artery velocimetry and cardiotocography of small-for-gestational-age fetuses. *Lancet* 340:936–40.

Arbeille, P., Body, G., Saliba, E., Tranquart, F., Berson, M., Roncin, A., and Pourcelot, L. (1988). Fetal cerebral circulation assessment by Doppler ultrasound in normal and pathological pregnancies. *European Journal of Obstetrics, Gynecology and Reproductive Biology* 29:261–73.

Arduini, D., Rizzo, G., and Romanini, C. (1992). Changes of pulsatility index from fetal vessels preceding the onset of late decelerations in growth-retarded fetuses. *Obstetrics and Gynecology* 79:605–10.

  (1993). The development of abnormal heart rate patterns after absent end-diastolic velocity in umbilical artery: analysis of risk factors. *American Journal of Obstetrics and Gynecology* 168:43–50.

Arduini, D., Rizzo, G., Romanini, C., and Mancuso, S. (1989). Fetal haemodynamic response to acute maternal hyperoxygenation as predictor of fetal distress in intrauterine growth retardation. *British Medical Journal* 298:1561–2.

Arndt, J. O., Klauske, J., and Mersch, F. (1968). The diameter of the intact carotid artery in man and its change with pulse pressure. *Pflügers Archive* 301:230–40.

Beattie, R. B., Hannah, M. E., and Dornan, J. C. (1992). Compound analysis of umbilical artery velocimetry in low-risk pregnancy. *Journal of Maternal-Fetal Investigation* 2:269–76.

Benthin, M., Dahl, P., Ruzicka, R., and Lindström, K. (1991). Calculation of pulse-wave velocity using cross correlation – effects of reflexes in the arterial tree. *Ultrasound in Medicine and Biology* 17:461–9.

British Institute of Radiology (1987). The safety of diagnostic ultrasound. *British Journal of Radiology* [Suppl. 20] 20:1–43.

Busse, R., Bauer, R. D., Schabert, A., Summa, Y., Bumm, P., and Wetterer, E. (1979). The mechanical properties of exposed human common carotid arteries in vivo. *Basic Research in Cardiology* 74:545–54.

Chandran, R., Serra, S. V., Sellers, S. M., and Redman, C. W. G. (1991). Fetal middle cerebral artery flow velocity waveforms – a terminal pattern. Case report. *British Journal of Obstetrics and Gynaecology* 98:937–8.

Cohn, H. E., Sacks, E. J., Heymann, M. A., and Rudolph, A. M. (1974). Cardiovascular responses to hypoxemia and acidemia in fetal lambs. *American Journal of Obstetrics and Gynecology* 120:817–24.

Dawes, G. S. (1968). *Foetal and Neonatal Physiology*. Chicago: Year Book.

Dawes, G. S., Fox, H. E., Leduc, B. M., Liggins, G. C., and Richards, R. T. (1972). Respiratory movements and rapid eye movement sleep in the foetal lamb. *Journal of Physiology* 220:119–43.

Dobrin, P. B. (1978). Mechanical properties of arteries. *Physiological Reviews* 58:397–460.

(1983). Vascular mechanics. In *Handbook of Physiology*, part 1, sect. 2, vol. III, ed. J. T. Shepard and F. M. Abbond (pp. 65–102). Baltimore: Williams and Wilkins.

Eik-Nes, S. H., Brubakk, A. O., and Ulstein, M. (1980). Measurement of human fetal blood flow. *British Medical Journal* 1:283–4.

Eik-Nes, S. H., Maršál, K., Brubakk, O., Kristoffersen, K., and Ulstein, M. (1982). Ultrasonic measurement of human fetal blood flow. *Journal of Biomedical Engineering* 4:28–36.

Eik-Nes, S. H., Maršál, K., and Kristoffersen, K. (1984). Methodology and basic problems related to blood flow studies in the human fetus. *Ultrasound in Medicine and Biology* 10:329–37.

European Association of Perinatal Medicine (1989). *Regulations for the Use of Doppler Technology and Perinatal Medicine. Consensus of Barcelona*. Barcelona: Instituto Dexeus.

Fitzgerald, D. E., and Drumm, J. E. (1977). Non-invasive measurement of human fetal circulation using ultrasound: a new method. *British Medical Journal* 2: 1450–1.

Fouron, J. C., Teyssiger, G., Maroto, E., Lessard, M., and Marquette, G. (1991). Diastolic circulatory dynamics in the presence of elevated placental resistance and retrograde diastolic flow in the umbilical artery: a Doppler echographic study in lamb. *American Journal of Obstetrics and Gynecology* 164:195–203.

Gennser, G., Lindström, K., Dahl, P., Benthin, M., Sindberg Eriksen, P., Gennser, M., and Lindell, S.-E. (1981). A dual high-resolution ultrasound system for measuring target movements. In *Recent Advances in Ultrasound Diagnosis 3*, ed. A. Kurjak and A. Kratochwil (pp. 71–5). Amsterdam: Excerpta Medica.

Gennser, G., and Stale, H. (1988). Aortic pulse waves in growth retarded human fetuses. In *Fetal and Neonatal Development*, ed. C. T. Jones (pp. 543–7). New York: Perinatology Press.

Giles, W. B., and Bisits, A. (1992). Clinical place of Doppler in high risk pregnancy. *Ultrasound in Obstetrics and Gynecology* [Suppl. 1] 2:106 (abstract).

Gill, R. W. (1978). Quantitative blood flow measurement in deep-lying vessels using pulsed Doppler with the Octoson. *Ultrasound in Medicine and Biology* 4:341–5.

Gosling, R. G., and King, D. H. (1975). Ultrasonic angiology. In *Arteries and Veins*, ed. A. W. Harcus and L. Adamson (pp. 61–98). Edinburgh: Churchill-Livingstone.

Gramellini, D., Folli, M. C., Raboni, S., Vadora, E., and Merialdi, A. (1992). Cerebral-umbilical Doppler ratio as a predictor of adverse perinatal outcome. *Obstetrics and Gynecology* 79:416–20.

Gudmundsson, S., Fairlie, F., Lingman, G., and Maršál, K. (1990). Recording of blood flow velocity waveforms in the uteroplacental and umbilical circulation –

reproducibility study and comparison of pulsed and continuous wave Doppler ultrasound. *Journal of Clinical Ultrasound* 18:97–101.

Gudmundsson, S., Huhta, J. C., Wood, D. C., Tulzer, G., Cohen, A. W., and Weiner, S. (1991). Venous Doppler in the fetus with non-immune hydrops. *American Journal of Obstetrics and Gynecology* 164:33–7.

Gudmundsson, S., and Maršál, K. (1988a). Umbilical artery and uteroplacental circulation in normal pregnancy – a cross-sectional study. *Acta Obstetricia et Gynecologica Scandinavica* 67:347–54.

(1988b). Umbilical and uteroplacental blood flow velocity waveforms in pregnancies with fetal growth retardation. *European Journal of Obstetrics, Gynecology and Reproductive Biology* 27:187–96.

(1991). Fetal aortic and umbilical artery blood velocity waveforms in prediction of fetal outcome – a comparison. *American Journal of Perinatology* 8:1–6.

Gustafsson, D., Stale, H., Björkman, J.-A., and Gennser, G. (1989). Derivation of haemodynamic information from ultrasonic recordings of aortic diameter changes. *Ultrasound in Medicine and Biology* 15:189–99.

Hallock, P. (1934). Arterial elasticity in man in relation to age as evaluated by the pulse wave method. *Archives of Internal Medicine* 54:770–98.

Hokanson, D. E., Mozersky, D. J., Sumner, D. S., and Strandness, D. E., Jr. (1972). A phase-locked echo tracking system for recording arterial diameter changes in vivo. *Journal of Applied Physiology* 32:728–33.

Imura, T., Yamamoto, K., Kanamori, K., Mikami, T., and Yasuda, H. (1986). Non-invasive ultrasonic measurement of the elastic properties of the human abdominal aorta. *Cardiovascular Research* 29:208–14.

Kawasaki, T., Sasayama, S., Yagi, S.-I., Asakawa, T., and Hirai, T. (1987). Non-invasive assessment of the age related changes in stiffness of major branches of the human arteries. *Cardiovascular Research* 21:678–87.

Kjellmer, I., Karlsson, K., Olsson, T., and Rosén, K.-G. (1974). Cerebral reactions during intrauterine asphyxia in the sheep. I. Circulation and oxygen consumption in the fetal brain. *Pediatric Research* 8:50–7.

Länne, T., Stale, H., Bengtsson, H., Gustafsson, D., Bergqvist, D., Sonesson, B., Lecerof, H., and Dahl, P. (1992). Noninvasive measurement of diameter changes in the distal abdominal aorta in man. *Ultrasound in Medicine and Biology* 18:451–7.

Laurin, J., Lingman, G., Maršál, K., and Persson, P.-H. (1987). Fetal blood flow in pregnancies complicated by intrauterine growth retardation. *Obstetrics and Gynecology* 69:895–902.

Legarth, J., and Thorup, E. (1989). Characteristics of Doppler blood-velocity waveforms in a cardiovascular in vitro model. II. The influence of peripheral resistance, perfusion pressure and blood flow. *Scandinavian Journal of Clinical and Laboratory Investigation* 49:459–64.

Lindström, K., Gennser, G., Sindberg Eriksen, P., Benthin, M., and Dahl, P. (1987). An improved echo tracker for studies on pulse waves in the fetal aorta. In *Fetal Physiological Measurements*, ed. P. Rolfe (pp. 217–26). Tonbridge, England: Butterworth.

Lindström, K., Maršál, K., Gennser, G., Bengtson, L., Benthin, M., and Dahl, P. (1977). Device for measurement of fetal breathing movements. I. The TD-recorder. A new system for recording the distance between two echogenerating structures as a function of time. *Ultrasound in Medicine and Biology* 3:143–51.

Lingman, G., Laurin, J., and Maršál, K. (1986). Circulatory changes in fetuses with imminent asphyxia. *Biology of the Neonate* 49:66–73.

Lingman, G., and Maršál, K. (1986). Fetal central blood circulation in the third trimester of normal pregnancy. Longitudinal study. II. Aortic blood velocity waveform. *Early Human Development* 13:151–9.

Luterkort, M., and Gennser, G. (1986). Cardiovascular dynamics in relation to presentation and postural changes in normal fetuses. *European Journal of Obstetrics, Gynecology and Reproductive Biology* 24:13–22.

McCallum, W. D., Williams, C. S., Napel, S., and Daigle, R. E. (1978). Fetal blood velocity waveforms. *American Journal of Obstetrics and Gynecology* 132:425–9.

Malcus, P., Kjellmer, I., Lingman, G., Maršál, K., Thiringer, K., and Rosén, K.-G. (1991). Diameters of the common carotid artery and aorta change in different directions during acute asphyxia in the fetal lamb. *Journal of Perinatal Medicine* 19:259–67.

Mandruzzato, G. P., Bogatti, P., Fischer, L., and Gigli, C. (1991). The clinical significance of absent or reverse end diastolic flow in the fetal aorta and umbilical artery. *Ultrasound in Obstetrics and Gynecology* 1:192–6.

Mari, G. (1991). Arterial blood flow velocity waveforms of the pelvis and lower extremities in normal and growth-retarded fetuses. *American Journal of Obstetrics and Gynecology* 165:143–51.

Mari, G., and Deter, R. L. (1992). Middle cerebral artery flow velocity waveforms in normal and small-for-gestational-age fetuses. *American Journal of Obstetrics and Gynecology* 166:1262–70.

Mari, G., Kirshon, B., and Abuhamad, A. (1993). Fetal renal artery flow velocity waveforms in normal pregnancies and pregnancies complicated by polyhydramnios and oligohydramnios. *Obstetrics and Gynecology* 81:560–4.

Mari, G., and Wasserstrum, N. (1991). Flow velocity waveforms of the fetal circulation preceding fetal death in a case of lupus anticoagulant. *American Journal of Obstetrics and Gynecology* 164:776–8.

Maršál, K., Gennser, G., and Lindström, K. (1976). Real-time ultrasonography for quantified analysis of fetal breathing movements in man. *Lancet* 2:718–19.

Maršál, K., Gudmundsson, S., and Stale, H. (1994). Doppler velocimetry in monitoring fetal health during late pregnancy. In *The Fetus as a Patient – Advances in Diagnosis and Therapy*, ed. A. Kurjak and F. Chervenak (pp. 455–76). London: Parthenon Publishing.

Maršál, K., and Ley, D. (1992). Intrauterine blood flow and postnatal neurological development in growth-retarded fetuses. *Biology of the Neonate* 62:258–64.

Maršál, K., Lindblad, A., Lingman, G., and Eik-Nes, S. H. (1984). Blood flow in the fetal descending aorta; intrinsic factors affecting fetal blood flow, i.e., fetal breathing movements and cardiac arrhythmia. *Ultrasound in Medicine and Biology* 10:339–48.

Maulik, D., Yarlagadda, A. P., Nathanielsz, P. W., and Figueroa, J. P. (1989a). Hemodynamic validation of Doppler assessment of fetoplacental circulation in a sheep model system. *Journal of Ultrasound in Medicine* 8:177–81.

Maulik, D., Yarlagadda, A. P., Youngblood, J. P., and Willoughby, L. (1989b). Components of variability of umbilical arterial Doppler velocimetry–a prospective

analysis. *American Journal of Obstetrics and Gynecology* 160:1406–12.

Mehalek, K. E., Berkowitz, G. S., Chitkara, U., Rosenberg, J., and Berkowitz, R. L. (1988). Comparison of continuous-wave and pulsed Doppler S/D ratios of umbilical and uterine arteries. *Obstetrics and Gynecology* 72:603–6.

Miller, M. W., Church, C. C., and Barnett, S. B. (1987). Bioeffects of Doppler ultrasound in the maternal-fetal context. In *Doppler Ultrasound Measurement of Maternal-Fetal Hemodynamics*, ed. D. Maulik and D. McNellis (pp. 105–14). Ithaca, NY: Perinatology Press.

Mires, G., Dempster, J., Patel, N. B., and Crawford, J. W. (1987). The effect of fetal heart rate on umbilical artery flow velocity waveforms. *British Journal of Obstetrics and Gynaecology* 94:665–9.

Morrow, R. J., Adamson, S. L., Bull, S. B., and Ritchie, J. W. (1989). Effect of placental embolization on the umbilical arterial velocity waveform in fetal sheep. *American Journal of Obstetrics and Gynecology* 161:1055–60.

Mulders, L. G. M., Muijers, G. J. J. M., Jongsma, H. W., Nijhuis, J. G., and Hein, P. R. (1986). The umbilical artery blood flow velocity waveform in relation to fetal breathing movements, fetal heart rate and fetal behavioral states in normal pregnancy at 37–39 weeks. *Early Human Development* 14:283–93.

Nicolaides, K. H., Bradley, R. J., Soothill, P. W., Campbell, S., Billardo, C. M., and Gibb, D. (1987). Maternal oxygen therapy for intrauterine growth retardation. *Lancet* 1:942–5.

Pearce, J. M., Campbell, S., Cohen-Overbeek, T., Hackett, G., Hernandez, J., and Royston, J. P. (1988). References ranges and sources of variation for indices of pulsed Doppler flow velocity waveforms from the uteroplacental and fetal circulation. *British Journal of Obstetrics and Gynaecology* 95:248–56.

Peeters, L. L. H., Sheldon, R. E., Jones, M. D., Makowski, E. L., and Meschia, G. (1979). Blood flow to fetal organs as a function of arterial oxygen content. *American Journal of Obstetrics and Gynecology* 135:637–46.

Pourcelot, L. (1974). Applications clinique de l'examen Doppler transcutane. In *Velocimetric ultrasonore Doppler*, ed. P. Peronneau (pp. 213–40). Paris: INSERM.

Rochelson, B., Schulman, H., Farmakides, G., Bracero, L., Ducey, J., Fleischer, A., Penny, B., and Winter, D. (1987). The significance of absent end-diastolic velocity in umbilical artery velocity waveforms. *American Journal of Obstetrics and Gynecology* 156:1213–18.

Satoh, S., Koyanagi, T., Fukuhara, M., Hara, K., and Nakano, H. (1989). Changes in vascular resistance in the umbilical and middle cerebral arteries in the human intrauterine growth-retarded fetus, measured with pulsed Doppler ultrasound. *Early Human Development* 20:213–20.

Sindberg Eriksen, P., and Gennser, G. (1984). Acute responses to maternal smoking of the pulsatile movements in fetal aorta. *Acta Obstetricia et Gynecologica Scandinavica* 63:647–54.

Sindberg Eriksen, P., Gennser, G., and Lindström, K. (1984). Physiological characteristics of diameter pulses in the fetal descending aorta. *Acta Obstetricia et Gynecologica Scandinavica* 63:355–63.

Sindberg Eriksen, P., Gennser, G., Lindström, K., Benthin, M., and Dahl, P. (1985). Pulse wave recording – development of a method for investigating foetal circulation in utero. *Journal of Medical Engineering and Technology* 9:18–27.

Sonesson, B., Hansen, F., Stale, H., and Länne, H. (1993). Compliance and diameter in the human abdominal aorta – the influence of age and sex. *European Journal of Vascular Surgery* 7:690–7.

Sonesson, S.-E., Fouron, J.-C., Drblik, S. P., Tawile, C., Lessard, M., and Scott, A. (1993). Reference values for Doppler velocimetric indices from the fetal and placental ends of the umbilical artery during normal pregnancy. *Journal of Clinical Ultrasound* 21:317–24.

Spencer, J. A., and Price, J. (1989). Intraobserver variation in Doppler ultrasound indices of placental perfusion derived from different numbers of waveforms. *Journal of Ultrasound in Medicine* 8:197–9.

Stale, H., and Gennser, G. (1991a). Aortic diameter pulse waves during fetal development. *Journal of Maternal-Fetal Investigation* 1:41–5.

——— (1991b). Fetal aortic diameter pulse wave response to changes in maternal position after membrane rupture. *Ultrasound in Obstetrics and Gynecology* 1:261–5.

Stale, H., Maršál, K., and Gennser, G. (1990). Blood flow velocity and pulsatile diameter changes in the fetal descending aorta: a longitudinal study. *American Journal of Obstetrics and Gynecology* 163:26–9.

Stale, H., Maršál, K., Gennser, G., Benthin, M., Dahl, P., and Lindström, K. (1991). Aortic diameter pulse waves and blood flow velocity in the small for gestational age fetus. *Ultrasound in Medicine and Biology* 17:471–8.

Stembera, Z. K., Hodr, J., Kittrich, M., and Janda, J. (1972). Fetoplacental circulation in the umbilical cord when coiled around the fetal neck. *Biology of the Neonate* 20:120–6.

Stuart, B., Drumm, J., Fitzgerald, D. E., and Diugnan, N. M. (1980). Fetal blood velocity waveforms in normal pregnancy. *British Journal of Obstetrics and Gynaecology* 87:780–5.

Thompson, R. S., and Stevens, R. J. (1989). Mathematical model for interpretation of Doppler velocity waveform indices. *Medical and Biological Engineering and Computing* 27:269–76.

Thompson, R. S., Trudinger, B. J., and Cook, C. M. (1986). A comparison of Doppler ultrasound waveform indices in the umbilical artery. I. Indices derived from the maximum velocity waveform. *Ultrasound in Medicine and Biology* 12:835–44.

Trudinger, B. J., Stevens, D., Connelly, A., Hales, J. R., Alexander, G., Bradley, L., Fawcett, A., and Thompson, R. S. (1987). Umbilical artery flow velocity waveforms and placental resistance: the effects of embolization of the umbilical circulation. *American Journal of Obstetrics and Gynecology* 157:1443–8.

Valcamonico, A., Dante, L., Soregaroli, M., Frusca, T., Abrami, F., Tibertis, A., and Zucca, S. (1992). Absent end diastolic velocity in umbilical artery and risk of neonatal brain damage. *Journal of Maternal-Fetal Investigation* 2:135.

van Eyck, J., Wladimiroff, J. W., Noordam, M. J., Tonge, H. M., and Prechtl, H. F. (1985). The blood flow velocity waveform in the fetal descending aorta: its relationship to fetal behavioural states in normal pregnancy at 37–38 weeks. *Early Human Development* 12:137–43.

van Eyck, J., Wladimiroff, J. W., van den Wijngaard, J. A., Noordam, M. J., and Prechtl, H. F. (1987). The blood flow velocity waveform in the fetal internal carotid and umbilical artery; its relation to fetal behavioural states in normal pregnancy at 37–38 weeks. *British Journal of Obstetrics and Gynaecology* 94:736–41.

Vyas, S., Nicolaides, K. H., Bower, S., and Campbell, S. (1990). Middle cerebral artery flow velocity waveforms in fetal hypoxaemia. *British Journal of Obstetrics and Gynaecology* 97:797–803.

Vyas, S., Nicolaides, K. H., and Campbell, S. (1989). Renal artery flow-velocity waveforms in normal and hypoxemic fetuses. *American Journal of Obstetrics and Gynecology* 161:168–72.

Weiss, E., Ulrich, S., and Berle, P. (1992). Blood flow velocity waveforms of the middle cerebral artery and abnormal neurological evaluations in live-born fetuses with absent or reverse end-diastolic flow velocities of the umbilical arteries. *European Journal of Obstetrics, Gynecology and Reproductive Biology* 62:93–100.

Wiggers, C. J. (1952). Physiologic studies. In *Circulatory Dynamics*. New York: Grune & Stratton.

Wladimiroff, J. W., Vosters, R., and McGhie, J. S. (1982). Normal cardiac ventricular geometry and function during the last trimester of pregnancy and early neonatal period. *British Journal of Obstetrics and Gynaecology* 89:839–44.

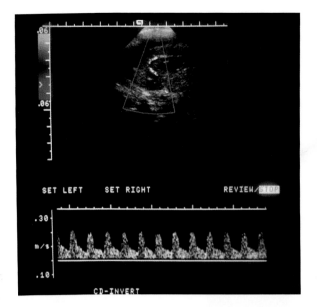

Figure 18.2. Spectral display of velocity tracings from the anterior cerebral artery and the corresponding image obtained through the sagittal plane.

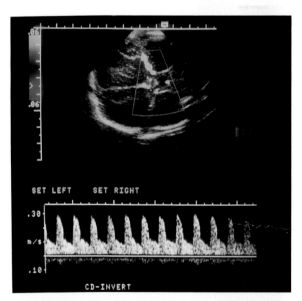

Figure 18.3. Spectral display of velocity tracings from the middle cerebral artery and the corresponding image from the axial plane.

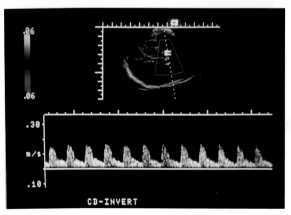

Figure 18.4. Spectral display of velocity tracings from the posterior cerebral artery and the corresponding image from the axial plane.

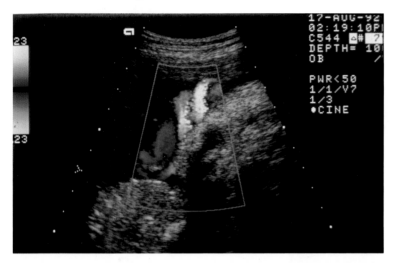

Figure 19.2. Color Doppler image of the umbilical cord: red, flow in the two umbilical arteries toward the transducer; blue, flow in the umbilical vein away from the transducer.

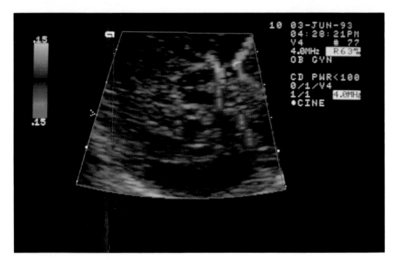

Figure 19.8. Ultrasound image of a transverse section through a fetal skull and a color Doppler image of the fetal circle of Willis and the middle cerebral artery.

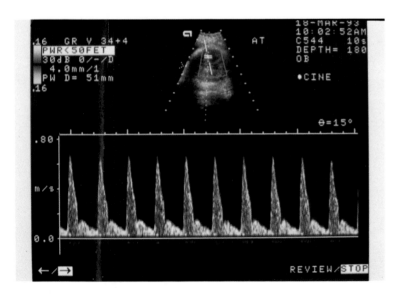

Figure 19.9. Velocity waveforms recorded from the middle cerebral artery of a 30-wk-old healthy fetus.

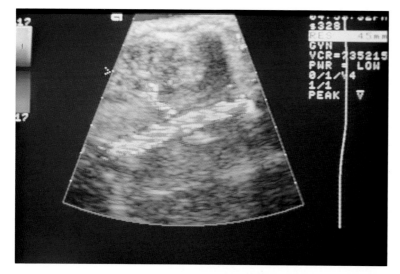

Figure 19.10. Color Doppler image of fetal descending aorta and renal artery.

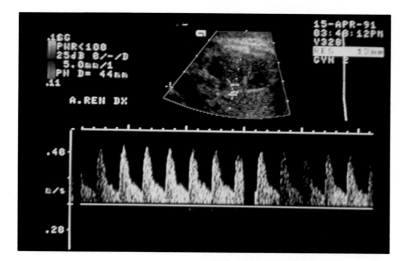

Figure 19.11. Fetal renal artery velocity waveforms.

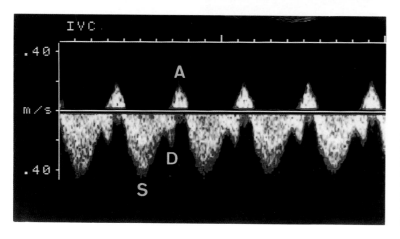

Figure 19.12. Doppler spectrum recorded from the inferior vena cava of a 36-wk healthy fetus: S wave, rapid atrial filling in ventricular systole; D wave, second atrial filling during ventricular diastole; A wave, backflow during ventricular end-diastole caused by atrial contraction.

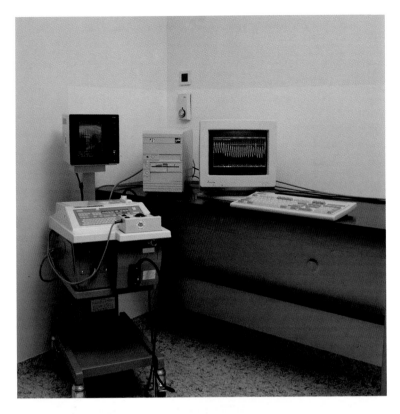

Figure 19.13. DIAMOVE: computerized ultrasound system for recording of vessel diameter pulse waves.

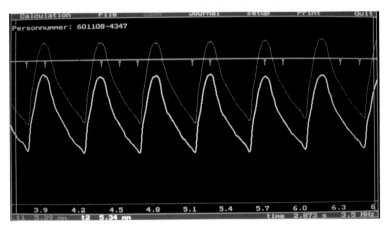

Figure 19.14. Vessel diameter pulse waves presented on the monitor.

PART VI

Hyperbilirubinemia

Noninvasive diagnosis and treatment of neonatal hyperbilirubinemia are discussed in this Part VI. Although the mechanisms of bilirubin neurotoxicity still are unclear, and relaxation of diagnostic criteria and therapeutic intensity is currently in vogue (at least for term infants), hyperbilirubinemia remains the most common reason for prolonged hospitalization of term newborn infants. The sheer magnitude of this problem makes it a major target for modern technology. Diagnosis of hyperbilirubinemia to date has relied on blood sampling, involving extensive utilization of hospital laboratories and their instrumentation, as well as technicians to draw blood, technicians to measure the plasma bilirubin concentration, laboratory directors, nurses, and so forth. The transcutaneous bilirubinometer (admittedly manufacturer-specific as discussed in this book, but Minolta was the pioneer in this technology) now offers the opportunity to avoid repeated heel pricks and all that goes with laboratory diagnosis.

Treatment, principally now by phototherapy, also has largely been confined to the hospital, although home phototherapy has gained a foothold. Phototherapy for neonatal hyperbilirubinemia is deceptively simple, because it works quite well and causes only modest complications, most of which are important only in extremely premature infants. It ought to be more usable at home. The major current limitation to home use is the absence of a much-needed combination: a phototherapy unit with instrumentation to measure and signal its own proper functioning and an accurate, noninvasive means to measure and report plasma bilirubin concentrations. Also, such units ought to use relatively "white" light; blue and green lights are noxious and interfere with visual assessment of skin color and thus blood oxygenation (addition of pulse-oximetry instruments to home phototherapy units would help, but probably would not be cost-effective or easy enough to use at home). The elements of this technology are well described in the two chapters in Part VI. Instruments to measure skin irradiance are available. All that is needed is to put it all together. Further additions, such as a servocontrolled thermoregulation unit, would make such a combined system safe, effective, easy to use, and profitable. Profitability could very easily be achieved by eliminating hospitalizations and the home visits by nurses and technicians now employed to make the necessary checks on instrument function and infant well-being.

20

Transcutaneous monitoring of bilirubin: Minolta jaundice meter

YOSHITADA YAMAUCHI, M.D.
AKIO YAMANISHI
ITSURO YAMANOUCHI, M.D.

INTRODUCTION

Virtually every case of jaundice in a neonate carries the risk that it could develop into a serious illness that could have harmful effects on the development of the neonate's brain and many other facets of life. Of course, if such abnormal change is detected at an early stage, there are established therapies that can be applied. Because of this, pediatricians, obstetricians, and other who treat neonates must be careful to check for jaundice.

The general procedure for examining a neonate for jaundice involves two steps: First, the color of the neonate's skin is examined with the naked eye. Then, if the yellow tint of the skin is judged to be high, a blood sample is taken and tested to allow an exact diagnosis. Although examination of skin color with the naked eye sounds simple, considerable experience is needed in determining the acceptable range of skin colors, and considerable skill is required to determine if the skin color of the neonate being examined is within the normal range. Because the safety of the neonate is at issue, the quality of the visual evaluation is extremely important, and as a result the frequency with which blood samples are taken has become high. At the same time, the taking of blood samples is a troublesome procedure; it also causes pain to the neonate and is accompanied by the risk of infection. It would thus be desirable to reduce, as much as possible, the frequency with which blood samples are taken.

It has long been desirable, therefore, to find an examination method that will be at least as convenient as visual evaluation but will provide better accuracy and will give results that will compare well with those obtained by blood testing. The Minolta jaundice meter (Yamanouchi, Yamauchi, and Igarashi, 1980) was developed to meet that need.

The Minolta jaundice meter uses optical-sensor technology to measure the difference in optical density for light in the blue- and green-wavelength regions of the spectrum and to determine the "yellowness" of skin tissue without taking blood samples. The meter was designed to be compact, lightweight, and extremely easy to operate. The result is an instrument that is only $16 \times 7 \times 3$ cm ($6\frac{1}{4} \times 2\frac{3}{4} \times 1\frac{3}{16}$ in.) in size and weighs only 300 g ($10\frac{9}{16}$ oz.). Figure 20.1 shows the jaundice meter in use.

MINOLTA JAUNDICE METER

This section will describe the structure of the Minolta jaundice meter and the calculations it performs.

Measuring principles

The Minolta jaundice meter determines the yellowness of the skin by measuring the difference in optical density for light in the blue- and green-wavelength regions. Light incidence on the skin is reflected, scattered, and absorbed by the epidermis and corium before reaching the subcutaneous tis-

$$\log \frac{I_0(\lambda_1)}{I(\lambda_1)} - \log \frac{I_0(\lambda_2)}{I(\lambda_2)} = \log \frac{F(\lambda_2)}{F(\lambda_1)} \qquad (20.2)$$
$$+ \ [\epsilon(\lambda_1) - \epsilon(\lambda_2)] \cdot C \cdot l$$

From this equation it can be seen that the difference in the optical densities of the two wavelengths can be expressed as the sum of a term describing the decrease in light (not including the effect of bilirubin) due to skin tissue (term 1) and a term proportional to the bilirubin concentration (term 2).

After the effects due to bilirubin have been separated from those due to skin tissue, the main element remaining is hemoglobin. A graph of the spectral absorption coefficients for hemoglobin (oxyhemoglobin and reduced hemoglobin) and bilirubin is shown in Figure 20.2. If the curves in the vicinity of 460 nm and those in the vicinity of 550 nm are considered, it is clear that there is a large difference in the absorption coefficients for bilirubin at these two wavelengths, but that those for hemoglobin are approximately the same. If these two wavelengths are chosen for measurement, the effect of the presence of hemoglobin in the first term is eliminated.

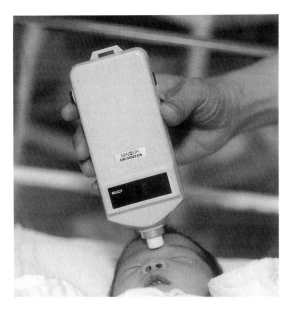

Figure 20.1. The Minolta jaundice meter in use.

sue. The fat in the subcutaneous tissue absorbs shorter wavelengths of light, according to the yellow tint of the unconjugated bilirubin present; the remaining light is scattered and reflected, and part of it passes through the skin surface again. If light is returned from an area distinct from the area to which light was applied, and if it is ensured that light reflected from the skin surface is not being received, then the received light is mainly that which reached the subcutaneous tissue and was reflected therefrom. The intensity (I) of this light as a function of wavelength (λ) can then be expressed in accordance with the Lambert-Beer law by the following formula:

$$I(\lambda) = I_0(\lambda) \cdot F(\lambda) \cdot 10^{-\epsilon(\lambda) \cdot C \cdot l} \qquad (20.1)$$

where $I_0(\lambda)$ is the quantity of incident light of wavelength λ, $F(\lambda)$ is the decrease in the quantity of light at wavelength λ due to skin tissue (excluding the effects of bilirubin), $\epsilon(\lambda)$ is the absorption coefficient of bilirubin for light of wavelength λ, C is the bilirubin concentration in subcutaneous tissue, and l is the effective optical path length for bilirubin in subcutaneous tissue. For two wavelengths λ_1 and λ_2 that have different bilirubin absorption coefficients, their respective optical densities, $\log[I_0(\lambda)/I(\lambda)]$, can be calculated using equation (20.1). Combining the formulas for the two optical densities into one, and rewriting, yields the following:

Probe construction

A simplified diagram of the probe that is placed against the skin of the neonate is shown in Figure 20.3. Light from the xenon tube in the main body of the probe is guided by optical fibers around the circumference of the concentric fiber-optic cable probe and is incident on the skin. The light that exits the skin surface again, after scattering and reflection within the skin tissue, enters the center fiber-optic cable and is guided into the main body.

Inside the main body, the light from the fiber-optic cable is divided into two beams (blue and green) by a dichroic filter that reflects blue light and transmits green. These two beams are then incident on silicon photocells equipped with filters; the filter for the blue light has a peak transmittance at 460 nm, and that for the green light has a peak transmittance at 550 nm. The silicon photocells convert the light into electric currents that are proportional to the intensity.

In order to ensure that the pressure on the skin at the time of measurement is uniform and that the skin is ischemic, the jaundice meter was constructed so that the measurement probe is movable in relation to the main body, as shown in Figure 20.4. The measurement probe moves along the guide slot of a mounting plate that is fastened to the main body in a fixed position. Outward force on the probe is sup-

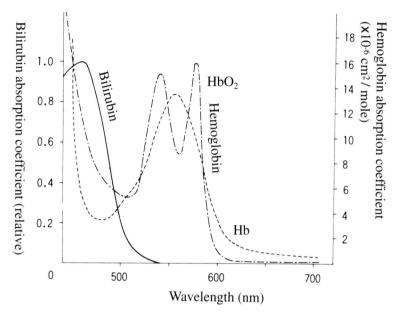

Figure 20.2. Spectral absorptions for bilirubin and hemoglobin.

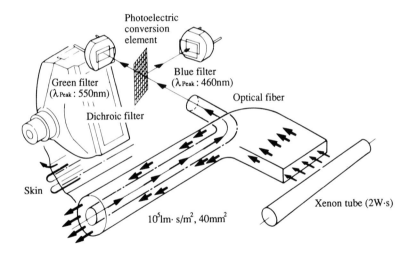

Figure 20.3. Optical system of the probe.

plied by springs and by the return force of the switch that triggers the xenon tube for measurement. When the probe is pressed against the skin, the skin resists the force of the springs and switch, and the probe moves into the main body. At a certain point in the motion of the probe, the switch is operated, and the xenon tube is fired to take a measurement. In this way, the pressure on the skin at the time of measurement is always uniform and forces the blood out of the measurement area to create an ischemic condition.

Meter construction

A block diagram of the jaundice meter (including the probe) is shown in Figure 20.5. Power from the rechargeable NiCd batteries (1) is distributed to the voltage-regulator circuit (2), which supplies power for the integrated circuits (ICs) in the meter, and to the step-up charging circuit (3), which supplies the power for firing the xenon tube (4).

Light emitted by the xenon tube (4) is guided to the skin surface by the probe's optical system (5)

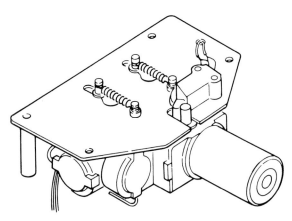

Figure 20.4. Probe structure.

and is incident on the skin; the light returning from the skin is collected and separated into two beams of different wavelengths by the probe's optical system (5). These two beams are converted into electric currents that are proportional to the light intensity and then into proportional voltages by the photoelectric conversion circuits (6). The green voltage then passes through a gain adjustment circuit (7) before being sent to the gate circuits (8); the blue voltage is sent directly to the gate circuits (8) from the photoelectric conversion circuits (6).

In the gate circuits (8), the difference in the times required (within the region where the light intensity is decreasing) for the respective outputs for blue light and green light to reach a specified level is determined. The logarithmic calculations in equation (20.2) can then be performed according to this time difference (see the following section).

The counter (10) counts the pulses output by the clock (9), and a numerical value based on the time difference is shown in the display (11).

The state controller (13) controls the voltage of the step-up charging circuit (3) and lights the "READY" indication when a specified voltage has been reached and measurement preparations are complete. The state controller (13) also controls the lighting of the display (11).

Calculation method

In the jaundice meter, logarithmic calculations must be performed to determine the difference in optical densities. In order to perform these calculations, a logarithmic conversion method was used to make the waveform of the light emitted by the xenon tube exponential in the region where light intensity is decreasing, and a simplified circuit was designed.

A xenon tube is fired, and light is instantaneously emitted, when a high voltage is applied to the trigger electrode, causing a high-voltage electric charge stored in a capacitor to be discharged through the xenon gas in the glass tube.

Graphs of the waveforms of the light emitted by the xenon tube are shown in Figure 20.6. The xenon tube, capacitor, and capacitor voltage are the same for both panels of the figure; however, because a resistor has been added in series with the xenon tube in the right panel, the light quantity and the waveform are very different from those in the left panel. If the resistor is chosen so that variations in the resistance r_{xenon} of the xenon tube can be disregarded, the circuit is equivalent to a resistance-capacitance (RC) discharge circuit during the period of

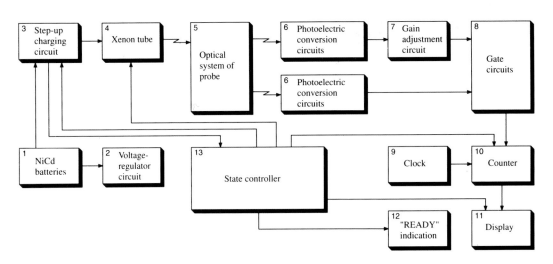

Figure 20.5. Block diagram of the Minolta jaundice meter.

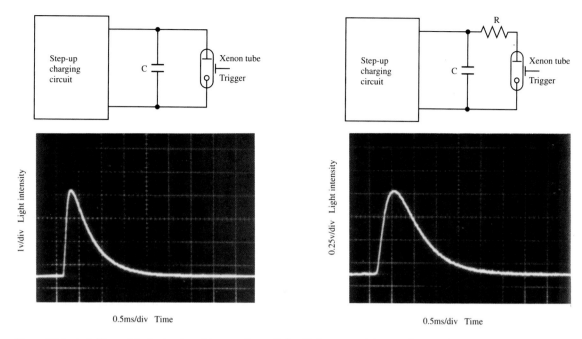

Figure 20.6. *Left:* Normal flash circuit and its waveform. *Right:* Flash circuit of the Minolta jaundice meter and its waveform.

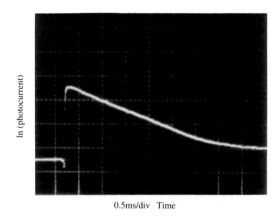

Figure 20.7. Results of logarithmic conversion of light intensity.

decreasing light intensity, and the voltage applied to the xenon tube decreases exponentially. The results of performing a natural logarithmic conversion on the light emitted by this xenon tube are shown in Figure 20.7. In this graph, it can be seen that the decrease in emitted light during the period when the intensity is decreasing forms a straight line, and thus the output contains a region where the emitted light is decreasing exponentially.

By controlling the waveform of the light emitted by the xenon tube so that the intensity decreases

exponentially, determining the difference in optical densities at two wavelengths becomes more convenient.

In Figure 20.8, the start of emission is set as zero on the time scale, and from point t_c onward, the light intensity decreases exponentially. If the output voltages from the photoelectric conversion circuits for wavelengths λ_1 and λ_2 are termed $V(\lambda_1)$ and $V(\lambda_2)$, respectively, then the output voltage at any time t within the exponential region is

$$V(\lambda_1) = V_c(\lambda_1) \cdot \exp[-(t - t_c)/\tau] \quad (20.3)$$
$$V(\lambda_2) = V_c(\lambda_2) \cdot \exp[-(t - t_c)/\tau] \quad (20.4)$$

where $V_c(\lambda_1)$ and $V_c(\lambda_2)$ are the voltage outputs from the photoelectric conversion circuits for wavelengths λ_1 and λ_2, respectively, at time t_c, and τ is the time constant for the region where the decrease is exponential.

If the times required for $V(\lambda_1)$ and $V(\lambda_2)$ to become equal to a specified voltage V are termed $t_{\lambda 1}$ and $t_{\lambda 2}$, respectively, then the following can be obtained from equations (20.3) and (20.4):

$$\ln[V_c(\lambda_2)/V_c(\lambda_1)] = (t_{\lambda 2} - t_{\lambda 1})/\tau \quad (20.5)$$

Meanwhile, if the coefficients (the products of the spectral transmission of the filter, the spectral sensitivity of the sensor element, and the gain of the circuit) of the photoelectric conversion circuits are termed $A(\lambda_1)$ and $A(\lambda_2)$, then

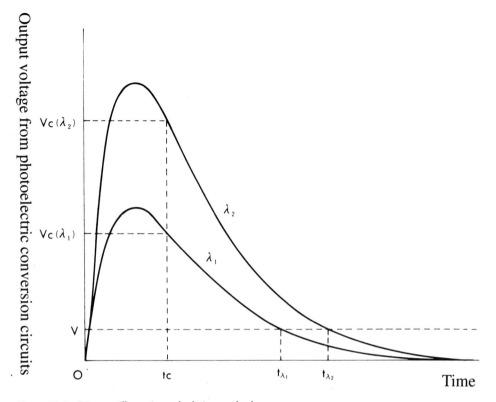

Figure 20.8. Diagram illustrating calculation method.

$$V_c(\lambda_1) = A(\lambda_1) \cdot I(\lambda_1) \qquad (20.6)$$
$$V_c(\lambda_2) = A(\lambda_2) \cdot I(\lambda_2) \qquad (20.7)$$

where $I(\lambda_1)$ and $I(\lambda_2)$ are the light intensities for wavelengths λ_1 and λ_2, respectively, at time t_c.

Using equations (20.6) and (20.7), equation (20.5) can be rewritten as

$$\ln\left(\frac{I(\lambda_2)}{I(\lambda_1)}\right) + \ln\left(\frac{A(\lambda_2)}{A(\lambda_1)}\right) = \frac{t_{\lambda_2} - t_{\lambda_1}}{\tau} \qquad (20.8)$$

If the gain is then adjusted so that for a white diffusion plate having equal reflectances at wavelengths λ_1 and λ_2, $t_{\lambda 1} = t_{\lambda 2}$, then

$$\ln\left(\frac{I_0(\lambda_2)}{I_0(\lambda_1)}\right) = -\ln\left(\frac{A(\lambda_2)}{A(\lambda_1)}\right) \qquad (20.9)$$

Using equations (20.8) and (20.9), equation (20.2) can then be rewritten as

$$\log\left(\frac{I_0(\lambda_1)}{I(\lambda_1)}\right) - \log\left(\frac{I_0(\lambda_2)}{I(\lambda_2)}\right) = \left(\frac{\log e}{\tau}\right) \cdot (t_{\lambda 2} - t_{\lambda 1}) \qquad (20.10)$$

Thus, the optical-density difference for two wavelengths of light can be determined from the difference in the respective times required (within the region of decreasing light intensity) for the outputs from the two wavelengths to reach a specified level.

Operating procedure

Set the power switch to "ON" and check that the "READY" indicator lights up. Holding the jaundice meter in the palm of the hand, place the tip of the measuring probe against the forehead (or other measuring point) of the neonate, as shown in Figure 20.1. Slowly and gently press the jaundice meter against the measuring point until a click is heard; at the same time, the light emitted by the xenon tube for measurement can be seen. The measured value will appear in the display. Remove the jaundice meter from the measuring point and read the displayed value. This completes one measurement cycle.

To take another measurement, press the "RESET" button of the jaundice meter. The displayed value will disappear, and the "READY" indicator will

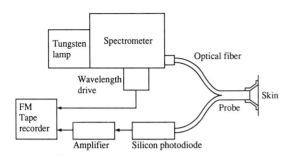

Figure 20.9. System used by Hannemann, DeWitt, and Wiechel (1978).

light up after a few moments, indicating that the next measurement can be taken.

RELATION BETWEEN SPECTRAL REFLECTANCE OF SKIN AND SERUM BILIRUBIN CONCENTRATION

Even before development of the Minolta jaundice meter, attempts were made to estimate serum bilirubin concentrations without taking blood samples: Brunsting and Sheard (1929) reported that it was possible to quantify the degree of jaundice using measurements of the spectral reflectance of skin at wavelengths from 400 to 700 nm. In a study of a mechanism for observing and treating jaundice in neonates, using measurements of spectral reflectance from skin at wavelengths from 350 to 700 nm, it was reported that the spectral reflectance from the skin of neonates with jaundice was reduced in the wavelength range from 430 to 520 nm (Ballowitz and Avery, 1970).

Hannemann, DeWitt, and Wiechel (1978) reported a method for determining serum bilirubin concentrations by measuring the spectral reflectance from the skin of neonates. The measuring equipment used in that research is shown in Figure 20.9. The light source is a tungsten lamp. A diffraction-grating-type spectroscope is used to obtain monochromatic light, which is then guided by an optical fiber to the skin surface. The light reflected by the skin surface enters a second optical fiber and is guided to the photodiode sensor. The electric-signal output of the sensor is amplified and then stored on magnetic tape, together with the wavelength of the incident light. The instrument was used to obtain measurement data from 30 white neonates. Computers were used to perform calculations on the data for various combinations of wavelengths; the correlation between the results of such calcula-

tions and the serum bilirubin concentrations determined from blood samples taken at the same time as the measurements was determined. The highest correlation coefficient ($r = 0.931$) was obtained from calculations using five wavelengths: 425, 460, 525, 535, and 545 nm.

In a later experiment by Hannemann et al. (1979), measurement data obtained for 58 white and 45 black neonates using the same method were subjected to various calculations. The correlation coefficients obtained are listed in Table 20.1.

In another experiment, Peevy et al. (1978) determined that the correlation coefficient between serum bilirubin concentrations and measurements of spectral reflectance from the skin at five wavelengths (424, 465, 511, 556, and 629 nm) for 14 white and 30 black neonates was 0.94 for both white and black neonates.

In all of those reports, the results were obtained by using a spectrometer for measurements and a computer for data processing; such systems are not practical for clinical use.

ACCURACY AND RELIABILITY OF THE MINOLTA JAUNDICE METER

The accuracy and reliability of the Minolta jaundice meter, as determined through clinical studies of healthy neonates and neonates with various diseases, will be discussed in this section (Yamanouchi et al., 1980; Hegyi et al., 1981a; Hegyi, Hiatt, and Indyk, 1981b; Betil et al., 1982; Goldman, Penalver, and Penaranda, 1982; Hannemann, Schreiner, and DeWitt, 1982; Heick et al., 1982; Maisels and Conard, 1982; Pereira and Gorman, 1982; Schreiner and Glick, 1982; Tan, 1982; Tudehope and Chang, 1982; Maisels and Lee, 1983; Schumacher, Thornbery, and Gutcher, 1985; Fok et al., 1986; Yamauchi and Yamanouchi, 1988b, 1989c).

Healthy neonates

The results of a study (Yamauchi and Yamanouchi, 1988b) of the reliability and accuracy of the Minolta jaundice meter, conducted on 336 full-term newborn infants, are shown in Table 20.2. In that study, values measured with the Minolta jaundice meter on the forehead, chest, and sternum were compared with serum bilirubin concentrations measured with an AO bilirubinometer (American Optical, Buffalo, NY); the correlation coefficient was found to be between 0.910 and 0.922. Moreover, the 95% confidence interval of ± 2.84 to ± 3.04 mg · dl^{-1}

Table 20.1. *Correlation coefficients between serum bilirubin concentrations and the results of analysis of spectral reflectance from skin for 58 white and 45 black neonates*

Analysis method	Number of wavelengths	Wavelengths (nm)	Correlation coefficient White	Black
Reflectance ratio	2	450, 520	0.81	
		480, 500		0.83
Multiple linear regression	6	410, 420, 440, 490, 520, 550	0.83	
	4	400, 490, 520, 590		0.88
Kubelka-Munk formula	3	420, 460, 520	0.78	0.87

Source: Data from Hannemann et al. (1979).

Table 20.2. *Correlation coefficients between serum bilirubin concentrations and TcB readings at different sites*

Site	Number of measurements	Correlation coefficient	Regression line $(y = ax + b)^a$	95% confidence interval $(mg \cdot dl^{-1})$
(1) Forehead	576	0.910	$y = 1.004x + 9.754$	±3.04
(2) Right upper chest	576	0.922	$y = 1.041x + 9.607$	±2.85
(3) Middle of sternum	576	0.922	$y = 1.001x + 9.418$	±2.84
(4) Right upper abdomen	576	0.890	$y = 0.884x + 8.657$	±3.36
(5) Upper back	576	0.888	$y = 0.837x + 9.752$	±3.37
(6) Lower back	576	0.883	$y = 0.766x + 8.826$	±3.44
(7) Sole	576	0.771	$y = 0.475x + 6.309$	±4.67
(8) Heel	576	0.763	$y = 0.493x + 6.257$	±4.74
$\frac{(1) + (2) + (3)}{3}$	576	0.930	$y = 1.015x + 9.587$	±2.68
$\frac{(1) + (2)}{2}$	576	0.928	$y = 1.023x + 9.674$	±2.73
$\frac{(1) + (3)}{2}$	576	0.929	$y = 1.002x + 9.583$	±2.71
$\frac{(2) + (3)}{2}$	576	0.926	$y = 1.021x + 9.511$	±2.78
Maximum (1, 2, 3)	576	0.924	$y = 1.028x + 10.160$	±2.81

[a] y = TcB reading; x = serum bilirubin concentration.
Source: Data from Yamauchi and Yamanouchi (1988b).

was very good. This accuracy is sufficient for screening and monitoring for jaundice in full-term newborn infants. When the infants were grouped according to age in days, it was found that the most reliable site for transcutaneous bilirubin measurement shifted from the forehead to the sternum with advancing postnatal age (i.e., forehead for infants up to 3 d old, chest for infants 4–5 d old, and sternum for infants 6 d old and older). Furthermore, there was a high correlation between the AO-measured serum bilirubin concentration and the overall

mean of values measured with the jaundice meter at the forehead, chest, and sternum, as well as for values measured at the forehead and sternum. Calculating the mean of values measured at such points reduced the width of the 95% confidence interval to ±2.68 mg · dl^{-1}, yielding better accuracy and reliability figures for transcutaneous bilirubin measurements. On the basis of that study, it can be stated that the Minolta jaundice meter is an excellent instrument for screening and monitoring for jaundice in healthy neonates.

Table 20.3. *Correlation coefficients between serum bilirubin concentrations and TcB readings for high-risk neonates*

Groups	Number of neonates	Correlation coefficient	p value	Regression line $(y = ax + b)$[a]
Respiratory distress syndrome, transient tachypnea of the newborn	63	0.905	0.001	$y = 1.299x + 7.242$
Asphyxia neonatorum	160	0.890	0.001	$y = 1.313x + 6.318$
Phenobarbital administration	44	0.959	0.001	$y = 1.402x + 5.045$
Meconium aspiration syndrome	113	0.947	0.001	$y = 1.244x + 6.669$
Congenital heart disease	100	0.845	0.001	$y = 1.125x + 7.109$
Surgery	149	0.824	0.001	$y = 0.952x + 9.431$
Others	75	0.907	0.001	$y = 1.049x + 8.454$
Hemorrhagic disease	60	0.853	0.001	$y = 1.019x + 8.651$

[a] y = TcB reading; x = serum bilirubin concentration.

Neonates with various diseases

There are few data available regarding the accuracy of the Minolta jaundice meter when used for measurements of neonates with various diseases. Table 20.3 shows the correlations between values measured with the Minolta jaundice meter and serum bilirubin concentrations for ill (mainly full-term) neonates who received treatment in the neonatal intensive-care unit (NICU) at Okayama National Hospital, grouped according to diseases. It can be seen that the coefficients range widely, from 0.824 to 0.960, for different diseases.

A comparison of the regression-line equations for neonates with various diseases is also shown in Table 20.3. These lines can be divided into two broad groups. The groups with approximately the same serum bilirubin concentrations (consisting of neonates with respiratory problems, those suffering from meconium aspiration syndrome, and those suffering from neonatal asphyxia) had relatively high skin bilirubin indices compared with the groups with other ailments. For the group not suffering from other combined ailments, the group undergoing surgical treatment, and the group with congenital heart disease, the regression lines are basically the same and, moreover, are nearly the same as the regression line for healthy neonates.

Thus, for neonates suffering from various diseases, as well as for healthy neonates, the Minolta jaundice meter can be used clinically for screening and monitoring for jaundice. However, because there are many factors that can affect measurements of neonates suffering from various diseases, the reliability is somewhat lower, and it is necessary to evaluate each patient group. Further detailed studies regarding the use of the Minolta jaundice meter for neonates of low birth weight or those born prematurely are needed.

Summary of supplementary results

Data received from various countries other than Japan are listed in Table 20.4. As in Japan, the data show a very good correlation for full-term newborn infants. However, the correlation coefficients, regression lines, and 95% confidence intervals vary between the testing institutions. The factors that can influence these variations include variations between individual Minolta jaundice meters and differences in the sites of measurement, the ages and races of the neonates, the individual performing the measurements and the methods of measuring serum bilirubin. In particular, aberrations in skin color and in the measurement of serum bilirubin (Schreiner and Glick, 1982; Maisels and Lee, 1983; Yamauchi and Yamanouchi, 1989c) can contribute greatly to these variations.

CLINICAL USE OF THE MINOLTA JAUNDICE METER

What kind of data can be obtained by using the Minolta jaundice meter for neonatal jaundice? Some possibilities for clinical use are listed in Table 20.5. At present, clinics are using the jaundice meter for very general applications, such as screening for hyperbilirubinemia in full-term neonates, monitoring of neonatal jaundice (Kivlahan and James, 1984; Yamauchi and Yamanouchi, 1989b), observing the progress of patients (Hegyi et al., 1981a), and predicting significant hyperbilirubinemia on the first

Table 20.4. *Selected data from previous studies*

Bilirubin test	Measurement site	Clinical details	Regression line $(y = ax + b)$[b]		Correlation coefficient
Japanese: birth weight (g)					
AO bilirubinometer	Forehead	>2,500	1.08	7.22	0.95
		2,001–2,500	1.13	11.92	0.89
		1,501–2,000	1.32	11.76	0.92
		1,001–1,500	1.46	11.65	0.98
		<1,000	1.24	16.23	0.71
Gestation (wk)					
White, Haidar, and Reinhold (1958)	Sternum	White, term	—	7.0	0.90
		Black, term	—	15.0	0.92
AO bilirubinometer or Gambino (1965)	Forehead	White, >38	1.25	9.63	0.90
		34–37	1.30	7.57	0.88
		Black, ≥34	0.97	13.49	0.71
Abbott bichromatic analyzer (ABA-100)	Forehead	White, >38	1.00	7.8	0.71
		33–38	0.76	10.2	0.52
		<33	0.45	12.5	0.32
		Black, >38	0.53	14.0	0.52
		33–38	0.53	14.9	0.57
		<33	1.70	6.6	0.91
Du Pont automatic clinical analyzer (ACA-III)	Forehead	White, term	1.33	7.96	0.93
	Sternum		1.35	7.44	0.93
Du Pont automatic clinical analyzer (ACA-II)	Forehead	White, term	0.91	9.25	0.74
(Method not stated)	Forehead	White, term	1.15	6.44	0.90
Du Pont automatic clinical analyzer (ACA-III)	Forehead	White, term	0.90	8.30	0.89

[a] y = TcB reading; x = serum bilirubin concentration.
Source: Data from Cassady (1983).

Table 20.5. *Clinical applications of TcB measurements*

1. Screening for hyperbilirubinemia
2. Prediction of hyperbilirubinemia
3. Observation of natural progress of neonatal jaundice
4. Analysis of factors affecting neonatal jaundice
5. Observation of dermal bilirubin kinetics
6. Estimation of serum bilirubin (bilirubinometer)

day after birth (Smith et al., 1985; Yamauchi and Yamanouchi, 1990).

Factors affecting transcutaneous bilirubin measurement

Bilirubin within the body can be broadly classified as that within the blood vessels and that outside the blood vessels. Because most of the bilirubin within the blood vessels is strongly combined with albumin, and the remainder is attached to red blood cells, platelets, or the cells of the inner surfaces of the blood vessels, there is very little unbound bilirubin. Meanwhile, the bilirubin outside the blood vessels is widely distributed throughout the skin

and various organs, especially the liver, and there is generally a uniform, balanced relation between the bilirubin within the blood vessels and that outside. The exceedingly good correlation between the bilirubin concentration in the skin and that in the blood has been demonstrated for humans and animals. This balanced relation indirectly confirms the good correlation between the values measured with the Minolta jaundice meter and the serum bilirubin determinations.

Of course, there are various factors that can influence this balanced relation between bilirubin within and outside the blood vessels, such as the blood pH, the reserve binding capacity of albumin, the concentration of bilirubin in the blood, the amount of subcutaneous fat, various circulatory conditions, and phototherapy (Lucey, Nyborg, and Yamanouchi, 1980; Brown et al., 1981; Vangyanichyakorn et al., 1981; Engel et al., 1982; Wu et al., 1982; Erenberg and Bhatia, 1983; Yamauchi and Yamanouchi, 1988a, 1989a, 1991a–c). Because there are many factors that affect the balance of that relation for neonates with diseases, there are cases in which skin bilirubin measured with the Minolta jaundice meter may not exactly reflect the serum bilirubin concen-

Table 20.6A. *Factors affecting TcB readings: factors resulting in high TcB/TB ratios*

Causes of increased TcB readings	Causes of reduced total bilirubin (TB)
Preterm, respiratory distress syndrome	Bilirubin decline
Hypoproteinemia	Exchange blood transfusion
Skin color (black)	
Hyperpigmentation	
Meconium-stained skin	
Drugs	

Table 20.6B. *Factors affecting TcB readings: factors resulting in low TcB/TB ratios*

Causes of reduced TcB readings	Causes of increased total bilirubin (TB)
Shock; heart failure	Dehydration
Phototherapy	Polycythemia
Natural light	Hemolytic jaundice
Baby's position	Severe jaundice
Measurement site (heel, sole)	Albumin administration
Birth trauma (ecchymosis, congestion)	
Crying	
Cyanosis	

tration. Analyzing and comprehending the factors that influence whether or not measurement of skin bilirubin will satisfactorily reflect the concentration in the blood, and determining in which cases such measurements are not satisfactory, is a suitable application for the Minolta jaundice meter that should also provide information for clinical use in the future.

The cases in which the values measured with the Minolta jaundice meter (transcutaneous bilirubin, TcB) do not accurately reflect the serum bilirubin concentrations can be broadly divided into those in which the measured value is high in relation to the serum bilirubin concentration and those in which it is low (Table 20.6).

Cases in which TcB measurements will be high

Increased bilirubin in the skin

Among premature neonates and those suffering from respiratory diseases (Yamanouchi et al., 1980; Wu et al., 1982; Erenberg and Bhatia, 1983), those suffering from low blood albumin will also have a low amount of subcutaneous fat. This results in an increased shift of bilirubin to the skin and outside the blood vessels because of increased transmission

from the blood vessels, increased blood flow through the skin, and so forth.

Effect of skin color

In the case of black neonates or those with pigmentation or meconium staining (Brown et al., 1981; Engel et al., 1981; Vangyanichyakorn et al., 1981), it is necessary to take extra care, because the value displayed by the instrument may seem high even though the concentration of total bilirubin in plasma is not.

Sudden decreases in serum bilirubin concentrations

When the serum bilirubin concentration decreases suddenly or within 24 h of an exchange transfusion, the measured skin value will remain relatively high.

Cases in which TcB measurements will be low

Decrease in bilirubin in the skin

Effect of phototherapy or natural light. Bilirubin in the skin decreases because it is converted to a hydrophilic form of bilirubin (configurational and structural isomers) as a result of the action of light energy, and it migrates rapidly into the bloodstream (Brown et al., 1981; Vangyanichyakorn et al., 1981; Yamauchi and Yamanouchi, 1988a, 1991a).

Incomplete circulation, acidosis. Bilirubin absorption by the skin decreases because of reduced blood flow through the skin.

Delivery wound (receiving or losing blood), crying. Under these circumstances, the measured value at the skin will be low; this is particularly noticeable for measurements at the forehead (Lucey et al., 1980; Yamauchi and Yamanouchi, 1991c).

Even for high-hematocrit blood in hypovolemia or dehydration, the measured value is relatively low because of the decrease in blood flow through the skin and the increased production of bilirubin (Yamauchi and Yamanouchi, 1989a, 1991b).

When the bilirubin concentration in the blood increases rapidly, as in the case of hemolytic disease, the measured skin index is relatively low, because several hours are required before the balance between the bilirubin in the blood and that in the skin returns to normal.

Because so many factors affect the measurement of skin bilirubin concentration, when there is a great change in the movement of bilirubin between the blood and the skin, it is important to determine whether the measured value is due to an effect of the instrument or to an imbalance between bilirubin in the skin and that in the blood.

THE FUTURE OF TRANSCUTANEOUS MONITORING OF BILIRUBIN

Elimination of the differences in indicated values for different races is one of the main areas for development in future instruments. Studies should continue in an effort to improve the measuring geometry and the calculation algorithm, as well as to determine the wavelengths or number of wavelengths to be measured.

However, because the clinical usefulness of the current system for determining the density difference at two wavelengths has been clearly demonstrated, for the time being the measuring principle of the Minolta jaundice meter should be applied and extended to develop an instrument that will be even smaller and will offer improved accuracy. It should be possible to build an instrument that could perform the logarithmic calculations with a microcomputer.

There is some controversy whether or not the onset of bilirubin encephalopathy can be predicted, and information useful in clarifying the onset mechanism can be obtained through clinical measurement of the skin bilirubin index (Knudsen and Brodersen, 1989). Further research in this area is anticipated.

REFERENCES

Ballowitz, L., and Avery, M. E. (1970). Spectral reflectance of the skin: studies on infant and adult humans, Wistar and Gunn rats. *Biology of the Neonate* 15:348–60.

Betil, B., Ballowitz, L., Goitia, E., Ludwig, R., and Wiese, G. (1982). Nicht invasive Bilirubinmessungen. *Paediatrie Praxis* 26:413–23.

Brown, A. K., Kim, M. H., Nuchpuckdee, P., and Boyle, G. (1981). Transcutaneous bilirubinometry in infants: influence of race and phototheraphy. *Pediatric Research* 15:653.

Brunsting, L. A., and Sheard, C. (1929). The color of the skin as analyzed by spectrophotometric methods. *Journal of Clinical Investigation* 7:575.

Cassady, G. (1983). Transcutaneous monitoring in the newborn infant. *Journal of Pediatrics* 103:837–48.

Engel, R. R., Henis, B. B., Engel, R. E., and Bandt, C. (1981). Effect of race and other variables on transcutaneous bilirubinometry. *Pediatric Research* 15:531.

Erenberg, A., and Bhatia, J. (1983). Transcutaneous bilirubinometry in the neonate: effect of gestational age. *Pediatric Research* 17:311A.

Fok, T. F., Lau, S. P., Hui, C. W., Fung, K. P., and Wan, C. W. (1986). Transcutaneous bilirubinometry: its use in Chinese term infants and the effect of haematocrit and phototherapy on the TcB index. *Australian Paediatric Journal* 22:107–9.

Gambino, S. R. (1965). Bilirubin (modified Jendrassik and Grof). *Standard Methods in Clinical Chemistry* 5:55–64.

Goldman, S. L., Penalver, A., and Penaranda, R. (1982). Jaundice meter: evaluation of new guidelines. *Journal of Pediatrics* 101:253–6.

Hannemann, R. E., DeWitt, D. P., Hanley, E. J., Schreiner, R. L., and Bonderman, P. (1979). Determination of serum bilirubin by skin reflectance: effect of pigmentation. *Pediatric Research* 13:1326–9.

Hannemann, R. E., DeWitt, D. P., and Wiechel, J. F. (1978). Neonatal serum bilirubin from skin reflectance. *Pediatric Research* 12:207–10.

Hannemann, R. E., Schreiner, R. I., and DeWitt, D. P. (1982). Evaluation of the Minolta bilirubin meter as a screening device in white and black infants. *Pediatrics* 69:107–9.

Hegyi, T., Hiatt, I. M., Gertner, I., Indyk, L. (1981a). Transcutaneous bilirubinometry: the cephalocaudal progression of dermal icterus. *American Journal of Diseases of Children* 135:547–9.

Hegyi, T., Hiatt, I. M., and Indyk, L. (1981b). Transcutaneous bilirubinometry. I. Correlations in term infants. *Journal of Pediatrics* 98:454–7.

Heick, C., Mieth, D., Fallenstein, F., Schubiger, G., Nars, P. W., and Amato, M. (1982). Transkutane Bilirubinmessung beim Neugeborenen. *Helvetica Paediatrica Acta* 37:589–97.

Kivlahan, C., and James, E. J. P. (1984). The natural history of neonatal jaundice. *Pediatrics* 74:364–70.

Knudsen, A., and Brodersen, R. (1989). Skin color and bilirubin in neonates. *Archives of Disease in Childhood* 64:605–9.

Lucey, J. F., Nyborg, E., and Yamanouchi, I. (1980). A new device for transcutaneous bilirubinometry. *Pediatric Research* 14:604.

Maisels, M. J., and Conard, S. (1982). Transcutaneous bilirubin measurements in full-term infants. *Pediatrics* 70:464–7.

Maisels, M. J., and Lee, C. (1983). Transcutaneous bilirubin measurements: variation in meter response. *Pediatrics* 71:457–9.

Peevy, K. J., Mumford, L., Bruce, R., and Gross, S. J. (1978). Estimation of serum bilirubin by spectral reflectance of the skin. *Pediatric Research* 12:532.

Pereira, C., and Gorman, W. (1982). Transcutaneous bilirubinometry: an evaluation. *Archives of Disease in Childhood* 57:708–20.

Schreiner, F. L., and Glick, M. G. (1982). Interlaboratory bilirubin variability. *Pediatrics* 69:277–81.

Schumacher, R. E., Thornbery, J. M., and Gutcher, G. R. (1985). Transcutaneous bilirubinometry: a comparison of old and new methods. *Pediatrics* 76:10–14.

Smith, D. W., Inguillo, D., Martin, D., Vreman, H. J., Cohen, R. S., and Stevenson, D. J. (1985). Use of noninvasive tests to predict significant jaundice in full-term infants: preliminary studies. *Pediatrics* 75:278–80.

Tan, K. L. (1982). Transcutaneous bilirubinometry in full-term Chinese and Malay infants. *Acta Paediatrica Scandinavica* 71:593–6.

Tudehope, D. I., and Chang, A. (1982). Multiple site readings from a transcutaneous bilirubinometer. *Australian Paediatric Journal* 18:102–5.

Vangyanichyakorn, K., Sun, S., Abubakar, A., and Glista, B. (1981). Transcutaneous bilirubinometry in black and hispanic infants. *Pediatric Research* 15:685.

White, D., Haidar, G. A., and Reinhold, J. G. (1958). Spectrophotometric measurement of bilirubin concentration in the serum of the newborn by the use of a microcapillary method. *Clinical Chemistry* 4:211–22.

Wu, P. Y. K., Edward, N. B., Chan, L., Lee, G., and Wareham, C. (1982). Transcutaneous bilirubinometry and factors affecting the transcutaneous bilirubin index. *Pediatric Research* 16:315A.

Yamanouchi, I., Yamauchi, Y., and Igarashi, I. (1980). Transcutaneous bilirubinometry: preliminary studies of noninvasive transcutaneous bilirubin meter in the Okayama National Hospital. *Pediatrics* 65:195–202.

Yamauchi, Y., and Yamanouchi, I. (1988a). Transcutaneous bilirubinometry: effect of irradiation on the skin bilirubin index. *Biology of the Neonate* 54:314–19.

(1988b). Transcutaneous bilirubinometry: evaluation of accuracy and reliability of a large population. *Acta Paediatrica Scandinavica* 77:791–5.

(1989a). Difference in TcB readings between full-term newborn infants born vaginally and by cesarean section. *Acta Paediatrica Scandinavica* 78:824–8.

(1989b). Transcutaneous bilirubinometry in normal Japanese infants. *Acta Paediatrica Japonica* 31:65–72.

(1989c). Transcutaneous bilirubinometry: interinstrumental variability of TcB instruments. *Acta Paediatrica Scandinavica* 78:844–7.

(1990). Clinical application of transcutaneous bilirubin measurement: early prediction of hyperbilirubinemia. *Acta Paediatrica Scandinavica* 79:385–90.

(1991a). Factors affecting transcutaneous bilirubin measurement: effect of daylight. *Acta Paediatrica Japonica* 33:658–62.

(1991b). Transcutaneous bilirubinometry: effect of postnatal age. *Acta Paediatrica Japonica* 33:663–7.

(1991c). Transcutaneous bilirubinometry: variability of TcB measurements on the forehead with crying. *Acta Paediatrica Japonica* 33:655–7.

21

Phototherapy: Mechanism and clinical efficacy

Dr. K. L. TAN

INTRODUCTION

Neonatal jaundice (NNJ) is a very common complication among infants, even healthy, full-term infants; this is especially so in colored ethnic groups (Friedman et al., 1978; Munroe et al., 1984). It is even more frequent and severe among Chinese neonates, in whom it is the commonest condition in the first week of life; about 9% of full-term healthy infants experience nonhemolytic hyperbilirubinemia exceeding 255 μmol $\cdot$ l^{-1} (Tan, 1981) in the first week of life. Fortunately, NNJ, if not too severe, is harmless and may even be beneficial (Lightner, 1982; Onishi et al., 1988). However, when it is severe, it can lead to damage and death, even for a healthy, full-term neonate (Tan, 1978). Premature (Tan, 1987) and sick infants (Linn et al., 1985) are even more prone to severe NNJ. Hence the need to ensure that all infants with NNJ be closely monitored, especially sick and/or premature infants.

Bilirubin formation

NNJ is caused by accumulation of unconjugated bilirubin in an infant. Bilirubin is a tetrapyrrole chain formed by the catabolism of heme (Figure 21.1), of which hemoglobin is the major source. The high turnover rate of fetal red blood cells in the neonate chiefly accounts for the rate of bilirubin formation being about twice that in the adult. Further aggravating factors are the slow rate of bilirubin conjugation, diminished intracellular bilirubin-binding (Y) protein, impaired canalicular excretion of organic anions, and ductus venosus patency, with diverted blood flow resulting in the unconjugated bilirubin bypassing the hepatocytes. The conjugated fraction of bilirubin is excreted into the gut, where it is acted on by the β-glucuronidase produced by the intestinal cells, especially in the jejunum, and is deconjugated. The resultant unconjugated bilirubin is recycled into the normal circulation to add significantly to the bilirubin pool (Poland and Odell, 1971). This enterohepatic circulation may be advantageous in utero, because the bilirubin can be eliminated by the mother.

Management of NNJ

When the plasma's albumin-binding capacity for bilirubin is exceeded, the excess bilirubin is capable of crossing the blood–brain barrier in its free form to cause dysfunction and, at higher levels, irreparable damage to the brain. This is more likely in a compromised or premature infant. Presently, the accepted methods of management are exchange transfusion and phototherapy.

Exchange transfusion

The management of severe NNJ originally involved exchange transfusion, a procedure not only inconvenient and expensive in terms of equipment and personnel time but also accompanied by significant morbidity and mortality (Tan, Phua, and Ang, 1976). Besides, the rebound usually is quite significant and rapid, with about 25% of bilirubin values at 6 h after exchange exceeding or equaling the preexchange values (Tan, 1975), necessitating a second

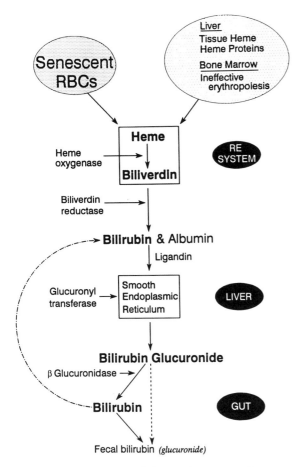

Figure 21.1. Bilirubin metabolism and excretion. The recycling of bilirubin via the enterohepatic circulation plays a significant role in causing NNJ.

exchange, with its accompanying increased morbidity and mortality. However, exchange transfusion was regularly practiced for want of a better substitute in the early days. In Singapore, it used to consume the greatest proportion of a pediatrician's time. It has largely been superseded by phototherapy.

PHOTOTHERAPY

With the first report, in 1958, of the use of light for management of NNJ (Cremer, Perryman, and Richards, 1958), phototherapy for NNJ was born. Since then, numerous publications have documented the efficacy, to varying degrees, of phototherapy. The noninvasive nature of the treatment, together with its ease and convenience and the apparent absence of severe side effects, has much to recommend it for general use. An important factor in an era of rising medical costs, especially in developing countries, is that it is inexpensive. It is therefore not surprising that it has gained almost universal acceptance as the treatment of choice for management of NNJ.

Mechanism of action

Phototherapy is effective because of its ability to remove bilirubin from the body by a series of processes that involve oxidation or isomerization. Observations of the phenomenon of bleaching of the jaundiced skin of newborns exposed to sunlight, later replicated in tests on serum, suggested the use of light for treatment of NNJ. This bleaching effect is due to photooxidation.

Photooxidation

Phototherapy results in the formation of several colorless, polar photooxidation products that subsequently can be isolated in the urine of infants exposed to phototherapy (Lightner, Linnane, and Ahlfors, 1982). This pathway does contribute toward the efficacy of phototherapy, but the process apparently is rather slow; hence it is currently believed to be a minor contributor, but the significance of its role has not been completely clarified.

Photoisomerization

The typical "native" bilirubin molecule is composed of four pyrrole rings linked by three carbon bridges, the outer two being double-bonded, and the middle single-bonded (Figure 21.2); the outer bonds follow the Z arrangement of the parent heme, resulting in a 4Z,15Z-bilirubin IXα configuration. The usual shape assumed is one rather angulated on itself, "concealing" the polar COOH and NH groups. This shape is stabilized by the hydrogen bonds, which though relatively weak individually are collectively strong. The hydrocarbon groups, instead of the polar groups, in this configuration are exposed, allowing them to interact with the surrounding solvent. Bilirubin is thus lipophilic rather than hydrophilic, a feature enabling it to cross biological membranes, this being beneficial to the intrauterine fetal status.

Phototherapy apparently is effective mainly because of photoisomerization, the bilirubin isomers being formed during exposure to light. Currently, two main forms of isomers have been described: the configurational or geometric, and the structural photoisomer.

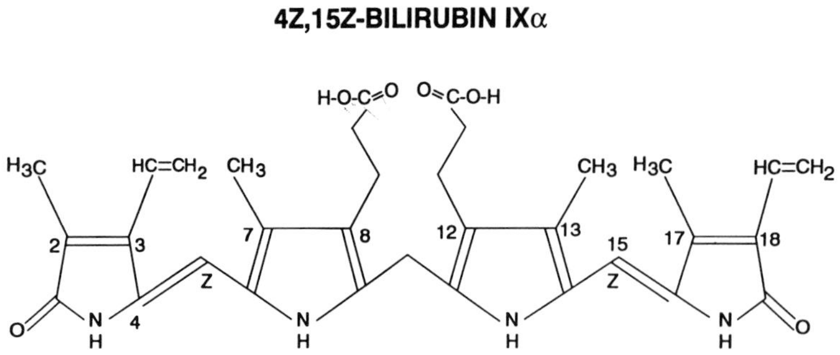

4Z,15Z-BILIRUBIN IXα

Figure 21.2. Usual planar representation of bilirubin, with the polar COOH and NH groups exposed.

Configurational or geometric isomerization

In geometric isomerization, one of the end pyrrole rings responds to light by undergoing a 180° turn, thus forming a 4Z,15E-bilirubin (Itoh and Onishi, 1985). Though theoretically the other C-4 bridge can also be rotated, or both ends together, for some unknown reason the 4Z,15E isomer seems to be the one favored during phototherapy; the 100-fold preference of human albumin for the configurational isomer (the double bond between C-15 and C-16 rather than that between C-4 and C-5) (McDonagh, Palma, and Lightner, 1982) may be a determining factor. This isomer is easily reversible in the dark; though its reversion seems to be very slow or to occur hardly at all in the plasma, it reverts back easily to the native bilirubin (4Z,15Z) in the bile. Thus, it is very likely that part of whatever geometric bilirubin excreted is recycled into the bilirubin pool. Though rapid formation occurs during phototherapy, excretion of this photoisomer is rather slow, leading to accumulation of the product in the plasma during exposure, and resulting in an equilibrium being reached; at that equilibrium, about 20% of the bile pigment is composed of this isomer.

Structural isomerization

The second photoisomer resulting from exposure to light involves a structural change in the bilirubin; hence it is more slowly formed during phototherapy. This structural photoisomer, lumirubin, is a result of the vinyl group (CH=CH$_2$) in the first pyrrole ring forming a new bond with its adjacent ring involving C-7, with creation of a new seven-sided ring (McDonagh et al., 1982); rotation of the C-4=C-5 carbon-carbon double bond simultaneously occurs (Figure 21.3) as a single-step process. A two-step process can also occur, with the bilirubin first being converted to the 4E,15Z-isomer (geometric isomer), followed by final cycling to lumirubin, with the for-

mation of the seven-sided ring (Itoh and Onishi, 1985). Configurational isomerization can also occur reversibly on the other end of the bilirubin molecule, leading to an E isomer. As many as four lumirubins are possible because of the two chiral centers. An optically active lumirubin, the product during phototherapy when bilirubin is bound to human albumin (McDonagh et al., 1986), would seem to be the most likely product during phototherapy in the human infant.

This structural isomer is much more stable than the geometric isomer and apparently can be excreted (via the liver, with no need for conjugation, being itself a polar compound) easily into the gut immediately after formation, with no reversion to native bilirubin. Continual formation therefore occurs during phototherapy, with no equilibrium occurring between the native bilirubin and the isomer. The rate of formation of lumirubin is thus determined mainly by the intensity of light of the correct wavelength, as well as its duration, increasing with increasing light intensity and period of exposure; it is apparently the principal isomer excreted during phototherapy.

Excretion of the photoproducts, which because of the exposure of their polar groups are hydrophilic, occurs through the biliary and urinary routes, with the former being the major route (Callahan et al., 1970); high-intensity phototherapy seems also to increase the concentration of lumirubin, with little effect on that of the configurational isomer (Costarino et al., 1985). Furthermore, lumirubin is the major component of bilirubin products in both the urine and duodenal bile aspirates of infants undergoing phototherapy (Onishi et al., 1980; Ennever et al., 1987).

These mechanisms of action of phototherapy on bilirubin and on excretion of the photoproducts (Figure 21.4), as presently understood, help to explain the efficacy of light for successful management of NNJ.

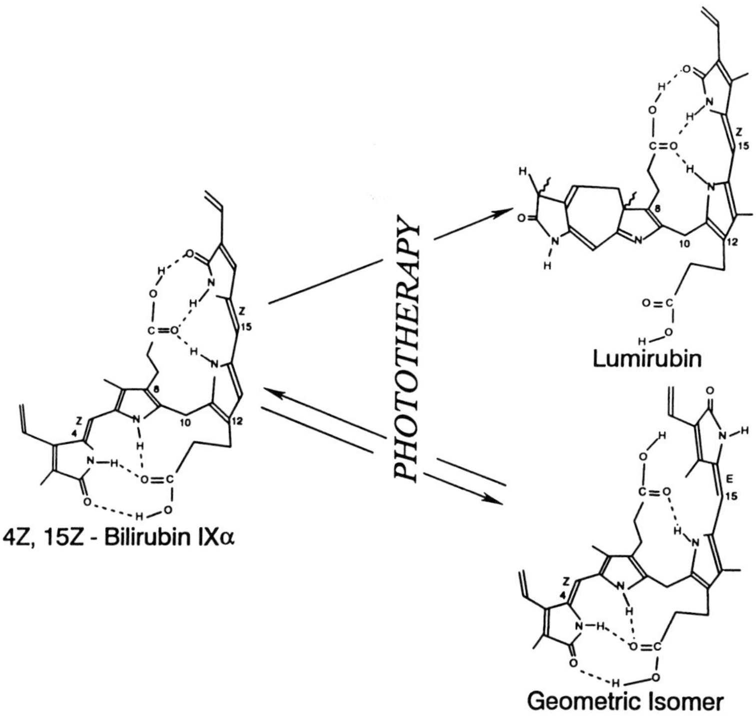

Lumirubin

4Z, 15Z - Bilirubin IXα

Geometric Isomer

Figure 21.3. The usual shape of bilirubin with its polar groups "concealed." Phototherapy causes isomerization; the isomers with their polar groups exposed are hydrophilic.

Advantages of phototherapy

The main advantages of the procedure are as follows:

1. Cost-effectiveness. Daylight fluorescent lamps cost little and last for relatively long periods without need for replacement, provided certain precautions are taken. Hence the initial and recurrent expenditures are very low.
2. Convenience. This procedure is about the most convenient in neonatology. The infant simply needs to be placed unclothed under the lights, with the bilirubin being monitored regularly. Hence, very little nursing or medical attention beyond the usual is required.
3. Safety. Being noninvasive, all the complications associated with an invasive procedure are avoided. When simple precautions are taken, no complication implicating phototherapy as the direct cause has ever been established. Our own experience with more than 20,000 infants of different weights and gestational ages confirms this observation.
4. Simplicity. The very simplicity of this procedure is appealing. Very few maneuvers are required to ensure adequate treatment. Hence, chances of the procedure being wrongly applied are minimized.

5. Efficacy. Though varying degrees of effectiveness have been reported, there is general consensus that the efficacy of phototherapy is beyond doubt.

Efficacy of phototherapy

Acceptance of phototherapy as the preferred mode of treatment for NNJ will depend mainly on its efficacy in the clinical situation. Hence the factors influencing its efficacy should be clearly defined. Our clinical experience has demonstrated quite clearly the important factors determining the effectiveness of phototherapy (Table 21.1).

Unconjugated bilirubin absorbs blue light in the process of becoming decolorized. Hence blue light is the main component responsible for the efficacy of phototherapy in NNJ. Sunlight, though able to bleach infant skin, is relatively ineffective for reducing bilirubin concentrations, mainly because of its relatively low blue content; hence, hyperpyrexia often occurs before any appreciable decrease in plasma bilirubin concentration is observed (Tan, 1976). Thus, solar therapy not only is ineffective but also can be dangerous, because the bleaching of the skin engenders a false sense of security, especially in laypeople.

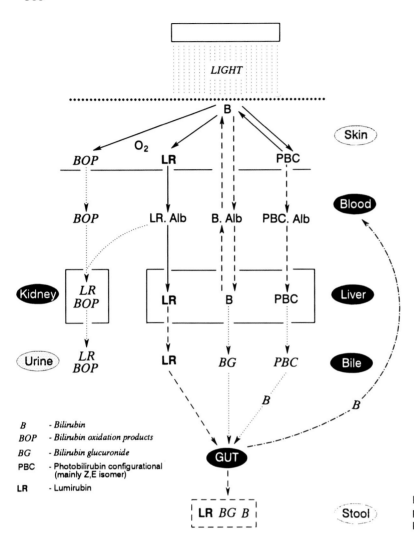

LIGHT

B

Skin

BOP O₂ LR PBC

Blood

BOP LR. Alb B. Alb PBC. Alb

Kidney LR BOP LR B PBC Liver

Urine LR BOP LR BG PBC Bile

B B

GUT

LR BG B Stool

B - Bilirubin
BOP - Bilirubin oxidation products
BG - Bilirubin glucuronide
PBC - Photobilirubin configurational
        (mainly Z,E isomer)
LR - Lumirubin

Figure 21.4. Mechanism of action of phototherapy. Lumirubin is the main product excreted.

Table 21.1. *Factors influencing the efficacy of phototherapy*

Postnatal age of infant
Gestational age of infant
Birth weight
Cause of NNJ
Bilirubin value
Light intensity
Emission spectrum

The differences in the effectiveness of phototherapy observed in numerous studies have mainly been due to varying birth weights and gestational ages for the infants studied, as well as the different types of lamps with different spectral emissions, and different intensities being used in those studies. Evaluation of the efficacy of phototherapy for 3,999 neonates exposed to daylight lamps (Tan and Boey, 1986) has demonstrated the importance of birth weight and gestational age in influencing the efficacy of phototherapy when the light intensity is uniform (Figure 21.5). The relatively greater surface area exposed by the extended posture of a small preterm baby, together with the thinner, more translucent skin, allows a relatively greater light dosage and greater penetration during phototherapy; hence its greater efficacy in preterms, especially the very small ones. However, very small but full-term infants (grossly growth-retarded infants) respond significantly more slowly to exposure, suggesting that the other factors of skin thickness and greater hematocrit, with a resulting greater rate of

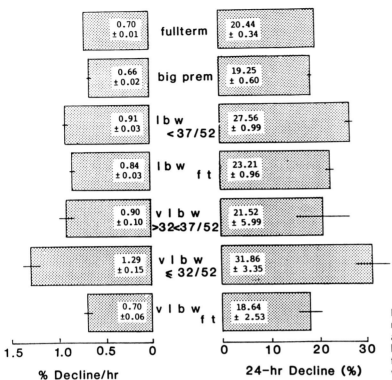

0.70 ± 0.01	fullterm	20.44 ± 0.34
0.66 ± 0.02	big prem	19.25 ± 0.60
0.91 ± 0.03	l b w < 37/52	27.56 ± 0.99
0.84 ± 0.03	l b w f t	23.21 ± 0.96
0.90 ± 0.10	v l b w >32<37/52	21.52 ± 5.99
1.29 ± 0.15	v l b w ≤ 32/52	31.86 ± 3.35
0.70 ±0.06	v l b w f t	18.64 ± 2.53

% Decline/hr —— 24–hr Decline (%)

1.5 1.0 0.5 0 | 0 10 20 30

Figure 21.5. Efficacy of phototherapy related to birth weight and gestational age. Preterm infants with very low birth weights respond the best, and full-term infants with very low birth weights respond the least.

bilirubin production, may be equally important or even more important. The flexed posture of a growth-retarded infant also reduces the surface area exposed. A large preterm infant will respond less well to phototherapy than will an appropriately small preterm peer, most likely because of the increased subcutaneous tissue, as well as large size, with the thicker barrier and relatively decreased light dosage thus reducing the efficacy of phototherapy.

Light intensity will determine the rate of bilirubin decline during phototherapy (Tan, 1982), with a dose–response relationship being demonstrated. An initial increase in response will occur with increasing light intensity, with the rate of increase in response declining as the light intensity continues to increase, until a "saturation" dose is reached, beyond which no further increase in response will occur with further increases in intensity. With bilirubin values greater than 225 μmol $\cdot$ l^{-1}, a 50% decline in bilirubin concentration in 24 h usually occurs in cases of nonhemolytic hyperbilirubinemia when lamps with a blue emission spectrum are used at "saturation dose" (Figure 21.6).

The response is also dependent on the initial bilirubin value at the commencement of exposure; a greater response will occur if there is a high bil-irubin concentration, with a decreasing response rate paralleling decreasing bilirubin levels, until 100 μmol $\cdot$ l^{-1}, below which no further decline will occur with further exposure (Tan, 1982). This observation explains the slow bilirubin increment observed despite prophylactic phototherapy until about 100 μmol $\cdot$ l^{-1}, after which no further increase is usually observed (Tan, 1978). Hence phototherapy is not indicated with bilirubin levels less than 100 μmol $\cdot$ l^{-1}; only when a bilirubin concentration is significantly raised should phototherapy be started.

The cause of the NNJ also influences efficacy, because in hemolytic conditions with rapid bilirubin production, the response to phototherapy is slower. ABO hemolytic NNJ usually responds to daylight phototherapy, even though the rate of response has been significantly slower, in our experience, as is also the case with infants deficient in glucose-6-phosphate dehydrogenase (G-6-PD) (Tan and Boey, 1993). However, in very severe hemolysis, as in rhesus hemolytic disease, the rate of bilirubin production and the resultant hyperbilirubinemia are too rapid to be adequately controlled by daylight phototherapy; only high-intensity phototherapy at "saturation dose" using "double-bank" blue light, with almost the same spectral emission as the bilirubin

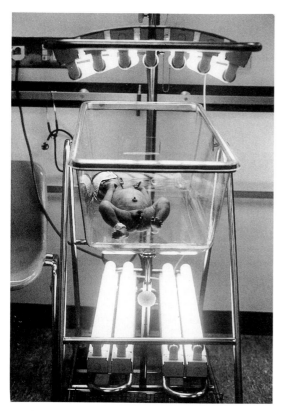

Figure 21.6. Phototherapy setup to provide "saturation" dose for optimal efficacy.

absorption spectrum, can be effective in that situation. Simple blood transfusion(s) can be administered for the resultant anemia, with minimal ill effects (Tan, 1984). This is especially useful because many such infants are not in optimal general condition. Fortunately, the efficacy of phototherapy does not seem to be influenced by the general condition of the infant (Tan, 1976).

The most effective spectrum of light for maximal effectiveness of phototherapy would seem to be that similar to the bilirubin absorption spectrum; our own experience has confirmed this. Some recent claims of equal efficacy for green light (Vecchi et al., 1986) in phototherapy could not be substantiated in our study (Tan, 1989), which demonstrated the obviously superior efficacy of blue light as compared with daylight or green light; the daylight lamps proved to be better than the green lamps for preterm infants, with equal efficacies for healthy full-term infants! The green lamps used in all these studies that have been discussed in fact contained some blue light.

Halogen lamps produce an intense light, far more intense than that of ordinary fluorescent lamps. However, the light is concentrated into a small area (Eggert and Stick, 1985), being not as uniformly spread as the light produced by fluorescent lamps. The halogen lamps also produce an appreciable amount of heat, which possibly could cause hyperpyrexia. Studies have not demonstrated an efficacy superior to that of the fluorescent lamps. Indeed, the uniform light produced by fluorescent lamps would seem more suitable for phototherapy; if the intensity for each individual lamp could be further increased, it would then be ideal.

Complications

Phototherapy, being a noninvasive procedure, is largely free of the major complications that can be associated with invasive procedures. However, there are some complications that can occur:

1. Fluid balance. During phototherapy, complete exposure of the infant's skin is necessary for maximal response. Increases in insensible fluid losses through the skin (Oh and Karecki, 1972) and via the stool (Wu and Moosa, 1978) will occur. Fluid loss will depend on the infant's size and maturity, the environmental humidity, and the light intensity, with about 20–60% loss occurring in 24 h.

2. Temperature status. With total exposure of the skin, increased loss of heat is inevitable. This usually is adequately offset by the heat produced by the phototherapy itself in a full-term infant. For a small premature infant, that will be inadequate, with resultant hypothermia. With double-bank phototherapy, overheating, with pyrexia, can occur in full-term infants.

3. Skin and eye complications. Skin rashes often occur because of overheating or exposure to ultraviolet (UV) light, which has the potential to cause skin and corneal burns, and possibly cataracts over the long term. Phototherapy has also been reported to cause premature aging of the retina in animals (Messner, Maisels, and Leure duPree, 1978). However, in the clinical situation, phototherapy is of relatively short duration, most probably too short to cause severe side effects.

4. Bronze baby syndrome. This syndrome, first reported by Kopelman, Brown, and Odell (1972), is characterized by bronzing of the skin during phototherapy, accompanied by black serum and dark-colored urine; spectroscopy of serum and urine will demonstrate an absorption band at 416

nm. In our experience (Tan and Jacob, 1982), hepatic dysfunction, coupled with direct-acting bilirubin, was observed in all affected infants. However, not all infants with hepatic dysfunction and direct-acting bilirubin will develop the bronze baby syndrome on exposure. Though alarming, this condition always fades within 3 mo, with clearing of the urine, but the characteristic spectroscopic absorption band is still detected in the serum even at 1 yr of age.

The complications of phototherapy are thus relatively mild and transient. That phototherapy is safe has indeed been documented in numerous studies.

Indications for phototherapy

Phototherapy is such a safe and easy procedure that often it has been unnecessarily used at the least excuse. Though such an attitude should be discouraged, it should also be realized that phototherapy has a more gradual, though prolonged, effect on bilirubin levels (Tan, 1975), and thus an adequate safety margin should be provided at the start of phototherapy. At least four factors should be considered before starting phototherapy:

General condition of the infant
Postnatal age
Cause of NNJ
Unconjugated bilirubin concentration
Residual bilirubin binding capacity (if possible)

These factors determine the need for phototherapy and the timing of its commencement. The general condition of the infant is influenced by prematurity and illness; these two factors compromise clinical status and perhaps albumin concentration, thus influencing the rate of bilirubin increase and the susceptibility to bilirubin toxicity. Electrolyte, acid–base, and metabolic disturbances often occur, further stressing the general condition of the infant and rendering the buffering of bilirubin less stable.

Increasing age results in increasing ability of the liver to eliminate the bilirubin load more efficiently. The peak bilirubin concentration at 4 or 5 d after birth in those with nonhemolytic hyperbilirubinemia testifies to the ability of an infant to deal more effectively with the bilirubin load after that age. The blood–brain barrier will also be more resistant to bilirubin encephalopathy.

Knowledge of the cause of the hyperbilirubinemia assists in the prediction of the subsequent bilirubin increment and the need for phototherapy. In severe hemolysis, a rapid increment in bilirubin is expected in the vast majority of cases, but with non-hemolytic NNJ, a more gradual rise, peaking at 4 or 5 d after birth, is usual. Hence, in hemolytic cases, phototherapy at lower bilirubin levels is preferred, a decision not warranted in nonhemolytic situations.

Unconjugated bilirubin is toxic to cells in vitro and in vivo, though the exact concentration that is toxic in the brain is yet to be determined (Karp, 1979). Albumin is an effective barrier because of its combination with the bilirubin (Ryall and Peake, 1982). Thus, the bilirubin concentration by itself is not a satisfactory indication for phototherapy. It must be considered together with all of the foregoing factors. The residual bilirubin-binding capacity of albumin, if it can be determined, will be helpful in making the decision.

The foregoing factors have been used in formulating our guideline regarding phototherapy:

Commencement of phototherapy: bilirubin > 255 μmol $\cdot$ l^{-1}
If < 48 h of life: bilirubin > 222 μmol $\cdot$ l^{-1}
High intensity (double-bank blue lamps): bilirubin > 300 μmol $\cdot$ l^{-1} (17.5 mg $\cdot$ dl^{-1})

Such a guideline takes into account the rate of bilirubin increment, together with the efficacy of phototherapy at different bilirubin levels. Because compromised as well as premature infants have a greater rate of bilirubin increment, phototherapy is usually required at the lower value of 222 μmol $\cdot$ l^{-1}. The safety margin is also adequately wide to allow for a greater response time. This margin is much narrower in the severe cases; hence the need for high-intensity exposure to ensure a more prompt and effective response. Though brain-stem auditory-evoked responses are prolonged at such levels, recovery occurs with decline in bilirubin values during phototherapy; the preceding guideline would thus appear to be safe. Lower levels are not necessary, because brain-stem auditory-evoked responses are not disturbed at levels below 200 μmol $\cdot$ l^{-1}, at least in full-term infants (Tan, Skurr, and Yip, 1992b). Besides, the efficacy of phototherapy at such levels is poor.

Termination of phototherapy should be considered only when bilirubin levels have reached physiological values. Hence the following guideline:

Termination of phototherapy

Bilirubin < 185 μmol $\cdot$ l^{-1} (11 mg $\cdot$ dl^{-1}) for two consecutive determinations
Minimum duration 24 h

This guideline takes into account the following factors:

1. The efficacy of phototherapy is dependent on the initial bilirubin value decreasing with decreasing values, until 100 μmol · l⁻¹, below which no further response will occur with further exposure (Tan, 1982).
2. Mean bilirubin values in Singapore are about 170 μmol · l⁻¹ (10 mg · dl⁻¹), a value that obviously does not affect the infants' well-being.
3. Diurnal variations in bilirubin values will be offset by the 24-h determination.
4. Two consecutive bilirubin measurements will minimize the likelihood of laboratory errors and the effects of diurnal variation.

Monitoring during phototherapy

Clinical monitoring of an infant during exposure to phototherapy is similar to that for infants not being treated. The extra monitoring required involves ensuring adequate exposure of the infant skin, temperature observation, and regular nursing and cleaning of the infant. In high-intensity phototherapy using blue light, monitoring of the infant's clinical status is not possible. Where close observation is necessary, electronic monitoring is indicated.

Bilirubin levels during phototherapy should be regularly monitored. In healthy infants, monitoring every 12 h is usually adequate; however, in infants who are premature or ill, monitoring every 6 h is advisable to detect bilirubin response trends early and thus permit prompt response. In high-intensity phototherapy, we monitor every 2 h for the first 6 h, and if the response is satisfactory, we monitor every 6 h thereafter. Failure of phototherapy is defined as increasing bilirubin values beyond the initial value in two consecutive samples. This has occurred only occasionally in our experience with daylight phototherapy; such infants are transferred to high-intensity phototherapy, with invariably good response.

Monitoring bilirubin values for 2 d after phototherapy will minimize the chances of a severe rebound being overlooked. However, rebound is usually mild, with infants exposed to high-intensity phototherapy having a slightly greater increase than those exposed to daylight lamps (Tan, Lim, and Boey, 1992a). Where rebound values exceed prephototherapy levels, a second exposure is required; this has occurred rarely in our experience, except in Rh hemolytic hyperbilirubinemia.

Measures to ensure efficacy of phototherapy lamps

Fluorescent lamps decay with usage; this rate of decay is accelerated with overheating (Sisson et al., 1972). However, if such lamps are kept adequately cool, they should be able to last 2,000 h, at which time their irradiance is about 75% of the original (Tan, 1991). Hence, adequate ventilation is necessary to maintain proper cooling of the lamps. Our solution is to leave the lamps exposed, with air spaces in between individual lamps to ensure adequate ventilation. Our experience with such a setup indicates that continual monitoring of their irradiance is unnecessary if these conditions can be met. It is important to stress the need for adequate ventilation for the setup; sheets and other materials should never be placed or draped over the spaced lamps.

Blue lamps can cause severe giddiness, headache, and nausea in attending personnel during phototherapy. To avoid such ill effects, "skirts" (Figure 21.7) can be placed around individual setups to confine the light to the infant. With the double-bank setup in high-intensity phototherapy, such an arrangement is no longer possible; the lamps have to be screened off. The infants, however, seem to tolerate such lamps with no difficulty; feeding is taken well, and behavior during such exposure does not differ from that of infants exposed to daylight phototherapy. Clinical monitoring of infants is not possible with blue light; color changes (e.g., cyanosis) are not detectable. Hence, medical and nursing personnel should be aware of these limitations during blue-light phototherapy.

Measures to maintain infant well-being during phototherapy

Such measures include the following:

1. Increased fluid intake. This will depend on infant size and maturity, as well as light intensity and environmental humidity. Usually, increased fluid intake of about 20–60% is all that is required during exposure.
2. Temperature maintenance. Although full-term healthy infants usually are able to maintain their body temperatures, small and especially premature infants need extra heating from a servocontrolled heater to maintain normothermia. Increased cooling may be required in full-term infants exposed to double-bank phototherapy.
3. Suitable lamps. Lamps with minimal UV light are

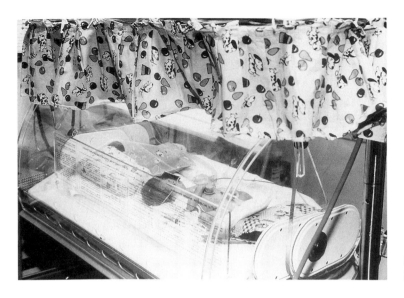

Figure 21.7. "Skirt" placed around phototherapy lamps to prevent glare.

mandatory. Our choice of the Philips TL54/18W daylight lamps, with little UV light, has resulted in efficacy, coupled with absence of tanning and skin burns. The Philips TL52/20W special blue lamps, with a spectral emission very similar to the bilirubin absorption spectrum, has been successfully used to control very severe or rapidly increasing hyperbilirubinemia, again with few side effects.

4. Adequate exposure. Maximal exposure is necessary for optimal response to phototherapy. Hence the need to keep the infant fully unclothed during exposure. Because of the relatively short period of exposure, eye complications are highly unlikely. However, to make "assurance double sure," it would be wiser to cover the eyes during phototherapy. The very superficial penetration of light into infant skin (Anderson and Parrish, 1981) makes the need for scrotal covering totally unnecessary.

No adverse effects have been observed in regard to albumin bilirubin-binding capacity (Cashore et al., 1975; Wolkoff et al., 1979), cholesterol, triglyceride (Hadjigeorgiou et al., 1978), cortisol, growth hormone (Bon Muhlendahl and Ballowicz, 1975), and riboflavin status (Tan, Chow, and Karim, 1978), or hepatic function (Tan et al., 1979); neither does it cause increased hemolysis in G-6-PD-deficient infants (Tan, 1977).

Since its inception in 1958, phototherapy has stood the test of time, with millions of infants being exposed, with no permanent or damaging side effects. Simple precautions are all that is required. The need for exchange transfusion has been greatly reduced and virtually eliminated because of high-intensity phototherapy using lamps arranged for optimal irradiance. Its main virtues of ease of application at little expense recommend it in an era of very expensive high-technology medicine.

REFERENCES

Anderson, R. R., and Parrish, J. A. (1981). The optics of human skin. *Journal of Investigative Dermatology* 77:13–19.

Bon Muhlendahl, K. E., and Ballowicz, L. (1975). Growth hormones and cortisol in neonates during phototherapy. *Zeitschrift für Kinderheilkunde* 119:53–8.

Callahan, E. W., Thaler, M. M., Karon, M., Bauer, K., and Schmid, R. (1970). Phototherapy of severe unconjugated hyperbilirubinemia: formation and removal of labelled bilirubin derivatives. *Pediatrics* 46:841–8.

Cashore, W. J., Karotkin, E. H., Stern, L., and Oh, W. (1975). The lack of effect of phototherapy on serum bilirubin-binding capacity of newborn infants. *Journal of Pediatrics* 87:977–80.

Costarino, A. T., Ennever, J. F., Baumgart, S., Speck, W. T., Paul, M., and Polia, R. A. (1985). Bilirubin isomerization in premature neonates under low and high intensity phototherapy. *Pediatrics* 75:519–22.

Cremer, R. J., Perryman, P. W., and Richards, D. H. (1958). Influence of light on the hyperbilirubinaemia of infants. *Lancet* 1:1094–7.

Eggert, P., and Stick, C. (1985). The distribution of radiant power in a phototherapy unit equipped with a metal halide lamp. *European Journal of Pediatrics* 143:224–5.

Ennever, J. F., Costarina, A. T., Polin, R. A., and Speck, W. T. (1987). Rapid clearance of a structural isomer of bilirubin during phototherapy. *Journal of Clinical Investigation* 79:1674–8.

Friedman, I., Lewis, P. J., Clifton, P., and Bulpitt, C. J. (1978). Factors influencing the incidence of neonatal jaundice. *British Medical Journal* 1:1235–7.

Hadjigeorgiou, E., Trilouri, D., Trichoupoulou, A., and Kaskorellis, D. (1978). Influence of phototherapy on serum lipids of jaundiced infants. *Pediatric Research* 12:690–4.

Itoh, S., and Onishi, S. (1985). Kinetic study of the photochemical changes of (ZZ)-bilirubin IXα bound to serum albumin. *Biochemical Journal* 226:251–8.

Karp, W. B. (1979). Biochemical alterations in neonatal hyperbilirubinemia and bilirubin encephalopathy: a review. *Pediatrics* 64:361–8.

Kopelman, A. E., Brown, R. S., and Odell, G. B. (1972). The 'bronze' baby syndrome: a complication of phototherapy. *Journal of Pediatrics* 81:466–72.

Lightner, D. A. (1982). Structure, photochemistry and organic chemistry of bilirubin. In *Bilirubin*, vol. 1, ed. K. P. M. Heirwegh and S. B. Brown (pp. 1–58). Boca Raton: CRC Press.

Lightner, D. A., Linnane, W. P., III, and Ahlfors, C. E. (1982). Bilirubin photo-oxidation products in the urine of jaundiced infants receiving phototherapy. *Pediatric Research* 18:696–700.

Linn, S., Schoenbaum, S. C., Monson, R. R., Rosmer, E., Stubblefield, E. G., and Ryan, K. J. (1985). Epidemiology of neonatal hyperbilirubinemia. *Pediatrics* 75:770–4.

McDonagh, A. F., Lightner, D. A., Reisinger, M., and Palma, L. A. (1986). Human serum albumin as a chiral template: stereo selective photo cyclization of bilirubin. *Journal of the Chemical Society. Chemical Communications*, no. 3, pp. 249–50.

McDonagh, A. F., Palma, L. A., and Lightner, D. A. (1982). Phototherapy for neonatal jaundice: stereospecific and regioselective photoisomerization of bilirubin bound to human serum albumin on NMR characterization of intramolecular cyclized photoproducts. *Journal of the American Chemical Society* 104:6867–9.

Messner, K. H., Maisels, M. J., and Leure duPree, A. E. (1978). Phototoxicity to the newborn primate retina. *Investigative Ophthalmology* 17:178–82.

Munroe, M., Shah, C. P., Badgley, R., and Bain, H. W. (1984). Birthweight, length, head circumference and bilirubin level in Indian newborns in the Sioux Lookout Zone, Northwestern Ontario. *Canadian Medical Association Journal* 131:453–6.

Oh, W., and Karecki, H. (1972). Phototherapy and insensible water loss in the newborn infant. *American Journal of Diseases of Children* 124:230–4.

Onishi, S., Isobe, K., Itoh, S., Kawade, N., and Sugiyama, S. (1980). Demonstration of a geometric isomer of bilirubin-IXα in the serum of a hyperbilirubinemic newborn infant and the mechanism of jaundice phototherapy. *Biochemical Journal* 190:533–6.

Onishi, S., Itoh, S., Isobe, K., Ochi, M., and Kondoh, M. (1988). Pathophysiological significance of bilirubin in neonatal jaundice as a defence mechanism against active oxygen during perinatal period. *Tanpakushitsu Kakusan Koso* 33:3005–16.

Poland, R. L., and Odell, G. B. (1971). Physiologic jaundice: the enterohepatic circulation for bilirubin. *New England Journal of Medicine* 284:5.

Ryall, R. G., and Peake, M. J. (1982). Theoretical constraints in the measurement of serum bilirubin binding capacity. *Clinical Biochemistry* 15:146–51.

Sisson, T. R. C., Kendall, N., Shaw, E., and Kechavarz-Oliai, L. (1972). Phototherapy of jaundice in the newborn infant. II. Effect of various light intensities. *Journal of Pediatrics* 81:35–8.

Tan, K. L. (1975). Comparison of the effectiveness of phototherapy and exchange transfusion in the management of nonhemolytic neonatal hyperbilirubinemia. *Journal of Pediatrics* 87:609–12.

— (1976). Phototherapy for neonatal hyperbilirubinemia in "healthy" and "ill" infants. *Pediatrics* 57:836–8.

— (1977). Phototherapy for neonatal jaundice in erythrocyte glucose-6-phosphate dehydrogenase deficient infants. *Pediatrics [Suppl.]* 59:1023–5.

— (1978). Some aspects on the management of neonatal jaundice in Singapore. *Journal of the Singapore Paediatric Society* 20:122–30.

— (1981). Glucose-6-phosphate dehydrogenase status and neonatal jaundice. *Archives of Disease in Childhood* 56:874–7.

— (1982). The pattern of bilirubin response to phototherapy for neonatal hyperbilirubinemia. *Pediatric Research* 16:670–4.

— (1984). Light dose–response relationship in phototherapy. In *Neonatal Jaundice – New Trends in Phototherapy*, ed. F. F. Rubaltelli and G. Jori (pp. 235–41). New York: Plenum Press.

— (1987). Neonatal jaundice in "healthy" very low birth weight infants. *Australian Paediatric Journal* 23:185–9.

— (1989). Efficacy of fluorescent daylight, blue and green lamps in the management of nonhemolytic hyperbilirubinemia. *Journal of Pediatrics* 114:132–7.

— (1991). Phototherapy for neonatal jaundice. *Clinics in Perinatology* 18:423–39.

Tan, K. L., and Boey, K. W. (1986). Efficacy of phototherapy in non-haemolytic hyperbilirubinaemia. *British Medical Journal* 293:1361–4.

— (1993). Efficacy of phototherapy in neonatal hyperbilirubinemia associated with G6PD deficient status. *European Journal of Pediatrics* 152:601–4.

Tan, K. L., Chow, M. T., and Karim, S. M. M. (1978). Effect of phototherapy on neonatal riboflavin status. *Journal of Pediatrics* 93:494–7.

Tan, K. L., and Jacob, E. (1982). The bronze baby syndrome. *Acta Paediatrica Scandinavica* 71:409–15.

Tan, K. L., Jacob, E., Chua, K. S., and Woon, K. Y. (1979). Phototherapy and neonatal liver function. *Biology of the Neonate* 36:128–32.

Tan, K. L., Lim, G. C., and Boey, K. W. (1992a). Efficacy of "high intensity" blue light and "standard" daylight phototherapy for non-haemolytic hyperbilirubinaemia. *Acta Paediatrica Scandinavica* 81:870–4.

Tan, K. L., Phua, K. B., and Ang, P. L. (1976). The mortality of exchange transfusions. *Medical Journal of Australia* 1:473–6.

Tan, K. L., Skurr, B., and Yip, Y. Y. (1992b). Phototherapy and the brain-stem auditory evoked response in neonatal hyperbilirubinemia. *Journal of Pediatrics* 120:306–8.

Vecchi, C., Donzelli, G. P., Sbrana, G., and Prateri, R. (1986). Phototherapy for neonatal jaundice: clinical equivalence of fluorescent green and special blue lamps. *Journal of Pediatrics* 108:452–6.

Wolkoff, A. W., Chowdhury, J. R., Gartner, L. A., Rose, L. A., and Biempiea, L. (1979). Crigler-Najjar syndrome (type I) in an adult male. *Gastroenterology* 76:840–8.

Wu, P. Y. K., and Moosa, A. (1978). Effect of phototherapy on nitrogen and electrolyte levels and water balance in jaundiced preterm infants. *Pediatrics* 61:193–7.

Index